STUDIES IN SCHIZOPHRENIA

A Multidisciplinary Approach to Mind-Brain Relationships

STUDIES IN SCHIZOPHRENIA

A Multidisciplinary Approach to Mind-Brain Relationships

BY THE TULANE
DEPARTMENT OF PSYCHIATRY AND NEUROLOGY

REPORTED BY:
ROBERT G. HEATH
Chairman

HAL C. BECKER
LEONA BERSADSKY
ROBERT M. CORRIGAN
ARTHUR W. EPSTEIN
WARREN L. FOUNDS
FRANCISCO GARCIA BENGOCHEA
CHARLES D. HENDLEY
ROBERT HODES
CHARLES HOGAN
H. E. KING
BYRON E. LEACH
RAEBURN C. LLEWELLYN
WALTER A. MICKLE
WILLIAM H. MILLER, JR.
FREDERICK F. MILLSAPS, JR.
RUSSELL R. MONROE
SAMUEL M. PEACOCK, JR.
T. DUANE PRICE
ERNEST SACHS, JR.
FLORENCE B. STROHMEYER
JOHN J. WEBER
KATHLEEN M. YOUNG

PUBLISHED FOR THE COMMONWEALTH FUND
BY HARVARD UNIVERSITY PRESS
CAMBRIDGE, MASSACHUSETTS, 1954

MANUFACTURED IN THE UNITED STATES OF AMERICA
LIBRARY OF CONGRESS CATALOG CARD NO. 54–8193

PUBLISHED FOR THE COMMONWEALTH FUND
BY HARVARD UNIVERSITY PRESS
CAMBRIDGE, MASSACHUSETTS

For approximately a quarter of a century THE COMMONWEALTH FUND, through its Division of Publications, sponsored, edited, produced, and distributed books and pamphlets germane to its purposes and operations as a philanthropic foundation. On July 1, 1951, the Fund entered into an arrangement by which HARVARD UNIVERSITY PRESS became the publisher of Commonwealth Fund books, assuming responsibility for their production and distribution. The Fund continues to sponsor and edit its books, and cooperates with the Press in all phases of manufacture and distribution.

Distributed in Great Britain
By Geoffrey Cumberlege,
Oxford University Press, London

Participants in the Project*

DON ALVARADO, A.B.
Artist

LUIS ALVAREZ, JR., M.D.

HAL C. BECKER, B.E. IN E.E.
Electronics Engineer

LEONA BERSADSKY, M.S.
Asst. in Psychiatry (Res. Psychol.)

GEORGE W. BURKE, M.D.

JOHN CANNAVAN
Electronics Technician

ROBERT M. CORRIGAN, M.A.
Asst. in Psychiatry (Res. Psychol.)

SOL IRVING COURTMAN, M.D.

LANFORD DE GENERES, M.D.

A. J. EHLERT, M.D.

MORTON L. ENELOW, M.D.

ARTHUR W. EPSTEIN, M.D.
Instr. in Psychiatry and Neurology

MURL FAULK, M.D.

OWEN FOSS, B.S.
Motion picture photographer

WARREN L. FOUNDS
Res. Asst.

DAVID A. FREEDMAN, M.D.

FRANCISCO GARCIA BENGOCHEA, M.D.
Asst. Prof. of Surgery (Neurosurgery) and Neurology

HOWARD WILLIAM GILLEN, M.D.

LEONARD H. GRUNTHAL, M.D.

ROBERT G. HEATH, M.D.
Prof. and Chrm., Dept. of Psychiatry and Neurology

CHARLES D. HENDLEY, PH.D.
Asst. Prof. of (Experimental) Neurology and Neurophysiology

JANICE HENDRICK
Executive Secretary

FREDERICK ROY HINE, M.D.

ROBERT HODES, PH.D.
Prof. of (Experimental) Neurology and Neurophysiology

CHARLES HOGAN, M.D.
Asst. in Psychiatry, Psychoanalytic Clinic, Columbia University

GEORGE JACOBSON, M.D.

STANLEY JOHN
Mechanician

H. E. KING, PH.D.
Asst. Prof. of Psychiatry (Res. Psychol.)

IRVIN A. KRAFT, M.D.

ROBERT LANCASTER, M.D.

†BYRON E. LEACH, PH.D.
Assoc. Prof. of Biochemistry and Neurology (Biochemistry)

RAEBURN C. LLEWELLYN, M.D.
Instr. in Neurosurgery and Neurology

FRANK THOMAS LOSSY, M.D.

PHILIP M. MANSON
Technician

†WALTER A. MICKLE, M.D.
Assoc. Prof. of (Experimental) Neurology and Neurophysiology

WILLIAM H. MILLER, JR.
Electroencephalographic Technician

FREDERICK F. MILLSAPS, JR., M.D.
Instr. in Radiology

RUSSELL R. MONROE, M.D.
Asst. Prof. of Psychiatry

JOHN MOOSSY, M.D.

VERA MOREL
Artist

*Affiliations and titles are given as of June, 1952, except as noted.
†Joined the Department after June, 1952.

BERYL O'REARDON, B.S.
Technician

SAMUEL M. PEACOCK, JR., M.D.
Instr. in Neurology (Neurophysiology)

T. DUANE PRICE, PH.D.
Asst. Prof. of Biochemistry and Neurology (Biochemistry)

MELVIN SABSHIN, M.D.

ERNEST SACHS, JR., M.D.
Asst. Prof. of Surgery (Neurosurgery) and Neurology

MARILYN SERPAS, B.S.
Technician

MARION DEWITT SHELTON, M.D.

EMASUE SNOW, M.D.

WILLIAM ROBERT SORUM, M.D.

WILLIAM H. STERNBERG, M.D.
Assoc. Prof. of Pathology

RICHARD L. STONE, M.D.

FLORENCE B. STROHMEYER, M.S.
Res. Assoc. in Neurology (Biochemistry)

ANDRE TOUZET, M.D.

ROY TRAHAN, B.A.
Motion picture photographer

GENE LEONARD USDIN, M.D.

JOHN J. WEBER, M.D.
Instr. in Psychiatry, Psychoanalytic Clinic, Columbia University

SPARKMAN WYATT, M.D.

KATHLEEN M. YOUNG, PH.D.
Asst. Prof. of Psychiatry (Clin. Psychol.)

Foreword

This monograph is in essence a transcript of a series of invitational meetings held in New Orleans, Louisiana, from June 11 to June 13, 1952, to present a review of the studies in schizophrenia conducted by the Department of Psychiatry and Neurology of the Tulane University of Louisiana School of Medicine. It is a description of work under way, a progress report on the thoughts and problems met in active research, rather than a final documentation of or recommendation for a particular type of psychosurgical therapy. The individual chapters were written by members of the research group, in which many and varied disciplines are represented. In order to give a thread of continuity to the presentation, a minimal amount of editorial comment has been inserted at various points in the monograph, in the hope that this will make it easier for the reader to see the manner in which each contribution fitted into the over-all research program.

In view of the large number of contributors, it was impractical to submit proofs of the entire monograph to each author. Individuals are therefore responsible only for the chapters to which their names are signed. Over-all responsibility is assumed by the Chairman of the Department.

Free discussions on all manner of topics took place throughout the meetings, which would have been difficult to report because of their conversational nature. The participants in these discussions included guests interested in various phases of the work, as well as members of the group responsible for the research. Most of the guests have, however, written summaries of their own impressions, suggestions, and criticisms, which have been included in Section V of this monograph.

During the time that elapsed between the date of the June 1952 meetings and the final preparation of the monograph, several additional significant studies were undertaken. Because of their direct relevancy to the topics of discussion, the reports of these studies have been included in the form of addenda, being presented in this way rather than incorporated in the chapters to which they pertain, since their content was not available to the discussants at the time of the meetings.

We have attempted to develop a unified approach to the understanding of behavior through utilizing the disciplines of psychiatry, psychology, physiology, biochemistry, neurology, and neurosurgery. We have developed a framework which we think gives some information regarding mind-brain interrelationships, and over the period during which our group has worked together, we have been able to test many of our theories concerning behavior.

In presenting our material, we shall not only give the actual data, but shall also discuss the reasons why the various steps in the work were undertaken—despite the fact that it is often considered impolitic to give a theoretical concept which goes more than a short distance beyond objective data. When we undertook the present project, we had a rather extensive, all-inclusive framework and relatively little data; now, as a result of our studies, some of the theoretical gaps have been filled. Although much that will be said here in the way of theory has not been proved, we feel that our theoretical concept is vital and that it may open the way to considerable extension of the work thus far undertaken. Throughout the report we shall attempt to demarcate established data from unproved theory. References to the literature will be given only when they are absolutely relevant to the material being presented.

It is not our purpose to announce a new treatment, though in working with schizophrenic patients and with the few nonschizophrenic patients included in the series reported in Section IV, our motivation has been therapeutic. We have obtained some therapeutic effects, but much work remains to be done in this regard. It will be readily apparent to the reader, as it was to those who attended the meetings, that no statistical evaluation of the therapeutic results is possible at this stage of development, owing primarily to variables in the therapeutic technique. The program has been, and will of necessity continue to be, extremely flexible. The difficulties of operative technique have, until recently, made it impossible to carry through exactly the same treatment from one patient to another. Considerable progress has been made in overcoming these difficulties as a result of recent technical improvements, and it is felt that the procedure may be stabilized in the very near future. If so, a series of patients may be comparably treated in order to evaluate therapeutic efficacy.

A brief historical note regarding the composition of our group is probably in order. Several of its members had worked together prior to the formation of this Department. Dr. Heath, Dr. King, and Dr. Young had worked on the first Columbia-Greystone Project; Dr. King and Dr. Young had continued to work on brain research programs for an additional year at the New Jersey State Hospital at Greystone Park and at Rockland State Hospital at Orangeburg, New York; and Dr. Garcia had worked on the second Greystone Project.

Moreover, the interests of various members of the research team who represented different disciplines considerably overlapped and one very much complemented the other. For some time prior to coming to New Orleans, Dr. Heath had been interested in studying the behavioral and metabolic changes following ablation of subcortical regions of the forebrain of animals, as well as in investigating the effects of frontal lobe surgery. Dr. King, while associated with the brain research projects in New York, had developed a marked interest in a psychophysiological approach to behavior and was working on techniques of motor measurements. Dr. Hodes had developed an interest in the physiology of the higher neural levels and wished to pursue further research in this area. Others who joined the staff somewhat later also had similar interests. Dr. Monroe, while at the Psychoanalytic Clinic, had shown a keen interest in correlating physiological findings with psychiatric data. As the research progressed in the Department, it became apparent that the biochemical aspects of the program had to be developed much more extensively. To accomplish this Dr. Price was added to the staff, and during the second year of the project he functioned as the biochemist of the group. Since the establishment of the Department, many other persons have worked into the research program. A full list of the participants is given on pages v–vi.

Several of us who had been previously concerned with problems centering about frontal lobe operations had developed similar feelings concerning that work. We felt first that the beneficial changes that were being obtained were minimal and that there was always something in the way of undesirable effects. Even when patients were considered to be benefited by the procedure, the changes could not be definitely related to the one piece of brain that had been removed. We therefore decided that it might be fruitful to study the results of altering the organism without destroying cortical tissue. Our immediate aim, then, was to determine what could be done by altering circuits within the intact person. The approach that was devised and the reasoning behind our concepts are presented in Chapter 1.

The research project was carried out in the Department of Psychiatry and Neurology of the Medical School and in the Tulane Neuropsychiatric Unit of the Charity Hospital of Louisiana in New Orleans. We thank Dr. Maxwell E. Lapham, Dean of the Tulane University of Louisiana School of Medicine, Dr. Robert Bernhard, Director, and Dr. Jacques Magne, Assistant Director, of the Charity Hospital of Louisiana, for their cooperation and assistance in providing facilities necessary for conducting this project. We also wish to express our gratitude to Sister Juliana, Supervisor of Psychiatry, and Mrs. Eve Long, Assistant Supervisor of Psychiatry, at the Charity Hospital, and the members of their nursing staff who worked with the patients included in this series.

The principal financial support was provided by the Commonwealth Fund. We wish to express our appreciation not only for this financial assistance, but also for many valuable suggestions from personnel of the Fund, which aided considerably in the development of the program. Additional financial support toward the basic neurophysiological aspects of the program was forthcoming from the Teagle Foundation and the United States Public Health Service. C. Mahlon Kline of the Smith, Kline and French Laboratories personally provided much-needed contingency funds, which made it possible to organize the meetings and the material for this publication.

R. G. H.

Table of Contents

Definition of the

SEPTAL REGION

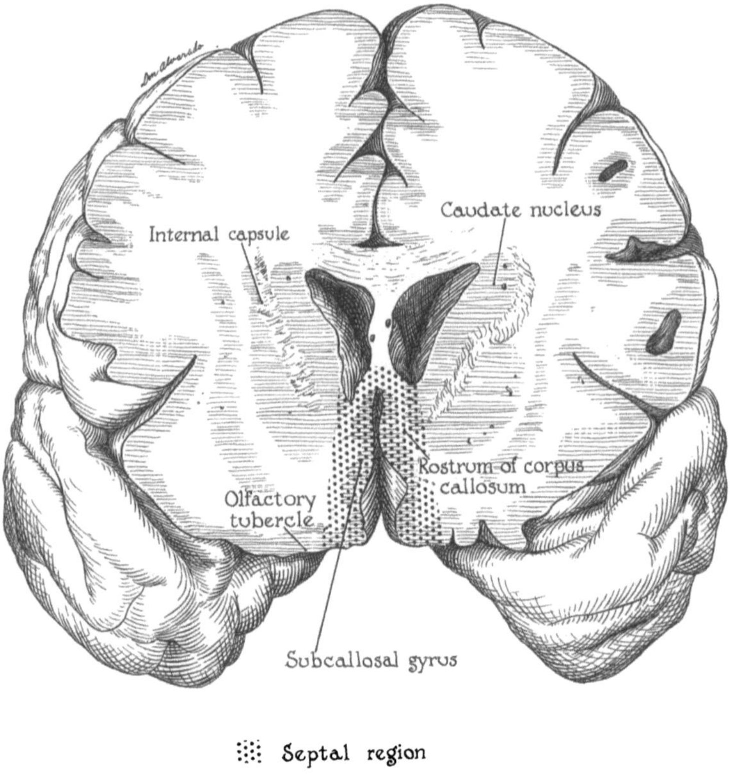

FIGURE 1. Outline drawing demarcating the septal region

Definition of the Septal Region

ROBERT G. HEATH

The term septal has been used throughout this monograph to demarcate the area in the brain most relevant to our studies. Since the meaning of the term is not consistent from one authority to another, a description of the area to which we apply it is given below. This is followed by a rationale for our application of the term to the region described.

ANATOMICAL DESCRIPTION

The caudal border of this region is formed by the anterior commissure; the rostral extent is the tip of the anterior horn of the lateral ventricle. It extends medially to the midline space separating the hemispheres. The dorsal extent is the septum pellucidum proper and the base of the lateral ventricles. It extends ventrally to the base of the brain and laterally about 5 mm. from the midline.

This region encompasses several different and distinct structures in the usual anatomical sense. Some of the structures included in the conventional anatomical texts are the subcallosal gyrus, rostrum of the corpus callosum, olfactory tubercle, septal nuclei proper, subcallosal fasciculus, pyriform cortex, and various olfactory pathways.

The known anatomical connections of the septum are as follows:

1. Afferents from the medial olfactory stria, hippocampus, and cerebral cortex (areas 9 and 11 of Brodmann).
2. Efferents to the hypothalamus, hippocampus, habenula by way of stria medullaris, and pre-optic region.
3. Pyriform cortex projects to the pre-optic area.

In summary, then, the septal region is part of the olfactory system. From its anatomical relationships it would appear to be a correlating structure interposed between the higher neocortical level and the diencephalic and midbrain structures.

RATIONALE

Just caudal to our septal region is the hypothalamus. Embryologically, however, the two regions are quite different. The septal region is derived from the rhinencephalon .division of the forebrain, whereas the hypothalamus is an elaboration of the primitive diencephalon. Although the anatomists have applied different names to several different nuclear masses within our septal region, these varied structures are developmentally part of the same system, namely, the rhinencephalon. Embryologically the rhinencephalon also includes those structures at the rostral end of the third ventricle. Our principal reason for rigidly demarcating the region we have called septal is that it appears to have particular functional qualities. This will become clear as the reader follows the various reports of our studies.

At times throughout the monograph we use the term septo-hypothalamic to designate the caudal aspects of the septal region. Since the septal region is very large in the rostro-caudal extent (approximately 2 1/2 cm.), we felt that this term would be useful in indicating that the electrodes were in the vicinity of the anterior commissure.

Some anatomical authorities (e.g., F. A. Mettler, *Neuroanatomy*, Mosby, St. Louis, 1948) refer to the septum as the ventral thalamus. This would seemingly imply that the region is related to the thalamus and therefore to the diencephalon. The only rationale for such a relationship is an architectonic one. This categorization is not in keeping either with the embryological development of the region or with our findings in regard to its function.

Figure 1 is an outline drawing of the brain showing that part of the forebrain which we have demarcated as the septal region. Figure 2 is a schematic drawing showing its embryological development. The references to embryology are from L. B. Arey, *Developmental Anatomy* (Saunders, Philadelphia, 1940, 4th ed.) and W. J. S. Krieg, *Functional Neuroanatomy* (Blakiston, Philadelphia, 1942).

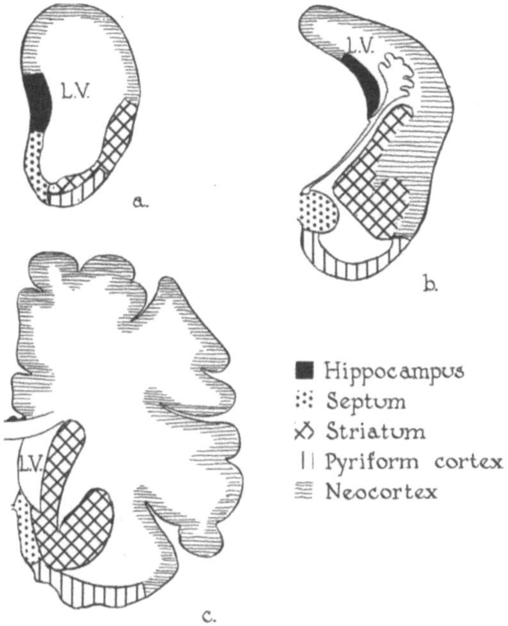

FIGURE 2. Diagrammatic representation of septal region in relation to other divisions of the cerebral hemispheres at various stages of development (a) embryo; (b) 50 mm. embryo; (c) adult. Adapted from Krieg

Section I

THEORETICAL CONCEPTS

CHAPTER 1

THE THEORETICAL FRAMEWORK FOR A MULTIDISCIPLINARY APPROACH TO HUMAN BEHAVIOR*

ROBERT G. HEATH

Interdisciplinary research in behavior disorders has long been considered an ideal method, but practically the results of this approach have been disappointing. At best, one could only make cross-interpretations. One reason why so little has been accomplished in this direction may be the lack of a satisfactory theory from which to develop experimental techniques.

The present monograph constitutes the report of a multidisciplinary investigation of the mind-brain relationships with primary reference to schizophrenia. The purpose of this chapter is to present our over-all theory and to integrate the results of our study, so that later chapters may be considered in the perspective of the total research.

THE THEORY IN BRIEF

The basis of life is metabolism. In all living organisms movement is directed toward the satisfaction of metabolic needs, but as organisms progress up the phylogenetic scale, movement or behavior becomes integrated through higher levels of the neuraxis. This produces more complex behavior patterns, with potentials for greater efficiency. It is in man, with the evolution of the highly developed cerebral cortex, that behavior is integrated by the activity of the mind, or thought.

In our theoretical formulation behavior was considered in terms of dynamic interaction between higher and lower levels of integration. We postulated that there were several dynamic levels of thought which might correspond with dynamic physiological interrelationships between different levels of the neuraxis. As a result of various observations, pri-

*The material in this chapter is essentially the same as that presented in the introductory paper read in New Orleans in June, 1952, although some changes in organization have been made in order to make it more suitable for publication.

marily from our own laboratories, the hypothesis was advanced that functional circuits existed in the brain, one which facilitated mental activity and bodily processes and another which inhibited such activity. As work progressed and the techniques developed in animal experiments were ultimately applied to human patients, evidence was collected within our conceptual scheme which added support to this hypothesis.

Schizophrenia was considered to be a disorder of the lower levels of integration. This was based upon clinical observations which indicated impairment of lower thought levels as well as upon various clinical and laboratory studies which suggested impairment of the subcortical levels of the nervous system. The clinical and laboratory evidence also combined to suggest that such impairment might involve the facilitatory mechanism. Application of this concept to schizophrenic patients revealed an apparent physiological abnormality in the region associated with the facilitatory circuit and techniques were designed to correct this. After the project was well under way clinical and laboratory data further suggested that alterations in the dynamic relationships between the two systems might be present in disease processes other than schizophrenia.

THE MIND-BRAIN PROBLEM

For several thousand years at least, man has speculated upon a possible relationship between the mind and the body. The search for the nature of this relationship still continues without success. Aristotle, Descartes, Spinoza, and many others considered this problem to be in the province of philosophy. During the height of the era of cellular pathology the discovery of spirochetes in the brains of paretic patients led to the assumption that all mental disorders might be the result of cellular lesions. The shortcoming of this approach was the failure to consider functional relationships of the cells as parts of a whole. In many ways this approach delayed progress in the understanding of behavior disorders. It served, however, to intensify investigative efforts in this field. Adolf Meyer first introduced a modern concept of scientific monism, but his approach lacked a satisfactory method of investigation. Psychobiology catalogued events in the patient's life but offered no means of appraising the meaning of these events to the patient. Sigmund Freud, in introducing the technique of free association, offered the first successful method of investigating activity of the mind, but formulations derived from utilization of his techniques offered no suitable framework for interdisciplinary research. In this connection it may be worth noting that Freud always considered data gathered through free association to be reflections of physiological and chemical activity of the brain; in fact, personal communiqués from his associates indicate that he was concerned lest physiological techniques should be introduced which would result in prompt therapeutic results and thus interrupt his investigations.[1, 2]

Representatives of many disciplines concerned with the study of behavior were included in the Department of Psychiatry and Neurology at Tulane in the hope that through a polyphasic approach it might be possible to integrate the data derived from introspection—i.e., reporting what the patient felt about himself—with evidence derived from the inspective techniques. In order to test our hypothesis it was of the utmost importance that a theoretical framework be established to relate activity of the mind and the nervous-humoral mechanisms. Observations from the field of evolution were therefore essential.

BASIC CONCEPTS

The word *mind* has vague connotations but is most specifically used to describe the governing factor in human behavior. The psychological concepts regarding mind and behavior to be presented here are largely derived from the adaptational approach of Dr. Sandor Rado[3] with some modifications of our own, derived principally from physiological experimentation. In this framework, behavior is basically related to survival or utility. The pleasure drive, long considered primary in psychoanalytic formulation, is relegated to a secondary role.

Schrodinger[4] advanced the concept that life is related to metabolism, and Sherrington[5] defined mind as the manager of muscle. We have attempted to trace the manner in which mind evolved as the integrator of behavior and to correlate behavioral characteristics with the evolution of the nervous system.

In our concept behavior is considered as follows. The basis of life is metabolic—i.e., survival requires the acquisition of that which is required to satisfy metabolic needs. This is motor activity. With the evolution of the mind in man behavior became integrated at several levels which can be roughly divided into thought, emotion, and feeling. I shall elaborate on this concept of the levels of integration after first considering the basic factor of movement, or drive.

One of the major contributions of psychoanalysis was the introduction of a concept of dynamics—the idea of a propelling force in behavior, which was described as *instinct*. In this early concept, however, instinct was tied to pleasure, the idea being developed that the inability to discharge the instinctual forces, or pleasure drive, led to a damming up of energy which was manifested clinically as neurosis. Multidisciplinary research through utilization of this framework is impossible. No opening is provided for utilization of the inspective techniques.

In the adaptational framework the propelling force (the basic metabolic, or biological, need) is related to survival of the self and the species. True satisfaction of a need is accompanied by pleasure proportionate to the motivational state. (For example, eating gives pleasure only if one is hungry, not after ingestion of a full meal.) This accompanying pleasure (usually considerably in excess of that required to satiate a need) may be regarded as one aspect of the law of physiological safety. In most biological functions related to survival there is an analogous overprotection; for instance, two kidneys are present though one is adequate, 10 per cent of the liver and one-half of one lung are sufficient for the load imposed by nature, and so on. This concept of the driving forces in behavior may be summarized thus:

Equilibrium (time 1) → need → activity → Equilibrium (time 2)
(tension) (pleasure)

Hence every individual is constantly moving from one equilibrium to another because of needs generated by metabolic requirements. Dispelling a disequilibrium that results from a need, or relieving tensions through activity, is accompanied by pleasure proportionate to the motivational state or need, and establishes a new equilibrium, but one which always differs from its predecessor owing to the passage of time. Here the moving force in behavior is related to basic metabolic processes and survival, and the vague, confusing concept of instincts included in the majority of psychoanalytic formulations is eliminated.

Levels of Integration. At each point on the phylogenetic scale we find increasingly complex patterns of behavior for dealing with the

TABLE I–1. Levels of behavior. Adapted from Rado

Relation of organism – environment	LEVEL					
	Neural.	Psychodynamic	Regulatory signal recording and anticipating benefit	Behavior	Regulatory signal recording and anticipating damage	Behavior
Intellectual cultural circuit	Cortical	Thought	Secure utility and pleasure avoid damage			
Sensory-nervous motor circuit	Thalamic distance receptors	Emotional	Love → Hope →	Hold-possess Catch-ingest Sustaining	Rage → Fear →	Combat Escape
Metabolic circuit	Reflex contact receptors	Hedonic (sentient)	Pleasure →	Absorption	Pain → Loss of pleasure →	Riddance Retrieval

basic drives. Movement, or motor activity, which we have considered basic in behavior, becomes integrated through different levels. In man, of course, the potentials for efficient adaptation are greatest.

In the lowest forms of life, in which the neuraxis is lacking, behavior is dependent upon direct contact and is limited to two responses—moving toward and withdrawal. Absorptive behavior must be related to stimuli of survival value (metabolic needs) and riddance behavior must be related to stimuli without survival value, or the species dies out. Since the basic pattern seemingly is related to sensations of pleasure and pain, the term *hedonic* (from Rado) will be used to describe this level of integration.*

The evolution of the nervous system and the humoral mechanisms (figuratively speaking, a telegraphic and a transportation system) occurs farther up the phylogenetic scale. This is accompanied by the development of sensory distance receptors, which make for a more efficient adaptive process in that the range of stimuli is extended. It is at this stage that *emotional* responses appear. The basic responses to pain and pleasure remain but the reactions to stimuli are integrated in a more complex way. For example, the emotion of love, which is "associated with anticipation of pleasure," produces the motor pattern of moving toward, or absorption, whereas the emotions of rage and fear, which are associated with anticipation of pain, produce the motor pattern of attack and flight—i.e., riddance.

All sensory perception is directly influenced by the motivational state or biological need. For example, in certain circumstances all sensory modalities—sight, smell, hearing, touch—selectively perceive stimuli related to food. In others all sensory modalities are at the service of sexual behavior. In short, the emotions mobilize the total organism in accordance with hedonistic principles.

The psychological responses just described are present in laboratory animals in which the midbrain is well established but in which there is minimal or no cortical development. With the evolution of the cerebral

*Although the term *hedonic* originally referred only to pleasure, it has been extended to cover both basic feelings (i.e., pain as well as pleasure). Only man is capable of reporting these subjective feelings. In the lowest animal forms the terms *pain* and *pleasure* are not applicable, but analogous motor activity may be observed.

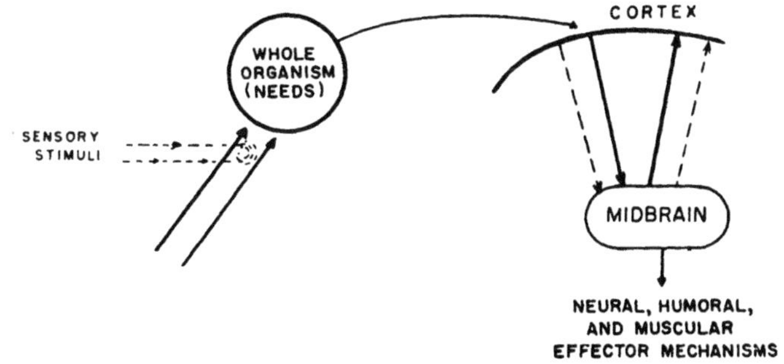

FIGURE I–1. Schematic representation of the cortex as the mediator between the needs of the whole organism and the efferent responses

cortex, on the highest level of the phylogenetic scale, psychological responses emerge with potentials for even more efficient adaptation. Here, as a result of memory, behavior is dependent upon past learning and the individual is able to anticipate the distant future. There develops the ability to defer immediate behavior for greater gain through planning. Basic drives or needs are met in terms of the higher levels of integration—i.e., in accordance with memory or learning experiences. These are the levels of thought.

In physiological terms all human behavior is dependent upon the activity of the cerebral cortex (see Figure 1), except for the relatively rare instances of the startle reflex responses resulting from activity of the distance receptors and the other familiar subcortically integrated reflexes. But even in man behavior characteristic of the more primitive levels of integration persists. Thoughts are accompanied to varying degrees by emotions and basically regulated by the principles of pain and pleasure in proportion to need. Thus during a strong alimentary motivational state it is difficult to concentrate on subjects other than food and during a strong sexual state all thinking is centered on sex. Similarly, all sensory modalities are brought into play in the service of the dominant basic metabolic need. It is only when needs are in a state of relative satiation that more abstract thinking can prevail.

Activity at Various Levels of Thought. Thus it is apparent that thought, the integrator of behavior in man, is a dynamic process, influencing and being influenced to a marked degree by the basic metabolic needs. In this framework it is convenient to describe this dynamic activity in terms of levels. Thought has been investigated most completely through the study of dreams in psychoanalysis, and the data presented here are largely derived from psychoanalytic observations. By way of generalization it may be said that:

1. There are many levels of thought, ranging from dream activity to concentration on problems in pure mathematics.
2. The highest levels are always conscious; the lowest levels are always unconscious. There is no clear dividing line between the conscious and the unconscious, but many shades and gradations of awareness. At any given time conscious thought represents only a small part of the activity of the mind.
3. The higher levels are more realistic and abstract with symbols approaching a one-to-one relationship to the referent; the lower levels more self-centered, wishful, and pervaded with emotion. Not all persons are capable of attaining the higher levels; there is a wide range of difference among individuals.
4. The higher levels are sometimes inactive, but not the lower levels.
5. Man must apply himself to attain the higher levels; even the greatest thinkers do not remain on the highest levels all day long. When tensions associated with biological needs increase, the activity of higher thought levels is impaired.
6. At any given time there is a top level of function, and activity above this ceiling is nonexistent. The best example of this is presented by sleep, when only the lowest levels are active.
7. Higher levels can, however, be re-instated according to need.

Freud first described the lower levels of thought, which he called *primary processes*. From the following summary it is apparent that the lower levels of thought and dream activity of the normal individual have much in common with the everyday thinking of the psychotic schizophrenic.

1. There is no negation—Opposites can appear side by side without contradiction.
2. Cathexis is mobile—The power of discrimination is lacking or very poor, closely related objects being treated as if they were the same. The common factor in such misidentification of loved, hated, or feared objects is always the associated emotion. As a result of this inability

to discriminate, there appear in dreams which characterize this lowest level of thought activity such factors as:

(a) Condensation—Many things with some resemblance are put together.

(b) Misplaced accent—For example, the child in the jewelry store is more intrigued with the fancy box than the expensive diamonds it contains.

(c) Timelessness—Experiences are related in spacial order but not in temporal order.

(d) Psychological reality versus actual reality—Hallucinations have the same value as reality.

Since mental aberrations are characteristic of behavioral disorders, detailed consideration of psychological levels of thought have important bearing on the problem of mind-brain relationships. If our "levels" scheme is correct, alterations in thought should be reflected in the physiological activity of the cortex. Thus electroencephalographic records indicating that the cortex is relatively inactive in sleep, when the higher levels of thought are inactive, were particularly relevant to our psycho-physiological studies of schizophrenic patients. In our preliminary studies such records helped us to circumvent the obstacle that subjective reports cannot be obtained in animal experiments. In this connection it was assumed that physiological procedures which altered states of awareness in animals would affect levels of thought if extended to man.

Disordered Behavior in the Adaptational Framework. Thus far the evolution of the higher levels of thought has been considered only as a potential for better, more efficient adaptation. It has been mentioned that this evolution is characterized by the ability to anticipate events in the distant future from complicated memories. Thus the manipulation of symbols in thinking is potentially more efficient than trial and error (motor activity), but retains a basic relationship to motor activity. But the same process wherein virtually all behavior is determined by learning experiences, can also result in undesirable effects. The major points in this concept may be summarized as follows:

1. Because of the long dependency period of man, the individual's relations with his parents are of the utmost importance in determining the manner in which he will react to any given situation.

2. Stresses in the everyday activity of modern man are virtually always related to memories and childhood experiences are particularly important.
3. Learning experiences can be such that the individual reacts inappropriately to ordinary life experiences. For example, adults who react to sexual feelings or temptations (biological need) with fear (stress) have been taught during childhood that sexual activity is dangerous. Individuals can adapt to stress with socially useful behavior or can respond with an inferior or maladaptive pattern.
4. Maladaptive or disordered behavior, or in usual terms, neurosis and psychosis, represent inferior attempts to relieve stress in faulty anticipation of the future based on painful memories.
5. Maladaptive psychological defenses against stress represent regressive behavior—i.e., repetition of childhood attempts to find safety.

In discussing the levels of the phylogenetic scale, emotional responses were correlated with the evolution of the midbrain,* and mental activity involving thought and memory was correlated with the evolution of the cerebral cortex. It was pointed out that, as the various levels of thought affect subcortical structures to greater and lesser degrees, emotional responses in turn affect the cortex. In accordance with this scheme the important dynamic physiological relationships occurring in response to stress may be stated as follows:

1. Of the greatest importance in a stress reaction is the integrated cortical activity. Activity in the cerebral cortex must play downward into the lower levels. The firing of these lower levels produces (in addition to somato-motor responses) peripheral activity such as tremor, sweating, and other phenomena characteristic of emotional response.
2. After the lower levels have been fired, they in turn play back on the cortex. Individuals react emotionally as well as physiologically, and thinking processes are altered. Moreover, with an inferior adaptation, the behavior that results from such stress is often quite childish, representing an attempt to use the earliest pattern laid down in the individual's developmental history. An interesting corollary to these

*As used here midbrain and subcortex also apply to the archicortex, whereas cortex refers to the neocortex.

observations is that patients with widespread organic disease of the cerebral cortex likewise adopt childish patterns of behavior.

Summarizing these observations from psychology and physiology, one could state that forces generated through biological needs, plus stimuli perceived over the distance receptors, are handled by each individual in accordance with his memories of past experiences (cortical activity). It is known that pleasant thought activity (for example, anticipation of reward) tends to produce increased efficiency. This is one of the major factors in the background of learning. Under such circumstances interaction between the cortical and subcortical levels results in cortical facilitation. On the other hand, if memories are such that biological needs create fear, the individual often reverts to childish patterns of behavior. Therefore, in situations of stress, interactions between the cortical and lower levels result in inhibition of the cortex.

In this framework, then, it is our thesis that emotional reactions are largely initiated by memory, and that painful emotion is the nuclear factor in disordered behavior in man. By means of the multidisciplinary approach it has been possible to examine the same process through different apertures. In presenting the results of our studies, we shall attempt to differentiate among objective data, logical reasoning, and unsubstantiated theory.

INVESTIGATIVE APPROACHES TO THE MIND-BRAIN PROBLEM

In keeping with the outline presented, there have been two key approaches to our study of mind-brain relationships.

The first was to demonstrate physiologically that stress is associated with activity of the nervous system, specifically influenced by activity of the cerebral cortex, and that production of stress could influence mental activity and be reflected by cortical activity. We hypothesized that mind, the integrator of behavior in man, is associated with development of the cerebral cortex and that emotional reactions are influenced by the cortex.

The second was to utilize motor measurements as a physiological tool which would reflect the activity of the cortex, this approach being based on the theory outlined—namely, that although the evolution of the cortex and the human mind have promoted greater efficiency, behavior remains basically motor. If this should prove to be the case, the common function of motor activity shared by man and animals might serve as a point of integration in experimental work.

Moreover, the inferior behavior patterns apparent on psychiatric study (introspection) should be reflected in motor tests, and physiological changes in the neural regions associated with emotion should affect motor activity and this should be reflected in behavior (i.e., in humans the reporting activity).

These approaches were considerably simpler than an attempt to understand mind-brain relationships through complicated studies of the neural basis of perception. It began at the endpoint with the idea that motor function should reflect alterations in the integrating machinery; then considered those factors which we felt were important in altering over-all integration.

Biochemical Aspects

Humoral Mechanisms in Stress. Obviously, from the review given above it can be seen that the primary obligation was to prove that emotional reactions were influenced by the cerebral cortex and that all the observations made on animals and humans during stress could be elicited by altering activity within the nervous system.

Previous studies of stress have largely been in terms of alterations in blood chemistry accompanying the emotions of fear and rage. The pioneer work was done by Walter B. Cannon,[6] who investigated primarily the bodily changes accompanying the emotions of rage and fear and who related these bodily changes to the release of hormones by the adrenal medulla. The bodily changes resulting from the circulating epinephrine of the adrenal medulla were found to be alterations in sugar metabolism, smooth and skeletal musculature, etc. These were considered homeostatic phenomena which enabled the animal to adapt to danger. Recently, considerable data have been presented to show that the endocrine system as a whole is involved in the process of adaptation, and greater emphasis has been placed on the interaction between the pituitary, with its tropic hormones, and the adrenal cortex. Selye has developed this thesis to the greatest degree.[7] Clear-cut bodily changes occur where extremes in function of the adrenal cortex are present. For example, extirpation of the adrenal cortex results in:

1. Alteration in electrolyte balance characterized by a drop in serum sodium and a rise in serum potassium—This is accompanied by increased excretion of serum sodium and decreased excretion of serum potassium, indicating that the adrenal hormone that influences electrolyte metabolism does so by acting on the kidney. The electrolyte changes are associated with the loss of large amounts of water.
2. Alterations in carbohydrate metabolism—Inability to store glycogen in the muscle and liver ultimately leads to hypoglycemia. There is also evidence to the effect that protein catabolism with respect to glycogen is impaired.
3. Listlessness, apathy, and hypothermia.
4. Ulcerations of the upper and lower gastrointestinal tract.
5. Lowered blood pressure.

A corollary observation is that persons with destructive diseases of the adrenal cortex (Addison's disease) are readily susceptible to intercurrent infections.

Several specific steroids have been isolated from the adrenal cortex which influence different aspects of metabolism. Some, principally desoxycorticosterone acetate, have been shown to have an effect on electrolyte metabolism, and others, dehydrocorticosterone and 17-hydroxy-11-dehydrocorticosterone, exercise a strong effect on carbohydrate metabolism; 17-hydroxy-corticosterone exercises a strong effect on carbohydrate metabolism and to some extent effects sodium retention. It is known that overactivity of the adrenal cortex also produces clinical disease syndromes. For example, Cushing's disease and tumors of the adrenal cortex produce definite clinical entities which are quite consistent.

It has been shown that the effects of the administration of secretions of the adrenal cortex are dependent upon the total state of the organism at the time they are administered; for example, desoxycorticosterone will produce salt retention and increase in blood pressure only if the adrenal cortex is normal or partially destroyed, whereas in the presence of overactivity of the adrenal cortex, as in Cushing's disease, the opposite effect, namely, a drop in blood pressure and loss of salt, occurs. This important factor, consideration of the state of the total organism when a specific stimulus is given, is something that must be taken into account in all our discussions. We have found similar considerations to be important in the physiological experiments.[8]

Selye[7] has built up a logical framework of general adaptation. In his theory the pituitary and adrenal cortex constitute the effector mechanism, and he postulates that under- and overfunction of the adrenals (or imbalances in secretions of various cortico-steroids) are related to some disease processes. He describes a general adaptation syndrome to stress and discusses clinical disorders associated with the altered humoral adaptation to stress. In one extreme, failure of the pituitary-adrenal mechanism in response to stress results in shock. Under such circumstances the resulting pathological changes are similar to those seen with extirpation of the adrenal cortex. The presenting clinical symptoms have already been described. In the other extreme, described as a resistance stage, pathological overactivity, or imbalance in the elaboration of various corticoids of the adrenals, produces syndromes of a different type. These are manifested clinically by such diseases as rheumatoid arthritis and hypertension. Selye has stressed the importance of this over-all adaptive mechanism of the organism in the maintenance of health. It has often been pointed out, particularly in recent years, that efforts of medical investigators have been directed toward discovering definite causative agents in illness without directing comparable effort toward understanding the other fundamental aspect of the disease, namely, the resistance or motivational state of the host. Selye speculates that the individual's susceptibility to disease or susceptibility to a causative agent is related to his humoral adaptation.

Many recent clinical studies tend to give support to the importance of the humoral mechanisms in the over-all adaptation of the individual, particularly in disease processes. To cite an example, it has been found that patients with ulcers of the gastrointestinal tract have lowered urinary excretion of 17-ketosteroids. This observation, along with the laboratory findings that ulcers of the gastrointestinal tract frequently follow extirpation of the adrenal gland, would suggest that ulcerations of the gastrointestinal tract are associated with underactivity of the humoral (adrenal) system. With the advent of ACTH and cortisone more interesting supportive data on the relationship between humoral activity and clinical disease have been forthcoming. Administration of various steroids has not always produced consistent or predictable results, but in many diseases improvement has often been rather dramatic. Most dramatically alleviated are symptoms of the collagen diseases and the overt allergies. Somewhat less improvement has been shown by patients with glomerulonephritis and the nephrotic syndrome, neoplastic diseases (particularly malignancies of breast and prostate), specific infectious diseases, cirrhosis of the liver, ulcerative colitis, pemphigus, and hyperthyroidism. Many of the diseases, particularly in the collagen group, which have been most affected (i.e., when the patients have improved with this treatment) are ones which Selye reasoned were produced by overactivity of the pituitary-adrenal mechanism or an imbalance in steroid excretion. Some patients receiving these drugs have developed behavioral disorders. Psychotic and neurotic complications have occurred most commonly in patients with overt allergies or collagen diseases who were successfully treated with these drugs. Minor changes in behavior, often referred to as steroid euphoria because of the general state of well-being, have been quite common. An interesting paradox is presented by the finding that patients who develop severe psychotic symptoms also show high serum potassium levels as a result of therapy. In this connection it will be recalled that increase in serum potassium often accompanies loss of sodium and that this is generally attributed to adrenocortical deficiency. Administration of ACTH and cortisone should logically produce the opposite effect. Here again, perhaps we are dealing with the factor of the resting state of the total organism. The presence of collagen diseases or overt allergies in schizophrenics is rare. There are many cases on file of patients who have had spontaneous complete remissions of allergic disorders and of collagen diseases with the inception of psychotic behavior.* These data suggest that the two disease processes may be antagonistic.

*These observations are referable only to the psychotic states characterized by retardation (i.e., catatonic and hebephrenic types of schizophrenia). Allergies and collagen diseases often coexist with paranoid psychosis and in several instances have been reported to begin with the onset of paranoid reactions. Several observations will be reported later in which the paranoid group has been found to differ from the other subgroupings of schizophrenia.

These data concerning the relationship between steroid activity and disease processes, both physical and mental, may be briefly summarized as follows:

1. Underfunction or absence of the adrenocortical steroids produces clear-cut disorders of the sort outlined above, whereas overactivity, either as a result of functional or histopathological abnormalities, produces clear-cut disease syndromes of a different type.
2. It has been demonstrated that administration of a steroid to a patient who is deficient in that particular substance results in a return to normal and that administration of excessive amounts results in symptoms resembling pathological overactivity of the adrenal cortex. However, if this same steroid is administered to a patient who already has pathological overproduction, the effect is not an additive one, but, instead, is characteristic of underproduction. Thus, the relationship between steroid activity and disease states does not appear to be a direct underactivity-overactivity relationship. Interesting correlations between clinical syndromes and steroid activity or steroid therapy have been made. To cite a few examples:
   (a) Patients with gastrointestinal ulcerations like those produced in animals with extirpation of the adrenal cortex show reduced output of 17-ketosteroids in the urine.
   (b) The collagen diseases and the overt allergies, supposedly characteristic of the resistance stage of adaptation and associated with increased activity of the adrenal cortex, are rarely observed in psychotic patients. Patients with these diseases when successfully treated with ACTH or cortisone sometimes develop complicating psychoses. The data on steroid activity in psychotic schizophrenics indicate that the majority are underresponsive and suggest specifically that the pituitary-adrenal mechanism is less responsive to stress in schizophrenics than it is in nonpsychotic persons. This relationship seems paradoxical, since the administration of steroids to patients with resistance diseases seemingly results in a process that appears to be characterized by underactivity of this stress mechanism.

Stress in the Intact Human. It was mentioned earlier that in the biochemical studies of stress in animals the stressful stimuli consisted of alterations in the external environment. From changes noted in the peripheral mechanisms of the animals, inferences were made in regard to intact humans living in our culture. In our basic animal studies the experiments centered about chemical changes resembling those seen with alterations of function in the pituitary and adrenal glands. Because similar chemical changes have been found in intact humans who were subjected to stress, it has been assumed by many that the important and basic factor in psychological stress in the intact human is altered adrenal function. It may well be that it is the pituitary-adrenal mechanism which is altered under stress, but the manner in which it is activated becomes an important research problem if the relationship between the mind and bodily function is to be understood.

It does not seem likely that either the pituitary or the adrenal cortex by itself would begin to throw out excessive or reduced amounts of hormones. In our concept it must be stimulated to do this. Because of the hypothalamic-pituitary relationships which have been described by several authors, it is often assumed that the hypothalamus is responsible for activating the pituitary, which in turn activates the adrenals. The manner in which the cerebral cortex is related to lower centers has not been extensively investigated. If our "levels" scheme is correct, however, the peripheral chemical changes associated with stress must be the result of the interpretation by the individual of a given stimulus in the context of past experience or cultural factors, and, therefore, must be influenced at the level of the cerebral cortex. This would suggest that there are efferent pathways from the cerebral cortex which influence the humoral adaptive mechanism. (Even though the endpoint chemical changes are similar to those noted with altered pituitary-adrenal function, it does not necessarily follow that the pituitary and adrenals are the effectors in psychological stress.)

Basic Experiments. As mentioned earlier, our present working hypothesis has evolved over the course of several years. Experiments were designed on the basis of theory, and theory has evolved and changed in accordance with the data derived from experimentation. The relevant data from various experiments as presented at the meetings held in New Orleans in June, 1952, are covered in detail in later chapters. Some of them will be briefly mentioned here in order to demonstrate the manner in which they influenced the evolution of various concepts and gave support to the contention that psychological, neural, and humoral changes represent different aspects of the same process.

Biochemical Changes Induced by Manipulation of the Neuraxis. In order to demonstrate that efferent pathways from the cerebral cortex could influence the humoral adaptive mechanism, a number of animal experiments were undertaken (see Chapters 2 and 3). In summarizing these, the following points may be stressed:

1. Destructive lesions in a specific subcortical region of the cat brain were followed by metabolic changes resembling those following adrenalectomy—namely, changes in electrolyte balance and glucose metabolism, consistent hematological changes, ulceration of the gastrointestinal tract, and loss of temperature control. Despite this Addisonian-like picture, the pituitaries and adrenals were normal or hypertrophied, suggesting that the neural mechanism might be primary (since the endocrine mechanism appeared to be normal).
2. The metabolic changes were consistently accompanied by marked hypokinesia and loss of affect.

These data on the effects of ablation were important in the light of our over-all theoretical framework, in that they demonstrated one of the key points—namely, that the chemical changes associated with stress could be produced by lesions within the neuraxis and, more particularly, from a region in the nervous system which was known from anatomical studies to be connected with the cerebral cortex. This, then, seemingly placed the humoral adaptation under the influence of the cerebral cortex.

Eventually, this same region, namely the base of the septum (pp. 1–5) was stimulated in schizophrenic patients. From the chemical studies on these patients, much supporting evidence has been collected. This will be presented in detail in Chapter 15. Here it is sufficient to note that in one case sodium retention resulted from stimulation over a fairly long period and in another case the development of an abscess in the septal region was accompanied by many of the same chemical changes that had appeared in animals with lesions placed in this region.

Studies of Motor Activity

On several occasions, particularly when developing the over-all theory of human behavior, reference has been made to the importance of motor activity. The implication was that behavior is basically motor, and that motor responses should therefore reflect alterations in mental activity, the integrator of behavior of man. (It was noted that response to stress—i.e., emergency behavior, was chiefly responsible for pathological alterations of mental activity in intact humans.) Considerable evidence, both basic and clinical, regarding the motor system has been collected within this framework.

Animal Experiments. In the basic animal studies, which will be described in detail in Chapter 4, the most relevant experiment was concerned with systematically exploring the subcortical regions of the forebrain of the cat for areas which would facilitate or inhibit cortical activity. The technique consisted of first inducing background motor activity by stimulation of the motor cortex. Concurrently with this, deep stimulation was applied to various parts of the forebrain through electrodes placed by the Horsley-Clarke stereotaxic apparatus. Since it was impossible to get psychological data from reported introspection, as in human studies, it was felt that the cortically induced motor activity would be the best reflection of integrated cortical activity. Points of facilitation and inhibition were outlined in this manner, facilitatory points by and large being located in the rostral midline structures, the septal region, and the rostral hypothalamus. Inhibitory points were also found at this rostral level, largely in the lateral aspect of the caudate nucleus.

Monkeys were stimulated through electrodes implanted in the subcortical sites which produced facilitation and inhibition (see Chapter 6). When stimulation was applied to the region associated with the facilitatory circuit, the animal became very alert. When stimulation was applied to the region associated with the inhibitory circuit, the animal became drowsy. It therefore seemed probable the cortically induced motor activity of the acute animal experiments was related to the awareness identified in the chronic animal experiments. It is worth noting at this point that the region in which stimulation produced facilitation corresponded closely to the region in which ablation produced the previously described metabolic changes resembling adrenalectomy, as well as loss of affect (see Addendum B for studies on chemical changes following stimulation of facilitatory and inhibitory circuits).

Clinical Studies. This basic motor data takes on more significance when considered in the light of clinical data gathered by Dr. King (see Chapter 16). Dr. King's test, in essence, centered about speed in simple motor acts. The great significance of this test was that it seemingly offered a tool—namely, motor response—which could be used to break down the barrier that heretofore had made translation of data from animals to humans difficult or impossible. It was designed entirely on the basis of observations in humans and was developed during the topectomy studies in 1948. Most of the patients tested were schizophrenics, although patients with other diseases were studied to a lesser extent. The schizophrenic group was found to be markedly slow on performance of this test. Some of the non-schizophrenics who scored well above normal on speed were found to be subject to clinical disease processes in the form of migraine and hypertension. These patients have been studied as psychosomatic problems. We have been impressed psychiatrically by their quick emotional responsivity.

Some speculative formulations are possible from the data thus far presented, which will be elaborated upon later. The points to be stressed here are that the greatest inhibition on motor performance was found among retarded schizophrenic patients. This is the group which showed chemical evidence of underactivity of the stress mechanism and which, when examined psychiatrically by introspective techniques, also showed a marked disturbance in basic affect. The clinical disorders which were characterized by increased speed on this preliminary survey were those in which the chemical data indicated overactivity of the stress mechanism and in which psychiatric examination indicated quick affective responsivity.

Other Approaches Contributing Data to the Over-all Formulations

Data derived through a variety of other studies contributed to the formulation of our hypothesis and the ultimate evolution of techniques utilized in human studies. Studies of human behavior after frontal lobe surgery contributed somewhat to our ideas of cortical function. Also, anatomical and physiological studies of cortical-subcortical interrelationships contributed to our formulations of the nature of the dynamic interaction between levels of integration in the brain.

Ablation of Cerebral Cortex in Humans. Since the advent of lobotomy and topectomy in the treatment of psychotic patients, it has been possible to observe the effects of injury to the frontal lobe on human behavior through utilization of the technique of reported introspection. In essence, the principal psychological change resulting from these surgical procedures seems to be a reduction in affective responses associated with painful memories. This has had some value in the treatment of certain types of patients, but it may also be accompanied by undesirable changes in behavior. Basically, the latter appears as a carefree attitude on the part of the patient, with a lessening in his concern for the future, and a tendency to live more for the here and now. These undesirable alterations in behavior are consistent with the observations from phylogeny that the ability to anticipate the future and plan far ahead is associated with the evolution of the cerebral cortex. Lack of concern for the future appears regardless of where the cortex is damaged within the frontal lobe, whereas lessening of emotional response to memories results only when specific areas of the prefrontal cortex or their connections are damaged. This statement is derived from data gathered in the Columbia-Greystone study. Kluver and Bucy[9] have also reported alterations of affective responses following damage to the temporal lobe.

In the Columbia-Greystone topectomy study operative removal of areas 9 or 10 or the orbital gyrus produced lessening in painful affect, whereas other removals in regions of areas 6 and 8 did not. It is noteworthy that some patients with fluctuating hypertension became normo-tensive after topectomy. The same has been reported following lobotomy. Very little alteration in metabolism has been reported following frontal lobe operations. Some of the Greystone patients showed temporary alterations in glucose tolerance but no changes in electrolyte balance. The evidence gathered from observations on lobotomy patients which is especially pertinent to our present framework may be summarized as follows:

1. Removal of specific areas of the frontal lobe—namely, 9, 10, and 11 and possibly 46, produced lessened affect from painful memories.
2. Damage to the cortex produced lack of concern for the future in proportion to the degree of cortex removed.

3. The minimal alterations in metabolism which occurred did not persist.
4. The basic schizophrenic process did not appear to be altered as a result of frontal lobe operations.

Anatomical and Physiological Studies of Cortical-Subcortical Connections. One important observation which emerged from the Columbia-Greystone topectomy study was that removal of cortical areas connected with the septal region of the forebrain produced the most consistent reduction in emotional overflow from memories. This was one of our reasons for directing attention to the septal region in attempting to make correlations between dynamic physiological activity and behavior. Observations on animals following ablation of the prefrontal cortex[10, 11] suggest that areas 9 and 11, which project to the septal region may exert some over-all inhibitory effect on motor behavior. It has been reported that, following removal of granular cortex, animals display spontaneous overactivity, some distractability, and a reduction in affective responses. Stimulation of the dorsum of the prefrontal cortex has given inconclusive results. But in our laboratories we have occasionally observed inhibition of background motor activity following stimulation of the rostral part of the prefrontal cortex.[8] Recordings during stimulation have indicated interconnections between the frontal cortex and the septal region and between the septal region and the frontal and temporal cortex. A more detailed review of the stimulation and recording work of others,[12] along with studies performed in our laboratories, will be given later. Our studies were conducted with animals in which electrodes were chronically implanted in specific subcortical regions and on the cortex.

In considering these physiological relationships it is important to point out that the cortex fires many subcortical regions other than the septal region and that many other subcortical regions fire the cortex. Our interest was particularly directed toward this site because it is the neural region which specifically affects the chemistry of stress and had been shown to have a pronounced effect on background motor activity.

To summarize—anatomical and physiological data derived from animal experimentation demonstrated that:

1. Stimuli to the prefrontal and temporal cortex (those parts which, when ablated in the human, produced lessened affect from painful memories) fire the septal region.

2. Stimuli to the septal region activate the cortex, especially the frontal and temporal lobes.

CONCEPTS OF THE FACILITATORY AND INHIBITORY CIRCUITS

Thus far I have outlined an operational hypothesis, derived largely from psychology and evolution, which suggested possible correlations between behavior and different levels of the neuraxis. Various procedures used to test some aspects of this hypothesis in animals have been described. Attention has been directed to dynamic interaction between the cortex and the septal region of the forebrain.

From this data we were able to postulate patterns of overactivity and patterns of underactivity. The overactivity we attributed to excitation of the facilitatory circuit and the underactivity to a deficiency in the facilitatory circuit or excitation of a hypothetical inhibitory circuit. These terms were picked up because they were in general use in neurophysiology. They were particularly appropriate in conjunction with motor measurements. Throughout our discussion they will be applied to the total state of the organism. This broad application seems justified, since we have been able to demonstrate that changes in specific regions concurrently affect motor activity, psychological activity, and the chemical homeostatic mechanisms. The term *facilitatory* then refers to acceleration of motor activity, increased chemical activity, and higher psychological levels of awareness, whereas the term *inhibitory* refers to slowing of motor activity, reduced chemical activity, and lower levels of awareness.

In our original formulation of human behavior we stressed the importance of the relationship between states of awareness and the reporting of the patient. Since animals cannot report, our basic experiments on psychological activity were limited to demonstrations that states of awareness could be altered. From these experiments, however, it was impossible to be certain that alterations of the neuraxis which produced either facilitation or inhibition would also produce changes in thought which could be observed through introspective reporting. The only way in which this could be determined was to carry out specific procedures on patients.

The only patients in whom such new and untried procedures would be justified were those in whom craniotomy was also justified as a therapeutic measure. The largest group of patients upon whom this appeared to be feasible was the hopeless schizophrenic group—that is, patients who were already undergoing drastic surgical procedures and who had failed to respond with remissions to existing therapy. Before operating upon the first patient we had the basic chemical data from animal experimentation, the findings on facilitation and inhibition against background motor activity, and psychological data on schizophrenics which indicated retarded motor activity. We therefore felt that we had sufficient evidence to undertake a new procedure.

The major points in the evolution of techniques involved in this procedure will be discussed after the presentation of our views on the clinical disorder of schizophrenia. In the following section emphasis will be placed on the manner in which available data on the disease fits into our over-all scheme of mind-brain relationships.

OUR OPERATIONAL CONCEPT OF SCHIZOPHRENIA

Little is definitely known in regard to schizophrenia. There is considerable disagreement about the nature of the disease among investigators and clinicians treating patients who have been diagnosed as schizophrenics, and even as to diagnosis different observers are in agreement only when overt psychotic symptoms are present. A brief outline of the operational concepts that we have found useful in working with patients presenting this clinical entity is therefore in order.

Although all the schizophrenic patients included in this report fall into the category of the Kraepelinian diagnostic definition, we consider schizophrenia as a much broader entity. Our concept includes the less clear-cut syndromes previously used to describe borderline conditions—namely, prepsychotic schizophrenia, preclinical schizophrenia, latent schizophrenia, schizothymic, schizophreniform, and so forth. Bleuler,[13] who originated the term *schizophrenia*, used the following definition in 1911: "Schizophrenia is characterized by specific kind of alteration of thinking and feeling and of the relations with the outer world that occurs nowhere else." Emphasizing that Kraepelin's dementia praecox was a secondary manifestation of a basic disease process, Bleuler continues: "In every case we are confronted with a more or less clear-cut splitting of the psychic functions. If the disease is marked, the personality loses its unity. At different times different psychic complexes seem to represent the personality. Integration of different complexes and strivings appear insufficient or even lacking. The psychic complexes do not combine in a conglomeration of strivings with a unified resultant as they do in a healthy person; rather one set of complexes dominates the personality for a time while other groups of ideas or drives are 'split off' and seem either partly or completely impotent. Often ideas are only partially worked out and fragments of ideas are connected in an illogical way to constitute a new idea. Concepts lose their completeness, seem to dispense with one or more of their essential components. Indeed, in many cases they are only represented by a few truncated notions."

As a result of experience in psychoanalysis and in intensive psychiatric observation and treatment, more persons are tending to accept Bleuler's concept that a primary disease process is present long before the Kraepelinian symptoms of dementia praecox appear. Several investigators are attempting to learn more about the nature of this basic disease process. Clinical observations, as well as increasing experience with unhospitalized patients, have made it quite apparent that disordered behavior begins very early—in fact, as far back as observations are valid. It is assumed by many that the disease process is either present at birth or results from early environmental trauma.

Because various workers in the field differ widely in the use of the term *schizophrenia*, I shall begin by defining two terms that will appear in the following discussion. The term *decompensated* will be used in reference to the Kraepelinian criteria for dementia praecox (or, in Bleuler's definition, the accessory symptoms) and the term *basic* will be used in reference to Bleuler's fundamental symptoms. Since little controversy exists as to the description of the decompensated schizophrenic, my remarks will be largely confined to observations on the nature of the basic defect and to the relationship between the accessory and the fundamental symptoms.

To us, the conventional psychoanalytic framework for the integration of the mind was not a satisfactory working hypothesis, since the organization of the mind into id, ego, and superego provided no basis for an understanding of the mechanism of schizophrenia. The formulations that we found most useful were the concepts of Rado and others who stress the importance of basic deficiencies in feeling from early infancy. Rado postulates that subsequent alterations in behavior arise primarily from a basic deficiency in pleasure. At the beginning of this presentation, it was stressed that the hedonic regulators remain in control of behavior, even with the superimposition of higher, potentially more efficient adaptation through the development of the emotional and psychological levels. Viewing behavior in the light of the adaptational theory of increasingly complex levels of development, one can readily see that impairment on the hedonic, or feeling, level would influence all subsequent higher levels of adaptation. An individual who has a basic deficiency in pleasure does not develop normally and is handicapped in his ability to respond in the manner of normal persons. It is postulated that many of the behavioral deviations which have been observed in schizophrenia result from such impairment. The basic deficiency is perceived by the interviewing clinician as a lack of empathy.

In psychiatric literature, and especially in psychoanalytic literature, there are many descriptions of the schizophrenic process and many attempts to explain schizophrenic behavior. While there is agreement on these observations, implications to the effect that certain factors are etiological cannot be supported. Explanations centered about the concept of withdrawal of libido have frequently appeared, but no evidence has been advanced to show that this is a causal factor or even that withdrawal takes place. There have been also consistent reports to the effect that ego development is impaired in schizophrenia, but this too must be considered as a result rather than a cause. Others have explained the schizophrenic reaction as an inability to interpret symbols properly, but this, too, we consider a symptom of a disturbance resulting from a more basic process. Symbols develop meaning in terms of feeling. If feeling is impaired, the meaning of symbols should be altered.

In our concept there is no implication that the impairment on the hedonic, or feeling, level is etiological. Our contention is rather that impairment represents a primary deficiency and that many of the reported observations on schizophrenia are secondary elaborations resulting from it. Our speculations on the possible cause will be presented after data from other disciplines have been reviewed.

Behavioral changes observed in patients with the diagnosis of basic schizophrenia appear to support the concept outlined above—namely, that impairment of the hedonic mechanism is primary. Mothers of schizophrenics frequently report that as far back as they can remember something has been lacking in the patients' relationships. As children they appeared to be "different." To summarize consistent descriptions, one could say that in general the mother describes a lack of resonance with the child. Frequently, the mother says that she noticed this while feeding the baby. Case histories indicate that self-awareness is impaired early. Self-awareness, or ego development, is largely based on feeling. We hypothesize that the impairment of feeling is responsible for the faulty awareness of self which develops and becomes more obvious as the individual enters into more complicated relationships.

The basic crippling is manifest in virtually every activity. It is apparent in sexual behavior at a very early age and becomes more striking in adolescence and adult life. Many writers have attributed the bizarre sexual practices of schizophrenics to an inability to integrate pleasure with sexual activity. Their lack of feeling, extensively described by Hoch[14] and others, may also be responsible for their consistently observed tendency to mimic or attach themselves to others. Reider[15] has used the term *pseudo-normality* to describe the schizophrenic's attempt to use intellectual control rather than spontaneous feeling as motivation in behavior.

Since Bleuler's early expression of opinion, there has been much in the way of general discussion on the schizophrenic's intellectual ability.

Many consider the intellect to be quite normal before the onset of the secondary process, or decompensated psychosis. By standard intellectual measurements, it is often the case that prior to or between decompensated psychotic episodes schizophrenics function at a very high intellectual level. However, close observation of the intellectual functions of such patients do reveal impairment even in those who are performing at a high level. This appears primarily in the sphere of their ability to use the intellect—to integrate it in the most useful manner. When oriented toward picking up this specific defect, perhaps psychological tests to measure intellect will yield more information.

Some tests now used in clinical psychology reflect patterns which are thought to be characteristic of basic schizophrenia. One of the outstanding features—namely, the lack of over-all integration on associating to the Rorschach patterns—indicates a tendency to see the pieces rather than the whole and failure to distinguish foreground from background. This accords well with clinical observation.

Subjectively, basic schizophrenics are often aware of their deficiencies. Many complain of having no aim in life and of not knowing exactly where they fit. This often leads to panic, during which they will consult the psychiatrist, complaining correctly of fears of "going crazy." They often remain in psychoanalysis for prolonged periods, hoping that in some magical way they will find themselves. The anxiety is considerably different from that seen in neurotic patients, and the basis clearly appears to be centered about limited awareness of self and concern about meeting the demands of society.

Psychoanalytic therapy with basic schizophrenics is often tragic. Many articles have lately appeared in which altered techniques are described; most authors favor a technique which aids repression and gives support, thus aiding the patient to find a way of meeting the vicissitudes of life. In sharp contrast, the common practice of directing therapy toward removing repression often precipitates a psychosis. As a rule the intense emotional stress which is associated with precipitation of the decompensated state is primarily due to panic developing within the individual because of internal awareness of basic deficiency. However, it is not meant to imply that stressful memories and environmental factors play an unimportant role. The fact that environmental stress is always prominent in the clinical symptoms of patients with decompensated psychoses makes its contribution clear. Such patients do not handle stress well; in an unconscious attempt to find security they regress to infantile patterns of behavior. The outside environment is distorted and is interpreted in unreal terms.

Psychological repair appears to be accompanied by markedly increased disintegration of emotionality. It is during this stage that there is consistent impairment at the intellectual level. Case histories often indicate that individuals who have performed quite well intellectually, despite the symptoms of basic schizophrenia, suddenly begin to perform poorly after the onset of decompensated psychosis. In our holistic concept we have found it necessary to consider basic schizophrenia not in terms of all or none but rather in terms of degrees. Persons with greater degrees of basic schizophrenia require less in the way of environmental stress (interpreted against past experiences) to precipitate decompensated reactions. When basic schizophrenia is minimal, overwhelming stress is necessary. Prognosis for recovery varies considerably. In general, patients who have shown the least in the way of basic schizophrenia during the prepsychotic period (i.e., before decompensation) have the most favorable prognosis.

Bleuler wrote that he had never seen a patient in whom the primary schizophrenic disease was cured. Most workers in the field today would agree with this statement of Bleuler's. Of all the treatments used in schizophrenia thus far, none has been shown to alter the primary, or basic, disease. It is true that some patients suffering from decompensated schizophrenia do improve, many spontaneously, and that treatment influences others toward better social adaptation. A close evaluation of the improvements resulting from psychotherapy inevitably leads to the conclusion that patients receive the greatest therapeutic benefit from support which helps them to strengthen their intellectual control in everyday behavior. There is no evidence that shock therapies alter the basic disease process. In studies of the effects of psychosurgery, one of the most consistent observations was that relief of stress from memories was the factor that benefited those persons who improved. Those in whom the basic disease process was strongest and in whom the degree of painful affect was minimal were least benefited by the operation. Consideration of this factor made it possible in many instances to prognosticate the type of patient who could be helped.

These observations on the nature of the basic disease process and the effect of other therapies constituted our rationale in selecting patients for electrical stimulation. We wanted to determine whether or not basic schizophrenia could be altered, and, therefore, selected patients in whom the affective component was minimal and the basic schizophrenia very marked. This will be discussed in greater detail when the patient population used in this study is surveyed (see Chapter 8).

BIOCHEMICAL STUDIES

In schizophrenic patients some humoral changes have been observed and reported. Most recent data regarding such changes[16] have been speculatively interpreted to indicate that the adrenal cortex does not respond properly to stress, possibly as a result of impairment of the pituitary-adrenal tropic mechanism. The data on which this conclusion was based were derived from measurements which reflect adrenocortical function—namely, urinary excretion studies of steroids, uric acid, electrolytes, etc.—plus measurements of lymphocyte and eosinophil changes under stress. Studies of carbohydrate metabolism were also used. However, the indirect evidence thus obtained offers no proof that pathological underactivity of the adrenal cortex is basic in schizophrenia or even that a defective response to stress is always involved.

Cleghorn[17] has reported a series of studies on psychotic patients in which he compared the adrenocortical activity resulting from electroshock with that induced by administration of ACTH. Many patients in the shock group had clinical remissions of psychosis, while the ACTH group showed no improvement, yet it was found that with the measurements he used the adrenals responded less to shock than to ACTH, indicating that it was not primarily activation of the adrenal cortex which produced the clinical improvement following electroshock. Likewise, some of the data regarding carbohydrate metabolism in schizophrenia, as outlined by the original investigators, does not appear to be too consistent. We have not been able to obtain these findings on our service here.

The principal conclusion to be drawn from biochemical studies in schizophrenia is that there appears to be less response to externally induced stress in the schizophrenic than in the normal, as determined by measurements which usually reflect adrenocortical activity but which need not reflect only such activity.

PSYCHOMOTOR STUDIES

In the previously mentioned motor tests devised by Dr. King marked slowing was consistently shown by all the schizophrenics in the catatonic-hebephrenic retarded group. Altered responses were consistently present in the very active, alert, rage-driven paranoid group, but to a lesser degree.

SCHIZOPHRENIA AND THE MIND-BRAIN CONCEPT

Although we have not attempted in the present investigation to deal with the manner in which schizophrenia begins, speculations on the genesis of the disease were essential to the development of our operational framework. As previously stated, it seemed to us that a basic deficiency on the hedonic level of integration was of primary importance and that this deficiency was manifested by defective self-awareness, faulty integration of emotional reactions, and a type of intellectual impairment. A good description of one very early stage of self-awareness has been given by William James,[18] who pointed out that awareness is first expressed in terms of motion related to breast-feeding. This early motion—namely, moving toward the breast and sucking—is obviously associated with the pleasure of satiating hunger. The subsequent stages of self-awareness will not be discussed in detail here. However, it seems logical to assume that they could be affected by difficulty at this very early stage. Persons who advocate the inheritance factor in mental disease would reason that abnormality is present before birth and that the early child-parent relationship is inconsequential as an etiological factor, but most workers in the field would agree that an interplay between the two factors is involved. In our concept we stress the genetic factor as well as the early parent-child relationship because of the observation that in schizophrenia defects can be traced as far back in the life cycle of the individual as observations are valid.

Recently attention has been increasingly directed toward early diagnosis ot schizophrenia, and a higher incidence of childhood schizophrenia has been reported, but diagnosis is still largely determined on the presence of decompensating psychotic symptoms. Many persons with symptoms of basic schizophrenia do not develop decompensating symptoms, and at present it remains difficult or impossible to predict accurately which ones will develop decompensating schizophrenia. Preliminary studies utilizing the psychomotor test designed by Dr. King indicate that slowing occurs in a lesser degree in basic, or compensated, schizophrenics; no work has been done with children to date. It is apparent from studies carried out thus far that the tests to determine activity of the humoral mechanism—that is, stress tests—are not conclusive before overt manifestations of psychosis appear.

In view of the relatively meager findings in schizophrenia we are largely limited at present to clinical observations, and the framework which we have utilized is conspicuously lacking in clear-cut data. Our concept, therefore, rests on the assumption that precipitating emotional factors, plus inherited predisposition, produce early alterations in the neural circuits which continue in effect and thereby influence subsequent psychological development. In accordance with the observation that decompensated schizophrenia appears in those who have had defects since childhood, we postulated that it is during the very vulnerable period of infancy, and then only in those with genic predisposition, that psychological trauma can produce such profound effects.

In the previous discussion of our ideas concerning schizophrenia, it has been pointed out that little or no intellectual impairment occurs before overt psychosis appears. It therefore seems certain that any physiological alterations that are present must be well under way by this time. Hence intellectual development must eventually become markedly affected. It is the usual observation that some children do well in school up to a certain point and then, with the beginning of decompensating symptoms, lose the ability to perform in class and to learn.

Since decompensating symptoms have much in common with states of reverie or sleep, we further postulated that there must be some inhibition of cortical activity during the decompensated period. Pathological delusions and hallucinations, which are among the decompensated schizophrenic's most characteristic symptoms, are manifestations of impaired self-awareness. Hallucinations occur when thoughts are not bound, when a part of the self seems to come from the outside. In sleep, reverie, or extreme fatigue, the normal individual may temporarily have similar symptoms, i.e., internal thoughts may appear to come from the outside. To illustrate—a normal individual, upon first awakening from a deep sleep might see a lamp shade and while still dazed might interpret it as a marauder, if the trend of the unconscious thought processes of his dream life happened to be threatening at the time. Upon full awakening, however, this misinterpretation would disappear.

These vague common characteristics between sleep and the schizophrenic psychosis led to a more thorough investigation of physiological activity in the form of recordings of electrical potentials. It is well-known from electroencephalographic studies that in normal sleep there is marked inhibition of brain activity, whereas in light sleep and in reverie the potentials begin to approach those found in the waking state. Hitherto schizophrenic records have not shown clear-cut abnormalities, although mild inconsistent changes have been reported, generally in the direction of minimal slowing of activity and temporal lobe spiking. The recording techniques, however, were admittedly crude, since they summed up the activity of the subcortex, cortex, muscle, scalp, and so forth. It therefore seemed to us that refinement in technique might reveal consistent electrical abnormality at the cortical level in decompensated schizophrenics. The various aspects of this problem and the results of our recordings will be discussed in detail in Chapter 11. Two points are worth highlighting here. The first is that vague slow-downs in cortical rhythm sometimes occurred when recordings were made between scalp leads and indifferent deep leads which did not appear on recordings taken simultaneously between scalp leads. The second is that in our series of schizophrenic patients all the abnormalities recorded were more marked during light sleep and periods of quiet and tended to lessen when attention on the part of the patient was focused on something real and external—for example, the drawing of blood for chemical tests.

To summarize our speculations in the light of the data presented—we hypothesized that physiological abnormalities beginning in early childhood or before interfere with emotional and, in varying degrees, intellectual development. The individual is thus unprepared to meet the vicissitudes of everyday life; at some time during his life cycle various stress-invoking situations can produce an intense over-reaction in the form of decompensated schizophrenia.

A description of the onset of decompensated schizophrenia in physiological terms according to our over-all theoretical framework would be as follows: Activity at the level of the cerebral cortex induces a markedly abnormal subcortical rhythm which in turn spreads back to cortex, producing additional physiological effects on the cortex which are reflected clinically as abnormalities in the thinking and learning processes.

Observations on the effects of frontal lobe surgery were important in our reasoning at this juncture. Such operations lessened the affect from painful memories, but failed to alter the primary schizophrenia. We, therefore, hypothesized that the abnormal reverberating subcortical circuit was activated by stressful stimuli received from the cortical level.

On the basis of clinical observations we assumed that the over-all effect in schizophrenia was one of cortical impairment. We therefore reasoned that if the subcortex was functioning abnormally as a result of cortical firing, then electrical stimulation to the basal part of the septal region might stir it into more normal activity, thus facilitating cortical activity and bringing the individual out of the sleep-like state of reverie and helping him to make a better interpretation of reality. It was hoped that the stimulation procedure might enable him to perceive his emotionally charged conflicts in terms of the here and now rather than in the infantile terms which the disease process had established.

The operative technique involved in the placement of electrodes required only a small unilateral incision in the ventricle, which we felt would result in less damage to the brain than the existing psychosurgical procedures and so would leave the patient more nearly intact. Nevertheless, in selecting patients for the new procedure we confined our choice to those who had not benefited by the established therapies given and who were not considered suitable for frontal lobe surgery.

At the meetings held in New Orleans in June, 1952, we presented a motion picture showing the pre- and postoperative course of the first patient who received stimulation in the basal part of the septal region. The outcome thus far has been favorable. In this particular patient one could argue, although the statistical odds are weighted as heavily as possible against it, that the effect of stimulation was nonspecific and that no proof was established that the subcortex had been truly impaired. Recordings were not made on this patient, but they were taken on subsequent patients and the results will be reported in detail later.

TECHNIQUES

All our techniques have been modified and considerably improved as the work has progressed. The major modifications will be mentioned, since all data must be considered against the background of the techniques employed.

SURGICAL TECHNIQUES

Initially, the electrodes were implanted through a unilateral opening in the prefrontal cortex and a small incision in the anterior horn of the lateral ventricle. The first two patients were stimulated in the operating room and the electrodes were withdrawn before closure of the wounds.

Beginning with the third patient, the leads attached to the electrodes were brought out through the bone and skin, so that recording and stimulation could be carried out a few hours after completion of the operation. In each of the first five patients only one pair of electrodes was embedded, but in subsequent patients operated upon by the open method three pairs were usually implanted. This technique left much to be desired, since placement was highly inaccurate and the electrodes could be left in place for only a relatively short period (24 to 54 hours). The incision into the ventricle damaged brain tissue and thereby made interpretation of the findings on recordings difficult. Also, the direct pathway from the skin into the ventricle increased the hazard of infection.

A closed method utilizing the stereotaxic instrument was therefore developed. At the time of the June 1952 meetings this procedure had been employed in a few patients. Subsequently, the original stereotaxic technique has been considerably improved. The latest method is described in Addendum C and has been reported elsewhere.[19] Improvements in surgical technique have made it possible to substantiate much of the earlier data that was open to question when reported at the meetings. Concern over some of the findings was justified at that time because of uncertainty as to the exact site of implantation of the electrode and the added variable of cortical damage caused by the open method.

RECORDING TECHNIQUES

Records were not obtained from the first two schizophrenic patients, since stimulation was done in the operating room. In the third case it was possible to record effectively for a short time. However, a mechanical defect soon developed with respect to the electrodes. In view of the fact that rather typical findings were found on the recordings from the first five patients, we decided that electrodes should be placed in structures other than the septal region. Accordingly, we attempted to place bipolar electrodes in the caudate nucleus and in the region of the anterior thalamus, as well as in the septal region. These placements made it possible to take electrical recordings, through what were thought to be different circuits, prior to administering the therapeutic stimulation.

An important finding on the recordings, as will be reported in Chapter 11, was that in all the patients in whom electrodes were satisfactorily placed, there appeared to be a definite abnormality through the facilitatory circuit in the septal region. At the time of the meetings, because of the above-mentioned problems in surgical technique, there was justification for questioning the significance of the recordings, especially the localization of the abnormality. However, subsequent technical improvements have substantiated our major findings. The abnormality reported at the meetings has been demonstrated in many schizophrenics to be restricted to a relatively small area in the septal region. As of this writing, electrodes have been placed in the hypothalamus, caudate, tegmentum of the mesencephalon a few millimeters ventral to the aqueduct, hippocampus, and amygdaloid nucleus. The only other structure from which the abnormality has been recorded is the hippocampus, where it has been of smaller amplitude. Even there it did not appear each time it showed in the septal region. With the new technique electrodes have been left in place for long periods (up to 9 months in one patient). It is clear now that the abnormality is not related to the acute trauma of surgery, since it persists as long as the behavioral disorders continue.

A few additional patients with disorders other than schizophrenia have recently been incorporated in our series. None of them showed a similar abnormality, and this is consistent with the findings in the small group of nonschizophrenic patients reported at the meetings.

A second important finding was that in many instances it was possible to record changes through the facilitatory circuit when patients were excited by questioning about problems which had been known to produce unpleasant feelings. On the second point there is some need for clarification. Occasionally, abnormalities of similar types appeared when patients were not being questioned. Although it was impossible to know what the patients were thinking at all times, some correlations were possible. These will be discussed more in detail in Chapter 11 and Addendum E.

Recordings taken during altered states of awareness induced by the administration of drugs have been quite interesting. Such studies were not reported at the June 1952 meetings but have since been reported.[20] There have been correlations between alterations in electrical recordings from different structures which tend to give support to the original psychological formulation regarding levels of awareness.

STIMULATION TECHNIQUES

Several problems arose in conjunction with the stimulation techniques designed to activate the facilitatory circuit, which was presumed to be somehow deficient. The first was that we had no way of knowing whether the passage of an electrical current would actually activate the circuit or not. This question is still not solved.

The second problem involved selection of the type of wave to use, the frequency of choice, and so forth. In the initial cases it was decided to use a rectangular voltage pulse of 1 millisecond duration, with repetition frequency of 100 cycles per second. This was arbitrarily chosen because it appeared to be the type of stimulus that most effectively facilitated background motor activity in animals. In all subsequent cases presented at the June 1952 meetings this type of stimulus was used exclusively. We are still by no means certain that it is the most effective way of influencing the circuit. It is known from animal experimentation that other frequencies do not influence cortical activity as favorably as is indicated by recorded electrical potentials, but it would be difficult to work out in animal studies alone the optimum type of stimulus. We feel this can be determined only by trial and error in humans, where it is possible to carry on the technique of reported introspection in conjunction with the stimulation. Since the June 1952 meetings we have altered the frequency and wave forms in stimulating some cases, but as yet we have no clear-cut evidence that other frequencies are more effective than 100 per second.

The third problem concerned the duration of stimulation. In the earlier cases we were limited by the fact that electrodes could not be left in over long periods of time because of the danger of infection. In no case in which the open technique was used were the electrodes in place over 54 hours. However, we felt that with the closed or stereotaxic technique, there would be less danger of infection. In the last patient in the reported series (Patient 25) electrodes were left in place for 18 days with no demonstrable ill effect. Findings over this period proved to be quite interesting. These will be reported in detail in Chapter 13. One of the highlights was the fact that subsequent stimuli had markedly different effects from the first few stimuli.

It is in the choice of the optimum type of stimulus that the greatest problems appeared to be and it is here that there is the greatest need for future research. The data gathered up to the time of the meetings on the effects of stimulation are reported in Chapter 13. We feel that the considerable variation in results was probably due to stimulation techniques. However, it may also reflect differences in the patients' illnesses.

Further investigation of stimulation techniques since the meetings has yielded important results. It now appears that some of the earlier stimuli may have been producing damage. For this reason certain changes have been made in the methods used. A full report of these alterations in technique and the reasons for such alterations is given in Addendum D. In patients stimulated since the meetings we have also tested to some extent the results of continuing septal stimulation for longer periods. Here the most important development was the tendency for abnormal paroxysmal activity to persist over long periods (up to a week) after discontinuation of the stimulus. This finding has recently been reported[19, 20] (see also Addendum E).

A consistent clinical observation has been that during stimulation of the septal region all patients have shown many similarities of response which can best be described as a type of awakening manifested by increased alertness, rapidity of speech, and clarity of thought. With longer follow-up periods some of the patients in the group have progressed, whereas others have failed to show continued improvement.

At the time of the original presentation the evidence on the postulated relationship between septal spiking and schizophrenia was admittedly inconclusive. It was felt, however, that the use of the stereotaxic technique, which makes it possible to keep electrodes in place over extended periods, might lead to a better understanding of this relationship. Electrodes have since been left in place for considerable periods. In the case of the patient who has had electrodes embedded over a period of nine months there has been a rather marked correlation between the increased frequency of the spiking and manifestations of psychotic behavior, and during periods of remission in psychosis the spikes are much less in evidence. A report with an illustration from the records is included in Addendum E.

The important results of the human studies may be summarized as follows in the light of the over-all theoretical framework:

1. It has been demonstrated through the application of recording and stimulating techniques, even though these techniques are somewhat crude, that there is some correlation between physiological abnormalities and pathological changes at the level of thought as determined by the patient's reporting.
2. The precipitation of stressful mental activity during interviews seemingly alters physiological activity through the facilitatory circuit of the brain.
3. Physiological activity induced by electrical stimulation of specific circuits in the brain is associated with alterations in levels of awareness and also with changes in thought as determined by the patient's reporting.

All these findings are as yet quite crude. We hope that with the refined techniques much closer correlations may be possible.

APPLICATION OF THE CONCEPT TO DISEASES OTHER THAN SCHIZOPHRENIA

Thus far, we have had only a few opportunities to put our over-all hypothesis to test in diseases other than schizophrenia. The principal limiting factor has been mentioned—namely, that testing the hypothesis requires a craniotomy, for which there is no precedent in most disease processes. Within the last few years, however, lobotomies have been performed for intractable pain. This provided us with a reason for craniotomy in the case of patients with far-advanced metastatic carcinoma. At the time of the meetings this operation had been performed on two patients with cancer (Patients 23 and 25), and since the meetings it has been performed on two other patients with cancer and on one patient with intractable rheumatoid arthritis. In addition, two psychotic patients with tuberculosis (Patients 18 and 21) have undergone the procedure.

These seven patients provided an opportunity to gather some preliminary observations on the manner in which altering the internal milieu of the body through stimulating the neural circuits would affect certain disease processes. The data on the application of our concept to diseases other than schizophrenia is meager but quite provocative. The rationale will therefore be given in brief. The tuberculosis patients will be discussed first.

TUBERCULOSIS

On the basis of data from various disciplines, we postulated that our concept of mind-brain relationships might be applied to tuberculosis along either of two lines of argument—namely, that inhibitory activity was dominant or that facilitatory activity was impaired. The reasons for this hypothesis are as follows:

1. Psychiatric observations—Several observers have described the tuberculous patient as showing a reduction in affective responsivity. One observer described this as "a tendency toward collapse."
2. Clinical psychological testing—It has been reported[21] that a very high incidence of tuberculous patients show schizophrenic characteristics on Rorschach testing.
3. Statistical survey—The incidence of tuberculosis is many times higher among schizophrenic patients than it is among the general population.
4. Electrolyte imbalance—Recent reports[22] indicate that there is frequently an alteration in electrolyte balance in tuberculosis, characterized by increased sodium and chloride excretion with corresponding diminution of sodium and chloride levels in the serum.
5. Co-existence of diabetes—Recent reports[23] speculate upon a relationship between diabetes and tuberculosis which could be logically explained by our data. In the animal studies impairment of the facilitatory circuit resulted in loss of sodium and inability to store carbohydrates.
6. In reviewing the subject of the role of the autonomic nervous system in immunity, Loumos[24] gives many references which suggest a relationship between the function of the nervous system and immunity. In particular, he notes that active patients, for example those with toxic goiter, are quite resistant to tuberculosis, whereas in retarded schizophrenic patients the incidence is extremely high.

These factors, when taken together, seemingly indicated that facilitatory activity is impaired in tuberculosis.

Very rapid progress toward healing appeared to follow stimulation in the case of Patient 18. This will be discussed in more detail on presentation of his case history. It is interesting to note that in a period of over 2 years he continued to improve in regard to tuberculosis but tended to relapse in regard to his psychosis, although initially his mental status had also improved.

In Patient 21 there was some evidence of improvement during the first 2 days. However, technical difficulties soon developed. This was the first patient in whom the stereotaxic technique was employed. On the second day he pulled out his electrodes; following this his mental status markedly deteriorated and much of the electrical activity characteristic of inhibition, namely slow waves, returned. In the course of the next 6 weeks he followed a downhill course and died. Prior to operation it had been predicted that he would die within 6 to 8 weeks if there were no improvement in his mental condition; it was the opinion of the internist who cared for him that the primary cause of death was not tuberculosis. To judge from animal studies, certain of the patient's symptoms (asthenia and loss of appetite) suggest injury to the facilitatory circuit. It was thought that this might have happened when he pulled out his electrodes. Unfortunately, he was transferred to another hospital within one week after operation and an adequate follow-up of the chemical studies was not made.

CANCER

Although there are a few psychiatric observations on the personality structure of patients developing malignancies, the findings are very inconsistent. Some interesting statistics, however, have been gathered on the incidence of carcinoma in psychotic patients as compared with that in the general population. The report made by Dr. Nolan D. C. Lewis[25] was especially interesting to us in view of the fact that he divided schizophrenics into over-reactors and under-reactors, the rage-driven paranoid patients being grouped as over-reactors and the retarded hebephrenics and catatonics as under-reactors. This classification is similar to our own —i.e., the rage-driven "facilitatory group" and the retarded "inhibitory group." There appeared to be a marked statistical difference between the two groups, the incidence of cancer being significantly higher in the over-reactor group and lower in the under-reactor group as compared with the expected incidence in the general population. Recent research has also focused on the role of steroid chemistry in cancer. Steroid therapy, especially with testosterone and estrogen, has induced temporary remissions in patients with metastatic cancer of the breast and prostate, and several patients with breast carcinoma are reported to have shown improvement after adrenalectomy with supplementary hormonal therapy.

In view of the recent finding[26, 27] that low antiproteolytic enzyme titers are associated with rapid tumor growth and high titers with retardation, it seemed to us that the antiproteolytic factor might give us an objective measure for judging the validity of our rationale in applying stimulation to cancer patients. So far we have obtained data from only one patient but we are planning to use this test more extensively in future investigations. In Patient 26, who was operated upon at the time of the June 1952 meetings, measurement of the antiproteolytic enzyme titer before and after stimulation indicated a rise from 55 to 88. In September 1952 Jacobs and others[28] reported studies on antiproteolytic enzymes in schizophrenia. Abnormally high rennin inhibitor titers were found only in very retarded patients.

The highlights of the results obtained on our four terminal cancer patients were that (1) none reported relief from pain as a result of the surgical operation itself, (2) all received relief from stimulation, and (3) all provided valuable controls for the schizophrenics in that none showed spiking during electroencephalographic recordings. Patient 23 was operated upon by the open method; the others were operated upon by the stereotaxic method. All were stimulated in the septo-hypothalamic region.

Patient 23 died on the third day following operation. She had been expected to die at any time. The cause of death was embolism from an abscess in the primary malignancy.

Patient 25, who had carcinoma of the breast with metastases involving virtually every bone in her body, lived for 18 days. The immediate cause of death was intestinal obstruction. At the time of operation it was recognized that she had many cerebral metastases, and she was not expected to survive the procedure. Nevertheless, some improvement was noted in her general condition following the first few stimulations.

She was more alert and responsive. The chemical data obtained on this patient are presented in Chapter 15. They are noteworthy in view of the fact that this was the first patient in whom the electrodes were embedded long enough to permit stimulation after the stress of the operation had worn off.

The third cancer patient to be stimulated likewise died 3 weeks after operation. Autopsy revealed a metastasis involving the inferior colliculus and mesencephalic tegmentum. Although this patient was semi-stuporous or stuporous during nearly all the postoperative period, after each septal stimulation she gained full consciousness for 45 to 60 minutes. During the periods when she was clinically alert the electrical activity characteristic of stupor which had been recorded before stimulation was consistently replaced by a desynchronized activity characteristic of a wakeful state. The records were shown at the American Neurological Association meetings in 1953.[19] The fact that we were able to facilitate a patient who was in stupor because of a lesion in the reticular activating system is relevant to the description by French[29] of stupor in patients with lesions in the mesencephalic tegmentum.

The fourth cancer patient to be stimulated underwent a striking remission during her three months' postoperative period, in which repeated stimuli were applied to the septo-hypothalamic region. Sample records of paroxysmal activity induced through prolonged stimulation were shown at the American Neurological Association meetings in 1953[19, 20] (see also Addendum E). Since striking chemical findings were obtained on this case, a detailed report is in preparation. The most notable biochemical change was in the level of serum cholesterol, which gradually dropped over a period of several months from a normal range to the low level of 20 to 30 mg. per cent. The patient was terminal at this time. Death resulted ultimately from pyelonephritis, which complicated a rectovaginal vesicular fistula. The thyroid and liver were normal at autopsy.

RHEUMATOID ARTHRITIS

Only brief mention will be made of the patient with chronic rheumatoid arthritis, since the case has been followed for but a short period of time. Symptoms had persisted in this patient without a complete remission for over 7 years, and the disease process had involved nearly every joint. There were osteoporotic changes, most marked in the right knee. Various medications, including salicylates, gold, and cortisone, gave partial relief. Without medication there was inevitably an immediate relapse.

This patient was stimulated in the septo-hypothalamic region on two occasions 5 weeks apart. Throughout the follow-up period* there has been no recurrence of the acute inflammatory process, but the mechanical defect in the right knee still markedly handicaps walking and weight-bearing produces pain in this joint. Otherwise the patient has been free from pain and has required no medication. His mental status has changed in that he has become somewhat euphoric. With each of the two stimulations there was a drop of 80 per cent in the lymphocyte count and a temporary drop of approximately 40 mg. per 100 cc. in serum cholesterol. Following the stimulations, new, and as yet unidentified, steroids appeared. This was determined by paper chromatography.

The working concept which we have used in regard to disease processes in general has been that the internal milieu of the individual is an important factor in diseases of all types. In infectious diseases, for example, it is necessary to consider the resistance of the host as well as the virulence of the invading organism. In the past the emphasis in research has been on discovering and combating the invading organism rather than on understanding factors which influence the resistance of the host. Many of these phenomena have not been adequately explained. Although the agents of disease may be generally present in a given environment, some individuals become ill and others do not. Likewise, a given individual who develops an infection becomes ill at a particular time in his life cycle. This is also true in neoplastic diseases. If some of the recent concepts that attribute neoplasms to humoral imbalance are correct, it is still necessary to ponder the mechanism by means of which this imbalance is brought about.

Since the advent of ACTH and cortisone a considerable fund of information has been built up regarding the role of the internal milieu of the individual in disease. The manner in which these compounds affect the course of the collagen diseases has been extensively studied. For example, it has been found that ACTH and cortisone can play an im-

* At the time of this writing 3 1/2 months after the first stimulation.

portant role in altering antibody formation. Some authors have hypothesized that sensitivity resulting from antibody formation is responsible for the collagen diseases. It has been shown in animal experiments that in some instances antibody formations can be inhibited by the administration of ACTH or cortisone, thereby reducing the incidence of the sensitivity reaction. The use of ACTH and cortisone as therapeutic agents in many of the so-called stress diseases has been highly informative.

SUMMARY OF FINDINGS IN PATIENTS WITH DISEASES OTHER THAN SCHIZOPHRENIA

All findings on patients in this group are preliminary. The number of patients in each category is too small to warrant any definite conclusions. The formulations presented here were largely suggested by reports in the literature of the effects of treatment on various disease processes with ACTH, cortisone, and other steroids.

Various reports suggest that the humoral factors play an important role in the prevention and alteration of many disease processes. We have demonstrated in animal experiments that the humoral mechanism can be altered by producing lesions in, or applying stimulation to, the neuraxis and in human studies have shown that a dynamic relationship exists between psychological activity and the physiological activity of the higher levels of the central nervous system. Studies in psychosomatic medicine indicate that consistent alterations in behavior due to stressful memories accompany certain somatic disease processes. Perhaps the integrated approach described here will contribute to the understanding of many diseases. Our tentative findings to date have been provocative. If our hypothesis is correct, further research may show that many of the alterations in the internal milieu of an individual which make him susceptible to somatic diseases and which can influence the progress of disease are influenced by the thought, or cortical, level of integration.

REFERENCES

1. Levy, David M. Personal communication.
2. Bond, Douglas A. Personal communication reporting on work of Anny Katan.
3. Rado, Sandor. Emergency behavior, in *Anxiety*, ed. by Paul Hoch and J. P. Zubin, pp. 150–176, Grune, New York, 1950.

4. Schrodinger, E. *What Is Life?* Macmillan, New York, 1945.
5. Sherrington, Charles. *Man on His Nature.* Cambridge Univ. Press, London, 1946.
6. Cannon, Walter B. *Wisdom of the Body,* rev. & enl. ed. Norton, New York, 1939.
7. Selye, H. *Stress,* 1st ed. ACTA Inc., Montreal, 1950.
8. Heath, Robert G., Robert Hodes, and Samuel M. Peacock, Jr. Cortical stimulation of induced motor activity, *Tr. Am. Neurol. A.,* 76:70–75 (1951).
9. Kluver, N. and P. C. Bucy. Preliminary analysis of functions of the temporal lobes in monkeys, *Arch. Neurol. & Psychiat.,* 42:979–1000 (1939).
10. Mettler, F. A. Extracortical connections of primate frontal cerebral cortex: corticofugal connections, *J. Comp. Neurol.,* 86:119–166 (1947).
11. Richter, C. P. and M. Hines. Increased spontaneous activity produced in monkeys by brain lesions, *Brain,* 61:1–16 (1938).
12. Stoll, J., C. Ajmone-Marsan, and H. H. Jasper. Electrophysiological studies of subcortical connections of anterior temporal region in cat, *J. Neurophysiol.,* 14:305–316 (1951).
13. Bleuler, Eugen. *Dementia Praecox or the Group of Schizophrenias.* International Univ. Press, New York, 1950.
14. Hoch, Paul. Unpublished seminar, Psychoanalytic Clinic for Training and Research, Columbia University.
15. Reider, Norman. The concept of normality, *Psychoanalyt. Quart.,* 19: 43–51 (1950).
16. Pincus, C. and H. Hoagland. Adrenal cortical responses to stress responses in normal men and in those with personality disorders: analysis of the pituitary-adrenal mechanism in man, *Am. J. Psychiat.,* 106:641–659 (1950).
17. Cleghorn, R. A., B. F. Graham, M. Saffran, and D. E. Cameron. A study of the effect of the pituitary ACTH in depressed patients, *Canad. M. A. J.,* 63:329–331 (1950).
18. James, William. *Principles of Psychology,* vol. 1, ch. 10. Holt, New York, 1890.
19. Heath, Robert G., Hal C. Becker, Samuel M. Peacock, Jr., Raeburn C. Llewellyn, Warren L. Founds, Jr., and William H. Miller. Some aspects of subcortical studies in man, *Tr. Am. Neurol. A.,* June 1953.
20. Heath, Robert G., Samuel M. Peacock, Jr., and William H. Miller. Induced paroxysmal electrical activity in man recorded simultaneously through subcortical and scalp electrodes, *Tr. Am. Neurol. A.,* June 1953.
21. Burke, William. Unpublished master's thesis, Department of Psychology, Tulane Univ.

22. Sims, E. A. H., L. G. Welt, J. Orloff, and J. W. Needham. Asymptomatic hyponatremia in pulmonary tuberculosis, *J. Clin. Investigation*, 29:1545–1557 (1950).

23. Ferrara, Michael A. The tuberculous diabetic patient, *New England J. Med.*, 246:55–56 (1952).

24. Loumos, S. The autonomic nervous system and immunity, *Arch. Neurol. & Psychiat.* 68:69–77 (1952).

25. Lewis, N. D. C. *Research in Dementia Praecox (Past Attainments, Present Trends, and Future Possibilities)*. National Committee for Mental Hygiene, New York, 1936.

26. West, P. M. and J. Hilliard. Proteolytic enzyme inhibitors of blood in relation to neoplastic diseases; preliminary report, *Ann. West. Med. & Surg.*, 3:227–234 (1949).

27. West, P. M., J. Hilliard, and A. C. Mietus. Serum antiproteases in normal pregnancy; comparison with changes observed in neoplastic diseases, *Surg., Gynec. & Obst.*, 92:209–212 (1951).

28. Jacobs, James S. L. and Clinton E. Tempereau. Studies on a proteolytic enzyme system in schizophrenia, *Arch. Neurol. & Psychiat.*, 68:388–392 (1952).

29. French, J. D., F. K. von Amerongen, and H. W. Magoun. An activating system in brain stem of monkey, *Arch. Neurol. & Psychiat.*, 68:577–590 (1952).

Section II

ANIMAL STUDIES

Ablation Studies

INTRODUCTION

ROBERT G. HEATH

Two reports are presented in the following section under the over-all heading of Ablation Studies. The first report is concerned with the metabolic changes observed in cats following destruction of certain subcortical structures connected anatomically with the cortex. These changes resembled the disturbances seen following extirpation of the adrenal cortex and occurred only with lesions in a rather restricted area, which we have called the septal region (see definition pages 3–4). The second report describes the outstanding behavioral responses observed in cats following destructive lesions in the same area.* The most pertinent findings were, first, that following operation the animals appeared affectless and did not respond to external stimuli and, second, that they were markedly hypokinetic. This reduction in motor activity is quite relevant when considered along with other observations on motor behavior which will be presented in subsequent sections (see Chapters 4 and 16).

*This paper was supplemented with a motion picture film when presented at New Orleans in June, 1952.

CHAPTER 2

METABOLIC CHANGES FOLLOWING DESTRUCTIVE LESIONS IN THE FOREBRAIN IN CATS*

ROBERT G. HEATH
†JOHN J. WEBER
†CHARLES HOGAN
T. DUANE PRICE

Reports in the literature present an unclear picture of the function of the subcortical structures of the forebrain. We were originally motivated to investigate the effects of destructive lesions in the forebrain of the cat by reports of severe alterations of behavior resulting from such lesions.[1] Somewhat later we became interested in conflictory reports regarding their effect on motor activity. It was during the course of investigating these phenomena that we became interested in the accompanying metabolic changes, many of which resembled the effects of adrenalectomy.

Because of reports in the literature, our attention was first directed to the region of the corpus striatum. A brief preliminary report of this work has already been published.[2] When the metabolic changes were first noted, it was thought that they resulted from destructive lesions in the caudate nucleus. As the work progressed, however, it was found that unless the lesions extended to neighboring structures, these changes did not occur. Accordingly, lesions were placed in various nearby structures in an attempt to determine a relationship between specific lesion and subsequent metabolic alterations.

METHODS

All experiments were performed on adult cats. The two sexes were almost equally represented. The lesions that were produced varied considerably until the Horsley-Clarke stereotaxic apparatus was employed,

*This work was begun at the laboratories of the College of Physicians and Surgeons, Columbia University, and continued in the laboratories of the Department of Psychiatry and Neurology, Tulane University School of Medicine.

†Psychoanalytic Clinic for Training and Research, Columbia University.

after the project was well under way. For this reason (viz., the operation variable) a statistical analysis of the series as a whole is impossible. One of us (J.J.W.) attempted such a statistical analysis on a group of nineteen cats operated upon by the open method. This suggested that the anterior thalamic nuclei were most consistently involved in the cats which developed metabolic effects. The results of this study were inconclusive because of variations in the lesions involving combinations of nuclei and pathways in the various animals. However, it did serve to give focus to the later, more specific procedure with the stereotaxic method. In this report some data from the large series of cats in which the open method was used will be presented as background information. The findings on individual cats with lesions placed by the stereotaxic apparatus will be presented without statistical analysis.

PREOPERATIVE STUDIES

Before operation each animal was weighed at least once, and a few were weighed daily over a long period. The regular animal-house diet was used. Fasting blood sugar specimens were obtained from one to fifteen times before operation on each animal in order to establish the preoperative fasting range; in most cases only two or three preoperative blood sugars were taken. The range of normal fasting blood sugars in the cat is approximately that of man, the majority falling within the range of 70 and 100 mg/100 ml. On a few occasions specimens were obtained which fell outside this range. Animals consistently outside the normal range were not used for the studies. In the earlier studies blood sugar determinations were made by the micro method of Benedict, using 0.1 cc. of fresh blood obtained by nicking the ear. The final values in the cats of this series were determined by the Klett-Summerson photoelectric colorimeter. In later studies (Cats 206 ff.) blood glucose was determined on 0.2 cc. of blood by the method of Nelson.[3] Non-glucose reducing agents were precipitated along with proteins in the first step of this procedure. Investigations into the effect of benzoic acid on glucose determinations by the Nelson method demonstrated that this compound does not interfere; it was, therefore, possible to compare samples with glucose standards prepared in *saturated* benzoic acid. These standards, in contrast to the widely utilized dilute solutions, were shown to be perfectly stable for at least six months.

Blood for serum sodium and potassium determinations was drawn from the femoral vein after a cutdown had been performed. At least one, but usually two or three, preoperative samples were taken from each animal. The preoperative serum sodiums varied over a fairly wide range from one cat to the other; the maximum plasma sodium concentration found in this series was 167 meq/L., the minimum 142 meq/L. There was likewise considerable variation in the plasma potassium levels, the maximum being 7.0 meq/L. and the minimum being 3.5 meq/L. In contrast to the variations noted from cat to cat, individual cats showed marked consistency from day to day. Several cats were followed for several months in order to detect possible periodic fluctuations. As a control, some of the animals were given widely differing diets in order to determine fluctuations in electrolytes. The maximum fluctuation in a given cat, despite extremes of diet ranging from pure water to a high sodium and potassium content, was 9.0 meq/L. for sodium and 0.9 meq/L. for potassium. The dietary factors are discussed below under Control Studies.

In all electrolyte determinations the flame photometer was used. The first specimens were analyzed in the laboratory of the College of Physicians and Surgeons of Columbia University. A group of later specimens was analyzed at the New Orleans Veterans Administration Hospital, and the last group was run on a Beckman flame photometer which was set up in the chemistry laboratory of the Department of Psychiatry and Neurology at Tulane. In the last twenty-seven animals electrolyte determinations were made on plasma instead of serum. The use of heparinized blood instead of serum and oxalated blood permitted us to make all our routine determinations from the same small blood sample (2 cc.). The sodium and potassium concentrations in the Upjohn heparin used were first adjusted to 140 and 4 meq/L., respectively. Sodium and potassium concentrations of such plasma samples are identical with those of serum separated simultaneously from the same untreated blood. To eliminate the "mutual excitation" error in photometric analysis, plasma and urine samples were diluted 200-fold; at this dilution the concentration of each element did not measurably influence the light emission of others. All specimens were analyzed by "bracketing" with standards of lower and higher mineral concentration than the diluted sample of unknown concentration.

Body temperatures were taken prior to operation.

Postoperatively, fasting blood sugar samples were drawn once a day and occasionally supplemented with nonfasting samples. Blood was taken for sodium and potassium determinations every two days (2 cc.), and weights were followed at irregular intervals.

OPERATIVE TECHNIQUES

Open Technique. The operations were performed under sterile conditions. With the animal under nembutal anesthesia, a midline linear incision was made in the scalp, which was then retracted laterally. Trephine openings were made in the skull bilaterally and extended somewhat with rongeurs; a midline bridge of cranium was left intact. The dura was carefully opened bilaterally and retracted. Incisions were then made through the cortex and the depths of the sulcus lateralis into the lateral ventricles. The cortical incisions were about 1 cm. in length. They were never extended rostral to the coronal sulcus or caudal to the level of the sulcus ectosylvius posterior. Through this approach to the ventricles, it was possible to visualize clearly the bulging surface of the caudate nucleus on the lateral side of the ventricle. With some medial retraction the septum became visible. By extending the incision slightly more caudally, it was possible to visualize the anterior thalamic nucleus. The choroid plexus, protruding through the foramen of Monro and extending along the septum and medial surface of the caudate nucleus, had always to be reckoned with while working in the ventricle, as *damage to it inevitably led to serious complications.* Destructive lesions to the pertinent structures under study were made by means of either a fine-tipped glass sucker or a small spoon. In this series of animals the procedure was always carried out bilaterally in a single operation, first on one side and then on the other. Unilateral lesions were ineffective in producing metabolic changes. After hemostasis, the cortex was allowed to fall together and the dura closed with fine, interrupted silk sutures. The overlying muscle, when present in sufficient quantity, was pulled together with heavy cotton sutures.

As the ventricular opening in the cat is quite small, it was very difficult to confine the destructive lesion to the desired structure, particularly when first using the open technique. Our early efforts were directed toward removal of the caudate nucleus, but inevitably we found that such lesions involved the neighboring structures—namely, the septal region, the adjacent gray matter at the base of the ventricle, and the anterior thalamus. In our early experiments many of the changes which we attributed to the striatal damage proved to be due to the involvement of a nearby structure. As our technique improved and lesions were confined to the caudate, no striking metabolic changes occurred. We attempted to locate the critical area by confining destructive lesions in control animals to sites (other than the striatum) in the vicinity of the head of the lateral ventricles. At best, however, these attempts at control were very crude, and under no circumstances could the lesions be confined to the part we intended to injure. This is understandable if one considers that different gray masses within the ventricle are contiguous with one another and that the suction technique is apt to pull out much more than anticipated. Making a specific lesion was also difficult because of inevitable bleeding, which obscured vision during the procedure.

Closed Technique. Lesions were placed in seven male cats in this series through utilization of the Horsley-Clarke stereotaxic apparatus. After apparatus was adjusted to the animal in the usual manner, coordinates were used which would place lesions in the rostral midline structures. According to plan, the lesions began 1 mm. rostral to the anterior commissure and extended forward about 4 mm., being carried laterally 4 mm. to each side of the midline. In the dorso-ventral extent the lesions began at H + 5 and were prolonged ventrally almost to the base of the brain, namely, H — 1. A series of electrolytic lesions was made. Each spot in which a burn was placed was 1½ mm. from the next. To make the electrolytic lesion a D.C. source delivering a current of 3 ma. for 30 seconds was used.

HISTOLOGICAL STUDIES

Animals were sacrificed when death seemed to be almost at hand. Those which did not regress rapidly were generally followed for two or three months before being sacrificed in order to check on the exact sites of the lesions. Postmortem histological studies were made on (a) liver, cardiac muscles, and striated muscle fixed in absolute alcohol for glycogen; (b) pancreas, pituitary, adrenals, spleen, liver, kidney, and pieces of the gastrointestinal tract fixed in 10 per cent formalin for H and E staining. The brain was fixed in 10 per cent formalin and stained either by the myelin sheath stains (Marchi and Weigert) and/or Nissl techniques. Serial sections were made on most of the brain in order to evaluate the actual dimensions of the lesions and volume of the particular nuclear mass destroyed.

RESULTS

As indicated in the introductory remarks, the subcortical lesions produced by the open techniques varied considerably and in every instance several different nuclei were injured. The cortical lesions likewise varied. Some of the animals showed consistent and profound metabolic changes, whereas others with equally large or larger lesions, also in propinquity to the lateral ventricles, showed no change. Studies of the brain suggested that disturbances in metabolism resulted when the gray matter at the base of the septum and lateral ventricles was destroyed. Inevitably there was also injury to the medial aspect of the caudate nucleus. The metabolic changes that occurred were similar to those observed after removal of both adrenals. Marked alterations were noted in blood sugar levels, electrolyte balance, and temperature regulation, as well as losses in weight and changes in the gastrointestinal mucosa.

As previously explained, by means of the set coordinates of the Horsley-Clarke apparatus it was possible to produce a series of lesions that varied little from one animal to the next.

METABOLIC DISTURBANCES

Changes in Blood Sugar. A temporary increase in the blood sugar level, which remained elevated up to seven days, was followed by a gradual decline—with some animals developing a profound hypoglycemia, usually between the fifth and twelfth days. When blood sugars reached extremely low levels in the region of 20 to 40 mg/100 ml., seizures or muscle irritability sometimes occurred. Slides of liver and muscle stained for glycogen consistently showed a complete depletion of glycogen stores. The blood sugars recorded through the pre- and post-operative periods on several animals operated upon by the open technique are shown on the accompanying figures (1, 2, 3).

Changes in Electrolyte Balance. Lesions in the septal region consistently produced alterations in electrolyte balance in many ways similar to those observed after the destruction of the adrenal cortex. The sodium levels fell consistently during the postoperative periods, preceding death; the drops ranged from 20 to 60 meq/L. Frequently a concomitant increase in serum potassium levels occurred. Occasionally, however, serum potassium remained quite constant. The electrolyte changes in a few animals are charted in Figures 1, 2, 3, and 4. Apparently, diet had some effect on the degree of sodium loss. This finding will be considered in detail under Control Studies (below) and in the individual reports on animals operated upon by the closed method. We were able to demonstrate that, although intact animals and animals with nonspecific lesions showed no significant drop in serum sodium, animals with septal lesions showed more precipitous sodium drops and more blood sugar changes when on low sodium diet.

Temperature Regulation. It was usual for the animals to show such marked poikilothermia during the first day or two following operation that an incubator was required; later the temperature generally settled within the normal range. Three to four days before death, however, the temperature invariably dropped below normal. This downward trend continued to levels of 85° F. or below. Temperature changes in two animals, which are typical, are shown in Figures 5 and 6.

Changes in Body Weight. In most instances, despite adequate caloric intake, the animals rapidly lost weight and at the time of death were very emaciated. As mentioned under Methods, the majority would eat spontaneously for at least two or three days following operation. During this period it was occasionally necessary to put the food in the animal's mouth by hand and to hold the pan of milk to its mouth. With some consistency, however, at the end of three or four days it would begin to refuse food even when placed in its mouth. It then became necessary to resort to tube-feeding. Losses usually were in the order of 30 per cent to 50 per cent of body weight.

Changes in the Gastrointestinal Mucosa. At postmortem examination

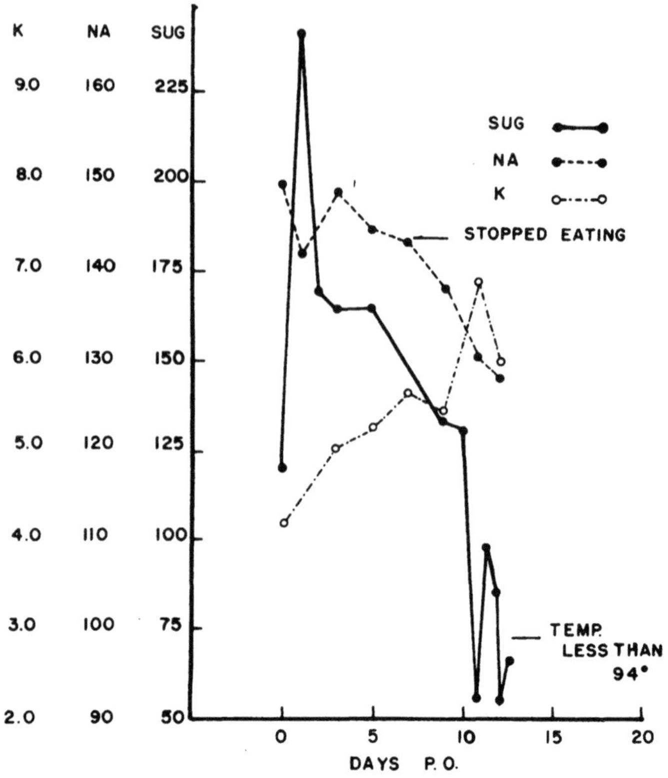

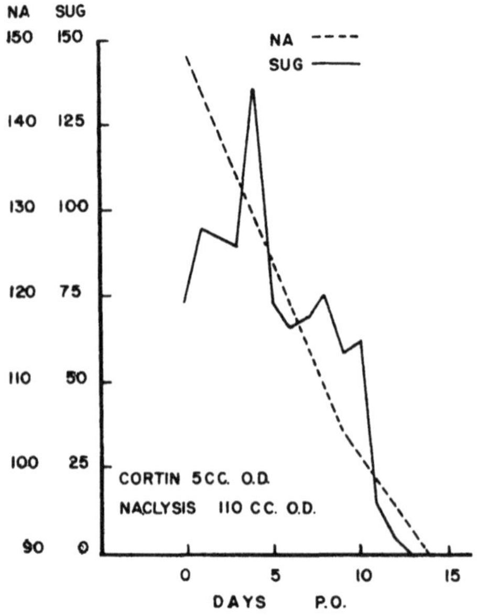

FIGURE II–1 (above). Metabolic changes in Cat 157

FIGURE II–2 (left). Sugar and sodium changes in Cat 536 during administration of supplemental cortin and sodium chloride

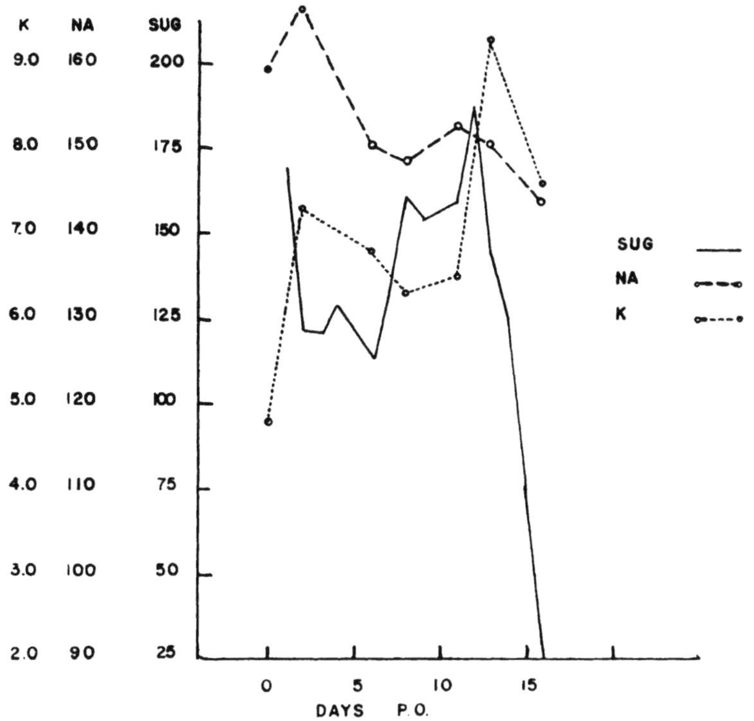

FIGURE II–3. Metabolic changes in Cat 709 after ablation of midline structures

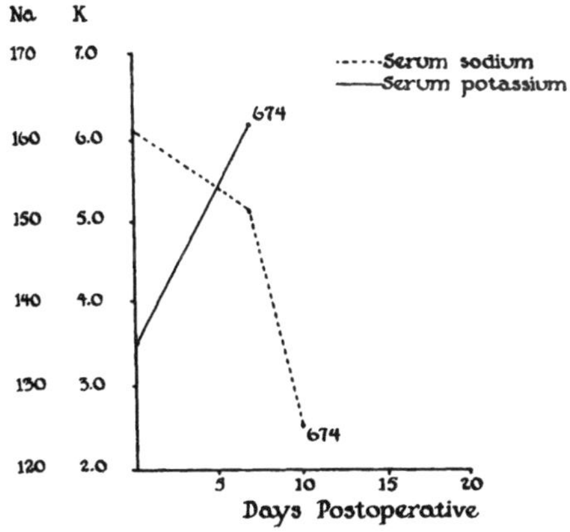

FIGURE II–4. Electrolyte changes in Cat 674 after ablation of septal region

all the animals in this group showed pathological conditions of the gastrointestinal mucosa. Some merely showed hyperemia, but others showed small hemorrhages or clear-cut ulcerations. These were found in both the duodenum and the colon.*

Hematological Changes. Drops in both red and white blood counts were frequently found in association with the other metabolic changes in animals with the septal lesions. The decrease in cellular constituents was considerably more marked than in the control animals. Figure 7 illustrates the changes in white blood count in Cat 229.

Specific Changes in Individual Cats:

Cat 219. The lesion in this cat (Figure 8) involved the base of the septum, orbital cortex, and to a slight extent the ventro-medial aspect of the caudate nucleus; the caudal aspect is rostral to the anterior commissure and extends forward several millimeters. It also involved the gray matter at the base of the lateral ventricles and implicated to a slight extent the ventral aspect of the caudate nucleus. The serum electrolyte and glucose studies on Cat 219 are shown on Figure 9.

Cat 229. Figure 10 shows lesions somewhat more rostrally placed than in Cat 219, but the destroyed region similarly encompassed the midline structures of the septal region and the gray matter at the base of the ventricles. Figure 11 shows the metabolic changes that followed this lesion.

Cat 231. It is to be noted in Figure 12 that the entire lesion is rostral to the anterior commissure, extending more laterally and involving more of the caudate nucleus than the lesions in Cats 219 and 229 but likewise implicating the gray matter at the base of the ventricle. Figure 16 indicates the specific metabolic changes in this cat, and Figure 13 shows multiple ulceration of the stomach.

Apparently, stomach changes, which were consistent and present to some degree in all the animals, take place quite quickly. Cat 228 had a brain lesion similar to that of Cats 229 and 231. By an error, it was not placed in the incubator immediately following operation. Its temperature dropped from a normal level of 101.5° F. to room temperature during the night, and it became moribund approximately 20 hours after

*Slides illustrating typical lesions were shown when this paper was read in New Orleans in June, 1952, but these are inadequate for publication.

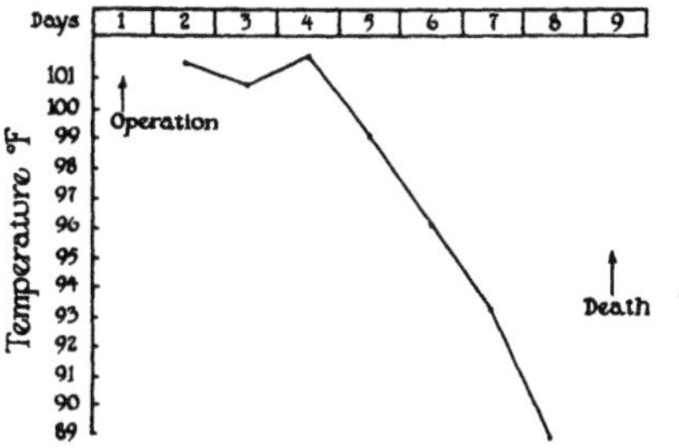

FIGURE II–5 (left). Postoperative temperature changes in Cat 231. The lesion was in the basal part of the septal region

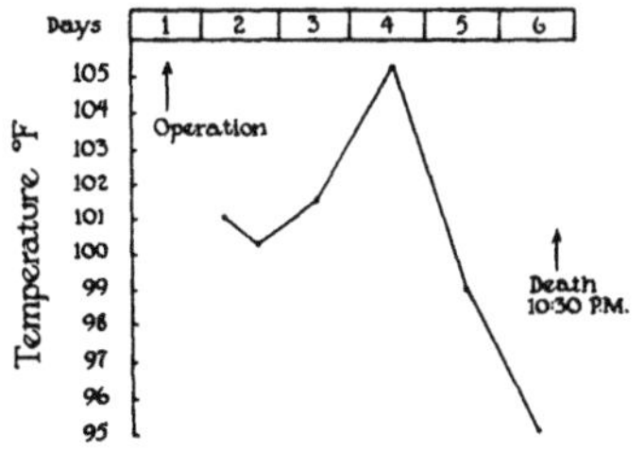

FIGURE II–6 (above). Postoperative temperature changes in Cat 229. The lesion was in the basal part of the septal region

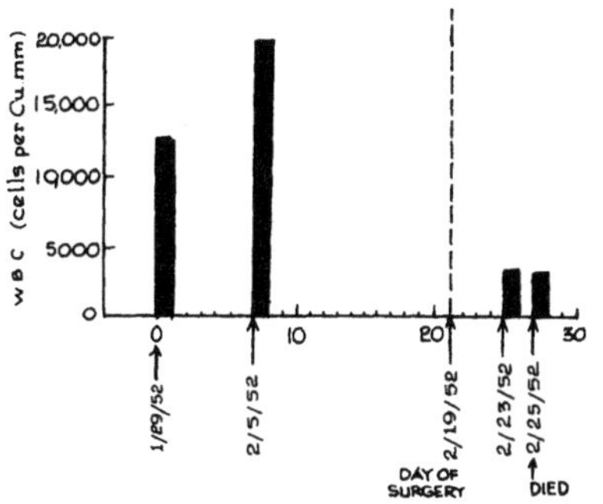

FIGURE II–7. White blood cell changes in Cat 229

operation. The animal was sacrificed then, and the stomach removed. The beginning stomach changes, with early ulcerations and multiple hemorrhagic areas, were already present.

CONTROL STUDIES

Several types of controls were devised to test our conclusions about the relationship between septal lesions and metabolic disturbances. The most important of these are discussed below:

Diet. As mentioned previously, a characteristic behavioral consequence of operation in the basal part of the septal region appeared to be the disappearance of appetite in two or three days. We therefore decided to study the effects of diet upon the plasma sodium and potassium and the blood glucose of (a) normal cats and (b) cats with lesions in other sites of the brain than the septal region. Under normal conditions all cats used in the ablation studies were maintained preoperatively on a diet of frozen horse meat and water. In our dietary tests solids were ruled out because they could not be given by stomach tube. The liquid diets

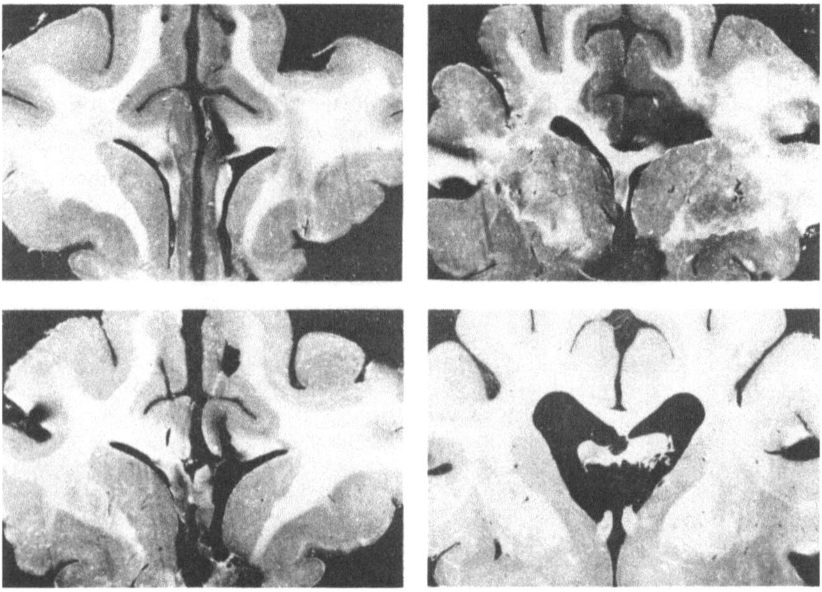

FIGURE II-8. Septal lesion in Cat 219

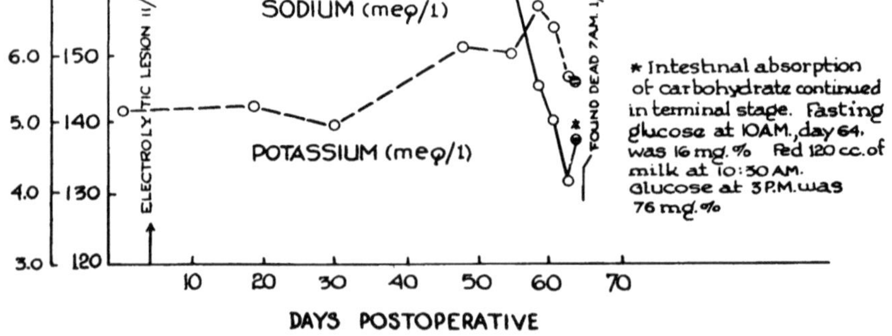

FIGURE II-9. Metabolic changes in Cat 219. The lesion was in the basal part of the septal region

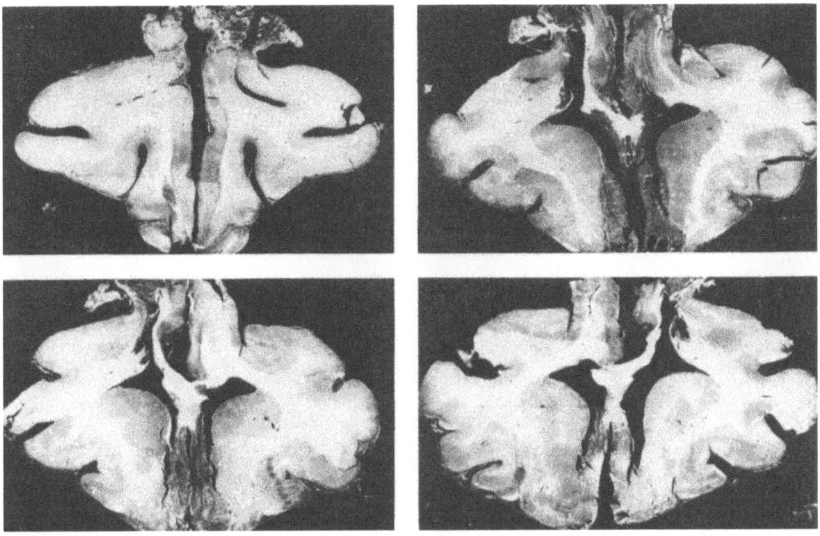

FIGURE II–10. Brain lesion in Cat 229

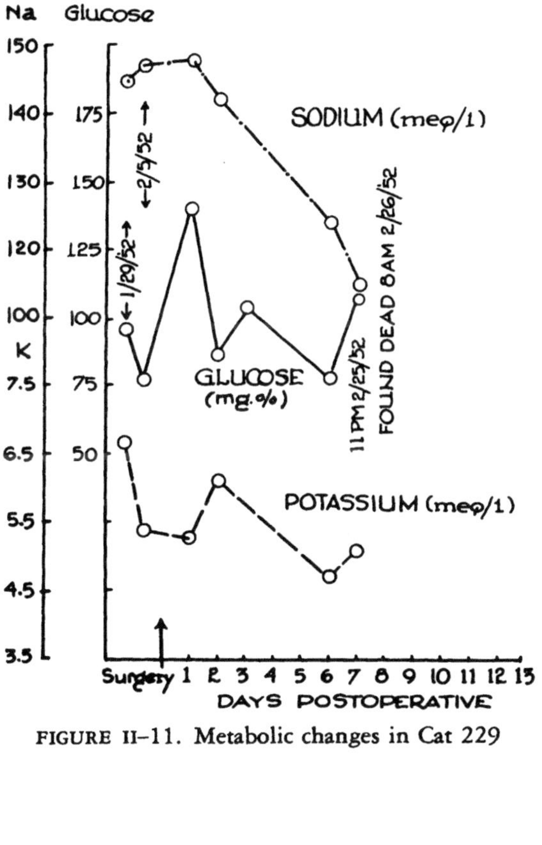

FIGURE II–11. Metabolic changes in Cat 229

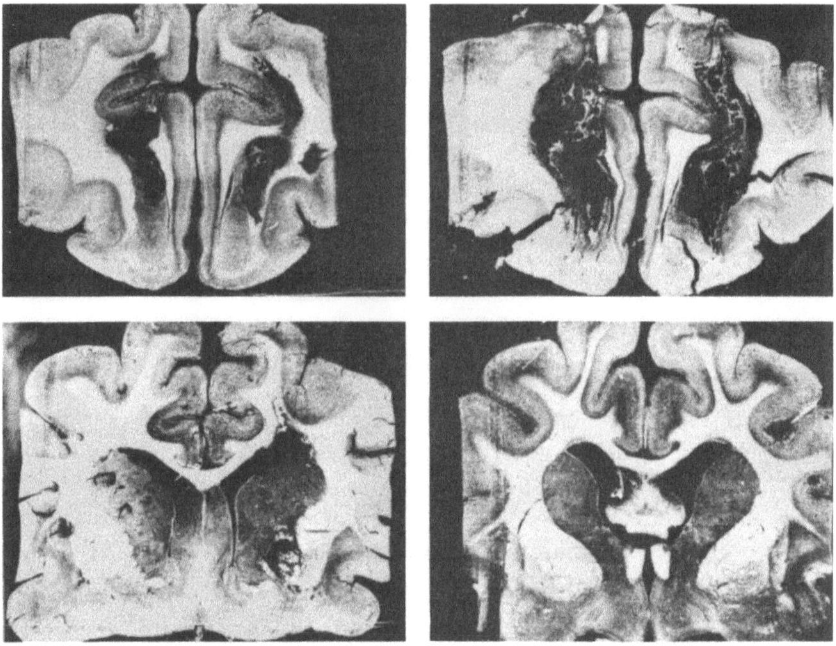

FIGURE II–12. Brain lesion in Cat 231

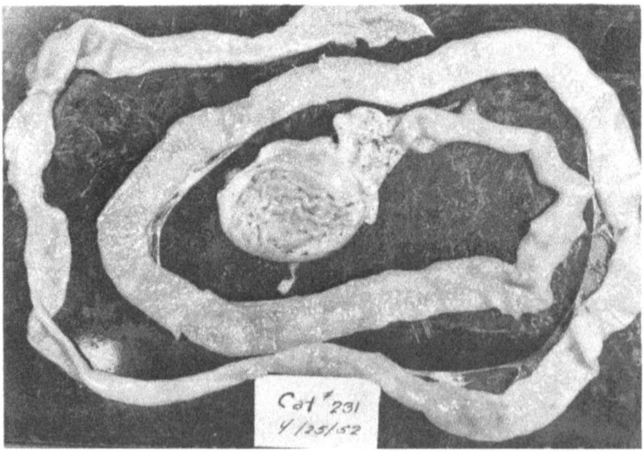

FIGURE II–13. Gastrointestinal tract of Cat 231

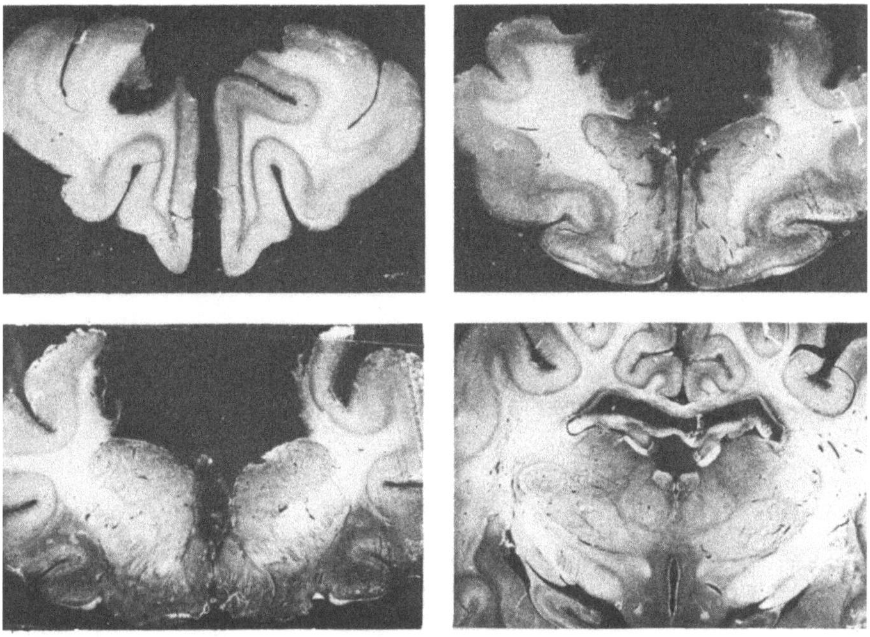

FIGURE II–14. Nonseptal brain lesion in Cat 232

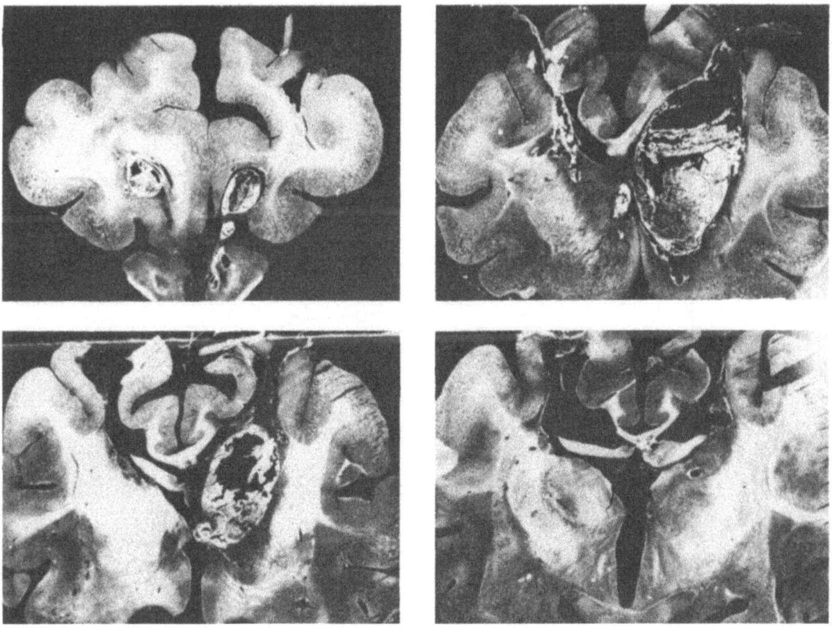

FIGURE II–15. Nonseptal brain lesion in Cat 222

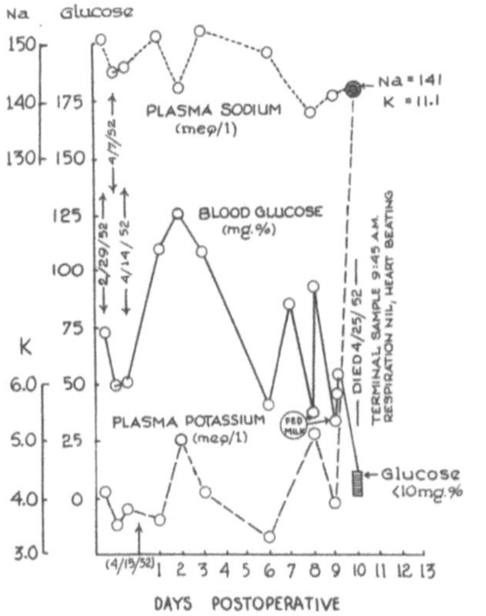

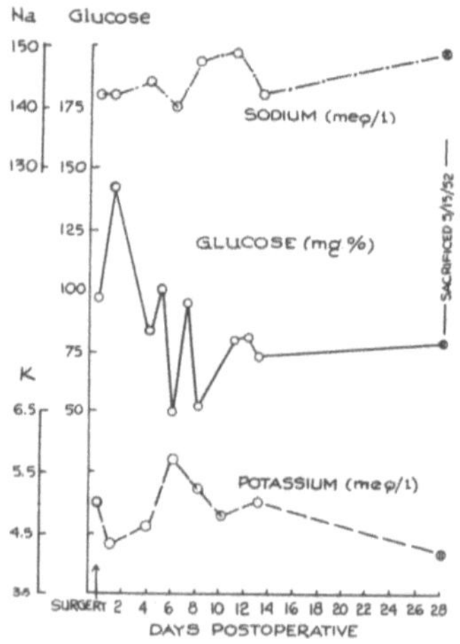

FIGURE II–16 (left). Metabolic changes in Cat 231

FIGURE II–17 (right). Chemistry findings in Cat 232 with nonseptal lesion

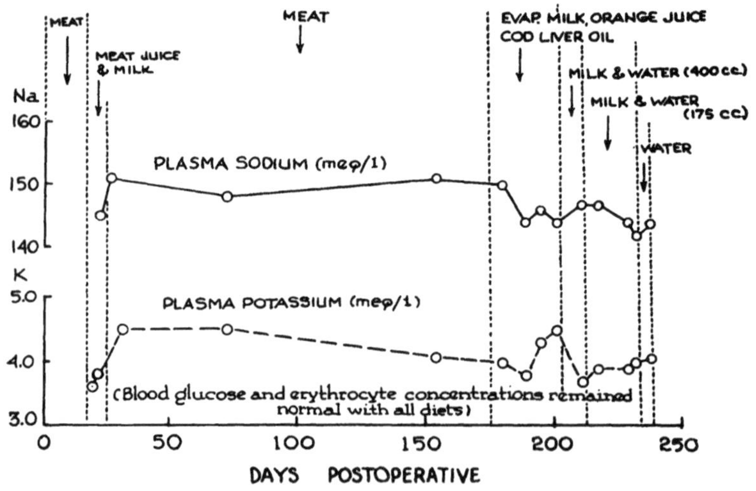

FIGURE II–18. Effect of dietary extremes on blood composition of Cat 209. This animal was used as a normal control

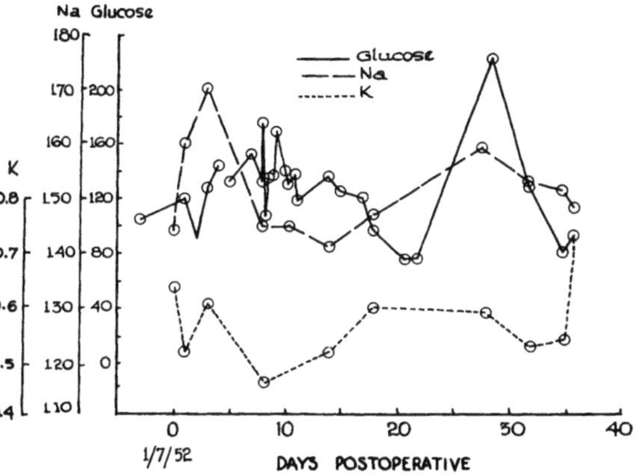

FIGURE II–19. Chemistry findings in Cat 222 with nonseptal lesion

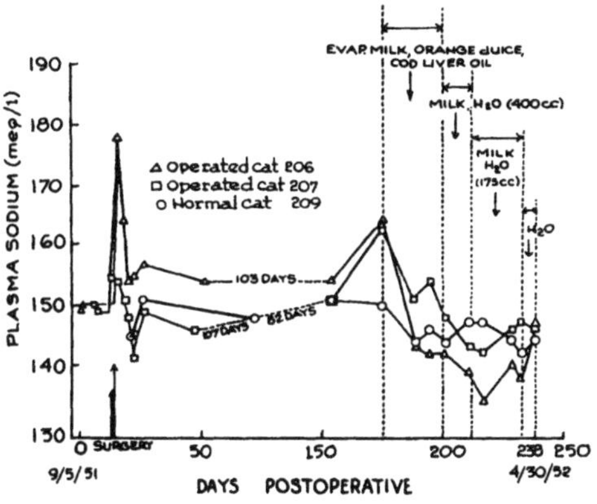

FIGURE II–20. Effect of various diets on plasma sodium of control cats

administered included meat juice and milk; evaporated milk, orange juice, and water; evaporated milk and water (1:1); and water. In normal cats under this regimen (e.g., Cat 209, Figure 18) the plasma sodium and potassium and blood glucose concentrations remained essentially constant, and in cats with nonseptal lesions postoperative recovery was uneventful—neither hypoglycemia nor decrease in plasma sodium occurred (see Figures 17, 19, and 20).

Size and Placement of Lesion. Because of the difficulty encountered in placing lesions even with the stereotaxic technique there were numerous instances in which extensive damage resulted in nearby structures without involvement of the target structure. In such cases the animal was always treated postoperatively in the same manner as those having the desired lesions, but in no instance did the above-described metabolic changes occur. The lesions and follow-up metabolic studies of two cats are shown for illustration. Cat 222 was operated on by the open method (see Figure 15), Cat 232 by the closed method (see Figure 14). In these animals as in many others which served as controls, no specific metabolic changes occurred (see Figures 17 and 19).

HISTOLOGICAL FINDINGS

The report of the histological findings will be limited to the positive findings. Slides stained for glycogen showed a complete depletion of sugar stores in the liver and muscle tissue of animals with septal lesions which had died in terminal hypoglycemia. Those animals which developed severe metabolic changes showed the most pronounced alterations in the adrenals; the histological sections of other organs were not remarkable or consistent. Animals with nonseptal lesions showed less pronounced changes.

The following report is a summary of the findings on several of the animals described above. This study was done by Dr. William H. Sternberg.*

Normal. In the adrenals of the normal cat there is a sharp delineation of cortical zones. Foamy cells are conspicuous in the zona glomerulosa and the outer two-thirds of the zona fasciculata.

Animals with Septal Lesions Followed by Metabolic Disturbances:

Cats 229 and 231, six days after operation. (The adrenals of these animals are very similar and are therefore described together.) The thickness of the cortex is about 1 1/2 times normal, most of the increase being attributable to the increase in the zona fasciculata. The delineation of zones is less sharp than in the normal cat, especially between the zona glomerulosa and the zona fasciculata. The lipids are depleted in both these outer zones, so that the cytoplasm of the cells appears acidophilic and granular in comparison with the foamy cells of the normal adrenal. However, small focal collections of foamy cells are present in the mid-portion of the zona fasciculata. The zona reticularis shows a somewhat greater vascularity but no other changes. Occasional mitoses are seen in the zona fasciculata.

The thickening of the adrenal cortex and the histological changes are interpreted as responses to severe stress—manifested as hyperplasia of the cortex and presumably increased output of cortical steroids.

*Associate Professor of Pathology, Tulane University School of Medicine.

Cat 219, sixty-five days after operation. The pattern is somewhat similar to that of Cats 229 and 231. The delineation of zones is even less sharp, and a distinct zona glomerulosa cannot be made out. The adrenal cortex appears thicker than normal but not so thick as in Cat 229. No foamy cells are present, and the cytoplasm is acidophilic, granular, and abundant. The zona reticularis appears narrower than normal and has a conspicuous vascularity.

Control Animals without Metabolic Disturbances:

Cat 222, twenty-one days after operation. The zonal pattern is fairly well retained, although the adrenal cortex is somewhat thicker than average. There is some disorganization of the zona fasciculata, owing to a patchy distribution of foamy cells, but much less lipid depletion than in the animals which showed the metabolic disturbance. The picture is compatible with fairly good recovery following stimulation of the adrenal cortex in association with nonspecific operative stress.

Cat 232, twenty-one days after operation. This animal's adrenal is almost normal histologically, except for a few minute foci of calcification in the cortex.

SUMMARY

Although lesions produced in the forebrain of the cat by the open method were extensive and involved incisions through the cerebral cortex, our findings suggest that metabolic changes occurred only if the damage was committed in a specific subcortical region which involved the septal nuclei and the gray matter at the base of the lateral ventricles, extending rostrally from the region of the commissure about 5 mm. and laterally into the ventro-medial aspect of the caudate nucleus. When larger lesions were produced in neighboring structures, these changes did not occur. The characteristic changes included depletion of body carbohydrate, as shown by blood glucose and tissue glycogen measurements, marked decrease in plasma sodium, and poikilothermia accompanied by a profound loss in body weight and ulcerations of the intestinal mucosa.

More discretely localized lesions were produced in later experiments by means of the Horsley-Clarke stereotaxic apparatus. The metabolic changes observed were similar to those following appropriate placement of lesions by the open method.

The metabolic changes were accompanied by a degree of adrenocortical hyperplasia strikingly similar to that seen in animals under several types of physiological stress. Though the disturbance sometimes simulated Addison's disease, it was certainly not the result of adrenocortical underfunction in any ordinary sense.

In the control animals (operated upon, but showing no metabolic disturbances) the adrenal cortex was correspondingly less hyperplastic. This is interpreted as the result of operative stress followed by moderate to almost complete recovery.

The observations of histological changes in the adrenals are based on study of a small group of animals and require additional confirmation.

DISCUSSION OF THE LITERATURE

There are very few reports to be found in the literature concerning the subject of metabolic changes with lesions of the forebrain. Raphael and Potter[4] noted low levels of creatinine in patients with striatal disease. Moore[5] and Mader[6] found that the temperature regulating function of the striatum produced opposite results from those we report. They reported that lesions in the striatum of rabbits produced fever. Reynolds and Spiegel[7] found that lesions in the striatum in rabbits produced fever and polyuria with a drop in the specific gravity of the urine. Tokay[8] described fever, polyuria, and increased salt output after stab wounds in the region of the caudate nucleus. The urinary output of salt increased to as much as six times the previous output, and the author points out that fever and diuresis did not necessarily accompany this extra excretion of salt. There is an occasional report in the literature of alterations in glycogen and electrolyte metabolism following lesions of the rostral part of the forebrain in man. Sweet and his colleagues[9] reported severe and fatal metabolic disturbances after lobotomy. Allott[10] reported five cases in which there was retention of sodium and chlorine in the presence of cerebral damage without kidney disease. However, the site of the lesions is not well described. Luetscher and Blackman[11] reported high serum sodium and chloride levels and persistent cerebral damage in association with injury to the kidneys following sulfathiazole administration. In this report, as in that of Allott, descriptions of lesions in the brain are incomplete, and it is therefore difficult to determine whether they are similar in any way to our experimental lesions.

REFERENCES

1. Mettler, F. A., and C. C. Mettler. Effects of striatal injury, *Brain,* 65: 242–255 (1942).

2. Heath, R. G., D. A. Freedman, and F. A. Mettler. Striatal removal without previous cortical ablation; release, disorientation, metabolic disturbance, *Fed. Proc.*, 6:126 (1947).
3. Nelson, N. Photometric adaptation of Somogyi method for determination of glucose, *J. Biol. Chem.*, 153:375–380 (1944).
4. Raphael, T., and F. G. Potter. Blood creatinine findings in five cases of corpus striatum disorder, *J. Nerv. & Ment. Dis.*, 55:492–496 (1922).
5. Moore, L. M. Relation of the corpus striatum to the regulation of body temperature, *Am. J. Physiol.*, 46:253–274 (1918).
6. Mader, A. Über die Bedeutung des Corpus striatum für die Wärmeregulation, *Jahrb. f. Kinderh.*, 103:287–294 (1923).
7. Reynolds, R., and E. Spiegel. Über die Wirkung von Stichverletzungen des Corpus striatum und seiner Nachbarschaft auf die Diurese, *Ztschr. f. d. ges. exper. Med.*, 70:504–512 (1930).
8. Tokay, L. Über die Wirkung von Stichverletzungen des Corpus striatum auf die Molenausscheidung mit dem Harn, *Ztschr. f. d. ges. Neurol. u. Psychiat.*, 136:47–61 (1931).
9. Sweet, W. H., G. C. Cotzias, J. Seed, and P. Yakovlev. Gastro-intestinal hemorrhages, hyperglycemia, azotemia, hyperchloremia, and hypernatremia following lesions of the frontal lobe in man, *A. Res. Nerv. & Ment. Dis., Proc.*, 27:795 (1948).
10. Allott, E. N. Sodium and chlorine retention without renal disease, *Lancet*, 1:1035–1037 (1939).
11. Luetscher, J. A., Jr., and S. S. Blackman, Jr. Severe injury to kidneys and brain following sulfathiazole administration; high serum sodium and chlorine levels and persistent cerebral damage, *Ann. Int. Med.*, 18:741–756 (1943).

CHAPTER 3

BEHAVIORAL CHANGES FOLLOWING DESTRUCTIVE LESIONS IN THE SUBCORTICAL STRUCTURES OF THE FOREBRAIN IN CATS

ROBERT G. HEATH

The observations on this subject reported in New Orleans in June, 1952, were illustrated by a motion picture film showing behavioral changes in Cat 219 following placement of a destructive lesion in the subcortical structures of its forebrain. A summary of the findings which were demonstrated in the film presentation is in preparation and will be published later by Heath, Hogan, and Weber. As pointed out at the meeting, the behavioral alterations in this cat were typical of those of a large series of animals in which the septal region was damaged. The accompanying metabolic changes have been described in Chapter 2.

All the lesions inevitably involved several anatomical structures, principally the caudate nucleus, septal region, and basal part of the olfactory cortex. Operations in which the open technique was used also resulted in damage to the cortex over the vertex. The technical approach in making these lesions has been described in Chapter 2 and therefore will not be repeated. However, one point should be stressed, namely, that when lesions were produced by the stereotaxic method the behavioral changes were essentially the same as those observed following use of the open method. Even though several anatomical structures were inevitably damaged, all the subcortical structures involved were derivatives of the rhinencephalon. It was difficult to detect any marked differences in the behavioral patterns when one of the structures involved was damaged more than another.

The behavioral changes observed were: (a) marked alteration in affective responses and (b) decided reduction in spontaneous motor activity.

ALTERATIONS IN AFFECTIVE RESPONSIVITY

Following operation, the cats were either completely affectless or showed a marked reduction in all emotional responses, i.e., fear and rage, as well as positive feelings toward the examiner. These findings were so gross that well-defined tests were not necessary. For example, the cats would lose their emergency responses to the presence of a dog and would react feebly to painful stimuli such as twisting the tail or pinching the ear. There was no arching of the back or purring with elevation of the tail in response to petting.

HYPOKINESIA

The alterations in motor behavior were inevitably quite pronounced. The animals seldom moved about spontaneously. They tended to posture, often assuming rather bizarre attitudes and holding them for long periods of time. In most instances it was possible to place the extremities in various peculiar positions, which the animals would maintain. This phenomenon closely resembled the "waxy flexibility" commonly seen in stuporous catatonic patients. One casual examiner looking at these cats described them as "immobile dopes." Such characteristic changes in behavior usually persisted throughout the relatively short postoperative survival period (generally ten days to two weeks).

When the lesions were so placed that the resulting metabolic changes did not culminate in death, the behavioral changes persisted over considerably longer periods. For example, a few animals were maintained for three months before being sacrificed. Throughout this long period there was never a complete return to normal affectivity, although in most instances the hypokinetic effects became somewhat less marked. There appeared to be no marked alterations in muscle tone as evaluated by adjustment of the animal's extremities. The tendency to assume peculiar postures appeared to be associated to some degree with a marked proprioceptive effect, since the cats with lesions in the caudate nucleus showed a persistent placing defect and those with "formes frustes" which lived for comparatively long periods continued to walk with a rather wide base, even though the hypokinesia became less marked. The righting reflex was not impaired.

Acute Experiments with Animals

INTRODUCTION

ROBERT G. HEATH

In Chapter 4 we present data, collected from acute physiological experiments with cats, which demonstrate the influence of subcortical structures on cortical activity. Responses induced by application of stimulation to the motor cortex were used as indicators of background motor activity. The data reported in Chapter 4 were gathered in 1950. Since the June, 1952, meetings Dr. Peacock has carried out further studies on the inhibitory system and on the parameters of electrical stimulation. His additional data were reported at the meetings of the American Neurological Association held in Atlantic City in June, 1953, and will appear in the *Transactions* for that year. A more complete report has been accepted for publication in the *Journal of Neurophysiology*. Because the data are reported elsewhere they are not included in the addendum.

The results obtained from rostral forebrain stimulation are of added interest when considered along with those of the ablation studies presented in Chapters 2 and 3. The septal region, in which stimulation facilitated somatic motor activity, corresponds to that in which ablation induced severe metabolic disturbances, affectlessness, lack of responsivity, and hypokinesia.

The abbreviations for nomenclature used in all figures are those adopted by Hodes and Magoun[1,2] and Jimenez-Castellanos.[3]

AC, Anterior commissure
AM, N. antero-medialis
ASG, Anterior suprasylvian gyrus
CC, Corpus callosum
CE, N. centralis, pars medialis
CL, N. centralis, pars lateralis
CN, Caudate nucleus
E, Entopeduncular nucleus
F, Fornix
GC, Gyrus cinguli

GP, Globus pallidus
HYPO, Hypothalamus
IAM, N. interantero-medialis
IC, Internal capsule
LGD, Lateral geniculate body, pars dorsalis
LOT, Lateral olfactory tract
LV, Lateral ventricle
MFB, Medial forebrain bundle
OC, Optic chiasma
OT, Optic tract
PUT, Putamen
PYR, Pyriform lobe
RE, N. reuniens
RH, N. rhomboidalis
RT, N. reticularis
SEP, Septal nuclei
SO, Supraoptic nucleus
SM, N. submedius
ST, Stria terminalis
TUB, Tuberculum olfactorium
VA, N. ventralis, pars anterior
VM, N. ventralis, pars medialis
3V, Third ventricle

In Figures 1 to 4 the following abbreviations are used for the kymographic recordings of knee jerks (rate = 1 per second) and cortically induced movement (rate = 2 per second):

RKJ and LKJ = right and left knee jerk, respectively

RFF and LFF = flexion of right and left foreleg induced by cortical stimulation

A scale denoting 5 and 30 second intervals and a signal marker denoting the period of stimulation are given below each kymograph.

The outline drawing beneath original records shows location of point whose stimulation caused the inhibition illustrated.

REFERENCES

1. Hodes, R., and H. W. Magoun. Autonomic responses to electrical stimulation of the forebrain and midbrain with special reference to the pupil, *J. Comp. Neurol.*, 76:169–190 (1942).
2. Hodes, R., and H. W. Magoun. Pupillary and other responses from stimulation of the frontal cortex and basal telencephalon of the cat, *J. Comp. Neurol.*, 76:461–473 (1942).
3. Jimenez-Castellanos, J. Thalamus of the cat in Horsley-Clarke coordinates, *J. Comp. Neurol.*, 91:307–330 (1949).

CHAPTER 4

INHIBITION AND FACILITATION OF MOTOR ACTIVITY FROM FOREBRAIN STIMULATION IN CATS

ROBERT HODES
SAMUEL M. PEACOCK, JR.
ROBERT G. HEATH

As explained in the introductory discussion of the nature of the schizophrenic process (Chapter 1) our over-all theoretical concept assumed that the fundamental disorder produces aberrations in the motor sphere as well as in the sensory and ideational spheres. Hence an important role for the phylogenetically recent cerebral cortex was postulated in manifestations of the disease. Reference has already been made to the fact that the effects of rostral forebrain stimulation on motor activity presented one line of investigation for the current studies. On the evidence of the data to be given below, it has been inferred that two neural circuits, apparently having opposite effects on motor response, are present in rostral forebrain structures.

In addition to providing supportive evidence for subcortical and cortical interrelationships in the motor sphere, this research provided maps of the cat forebrain which localized facilitatory and inhibitory areas. The regions designated facilitatory were roughly similar to those which, when ablated in the cat brain, produced certain changes in metabolism. For these and other reasons, the facilitatory region was ultimately selected as the area for stimulation in our series of schizophrenic patients.

Many distinguished neurophysiologists, whether they be officially classified as anatomists, surgeons, neurologists, or physiologists, have added significantly to our current knowledge concerning those central neural mechanisms which control the force of muscular contraction. To name but a few—Bucy, Dusser de Barenne and McCulloch, Hess, Hines, Magoun, Mettler, Ranson, and Tower have all made contributions on the central motor economy which are too well known to need repetition here. Summaries of much of the work of the above writers are given by Magoun and Rhines.[1]

The experiments to be described were undertaken after it became clear to us that large expanses of the nervous system rostral to the diencephalon and adjacent to the striatum had not been previously reported to contain elements which influenced the central inhibitory or facilitatory outflow. For example, Lindsley, Schreiner, and Magoun's diagrammatic summary of facilitatory regions[2] indicates no augmentor areas rostral to the diencephalon. The lack of evidence in regard to consistent or numerically impressive effects resident in the most rostral structures attests either to the absence of such effects or to the fact that the most rostral area of the neuraxis had not been examined as exhaustively or as effectively as had the more caudal areas. What scanty data existed in the literature and our own preliminary evidence pointed to the latter conclusion. The following intensive and systematic exploration of the forebrain was therefore begun in the hope of filling in some of the gaps in our present knowledge of the inhibitory and facilitatory moderators of motor response.

Details of the experiments establishing the inhibitory and facilitatory influences of rostral subcortical structures on somatic motor activity have been given elsewhere by Hodes and others,[3–6] and will be merely summarized here.

METHODS

The basic plan of the experiments was to set up somatic motor activity and to note the effects thereon of subcortical stimulation—a fruitful technique introduced by Mettler and others in 1939.[7] In some thirty cats under nembutal both knee jerks were elicited simultaneously once per second by solenoids carrying reflex hammers. Foreleg flexions were evoked by unilateral or bilateral electrical stimulation of the motor cortex. This motor activity was recorded by the multichannel autosyn recorder developed in this laboratory.[8] During the production of such a background of reflex and cortically induced movement, structures lying deep within the brain were stimulated for periods of 10 to 30 seconds through electrodes inserted into the desired regions by means of the Horsley-Clarke stereotaxic apparatus. The stimulation routinely employed was a rectangular wave pulse of 1 millisecond duration, 100 cycles per second frequency, and 14 volts intensity. Other pulse durations, frequencies, and intensities had been employed in several preliminary experiments. When the probing electrode was in an area which produced good effects on the recorded responses, such variations in the parameters of stimulation had little effect within fairly wide limits. The points whose stimulation caused inhibition or facilitation of motor activity were located after the termination of the experiment by examination of histological sections of the brain through the plane of the needle tracks. The points from which effects had been obtained on the test movements were then plotted on standard outline drawings at appropriate levels through the brain.

RESULTS

Left-sided stimulation of structures lying deep within the brain caused two types of inhibition of somatic motor activity: (a) inhibition of the response only on the right side of the body, and (b) inhibition of responses on both sides of the body.

Figure 1 shows the diminution in the force of the right knee jerk and the abolition of right foreleg flexion when the rostral portion of the left globus pallidus was excited. Although Figure 1 does not record the response of the left foreleg, other experiments indicate that the effects of such stimulation are limited strictly to the right side.

An example of bilateral inhibition of motor response is presented in Figure 2. This effect was produced by stimulating a point contiguous to the dorso-lateral hypothalamus, the internal capsule, and the internal division of the pallidum at the level of the tuber cinereum.

Unlike the inhibitory responses, facilitation was always expressed bilaterally, as seen in Figure 3. The increase in the vigor of the motor responses shown in the records resulted from exciting a point in the middle of the hypothalamus about 1 mm. lateral to the third ventricle. In a considerable number of placements, stimulation resulted in profound enhancement of the cortically evoked movement without any effect on the amplitude of the reflex response. This reaction (shown in Figure 4) resulted from stimulation in the region of the small antero-dorsal nucleus of the anterior portion of the thalamus.

When the results of several thousand stimulations are collected, maps

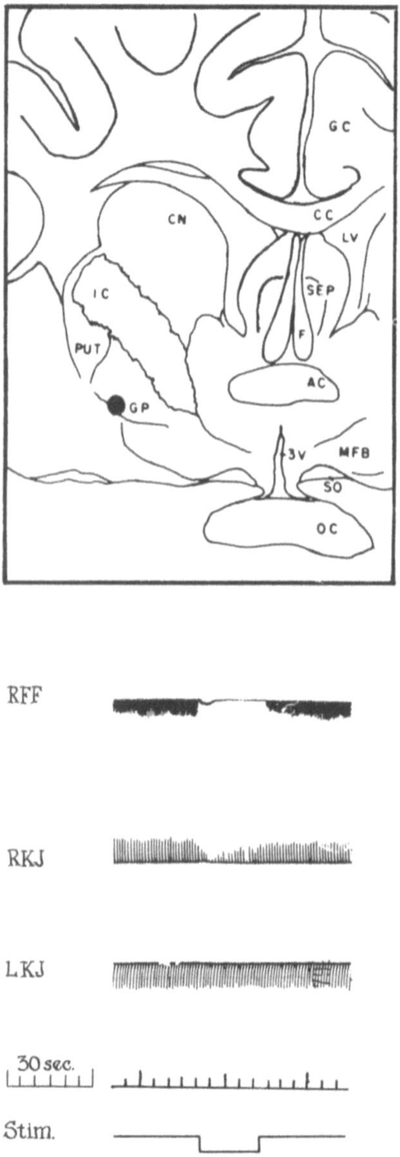

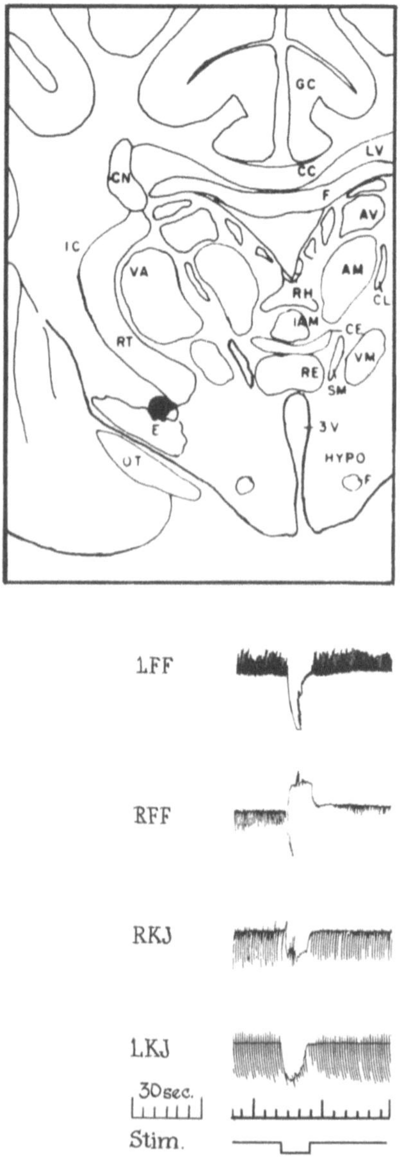

FIGURE IV–1 (left). Inhibition of background motor activity on right side from left-sided stimulation of subcortical structures

FIGURE IV–2 (right). Bilateral inhibition of motor activity from left-sided stimulation of structures lying deep within the brain. See text for further details

NOTE: Outline drawings show points to which stimulation was applied. See Introduction to Acute Experiments with Animals for the key to the abbreviations

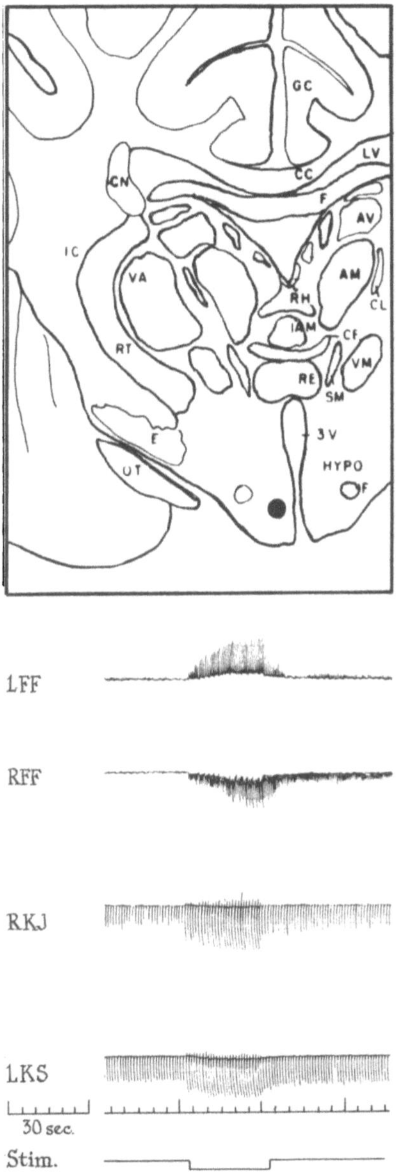

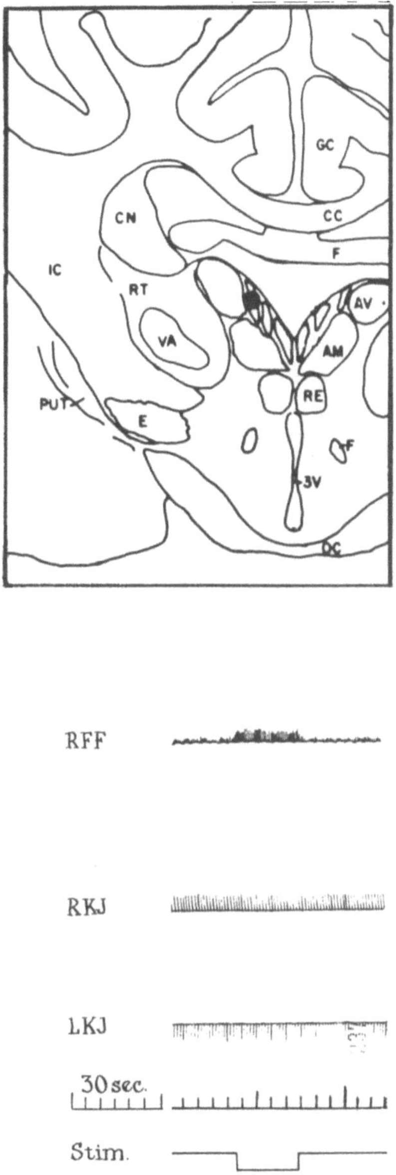

FIGURE IV–3 (left). Bilateral facilitation of cortically evoked activity (upper two records) and knee jerks (lower two records) from hypothalamic stimulation

FIGURE IV–4 (right). Kymographic tracings showing enhancement of cortically evoked movement (upper record) and no effect on reflexly produced responses (lower two records)

SEE NOTE on opposite page

of the brain can be constructed to show the location of the neural elements whose excitation causes positive or negative influences on somatic motor activity. This has been done for many levels of the brainstem, two such levels being illustrated in Figure 5. These levels through the forebrain were selected not only because they demonstrate the method of mapping but also because they show the striking differences in the distribution of reactive points for enhancement of cortically initiated and reflex motor responses which are described above and illustrated in Figures 1–4.

DISCUSSION

From anatomico-physiological maps similar to those of Figure 5 and from physiological and anatomical studies indicating the interconnections of various neuronal masses, it is possible to suggest some of the pathways by which central inhibitory or facilitatory influences reach their ultimate destination—the motor horn cells of the spinal cord. The reasons for suggesting the interconnections of the various nuclei or the ways by which inhibitory or facilitatory influences are directed caudally to the horn cells will not be discussed, since they have already been published in detail.[5–7] Instead, the major conclusions will be stated briefly.

The diagrams of Figures 6 and 7 indicate that there are two pathways by which inhibitory influences are sent to the cord, and also that two pathways may be utilized to send facilitatory influences to the final motor neuron. In each case, one circuit may be designated "ascending," the other "descending." The chief reason for calling the former "ascending" (Figures 6A and 7A) is that these circuits, originating in the cortex, eventually send their effects into the thalamus and from this neuronal mass inhibitory and facilitatory influences are presumed to be directed rostrally to the motor cortex. The activity of this cortex is then either inhibited or facilitated and consequently the barrage of impulses reaching the lower motor neuron by way of cortico-spinal tracts is either reduced or increased.

The "descending" circuits (Figures 6B and 7B), which may start in the cortex or diencephalon, appear to pass through or be collected in the hypothalamus and from there make their way caudally to the reticular formation of the bulb, whence they are distributed to both sides of the cord by the reticulo-spinal tracts.

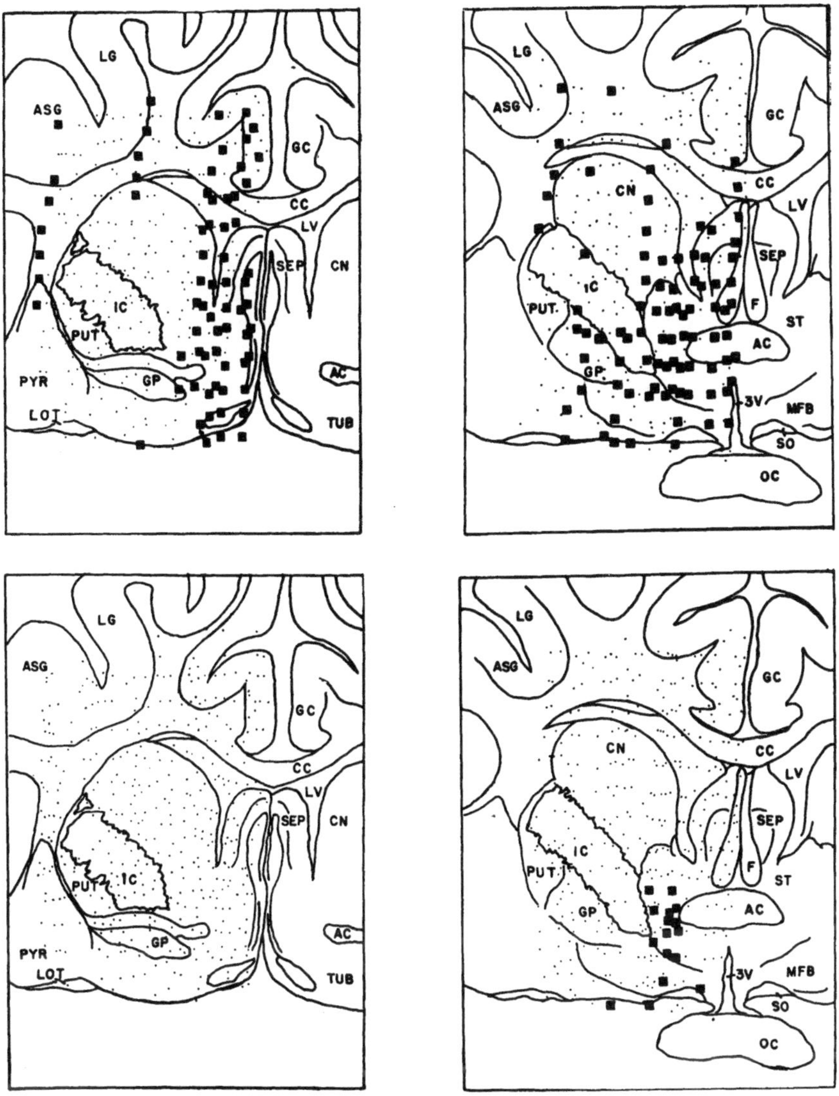

FIGURE IV–5. Sample maps of the brain cut in the frontal plane of the Horsley-Clarke apparatus. In the upper drawings the points causing facilitation of cortically evoked movements are shown by the filled squares, those not affecting the vigor of the test response are indicated by the dots. In the lower drawings, representing the same levels as the upper drawings, the points causing facilitation of the knee jerk are indicated by the filled squares. Note the complete absence of such points in the first level and their scarcity in the second level when compared with the corresponding maps in the upper drawings. For further discussion see text

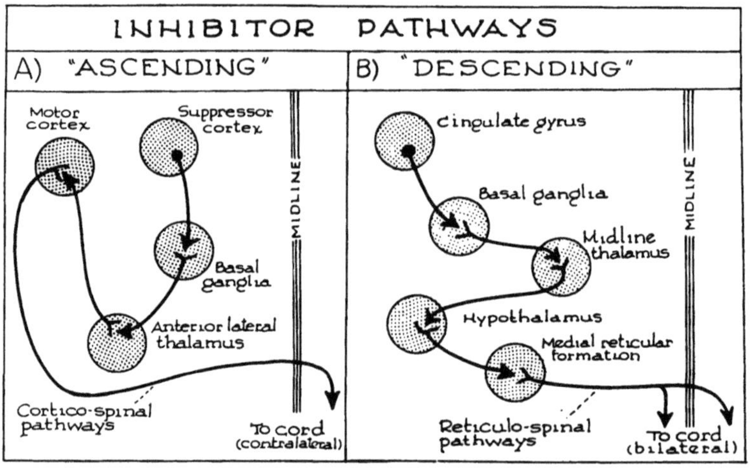

FIGURE IV–6. Schema of the postulated "ascending" and "descending" inhibitor pathways

The possibility is of course present that the "ascending" paths may send collaterals to the "descending" connections and so influence motor activity in an additional manner to that illustrated. The essential feature which distinguishes "ascending" from "descending" circuits in our formulation is that the former are arranged in neural loops extending from cortex to subcortex to cortex, whereas the latter are arrayed so as to pass their influences to progressively more caudal sites.

SUMMARY

Stimulation has been applied to the forebrains of anesthetized cats and its effects on somatic motor activity recorded kymographically. Thus forebrain structures not previously known to influence motor responses have been shown to inhibit or facilitate such activity.

When added to previous anatomical and physiological evidence, the present data allow the postulation of pathways by which central inhibitory and facilitatory influences are distributed to the motor centers of the cord. It may be that both the inhibitory and the facilitatory influences reach the cord by two separate pathways. In each case, one such circuit is designated "ascending," the other "descending." It is suggested (a) that the "ascending" pathways originate in the cerebral cortex, extend

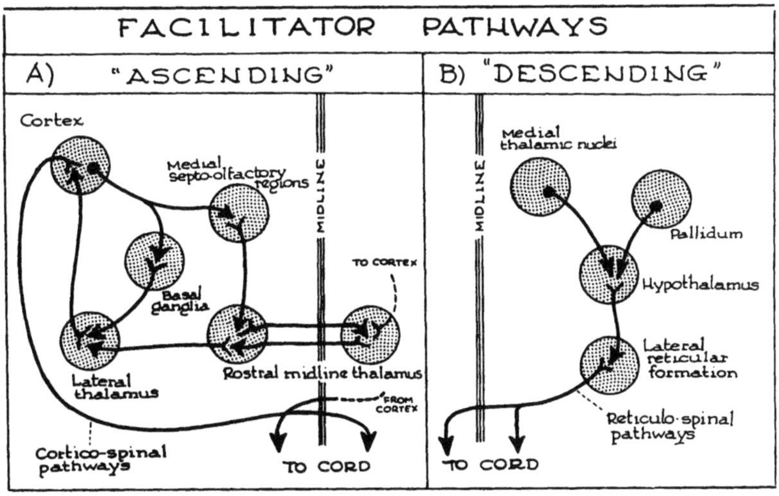

FIGURE IV–7. Schema of the postulated "ascending" and "descending" facilitator pathways

caudally into the rhinencephalon (septal region) and some rostral diencephalic structures, and return thence to the cortex, and (b) that the "descending" pathways, taking a different course, proceed in a continuous fashion caudally, through the diencephalon, midbrain, and bulbar reticular formation to their ultimate destination in the cord.

For reasons already noted in Chapter 1, portions of the ascending facilitatory system were stimulated in schizophrenic patients (see Chapters 12 and 13).

REFERENCES

1. Magoun, H. W., and R. Rhines. *Spasticity: the Stretch-Reflex and Extrapyramidal Systems.* Thomas, Springfield, 1948.
2. Lindsley, D. B., L. H. Schreiner, and H. W. Magoun. An electromyographic study of spasticity, *J. Neurophysiol.*, 12:197–205 (1949).
3. Hodes, R., S. M. Peacock, Jr., and R. G. Heath. Somatic and visceral effects from stimulation of the forebrain of the cat, *Tr. Am. Neurol. A.*, 75:194–198 (1950).
4. Hodes, R., S. M. Peacock, Jr., and R. G. Heath. Influence of the forebrain on somato-motor activity, I: Inhibition, *J. Comp. Neurol.*, 94:381–408 (1951).
5. Peacock, S. M., Jr., and R. Hodes. Influence of the forebrain on somato-motor activity, II: Facilitation, *J. Comp. Neurol.*, 94:409–426 (1951).

6. Hodes, R., and S. M. Peacock, Jr. Influence of the forebrain on somatomotor activity, *Bull. Tulane Univ. Med. Faculty*, 11:21–33 (1951).
7. Mettler, F. A., H. W. Ades, E. Lipman, and E. A. Culler. The extrapyramidal system, *Arch. Neurol. & Psychiat.*, 41:984–995 (1939).
8. Becker, H. C., R. Hodes, W. Founds, Jr., and S. M. Peacock, Jr. An application of autosyns to multi-channel physiological recording, *Proc. Soc. Exper. Biol. & Med.*, 76:761–763 (1951).

Chronic Experiments with Animals

INTRODUCTION

ROBERT G. HEATH

In the animal studies reported in Chapters 2 to 4 it has been demonstrated that metabolic changes similar to those following adrenalectomy could result from lesions in a specific region of the forebrain and that electrical stimulation in this same region would facilitate somatic motor activity. Stimulation of other areas of the rostral forebrain inhibited somatic motor activity. Because of technical difficulties it was impossible to ablate the inhibitory areas discretely. Up to this point our data had been derived from acute experiments with cats. It now became necessary to demonstrate as clearly as possible subcortical-cortical interrelationships through chronic experiments with intact animals. We therefore decided to implant electrodes in the brains of two Rhesus monkeys, one a male and the other a female, and to apply periodic stimulation over a period of several months.

The literature includes several descriptions of the interrelationships between the cortex and the olfactory zones of the forebrain and, of course, innumerable descriptions of connections between the cortex and other subcortical structures. Chapter 5 will include references to reports on the septal connections, since these have particular relevance to our research program. The principal technique by which these connections have been shown to affect the cortex is through electrical potentials. Jasper and his colleagues were able to demonstrate that application of stimulation to the septum produced potentials at the tip of the temporal lobe; they were likewise able to demonstrate that strychnine, implanted in the septum, would produce reflected spiking in the temporal region of the cortex. We have also been able to pick up potentials by applying stimuli in the septal region.*

The importance of temporal-lobe electrical abnormalities in behavioral disorders will be discussed, along with the presentation of the data on patients (Chapters 11 and 14). However, it may be said here that spikes in the tip of the temporal lobe have been found in many persons displaying behavioral disorders very similar in clinical picture to the endogenous psychoses. In reviewing material from our electroencephalographic laboratories, we have found a very high incidence of temporal lobe spiking in patients who were clinically diagnosed as schizophrenic. Because of the electrical abnormality, most workers in the field of electroencephalography would call these patients psychomotor epileptics, even though the presenting clinical picture was that of schizophrenia.

The literature includes several reports which are relevant in our consideration of this specific subcortical-cortical relationship. The most consistent findings in patients with organic lesions in the region of the foramen of Monro, fornix, and septum were abnormal electrical potentials in the region of the temporal lobe.[1, 2] Although the investigators were primarily concerned with the electroencephalographic abnormalities, they also report that paroxysmal disorders in many ways resembling psychotic behavior are sometimes found in patients having such lesions.

For the documentation of our over-all thesis it was also important to discover whether stimulation of the cortex would activate subcortical structures. Although there are many anatomical data to indicate that the cortex is connected to the midline septal region, a complete review of the literature will not be attempted. In man the principal afferents to the septal regions from the frontal cortex are from areas 9 and 11; area 6 likewise projects to this region. The septum is also anatomically related to the hypothalamus. In one of our Rhesus monkeys we were able to demonstrate that stimulation of the cortex can result in firing of the septal region. The physiological relationship, which Stoll, Jasper, and Ajmone-Marsan have described in their papers[3, 4] will be discussed in Chapter 5.

Chapter 6 reports the manner in which alterations in the inhibitory

*This study originated elsewhere; the experiments were repeated at Tulane because of their relevance to our over-all theoretical concept.

and facilitatory circuits influence the over-all behavior of the intact animal. The extremes in awareness thus produced were illustrated by a motion picture film when our results were presented in New Orleans in June, 1952. At that time our data on the biochemical changes resulting from stimulation of the different circuits were incomplete. However, in the presentation of our over-all thesis we had postulated that behavior, physiology, and body chemistry should all be reflections of the same process. Since the meetings we have obtained new data on the biochemical effects of stimulation. In as much as they are relevant to our concept, they will be reported in Addendum B.

Chapter 7 is concerned with electrical recordings made while the animals passed into and awakened from sleep. The data therein presented further clarify the effect of subcortical-cortical relationships on different types of behavior.

REFERENCES

1. Hunter, J. Further observations of subcortically induced epileptic attacks in unanesthetized animals, *Electroencephalog. & Clin. Neurophysiol.*, 2:193–201 (1950).
2. Lennox, M., and B. S. Brody. Paroxysmal slow waves in the electroencephalograms of patients with epilepsy and with subcortical lesions, *J. Nerv. & Ment. Dis.*, 104:237–248 (1946).
3. Ajmone-Marsan, C., and J. Stoll, Jr. Subcortical connections of the temporal pole in relation to temporal lobe seizures, *Arch. Neurol. Psychiat.*, 66:669–686 (1951).
4. Stoll, J., Jr., C. Ajmone-Marsan, and H. Jasper. Electrophysiological studies of subcortical connections of the anterior temporal region in the cat, *J. Neurophysiol.*, 14:305–316 (1951).

CHAPTER 5

CONNECTIONS BETWEEN THE CORTEX AND THE SEPTAL REGION IN RHESUS MONKEYS

CHARLES D. HENDLEY
ROBERT HODES
ROBERT G. HEATH

In our investigation of the problem of physiologically possible pathways from the septal region to the cortex and from the cortex to the septal region, we were particularly interested in the frontal association areas and the anterior portion of the temporal lobe. Mettler[1] had shown anatomically that frontal areas 9 and 11 project to the septal region, but anatomical methods had not revealed such connections for the anterior temporal cortex. Soon after we started our investigation, however, two papers were published by Stoll, Ajmone-Marsan, and Jasper.[2,3] These demonstrated physiologically many subcortical connections of the anterior temporal region in cats with "cerveaux isolés" and anesthetized monkeys. Subsequently we obtained some data from electrical stimulation which indicate a connection between area 9 and the septal region in the monkey.

Turning first to the experiments of the Montreal group, we show in Figure 1 recordings of electrical activity in a cat with "cerveau isolé." Stimulation of the left anterior temporal region has produced a pronounced after-discharge in the septum, as well as the nearby postsylvian gyrus and the contralateral temporal tip. On the other hand, a distant region of the cortex (auditory area) shows no after-discharge, and the response in the caudate is not striking. The recording electrodes were implanted on the left side, very close to the midline of the septum, above the anterior commissure.

Figure 2 indicates a connection between the diagonal band of Broca at the base of the septum and the temporal tip in an anesthetized monkey. The arrow on the section points to the region where the recording electrodes were placed in the septum. At the right of the figure are shown the results of strychninization of the left temporal tip. There are pro-

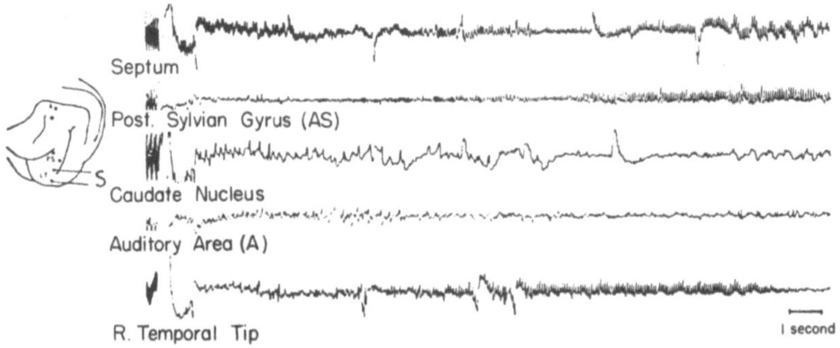

FIGURE V–1. Recording of electrical activity in a cat with the brainstem sectioned at the intercollicular level (cerveau isolé preparation). "Record showing example of after-discharge in septal region following a repetitive stimulation (3 V., 25 c/sec., 4 sec.)." From Stoll, Ajmone-Marsan, and Jasper, *J. Neurophysiol.*, 14: 308 (1951)

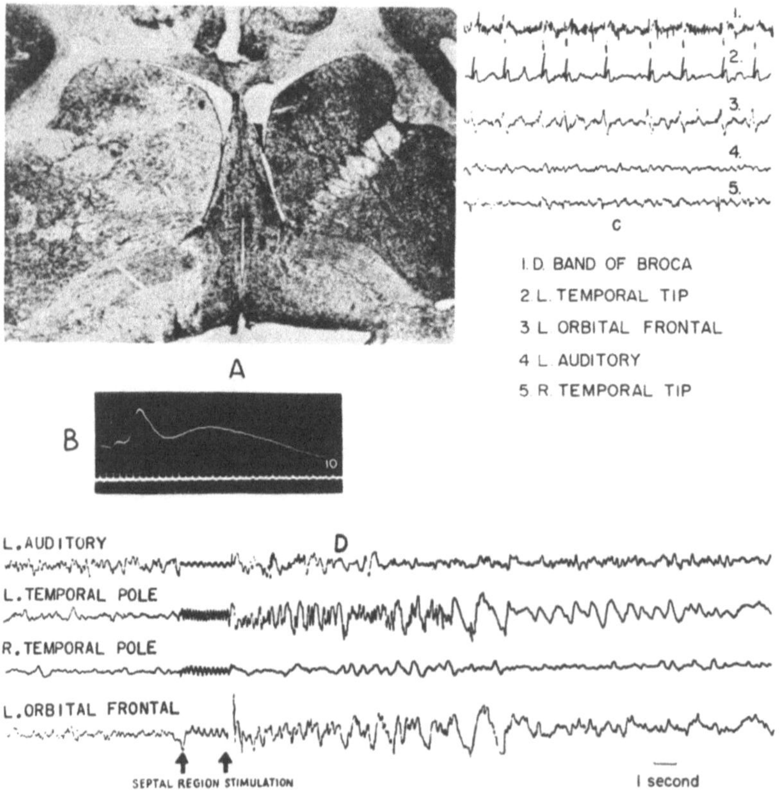

FIGURE V–2. Connections between septal areas and the temporal tip in the monkey (see text for description). From Ajmone-Marsan and Stoll, A.M.A. *Arch. Neurol. & Psychiat.*, 66:672 (1951)

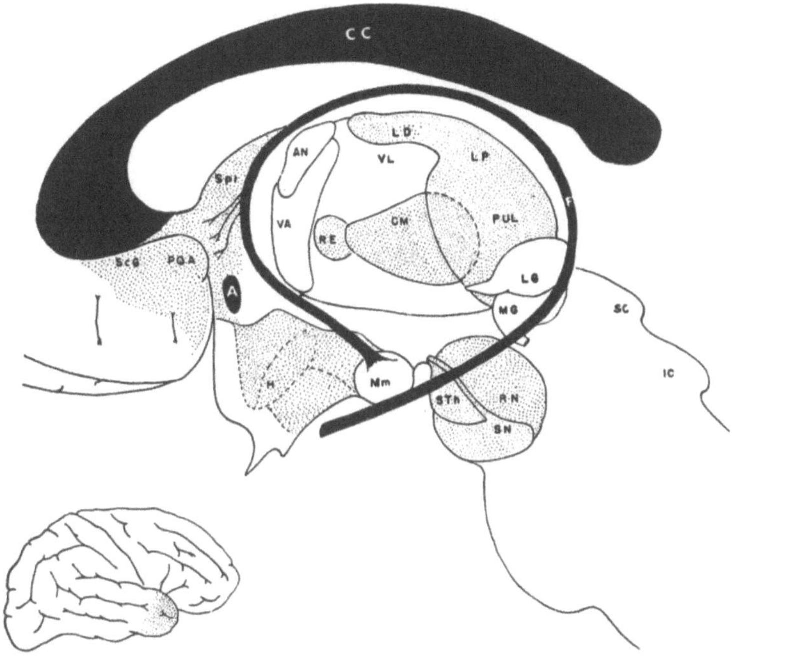

FIGURE V–3. Schematic drawing showing in outline (dotted areas) principal subcortical structures found to be functionally related to the temporal pole in the monkey. "*A* indicates anterior commissure; *AN*, anterior nuclei of thalamus; *CC*, corpus callosum; *CM*, centrum medianum of thalamus; *F*, fornix; *H*, hypothalamus; *IC*, inferior colliculus; *LD*, nucleus lateralis dorsalis of thalamus; *MG*, medial geniculate body; *Mm*, mammillary body; *POA*, paraolfactory area; *Pul*, pulvinar; *RE*, nucleus reuniens of thalamus; *RN*, red nucleus; *SC*, superior colliculus; *SCG*, subcallosal gyrus; *SN*, substantia nigra; *SPt*, septal areas; *STh*, corpus Luysi; *VA*, nucleus ventralis anterior of thalamus; *VL*, nucleus ventralis lateralis of thalamus." From Ajmone-Marsan and Stoll, A.M.A. *Arch. Neurol. & Psychiat.*, 66:681 (1951)

nounced strychnine spikes in the diagonal band of Broca. These are much larger than the spikes in any other region. The small oscillograph tracing labeled B shows an evoked response with long latency in the temporal tip following single pulse stimulation of the septal region. The latency in this case is about 25 milliseconds. The four tracings at the bottom show an after-discharge in the temporal tip and orbito-frontal cortex after repetitive stimulation of the septal region at 25 cycles per second. Figure 3 is a schematic drawing showing the subcortical structures found to be connected with the temporal pole in the monkey; the dotted areas in which connections were found extend from the subcallosal gyrus back to the red nucleus and the substantia nigra.

METHODS

In our own laboratory deep electrodes were implanted in two Rhesus monkeys under nembutal anesthesia. In the experiment reported here placement was made with the Horsley-Clarke stereotaxic apparatus. The electrodes were .25 mm. in diameter and 2 mm. long and were made of flexible copper wire with a sharp hook at the end. A stiff needle-carrier was used to insert the electrodes in the brain. When the needle-carrier was withdrawn, the electrodes remained in place by virtue of the fine hook catching in the brain tissue. Two electrodes, each consisting of one pole, were inserted close together, so that bipolar recordings from specific subcortical structures could be made. In all, seven pairs of deep electrodes were implanted, some on either side of the midline. Attempts were made to place them in the caudate nucleus, septal region, hypothalamus, and thalamic nuclei. In addition, eight electrodes were inserted in the cortex—one on each frontal, parietal, occipital, and temporal lobe—the contact point being a small flat disk. It was then possible to make repeated recordings over an extended period of time, and also to administer stimuli through specific subcortical or cortical regions. Recordings were continued for four months after operation. The necessity for anesthesia was avoided by the development of a special chair, which enabled the animal to feed himself but prevented him from displacing the electrodes (see Figure 4).

The approximate locations of the subcortical electrodes with which we are presently concerned is shown in Figures 5 and 7. The septal electrodes are shown in Figure 5, and it will be seen that one of these was actually implanted in the caudate at the border of the septum. Figure 7 shows the lesions made by electrodes in the posterior caudate region, and in the fornix right at the top of the thalamus. The stimuli were single pulse square waves of 1 volt intensity and 1 millisecond duration delivered through a subdural electrode. Stimuli were usually delivered 2 to 10 seconds apart.

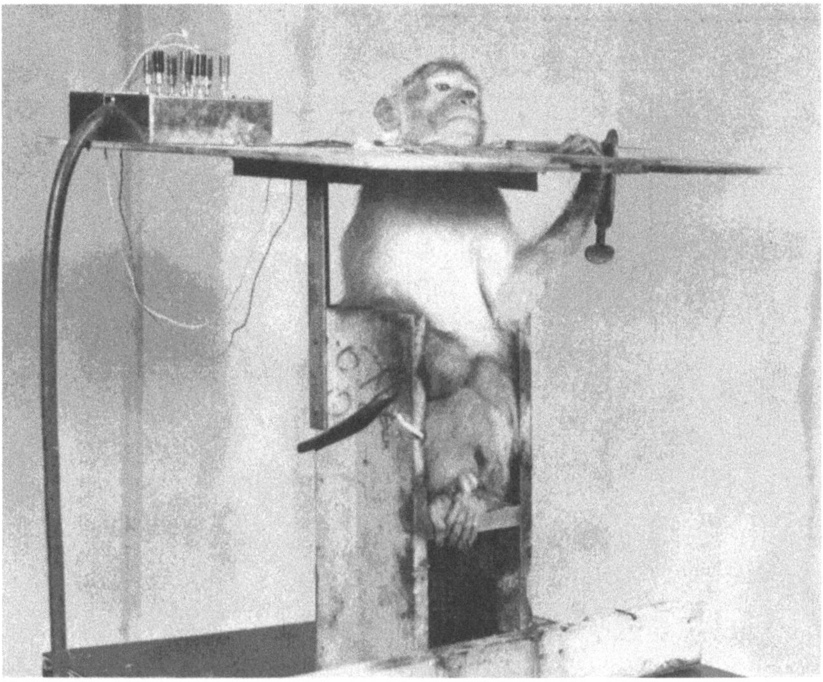

FIGURE V–4. Chair designed to permit long-term studies after implantation of electrodes in monkey brain

RESULTS

The pertinent results are summarized in the next two figures. Figure 6 shows the results of stimulating the right frontal region anterior to the arcuate sulcus at the posterior border of area 9. An evoked response was obtained in the left parietal and right occipital region, but that obtained in the right temporal was not very striking. After a long latency a large slow wave was evoked from the septal lead; this response is not seen in the others. Owing to the compression of our time base, we were unable to tell whether there were any short-latency primary responses, but secondary responses with a latency of about 70 milliseconds were found fairly consistently upon stimulation of the frontal lobe with weak single shocks. We were never able to obtain this response from other deep forebrain structures. Figure 8 shows a similar response, obtained from stimulating the left frontal electrode, also in area 9. Again, the evoked response was most prominent in the septum. This time the response was

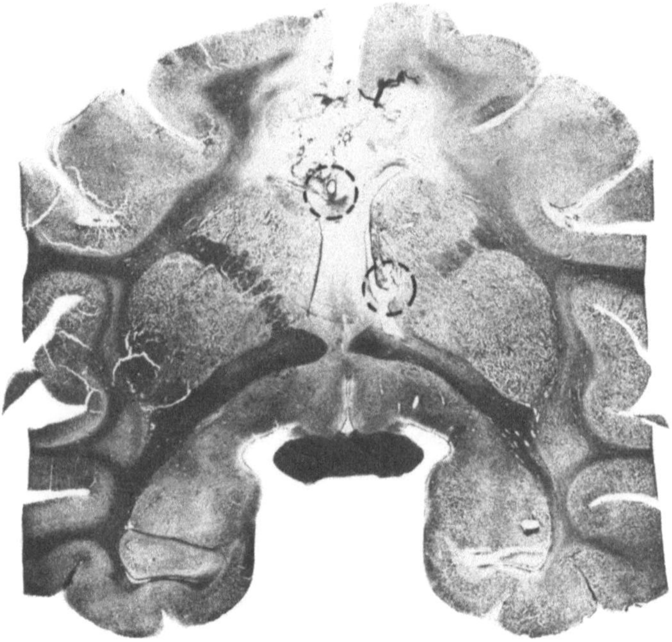

FIGURE V–5. Frontal section of brain showing placement of septal electrodes, (indicated by the circles). The left side of the brain is on the right of the figure

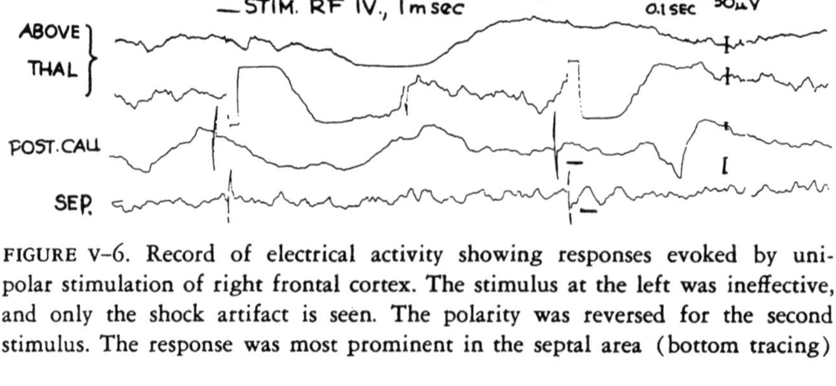

FIGURE V–6. Record of electrical activity showing responses evoked by unipolar stimulation of right frontal cortex. The stimulus at the left was ineffective, and only the shock artifact is seen. The polarity was reversed for the second stimulus. The response was most prominent in the septal area (bottom tracing)

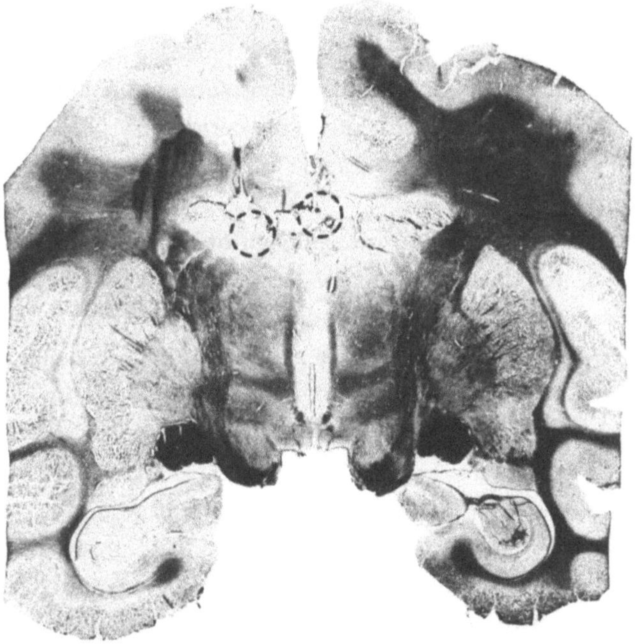

FIGURE V–7. Frontal section of brain showing placement of electrodes in the tail of the caudate nucleus (circle at left) and in the fornix (circle in the midline). The left side of the brain is on the right of the figure

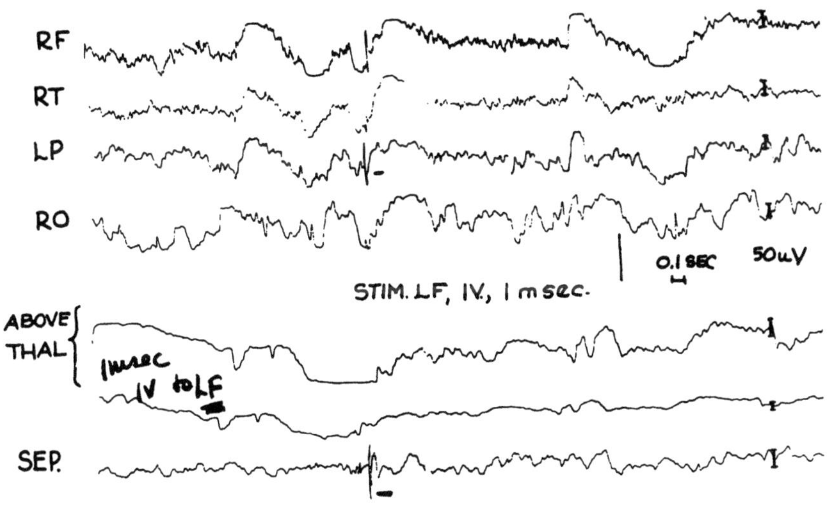

FIGURE V–8. Record of electrical activity showing responses evoked by unipolar stimulation of left frontal cortex

a double one; the usual large, slow wave had a latency of about 40 milliseconds. This long-latency slow wave was preceded by a much sharper one with a latency of about 10 milliseconds. That we obtained this result only when stimulating the left side of the cortex may be due to the fact that one of our "septal" electrodes was on the left side at the border of the caudate nucleus.

The short-latency response was obtained only a few times. The long-latency response, however, was very reproducible. It was obtained only from the septal electrodes—the other subcortical electrodes did not record it. For this reason we feel we are dealing with a definite, though circuitous pathway, in spite of the very long latency of the response.

SUMMARY

We now have good evidence from the Montreal group for connections from the septal region to the temporal lobe, and from the temporal region back to the septum. Our own results give some physiological evidence for pathways from the prefrontal cortex to the septal region that had already been established anatomically. Chapters 6 and 7 will describe in further detail how the septal region plays back upon the cortex.

REFERENCES

1. Mettler, F. A. Extracortical connections of the primate frontal cerebral cortex, part II: Corticifugal connections, *J. Comp. Neurol.*, 86:119–166 (1947).
2. Stoll, J., Jr., C. Ajmone-Marsan, and H. Jasper. Electrophysiological studies of subcortical connections of the anterior temporal region in the cat, *J. Neurophysiol.*, 14:305–316 (1951).
3. Ajmone-Marsan, C., and J. Stoll, Jr. Subcortical connections of the temporal pole in relation to temporal lobe seizures, *Arch. Neurol. Psychiat.*, 66:669–686 (1951).

CHAPTER 6

EFFECTS OF STIMULATION WITH ELECTRODES CHRONICALLY IMPLANTED IN RHESUS MONKEYS

ROBERT G. HEATH
ROBERT HODES

On the basis of the ablation studies reported in Chapters 2 and 3 and the stimulation experiments reported in Chapter 4, we reasoned that additional physiological information could be gathered, and also that further observations on behavior could be made, if the stimulation techniques applied in our earlier studies could be adapted to chronic experiments. As previously explained, deep electrodes were implanted in two Rhesus monkeys and the effects of stimulation were observed and recorded over a period of four months.

METHODS

The first animal was operated upon by the open method. A transcortical incision was made through the right prefrontal cortex into the anterior horn of the right lateral ventricle. One bipolar electrode was implanted in the medial aspect of the caudate nucleus and another was implanted in the midline septal region. After the dura was closed, the electrodes were sealed to the bone by means of dental cement and then brought out through the skin on the back of the head. The animal was kept in a specially constructed chair, which permitted him to feed himself but prevented him from displacing the electrodes (see Chapter 5, Figure 4).

RESULTS

The results presented here were obtained from stimulation of electrodes implanted by the open method.* When low current was applied at a frequency of 3 stimuli per second to the caudate lead, the monkey became drowsy and soon dozed off into a state of diminished awareness resembling

*A motion picture film (M.M.1) was shown in connection with the original report of this experiment (New Orleans, 1952).

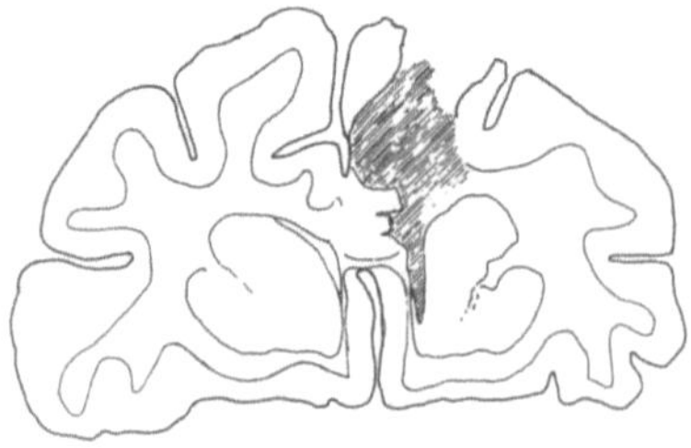

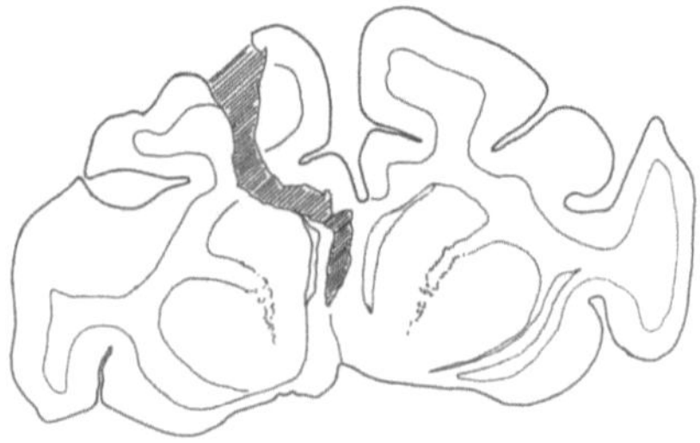

FIGURE VI–1 (left). Tract of caudate electrode in monkey brain (section)
FIGURE VI–2 (right). Tract of septal region electrode in monkey brain (section)

deep sleep. But when stimuli were applied to the electrode in the midline septal region, a sharply different response was elicited in that the animal's alertness was actually increased. Figures 1 and 2 show the areas in which the electrodes were placed.

Figure 3 shows the location of an electrode which was fortuitously placed in the lateral wall of the left ventricle of a schizophrenic patient under therapeutic treatment (for the operative procedure see Chapter 9). When a current of 4 ma. was applied for 2 minutes in square wave pulses of 1 millisecond duration and 100 cycles per second frequency, the patient became so drowsy that it was difficult to arouse him. This condition persisted for a few minutes after cessation of stimulation.

Observations of the monkey's behavioral responses were, of course, limited for the same reason that all animal psychological observations are limited—namely, that subjective information cannot be obtained. However, our findings suggest that stimulation of the area which facilitated somatic motor activity also produced increased alertness. It was impossible in this preparation to follow chemical changes systematically because of difficulties encountered in the management of the monkey. Blood samples could not be taken regularly, and it was impossible to get the necessary urine samples. Blood pressure, however, was taken with cuff measurements during stimulation. With application of higher intensities of current to the facilitatory area, very marked increases in blood pressure occurred. In fact, it rose higher than the manometer registered —the systolic rising above 310 and the diastolic as high as 130. This indirect observation seemingly gives some support to the concept that the chemical stress mechanism was activated.

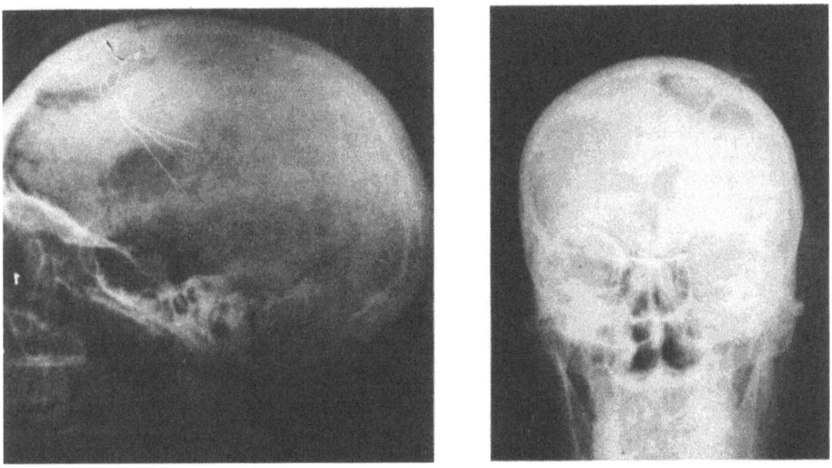

FIGURE VI–3. Lateral and anterior-posterior x-ray view showing electrodes in place in a schizophrenic patient (Patient 12)

Over the four months' period in which it was possible to make recordings from scalp, cortical, and subcortical electrodes, many observations were made on both monkeys at different stages of awareness. Changes came about as a result of spontaneous sleep, administration of nembutal, and external stimuli—particularly the presence or absence of observers in the room at the time the recordings were made. Such recordings represent an attempt to make correlations between neurophysiological activity and behavior.

SUMMARY

Markedly different effects were obtained by stimulation through two bipolar electrodes implanted respectively in the caudate nucleus and the septal region of a monkey's brain. Since the electrodes were only a few millimeters apart, these effects would seemingly indicate markedly different functions in the two regions. Stimulation of the midline septal region produced an alerting effect, whereas stimulation in the medial aspect of the caudate nucleus produced a state of diminished awareness. Stimulation through a bipolar electrode fortuitously placed in the lateral wall of the ventricle in the schizophrenic patient undergoing a therapeutic procedure likewise produced a state of diminished awareness. The marked increase in blood pressure during stimulation of the facilitatory area indirectly suggested that the chemical stress mechanism was involved.

CHAPTER 7

CORTICAL AND SUBCORTICAL ELECTRICAL ACTIVITY IN SLEEP

ROBERT HODES
ROBERT G. HEATH
CHARLES D. HENDLEY

Researches on the nature of sleep should offer important correlative adjuvants to a program devoted to studies of the schizophrenic process. For sleep is a normal and reversible—yet dramatic and qualitatively distinctive reduction of consciousness which in many ways resembles such morbid states as stupor, epilepsy, some of the common dementias, and even schizophrenia itself. A feature common to all these states is a reduced awareness of the external world. In sleep, as in the pathological conditions mentioned above, the individual appears to be out of touch with his environment, so that he does not react, in a fashion appropriate to the conscious state, to the ordinary provocations arising therefrom.

Theories regarding the nature of sleep probably rival in antiquity the very existence of man. Current concepts of the causation and maintenance of sleep are effectively summarized by Best and Taylor.[1] Until recently, neurophysiological theories of sleep have been concerned with the depression of cortical activity. Most researchers in this field agree to a correlation between an individual's cortical activity and his stage of awareness. Depression of the acuity of the cortex has been explained by various mechanisms. The diminution of corticipetal impulses[2-5] and the invasion of the cortical analyzers by conditioned inhibition[6,7] are two of the major mechanisms advanced to account for the decline of cortical hegemony.

Countless experiences of everyday living support the physiological concept of reduced cerebral activity as a prelude to slumber. We generally go to sleep at night when visual stimuli are reduced, when the hustle and bustle of the day are over, when the sounds of the city street or countryside are in abeyance, and when the time for retiring (to a large extent a conditioned response) approaches.

That noncortical areas are also concerned in the control of sleep has become clear from many types of observations. Hypersomnia is frequently noted in patients suffering from a variety of morbid processes involving basal diencephalic or midbrain regions. Cortical neurons are not grossly affected in some of these instances, nor are pathological conditions of the thalamic relay nuclei apparent.[8, 9] Experimental lesions of the hypothalamus[10, 11] have produced akinetic, expressionless, or hypersomnolent animals. Hess and his collaborators[12–16] and others[17, 18] believe that stimulation of certain subcortical masses causes sleep or sleeplike states.

It should be clear that both cortical and subcortical activity are prominent determinants of the conditions under which sleep envelops the organism. Recent attempts to reconcile diverse observations and concepts concerning the role of cortex and subcortex in the induction and persistence of sleep[9, 19] are useful, for only continual emphasis on the organization of the parts of the nervous system into an interrelated and integrated whole will reduce the unfortunate current tendency to isolate the cortex and the lower centers into independent units of function.

The above considerations led to the preliminary experiments to be reported now. Many previous studies on sleep had been performed on anesthetized animals subjected to various experimental procedures, on surviving animals in which portions of the neuraxis had been destroyed, or on patients with damage to different regions of the brain or brainstem. All these methods are valuable; all of them provide information to be synthesized ultimately into rational and comprehensive theories of the causation of sleep and perhaps, by extension, into more adequate physiological ideas concerning consciousness and its aberrations. However, in order to get closer to the functional and dynamic interrelationships which we felt must be attacked in the last analysis, we chose to make a preparation in which few of the complications inherent in the above kind of material would be present. The unanesthetized, restrained yet alert monkey, from which cortical and subcortical recordings could be obtained at will, appeared to us to be a subject on which experiments and observations could be made in states not too far removed from normal. In such an animal the electrical concomitants of *spontaneous* sleep could be observed.

METHODS

Two Rhesus monkeys were operated on under nembutal anesthesia. In the first operation (see Chapter 6) two bipolar electrodes were inserted under direct vision into the caudate nucleus and the basal part of the septal region. In the second operation (see Chapter 5) eight unipolar electrodes were placed in various subcortical regions by means of the stereotaxic apparatus; the method of implantation was essentially the same as that later described for the placement of electrodes in schizophrenic patients (see Chapter 10). The chief difference was that the positions in which subcortical electrodes were placed were selected by reference to a monkey brain atlas* rather than to the air ventriculogram used when humans were involved. In the second operation solder disk electrodes were also placed over the pia and their leads brought to the surface. In each instance the electrode leads were cemented to the skull and brought out through the skin.

After implantation was completed, the animals were placed in a special chair (see Chapter 5, Figure 4) which was so arranged that they could feed themselves but were prevented from reaching and pulling at the electrode wires. The leads were brought either directly to the electrode box of an eight-channel Grass electroencephalograph or to connections in a plastic cap screwed into the skull. From these terminals, connection was then made to the EEG instrument (Figure 1).

The animals lived their entire postoperative existence of approximately four months each in the chair. After a few weeks of becoming accustomed to the restraint, the chair, the laboratory sights and sounds, and the experimenters, they became quite tame. When fed or petted and soothed by the observers, the monkeys would frequently doze off into light sleep for short periods of time.

RESULTS

Electrical signs of drowsiness were unmistakably present in the deep leads at the onset of a bout of spontaneous slipping from consciousness. Such activity consisted of bursts of 1–3 per second high voltage waves, with occasional 8–10 per second peaks superimposed on the slow fluctuations. These evidences of drowsiness were more striking in the subcortical leads than in the simultaneous samplings from the cortical leads. Indeed,

*Kindly supplied by Dr. H. W. Magoun.

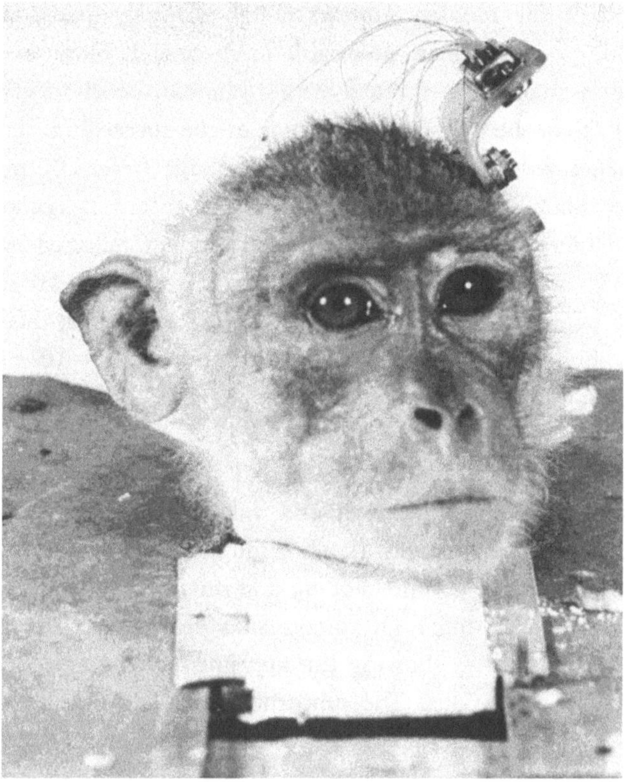

FIGURE VII–1. Monkey seated in chair. The wires from the electrodes are soldered to terminals in a plug mounted in a lucite holder which is screwed to the skull. A female plug with wires attached (not shown) is used to make connection with the EEG instrument

the synchronized subcortical bursts were often noticeable before such activity was apparent in the cortical leads.

Figure 2 shows a typical sequence of superficial and deep recordings as the animal progressed from quiet awareness (record 1) to drowsiness (records 2–5) to awareness (record 6). Such recordings were repeated on many occasions on both animals, and the observers became familiar enough with the features of the subcorticograms to tell the animal's state of awareness without looking at him. The first two channels of each record represent EEG's from the left frontal area and right parietal area, respectively. The others represent subcorticograms, channels 4–6 showing activity of electrodes in the caudate nucleus.

In record 1 the monkey appears to be relatively quiet, but muscle artifacts due to grimaces are noticeable in channel 1. Slow waves can be recognized in channels 4–6 but these are random, poorly organized, and less distinct than the slow waves of some of the succeeding figures. Even though the animal is still grimacing, high voltage (over 200 microvolts) slow waves, about 1 or 2 per second, appear in record 2. Record 3 shows the animal quiet; facial movements are no longer reflected in channels 1 and 2. To the right, in the subcorticograms small 8–10 per second waves are superimposed on well-defined 1.5 per second high voltage responses. Similar activity, with more pronounced 8–10 per second waves, is notable in the subcorticograms of record 4. When this recording was made, the animal's eyes were open. But it was apparent from his heavy-lidded, expressionless stare that he was in the vague intermediate state between partial sleep and wakefulness. His appearance was similar to that of an individual who, momentarily aroused, opens his eyes without seeing or comprehending and then promptly falls back into sleep. Baseline sway and high voltage slow waves occur in channels 1 and 2 of record 5, thus showing the first unequivocal evidence of sleep in the cortical derivations. The subcorticograms continue to show slow waves, 8–10 per second bursts and possible sleep humps. In record 6 grimacing is reflected again, about as in the first sample. The residual deep-seated slow wave patterns are of lesser amplitude and lack the bursting, organized character of the preceding records.

That the subcorticograms of Figure 2 were indeed related to the animal's state of awareness was noted in another type of experiment on several occasions. After the monkey had dozed off and was presenting the typical activity of sleep, one of the observers would stroll quietly into the room, or if already in the room, would quietly change his position or approach the drowsy animal. The animal would thereupon open his eyes and become momentarily alert. Then, apparently reassured by the sight of a familiar person and obvious lack of danger or need for vigorous attentiveness, he would close his eyes and slip back toward sleep. Such a sequence is shown in the record of Figure 3. The drowsy patterns, cortical and subcortical, are abruptly abolished following the startle response (arrow) to the observer's entry. The monkey would remain alert for about 20 seconds, and during this time the potentials would be

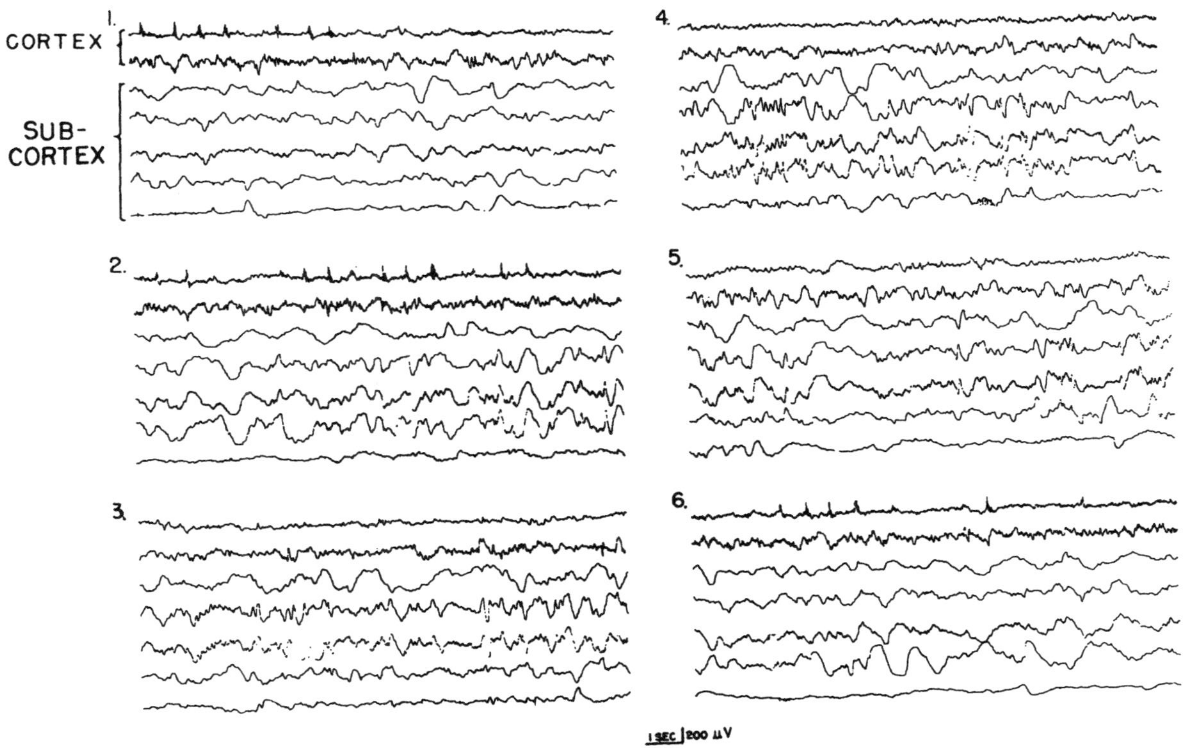

FIGURE VII–2. Recordings of electrical activity from cortex and subcortex, showing a progression from awareness (1) to drowsiness (2–5), then back to awareness (6). For description see text

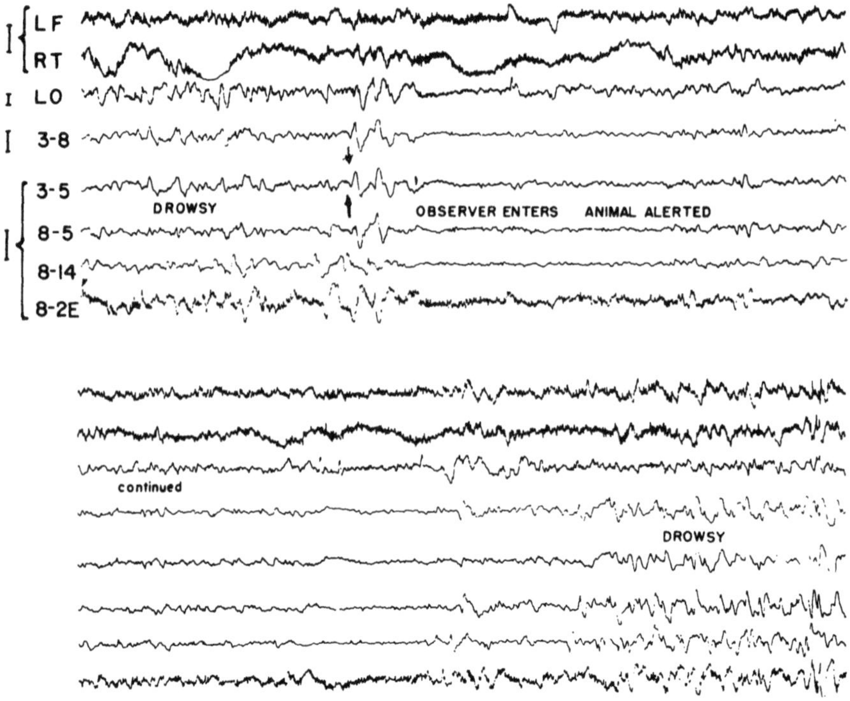

FIGURE VII–3. Tracings of cortical and subcortical activity, showing a drowsy record, a startle response when the observer enters, followed by an abrupt change in the record when the monkey became alert. At the end, the record again indicates drowsiness

significantly faster and flatter than during the period of dozing. With the wearing off of alertness there would be a reappearance of the electrical patterns already described as typical of sleep.

DISCUSSION

We have thus shown that electrical activity typical of sleep is recordable from the subcortex as well as from the cortex in natural sleep. The occurrence of recognizable electrical activity characteristic of sleep in the subcortex before it is recorded in the cortex requires some comment. The phenomenon may be due to the subcortical origin of this electrical activity, which only gradually suppresses the more rapid and less synchronous cortical activity. On the other hand, we may be dealing here with what is essentially an artifact of our crude recording methods. For, with the diffuse leads employed in routine electroencephalography and an almost simultaneous and equal involvement of most of the cortex in sleep, one would expect considerable cancellation and distortion of true sleep potentials. Probably both these factors—subcortical driving of the cortex and the artifacts of conventional recording—contribute to an explanation of our results, but further work is obviously necessary to clarify these points.[20]

From the data presented we cannot say which, if any, of the subcortical masses we have thus far examined are primarily involved in the production and maintenance of sleep; however, the recordings presented in this chapter and the stimulation experiments described in Chapter 6 do seem to implicate the caudate nucleus as one of the important neural masses concerned with the sleep process.

This conclusion would agree in a broad sense with the effects of stimulation of the caudate nucleus on motor activity—that is, reduction of motor response[21, 22]—and also with the recording therefrom of nembutal spindles, recently shown by Starzl and Magoun.[23]

REFERENCES

1. Best, C. H., and N. B. Taylor. The Physiology of Sleep, *in The Physiological Basis of Medical Practice,* pp. 1050–1055. Williams & Wilkins, Baltimore, 1950.
2. Bremer, F. Cerveau "isolé" et physiologie du sommeil, *Compt. rend. Soc. de biol.,* 118:1235–1241 (1935).
3. Bremer, F. Quelques propriétés de l'activité électrique du cortex cérébral "isolé," *Compt. rend. Soc. de biol.,* 118:1241–1244 (1935).
4. Bremer, F. Nouvelles recherches sur le mécanisme du sommeil, *Compt. rend. Soc. de biol.,* 122:460–464 (1936).
5. Bremer, F. Activité électrique du cortex cérébral dans les états de sommeil et de veille chez le chat, *Compt. rend. Soc. de biol.,* 122:464–467 (1936).
6. Pavlov, I. P. *Conditioned Reflexes; An Investigation of the Physiological Activity of the Cerebral Cortex.* Oxford Univ. Press, London, 1927.
7. Pavlov, I. P. *Lectures on Conditioned Reflexes,* vol. II: *Conditioned Reflexes and Psychiatry.* Int. Pubs., New York, 1941.
8. Bailey, P. *Intracranial Tumors,* 2nd ed. Thomas, Springfield, 1948.
9. Magoun, H. W. Caudal and cephalic influences of the brain stem reticular formation, *Physiol. Rev.,* 30:459–474 (1950).
10. Ingram, W. R., R. W. Barris, and S. W. Ranson. Catalepsy; an experimental study, *Arch. Neurol. Psychiat.,* 35:1175–1197 (1936).

11. Ranson, S. W. Somnolence caused by hypothalamic lesions in the monkey, *Arch. Neurol. Psychiat.*, 41:1–23 (1939).

12. Hess, W. R. Relation between psychic and vegetative functions, *Schweiz. Arch. f. Neurol. u. Psychiat.*, 15:260–277 (1924).

13. *Ibid.*, 16:36–55 (1925).

14. *Ibid.*, 16:285–306 (1925).

15. Akert, K., W. P. Koella, and R. Hess. Sleep produced by electrical stimulation of the thalamus, *Am. J. Physiol.*, 168:260–267 (1952).

16. Akert, K., and B. Andersson. Experimenteller Beitrag zur Physiologie des Nucleus caudatus, *Acta physiol. Scandinav.*, 22:281–298 (1951).

17. Kaada, B. Personal communication.

18. Heath, R. G., and R. Hodes. Induction of sleep by stimulation of the caudate nucleus in Macacus rhesus and man, *Tr. Am. Neurol. A.*, pp. 204–210 (1952).

19. Hodes, R. On Sleep-Wakefulness, *in* chapter by H. Haymaker of A. Baker and others, *Handbook of Neurology*. Hoeber, New York, 1954.

20. Hodes, R., R. G. Heath, and C. D. Hendley. Cortical and subcortical electrical activity in sleep, *Tr. Am. Neurol. A.*, pp. 201–203 (1952).

21. Mettler, F. A. Relation between pyramidal and extrapyramidal function, *A. Res. Nerv. & Ment. Dis., Proc. (1940)*, 21:150–227 (1942).

22. Hodes, R., S. M. Peacock, Jr., and R. G. Heath. Influence of the forebrain on somato-motor activity, Part I: Inhibition, *J. Comp. Neurol.*, 94: 381–408 (1951).

23. Starzl, T. E., and H. W. Magoun. Organization of the diffuse thalamic projection system, *J. Neurophysiol.*, 14:133–146 (1951).

Section III

HUMAN STUDIES

CHAPTER 8

DESCRIPTION OF THE PATIENT GROUP

RUSSELL R. MONROE
ROBERT G. HEATH

The group of patients selected for electrical stimulation included twenty who were diagnosed as unquestionably schizophrenic and three others who were not schizophrenic. Two of the three patients in the latter category were terminal cancer cases being treated for intractable pain. The other was a middle-aged man with an agitated depression in association with far-advanced tuberculosis. It was hoped that the stimulation procedure would alleviate his depression and agitation without aggravating his tuberculosis. These three patients were also controls for the schizophrenics. The rest of this chapter will be devoted to description of the twenty schizophrenic patients and will not include the terminal cancer cases or the psychotic agitated depression.

METHOD OF SELECTING SCHIZOPHRENIC PATIENTS

At first, the sole criterion for selecting patients for stimulation was the consensus of the attending physicians that prognosis for improvement under any therapeutic regimen was extremely poor. All but one had received somatic treatments (in six cases supplemented by psychotherapy), and all were considered unlikely to gain from psychosurgery. No patient who met the above criterion was rejected because of organic impairment or mental deficiency even when his case was unsuitable for evaluation by one of the cooperating disciplines; since it was felt that, though some of our data would be statistically incomplete, the fewer the criteria used in the selection of the group the more representative it would be as a sample.

Later, as it became apparent that a long rehabilitative procedure would be necessary and as the hospital itself had no rehabilitative facilities, patients were not accepted unless their families were in a position to offer extensive supervision for a sustained period.

STATISTICAL SURVEY

GENERAL DATA

The schizophrenic section included eleven males and nine females; seventeen patients were white and three colored (Table 1). The relatively small number of colored patients is explained by the inability of colored families to provide rehabilitative facilities. The age range varied from 17 to 56. Two patients were under 20, eight between 20 and 29, seven between 30 and 39, and three over 40. In view of the fact that all the schizophrenics were chronic cases, this age distribution seems to be characteristic of the expected age distribution for schizophrenia in general.

DIAGNOSIS AND LENGTH OF ILLNESS

There was no doubt among any observers that these patients were psychotic, nor was there any doubt that the predominant symptomatology was schizophrenic as described by Bleuler. Seven were diagnosed as hebephrenics, seven as paranoids, and six as catatonics. Five of the non-catatonics occasionally showed catatonic symptomatology. In general, the diagnosis was made on the basis of predominant symptomatology, the diagnosis of mixed schizophrenic reaction being avoided. Seven patients gave evidence of deterioration, in the form of sensorial or intellectual defects.

The length of illness in this section varied from 1 1/2 years to 32 years. Actually, in many cases, it had probably been of much longer duration. Thirteen patients had been sick 5 years or under, while seven had been psychotic for longer than 5 years. The actual breakdown is as follows:

NO. OF PATIENTS	DURATION OF ILLNESS
3	1 1/2–2 years
2	2–3 years
4	3–4 years
3	4–5 years
3	5–10 years
3	10–20 years
2	20 years or over

TABLE VIII–1. Group of twenty schizophrenic patients selected for stimulation

Patient	*Race Sex*	*Age*	DX	*Yrs. ill*	*Personality*	*Family history*	*Assoc. illness*	EST	*Insulin*	*Psycho-therapy*
1	WF	38	Heb.	1½	Obsess.	—	—	x	x	
2	WF	17	Cat.	3½	Schiz.	Psychosis	Anor. nerv.	x		x
3	WF	20	Heb.	3	"	?Psychosis	?Cushing's	x	x	x
4	WF	26	Cat.	1½	"	—	—	x		
*5(24)	WF	23	Cat.	4½	Unstable	Ment. def.	—	x		
†6	WM	28	Heb.	4½	Schiz.	—	—	x	x	x
7	CM	35	Par.	1½	"	—	Asthma	x		
*8(15)	WM	41	"	6	Par.	—	—	x	-x	x
9	WM	39	Heb.	20	Norm.	—	Cer. atrophy	x		
10	WM	56	"	18	Schiz.	Psychosis	Hyperten. & diabetes			
11	CM	19	"	3	"	?Psychosis	—	x		
12	WM	23	Cat.	4	Passive	—	—	x		
13	WM	35	Heb.	7	Obsess.	—	—	x	x	
14	WM	22	Par.	3	Depend.	Neurosis	—	x	x	
16	WF	47	"	32	Obsess.	Psychosis				x
17	WF	26	Cat.	2	Schiz.	—	?Ment. def.	x		x
18	WM	39	Par.	12	Obsess.	—	T.B.	x		
19	WM	32	"	10	Schiz.	—	Hyperten.		x	
20	WF	37	"	8	"	Neurosis	Obesity	x		
22	CF	21	Cat.	2½	Norm.	Psychosis	?Ment. def.	x		

*2 Stimulations †Topectomy

PREDISPOSING FACTORS

Only two patients were considered to have had normal personalities prior to the onset of their psychosis. Ten patients had distinctly schizoid personalities and four had shown predominantly obsessional traits. Four others had shown emotional disturbances of one kind or another. In the case of four patients one or more members of the immediate family were reported as overtly schizophrenic, and in the case of five patients members of the immediate family were reported as severely disturbed and probably psychotic. Ten of the patients had concurrent illnesses: one probably had tuberculosis, one had hypertension, one had asthma, one had diabetes and hypertension that had remitted somewhat during hospitalization, one had symptoms suggestive of Cushing's syndrome, one was mentally deficient, one was possibly mentally deficient, one had cerebral atrophy, one had anorexia nervosa, and one was markedly obese.

SPONTANEOUS REMISSIONS

Of the twenty patients only three had given any evidence of spontaneous remission in their symptoms, and in each case this was questionable. Patient 8 (15) had had a homosexual panic while courting his first wife but had had no contact with psychiatry between 1931 and 1938. However, during this interval he had experienced tremendous anxiety, his sexual performance had been inadequate, and he had spent many hours delving into sexual books and psychoanalytic literature to discover whether he was a "latent homosexual." Patient 16 had had symptoms suggestive of anorexia nervosa in 1918. She recovered after a short hospitalization but subsequently developed marked obsessional traits for which she was not rehospitalized until 1927. Patient 1 had reactive depressions in 1933 and 1939 following the death of close members of her family. Although she recovered from these episodes spontaneously, in retrospect one would certainly question the diagnosis, as she showed numerous schizophrenic symptoms during both these illnesses. Most of the patients were given sodium amytal at some time during the course of their hospitalization, but only three showed "normalizing" reactions.

Seventeen of the twenty patients had had full courses of electroshock therapy. Six had had electronarcosis as well as EST. Six had had insulin-coma therapy as well as EST (of these one had escaped from the hospital in 1938 before adequate treatment could be given). One had had metrazol and insulin-coma therapy as well as EST. One had had EST, insulin-coma therapy, and a topectomy. One had had a full course of insulin-coma therapy (61 treatments) but no EST. Only one patient in the entire group had received no somatic treatments; but this patient had been in custodial care for 18 years.

Only four of these patients had shown any significant improvement under any of these therapeutic regimens. Patient 8 (15) responded to metrazol in 1939 and to EST in 1945 but failed to respond to later somatic therapy. Patient 18 responded to electroshock therapy in 1939 but likewise failed to respond to subsequent courses of EST. Patient 14 responded to electroshock therapy in 1948 but failed to respond to similar therapy in 1950. Patient 19 responded temporarily to insulin-coma therapy but relapsed in nine months.

Six patients had received psychotherapy over significant periods. Patient 8(15) was seen in almost daily sessions during the six months prior to operation. Patient 16 had psychotherapy from 1935 through 1940; for several years she was seen in daily therapeutic sessions. Patient 2 was followed in the outpatient clinics of the Medical School for a six months' period prior to hospitalization. Patient 6 received two months of intensive psychotherapy while hospitalized in 1951. Patient 3 and Patient 17 were seen by private therapists for eight and three months, respectively, on an outpatient basis. None of these patients showed more than slight or transitory improvement under this regimen.

Six of the patients had been subjected to previous research projects, in which the effects of electroshock and electronarcosis were compared. This had involved special psychiatric interviews, as well as unusual attention and testing from the psychology department.

DISCUSSION

On the basis of the above data can we make any predictions as to the number of patients who might have shown improvement or left the hospital under purely custodial care or who might have responded to the total push of the experimental situation? It seems to us there are three ways to approach this question. One is to base our predictions on the statistics obtained for large groups of patients in the hope that our small group of 20 patients follows the same pattern. The second is to compare our group with groups subjected to similar experiences—namely, the total push that is involved when any patient is under experimental investigation—to try to find out what the total push alone will do to the course of the patient's psychosis. The third approach, which is more subjective but perhaps equally valuable, is to examine the group of 20 patients with the view of determining which, if any, might have been able to leave the hospital without benefit of a special procedure.

It has been noted that the literature contains all too few long-term evaluations of the natural course of institutionalized schizophrenics. Many of the reports that are available give no indication as to what happens to the patients who have been ill 2, 3, 4, or 5 years. One of the few reports containing such information is that by Rupp and Fletcher, who studied 641 institutionalized schizophrenics for periods of 4 1/2 to 10 years after admission to a state hospital for mental patients.[1] Selecting the data which fit our problem, we find that 206 cases in this series had symptoms of 2 years' duration before hospitalization. In this group only 16 per cent improved. Of the patients who had been hospitalized between 2 and 5 years, only 14 per cent improved, and of those hospitalized over 5 years, only 4 per cent improved. Again breaking down some of their data, we find that after 2 years of hospitalization only 4.5 per cent were returned to the community, and after 5 years of hospitalization only 1.7 per cent were returned to the community. On this basis it would seem that of the 20 schizophrenics in our group not more than 1 would be out of the hospital and only 4 would have shown slight improvement in the usual course of events.

A comparable group of patients, likewise subjected to the total push of an investigative program but given no specific treatment, is the one used as a control in the first Columbia-Greystone project.[2] Several of the present contributors helped to select the cases for that project, and all feel that the Columbia-Greystone patients had a better prognosis than those in the Tulane group. Yet according to the latest report only 4 out of the 24 Columbia-Greystone controls left the hospital.

If one examines the protocols of our patients, some prediction as to the possibility of discharge from the hospital can be made. It is our impression that very ill psychotic patients remain unhospitalized here in Louisiana more often than in the eastern states, probably because of the poor facilities for handling mental patients and hence the relatives' reluctance to institutionalize them. Six of our twenty patients might have been taken out of the hospital and tolerated by their families.* Patient 6, although obviously psychotic, was called into the hospital especially for the stimulation procedure. Patient 12, again obviously psychotic, was referred to the hospital for diagnosis because of organic symptoms. Patient 15, although making a marginal adjustment on the outside, was also called into the hospital for specific therapy at the request of the family. Patient 17 had been awaiting hospital admission for a number of months prior to her final admission; although tolerating her presence, her relatives were seriously considering commitment elsewhere if we did not have a bed available. Patient 18, idle and seclusive at home, was recalled into the hospital for this special procedure, which her family had requested some months previously. Patient 19 had been admitted to the surgical service because of hypertension. He did not come to the hospital because of a psychosis, nor did his relatives insist that he be hospitalized, although they had recognized for some time that he was psychotic. However, five of these six patients had been committed to mental institutions by their families some time in the recent past but, conceivably, might have returned temporarily to the community in the not too distant future even if their symptoms remained unchanged.

RESULTS

In actuality, of the 19 patients left in the group after 1 death, 10 are now out of the hospital—although to report the total at this point anticipates the data presented in later chapters. The patient who died was included in the group of 6 mentioned above who might have been able to leave the hospital in the natural course of events. Three of the remaining 5 in this group are now out of the hospital as opposed to 7 of the remaining 14 in the group for whom hospitalization was absolutely necessary. These figures do not indicate that the group of patients who

*At least temporarily without any real change in their psychotic symptoms.

had been tolerated outside the hospital contributed much more than their share of the subsequent therapeutic improvements.

CONCLUSIONS

It was pointed out above that many psychotic patients leave hospitals in the State of Louisiana who would not be tolerated at home if they lived in one of the larger eastern states, nor would they be considered for parole by hospital officials. Despite this, it is felt that the most optimistic appraisal that one could have made in regard to the 20 chronic schizophrenics selected for study was that no more than 3 or 4 patients would have left the hospital or would have shown significant improvement without specific therapy. All but 2 of the patients had undergone the usual somatic treatment without benefit, and it appeared unlikely that any in the group would have responded to conventional psychosurgery. Reference will be made to these conclusions when the therapeutic results are evaluated.

REFERENCES

1. Rupp, C., and E. K. Fletcher. Five to ten year follow-up study of 641 schizophrenic cases, *Am. J. Psychiat.*, 96:877–888 (1940).
2. The Columbia-Greystone Associates (second group). *Psychosurgical Problems,* edited by F. A. Mettler. Blakiston, New York, 1952.

Surgical Technique

INTRODUCTION

ROBERT G. HEATH

Several changes in surgical technique occurred during the period of this project, and there were also changes in surgical personnel. For these reasons, the report was subdivided and presented by a variety of authors.

The first two patients were stimulated under local anesthesia on the operating table, thereby making satisfactory electrical recording impossible. We therefore decided to implant electrodes through an opening into the anterior horn of the lateral ventricle on one side. At first only one bipolar electrode was implanted; then the number was increased to three. But as the work progressed, several difficulties were encountered with this technique.

1. The incision into the ventricle caused some brain damage.
2. Accurate placement of the electrodes by the visual method was often impossible.
3. The electrodes were often accidentally removed from the positions in which they were implanted during the operative closure.
4. Electrodes implanted by the original method necessitated a rather large open tract into the ventricles and thus provided a pathway for infection. For this reason, the electrodes could not be left in place for a prolonged period.

The next major change in technique was a shift to the stereotaxic, or closed, method. This made for improved placement with more accuracy and considerably less brain damage. Moreover, the electrodes could be left in place over a longer period of time. But with the adoption of the stereotaxic technique many new technical problems were encountered. These included the selection of a wire, first of all, with the proper tensile strength (i.e., one that was flexible enough to absorb the pulsations of the brain without creating damage); second, with insulation that would not break; and third, with insulation that would not irritate tissue. A fourth major problem was the difficulty encountered in anchoring the implanted electrodes to the bone, so that they could not move. The paper on the closed technique which was delivered during the meetings is included as Chapter 10 of this section. Since its presentation, considerable progress has been made in solving technical difficulties encountered with use of the stereotaxic technique. Our recent developments include: a method of implantation giving much greater accuracy in placement, a more satisfactory technique for anchoring wires at the bone, and more satisfactory types of wire and electrode. As these are important developments and give promise of eliminating the technical variable that plagued us throughout the initial series, a description of the new technique will be included in Addendum C.

CHAPTER 9

IMPLANTATION OF SUBCORTICAL ELECTRODES IN MAN BY THE OPEN METHOD

FRANCISCO GARCIA BENGOCHEA
ERNEST SACHS, JR.
RAEBURN C. LLEWELLYN

In a series of nineteen schizophrenic patients (one of whom had two operations),* electrodes were inserted at craniotomy by a transcortical, transventricular operation into various subcortical structures. Of these twenty open-method operations Dr. Garcia performed the first ten, and Dr. Sachs the last ten. In our first case, a concentric bipolar electrode was inserted into the right anterior thalamus and stimulation was carried out on the operating table while the wound was still open. No changes were observed during or following stimulation. Later, on the basis of experimental physiological information, it was felt that the region of the septal nuclei (located at the base of the anterior portion of the septum pellucidum near the junction with the floor of the ventricle) was a critical point to attack.

The aim of the procedure, then, was to insert a small sterilized bipolar wire electrode into the region of the septal nuclei just anterior and inferior to the foramen of Monro. In our second case, a concentric bipolar electrode was placed 12 mm. anterior to the foramen of Monro in the most ventral portion of the septum and stimulation was carried out on the operating table with the patient under local anesthesia. In the rest of the cases, the electrodes were left in place from thirteen to fifty-four hours. After the patients reacted from anesthesia, electrical stimulation was then given with every effort made to prevent any damage or destruction of tissue, as described elsewhere in this monograph. Great care was taken electrically and electronically to prevent any polarization at either pole of the electrode, in order to prevent undue heating of the tissue,

*The twentieth patient in the original schizophrenic series (see Chapter 8, Table 1) was operated upon by the closed method. The latter method was also used in the case of the demonstration patient (see Addendum A).

electrocoagulation, or other damage. This idea was energetically pursued throughout the series in an effort not only to reduce complications, but also to prevent the undesirable consequences of destructive psychosurgical procedures. In other words, stimulation of the subcortical structures was performed in an effort to bring about activation of the "normal" influence of these mechanisms, as nearly as is possible by external stimuli.[1]

It is believed that this is the first time such stimulation has been performed in man.* Electrical stimulation of the brain, of course, dates back to the experiments of Fritsch and Hitzig, and studies of the effect of cortical stimulations have been made by many investigators. The interpretation of such results has been thoroughly discussed by Fulton and Walshe. The various steps in our procedure are documented below.

METHODS

An extensive series of tests and laboratory studies was carried out on all patients; these are described in the chapters devoted to physiological, chemical, psychological, and clinical data. Each patient also had preoperative and postoperative neurological examinations by at least two different observers, one of whom was always the neurosurgeon.

THE FIRST TEN CASES (DR. GARCIA'S)

Preoperative Routine. Almost all patients had a cleansing enema the night before operation and preoperative barbiturate sedation the night before operation as well as the morning of surgery. Usually 1 1/2 grains of phenobarbital and 1/150 grain of atropine were given an hour before anesthesia, though seconal or morphine and scopolamine were used in some cases. All patients except Patient 2 received general anesthesia. The operation on this patient was performed under local anesthesia, but, because of a series of convulsions on the operating table when stimulation was applied, the procedure was discontinued. As a rule, a combination of nitrous oxide, oxygen, and pentothal was used for general anesthesia; in addition, the scalp was injected with a 1 per cent novocaine

*In 1948 J. L. Pool (personal communication of unpublished work) placed electrodes in the brains of two patients with leads in the caudate nucleus and cingulate gyrus, respectively. A primary inductance coil was held outside the skin over a secondary coil implanted in the skull, with the idea that this would produce stimulation. See also p. 142 for reference to work reported by Delgado in 1952.

solution. However, some of the earlier operations were done under ether. After the patient had been put to sleep, the throat was sprayed with cocaine and an endotracheal tube was inserted (except in the case of Patient 1). Because it was desired that the patient wake up as soon as possible after implantation of the electrodes, every effort was made to reduce the amount of pentothal anesthesia to the minimum requirement; the amount of pentothal varied from slightly less than 0.5 gram to 1.8 grams. The actual surgery lasted from two and a half to four hours; the length of anesthesia varied from 3 1/2 to 5 1/2 hours.

Operative Details. In each case the patient was operated upon in the dorsal recumbent position, with head considerably flexed on a head-rest. The entire head was shaved and surgically prepared with soap, sterile water, ether and alcohol, or ether and phisoderm, and was then draped for a frontal craniotomy. The right, nondominant side was operated upon in the first ten patients; a coronal or a small elliptical incision was made behind the hair line, with the base toward the forehead. The medial limb of the ellipse was at the midline and the lateral limb in the temporal area. In all cases either a 1 1/2-inch or 2-inch Becker-Poppen trephine was used to open the skull. The posterior rim of the trephine was placed just at or anterior to the coronal suture, and the medial rim of the trephine just lateral to the midline. The usual form of dural flap was made with the base toward the midline, and a transcortical incision was then made down into the anterior portion of the right lateral ventricle.

The foramen of Monro was identified by the choroid plexus running anteriorly into it. The caudate nucleus and the septum pellucidum were well identified. In the case of Patient 1 the right anterior thalamus was stimulated under direct vision. In the rest of the cases one electrode was placed from 5 to 15 mm. anterior to the foramen of Monro in the basal part of the septal region, and in the last five cases two other electrodes were implanted, one in the head of the right caudate nucleus and one in the anterior part of the right thalamus. Keeping these electrodes in the proper position during the closure of the dura, replacement of the bone button, and closing of the scalp proved to be quite a task.

In nearly all cases the electrodes used were made of fine silver wire. Some were nylon wrapped and insulated except for a few millimeters

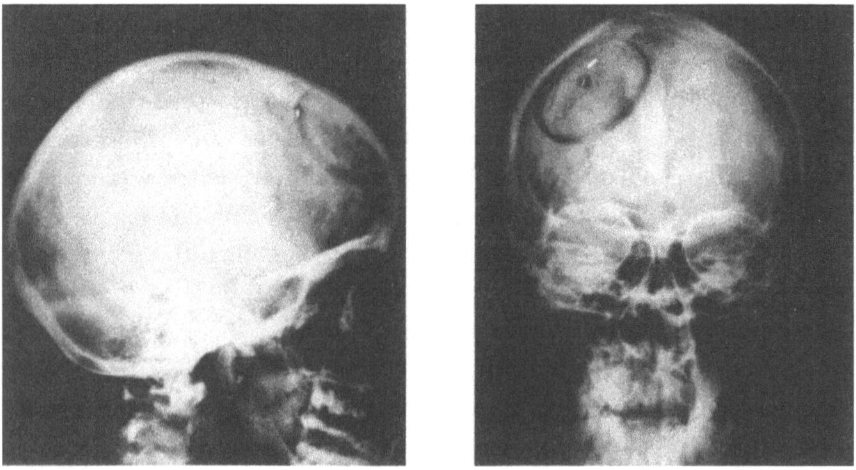

FIGURE IX–1. Postoperative x-ray films (lateral and anterior-posterior views) of Patient 3 showing one electrode in place

at the tips; a small cuff was made on the rest to facilitate their handling with surgical forceps. All electrodes were sterilized by soaking in 1:1,000 zephiran chloride solution. Once the electrodes were inserted in what were felt to be the desired positions, the dural flap was closed as tightly as possible with fine black silk or cotton, though this was somewhat difficult with the electrodes projecting from it. To make removal of the electrodes easy the bone button and the skull were notched before the button was replaced. The electrodes were then brought out through a separate stab wound beyond the area of the scalp incision. The scalp was then carefully closed in layers. A dry sterile dressing was applied to the scalp, and the wire electrodes were brought out through the center of the dressing and separately wrapped in an unsterile gauze pad.

Postoperative Routine. Administration of anesthesia was discontinued as soon as the operative procedure was completed. The patient was then taken to the x-ray room for localization films. He was then moved to the recovery room, where he was allowed to react from the anesthesia. As soon as he was awake and cooperative, he was moved to the special room prepared for the stimulation procedure. When patients were sufficiently recovered to be interviewed, they were released by the surgery and anesthesia departments.

All patients were kept quiet until they had fully reacted and were turned in bed by attendants until they were able to turn themselves. No sedation was administered postoperatively. Intravenous fluids were given until the patient was able to take adequate nourishment by mouth. Most patients reacted fully within a relatively short time, the periods varying from 2 or 3 hours to 10 or 12 hours. The electrodes were left in place from 13 to 54 hours. Neurosurgically, it was always considered advisable to remove the electrodes as soon as possible because of the danger of infection, which did occur in a few cases. The criteria for determining the time of removal will be discussed elsewhere. Neurosurgically speaking, however, the longer electrodes are left in place, the greater the danger.

The electrodes were removed by gentle pulling, after cutting any skin sutures that had been used to anchor them in place. They came out easily, like any surgical drain, and no hemorrhages or other undesirable consequences occurred relative to their removal. Considerable worry attended this procedure because of the potential danger of tearing vessels. However, great care had been taken at the time of operation to prepare the tract through which the electrodes went, so that no vessels would remain in their paths. As already mentioned, in the first ten cases electrodes were implanted in the right side only.

Postoperative Complications. Among the first ten cases no deaths resulted from this procedure. Two patients had convulsions in the early postoperative period, but these were readily controlled with phenobarbital and the patients experienced no convulsions thereafter. Wound infection occurred in two cases. One responded to removal of the bone button, and the other to débridement and closure of a draining sinus.

THE SECOND TEN CASES (DR. SACHS')

Preoperative and Postoperative Routines. The same routines were followed in the second ten cases as in the first ten cases (see above).

Operative Details. The operative procedure in the second ten cases was the same as in the first ten, except for the following operative details, which should be mentioned:

1. A 5-inch linear scalp incision was used instead of a curved incision. This incision was in line with the pupil of the eye, parallel to the

midline, extending just anterior to the hairline and posteriorly to the coronal suture.

2. A Patton self-retaining nasal speculum was used to hold open the transcortical incision into the ventricle.
3. The operator wore a headlight to improve illumination.
4. In Patients 12 and 13 (Figure 2) very fine copper wire electrodes were used in order to reduce the size of the wire to be handled at surgery. These electrodes were so fine, however, that they advanced readily into the brain past the structures for which they were intended.
5. To aid in the postoperative localization of the electrodes pneumoencephalography was performed immediately following surgery in nine cases.
6. Unfortunately, the ventricles did not always fill, and so in one case (Patient 20) a silver clip was placed on the border of the foramen of Monro to mark the position of this structure (Figure 3).
7. In the case of Patient 12 electrodes were implanted through the left ventricle.

Postoperative Complications. In the second ten cases two deaths resulted from this procedure. Both deaths were related to brain abscesses, one occurring five weeks and the other six months following operation. One patient developed a nonfatal infection postoperatively. Two patients had convulsions, one during stimulation and one in the immediate postoperative period, which were controlled with medication. Patient 11 developed a transient hemiparesis, which cleared in about seven days, and Patient 16 developed a transient left central facial weakness.

A NONPSYCHOTIC CASE (DR. LLEWELLYN'S)

Postoperative Complications. The open method was also used in operating upon Patient 23, a nonpsychotic with metastatic carcinoma. This patient expired forty-eight hours later; the nature of the complications is further described in Chapter 18.

REFERENCE

1. Walshe, F. M. R. *Brain,* 74:249 (1951).

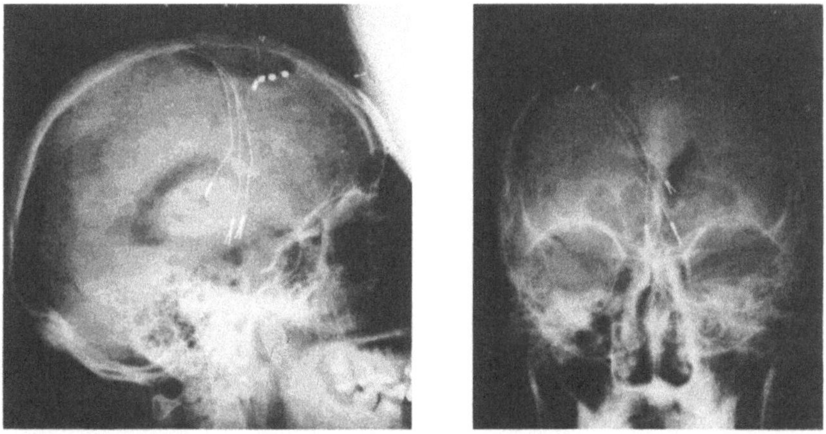

FIGURE IX-2. Postoperative x-ray films (lateral and anterior-posterior views) of Patient 13 showing three electrodes in place and air in the ventricles

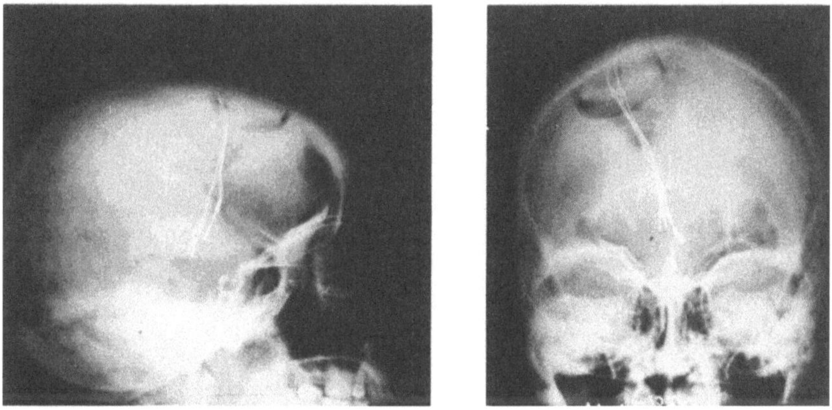

FIGURE IX-3. Postoperative x-ray films (lateral and anterior-posterior views) of Patient 20 showing two electrodes in place and a silver clip (barely visible) in the anterior rim of the foramen of Monro

CHAPTER 10

IMPLANTATION OF SUBCORTICAL ELECTRODES IN MAN BY A STEREOTAXIC METHOD

ROBERT HODES
ROBERT G. HEATH
WARREN L. FOUNDS
RAEBURN C. LLEWELLYN

In 1906 Clarke described with Horsley[1] an apparatus for inserting electrodes into the hidden substance of the neuraxis of animals without major surgical insult to the cerebral cortex or subjacent structures. It is clear that Clarke's purpose in developing this technique was to perfect its use in animals and then to apply the method to human patients requiring various kinds of neurosurgical intervention. This hope was not realized by Clarke, and although his original work has been advanced by many investigators it remained for Spiegel and others[2] to describe the first use of the stereotaxic technique on a psychotic patient in 1947. Since that time several reports have detailed the use of various types of human stereotaxic instruments. These reports include papers by Wycis and Spiegel,[3] Hayne and Meyers,[4] Talairach and others,[5] and Bailey and Stein.[6] At the meetings of the American Electroencephalographic Society held in June 1949 Jasper and Hunter[7] demonstrated their model of the human stereotaxic instrument. At the May 1952 meetings of the American Neurological Association Rémond[8] exhibited a new instrument, which appeared somewhat simpler and less expensive than many of the previous models.

Because of the well-known individual variability of the human brain and the inconstant relation of brain structures to external bony landmarks, it has been apparent for a long time that precautions beyond those necessary for accurate electrode placements in cat and monkey would be required when dealing with human patients. The deterrents to accuracy, imposed by brain variability, have been partially overcome by referring to brain atlases, composed of sections of the human brain cut in the planes of the particular type of stereotaxic instrument whose use is contemplated. Thus, Talairach and others[9] published a preliminary line-drawing atlas of the basal ganglia and diencephalon in 1950, and one can anticipate that the French workers will complete and reproduce the human sections in due course. Bailey and his collaborators[6] are also engaged in the preparation of a human brain atlas. Spiegel and Wycis' monograph, *Stereoencephalotomy*,[10] in addition to describing the authors' latest improvements in instrumentation, also presents an atlas with actual photographs of human brain sections cut in appropriate planes.

Another attempt to increase the accuracy of localization in the human patient has been the reliance on the reasonably constant anatomical relationship of certain intracranial structures (e.g., the pineal body[10]) to other neural elements. In addition, air encephalograms and ventriculograms have been considered[6] and used[9, 10] as adjuvants to an adequate placement of subcortical electrodes by stereotaxy.

The modifications of earlier techniques to be presented in this chapter were designed chiefly to make use of the aids to localization afforded by air ventriculography, and to devise means by which subcortical electrodes could be implanted and allowed to remain for prolonged periods of time within the brain. The latter technique, if successful, would present the possibility of recording and stimulating for extended intervals and would seem to be of considerable value in many types of neurological, neurosurgical, and psychiatric investigations.

The methods finally evolved permitted air studies and electrode placements to be accomplished at one operation, rather than in two stages as required by previous procedures.[5, 10] The implantation of in-dwelling electrodes in subcortical structures by stereotaxic means was also achieved. Delgado and his collaborators have also recently succeeded in placing, under direct vision, electrodes which have remained in human patients for a considerable period. The details of the methods worked out in animals were published[11] and applications to human problems were presented to the Electroshock Research Association in 1952.[12]*

APPARATUS

The stereotaxic apparatus used by us has been described by Bailey and Stein.[6] The instrument is manufactured by Lab-Tronics, Inc., of Chicago. Figure 1 shows the general arrangement of the instrument and the way in which the skull is centered and fixed by means of the ear bars,

*See also reference 13 at the end of this chapter.

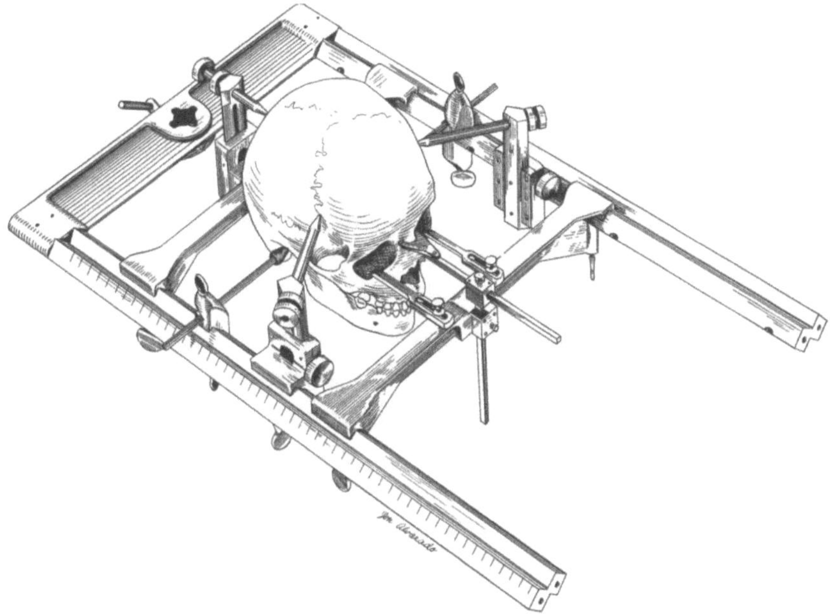

FIGURE X–1. Method of orienting the skull in horizontal plane by means of the Horsley-Clarke stereotaxic apparatus

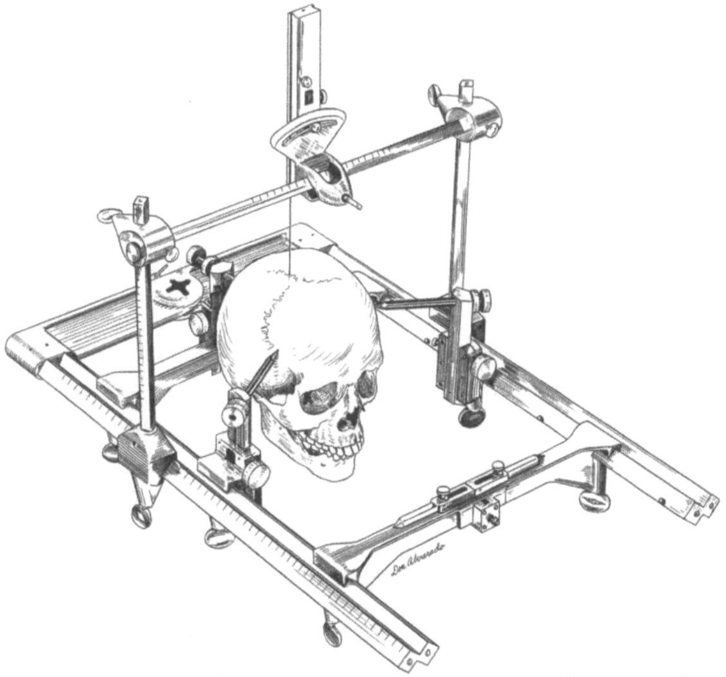

FIGURE X–2. Horsley-Clarke stereotaxic apparatus with ear bars, eye pieces, and nose piece removed and electrode-carrier in place on the superstructure

eye pieces, nose piece, and lateral and occipital fixation screws. Figure 2 shows the superstructure, consisting of the vertical sliding uprights, the horizontal bar, which is capable of rotation in a plane parallel to that of the vertical uprights, and the electrode carrier and protractor for measurement of the angle of rotation in the plane parallel to that of the horizontal bar. As indicated in Figure 2, after the fixation screws are inserted into the skull, the ear bars, eye pieces, and nose piece are removed to reduce postoperative discomfort to the patient.

We have modified the basic instrument to fit the needs of ventriculography, which is performed at the time of operation. The presence of air in the ventricles is an important aid in determining the coordinates and in verifying the placement of the electrodes, most of which are intended for structures in propinquity to the anterior horn of the lateral ventricle and the foramen of Monro. The final design of the instrument (Figure 3) allows for much freedom of movement of the superstructures and the fixation screws on the horizontal lateral bars and affords an x-ray film measuring 5 x 7 inches. This small film does not visualize the entire ventricular system or skull, but it does include the foramen of Monro and the subcortical structures of importance to this study. The cassette holder for the lateral x-ray film can be seen attached to the lateral horizontal bar, while the cassette holder for the antero-posterior film is attached to the second superstructure for support. The modifications required for ventriculography made it necessary to dispense with the occipital fixation screw and to use in its place two postero-lateral screws to fix the head posteriorly. The bakelite cover of the cassette was engraved with vertical and horizontal rulings, 1 cm. apart, made radio-opaque with lead paint. On the processed x-ray film the skull, ventricles, and centimeter grid were visible. The latter proved useful, for it obviated the necessity for measuring directly on the film the values required for setting the instrumental coordinates preparatory to electrode placement.*

*We wish to express our gratitude to Moore Saucier, Edward LaBarre, and Edward Dering, of the New Orleans Charity Hospital x-ray staff, and George A. Welman, of the New Orleans office of the Picker X-ray Corp., for much valuable assistance with some of the details and modifications required for securing adequate x-ray records.

ELECTRODES

Each electrode consisted of a 1-to-2 mm. sphere of silver solder into the center of which was inserted a thin wire 30 cm. long. The wire was made of 36-gauge stainless steel having extremely high tensile strength. Except for the end, which was inserted into the sphere of semifluid solder, the wire was insulated with teflon.* The insulation was routinely tested by immersing the electrodes in salt solution and checking the resistance between the wire and the solution. The electrode wire was threaded through a 15 cm.-length of 19-gauge thin-walled stainless steel hypodermic tubing. The spherical end of the electrode, being larger than the internal diameter of the guide tube, formed the penetrating tip when the tube and electrode assembly were advanced together by the ratchet and pinion of the electrode carrier into the chosen area of the brain. The guide tube, which was securely fixed in the electrode carrier, was removed from the brain when the direction of travel of the carrier was reversed. The ball and proximal part of the electrode wire, however, remained buried within the depths of the brain.

Five patients of this series underwent operation by the technique described. They were Patients 21, 22, 24, 25, and 26.

OPERATIVE PROCEDURE

Surgery was performed with the patient under intratracheal nitrous oxide anesthesia supplemented by intravenous sodium pentothal. The patient remained seated on an adjustable operating table throughout the procedure. The entire scalp was shaved and prepared in a sterile fashion and routine occipital trephine openings were made to allow ventriculography. The autoclaved instrument was secured to the operating table by means of two large C-clamps, and while an assistant supported the patient's head the apparatus was carefully adjusted (see Figure 1). The ear bars, eye pieces, and nose piece were then brought into position by one assistant while a second gently rotated the head to facilitate their placement. When the head was accurately centered by these guides,

*This inert material, similar to nylon, can be autoclaved without damage. The steel wire was especially prepared for us with four coatings of teflon by the Warren Wire Co., of Pownal, Vermont.

the four fixation screws were advanced far enough to make indentations upon the sterile scalp. (The non-sterile assistants had meanwhile carefully avoided contact with the tips of the fixation screws.) Individual stab incisions of the scalp were made at these points, and the outer table of the skull was perforated with a small drill to afford absolute fixation of the skull by means of the four screws. After the fixation screws were in position and the patient's head was considered immobile the ear bars, eye pieces, and nose piece were removed.

Air was introduced into the ventricles through the previously fashioned occipital trephine openings, and the anterior-posterior and lateral cassette holders were clamped into position. A marker electrode was placed on the surface of the scalp in the midline by means of the electrode carrier attached to the superstructure (see Figure 3). The readings on the vertical uprights along the horizontal bars as well as those on the scale of the electrode carrier were noted for further calculations. Anterior-posterior and lateral films were then taken from a distance of 6 to 7 feet in an attempt to approximate parallel rays. After the films were developed (about 10 minutes after exposure), the proper settings of the instrument for the insertion of the electrodes into the various subcortical structures were quickly calculated from the previously mentioned 1-cm. grid lines and the visible ventricular system.

Although we intended to implant most of our electrodes within a few millimeters of the midline and none more lateral than 1.5 cm., it was not possible to insert the electrodes perpendicular to the horizontal (interaural) plane because of the sagittal sinus. Consequently the electrode carrier was brought sideward and set at an angle. The angles were calculated to be such that the electrodes would penetrate the dorsum of the cerebral hemisphere about 3 cm. lateral to the midline and would continue medially and ventrally to the subcortical neural masses near the midline.

As the x-ray films were being developed and the requisite calculations being made, a 6-cm. linear incision was made in the right frontal area of the scalp. This incision was parallel to the sagittal suture approximately 3 cm. lateral to the midline extending posteriorly to the coronal suture. A trephine opening in the skull was enlarged by rongeurs to form a defect approximately 4 cm. in length and 1.5 cm. in width. The under-

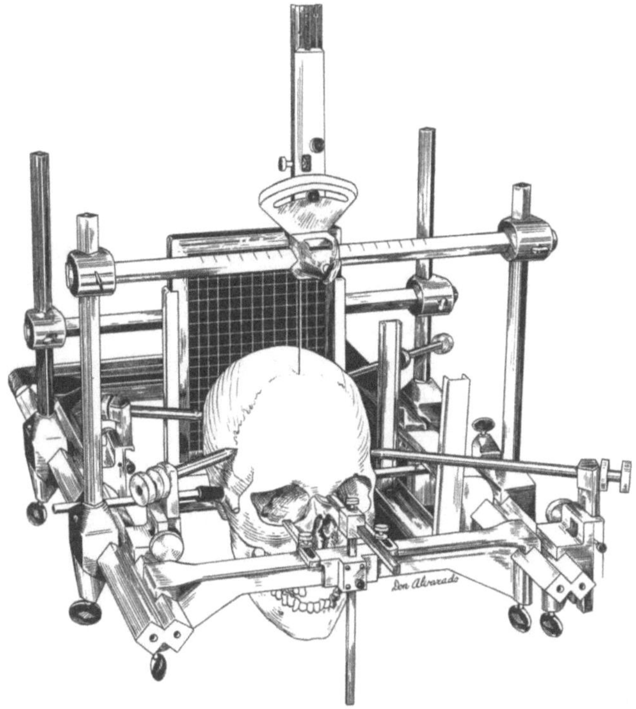

FIGURE X-3. Modified Horsley-Clarke apparatus with cassette holders for x-ray film in place

lying dura was opened and the cortical vessels coagulated. The electrodes were then inserted by means of the electrode carrier according to calculations previously made from the x-ray films.

The thin, flexible electrode wire was cemented to the skull defect at the point of exit from the brain. The cement used was quick setting dental wax (Baker's sticky wax). It was found advisable to cement the electrodes to the skull as soon as the guide tube was withdrawn, as the slightest tug tended to displace the electrodes dorsally from their intended positions. When all electrodes were placed, x-rays were again taken to verify their position. If an electrode was more than a few millimeters from its calculated position it was removed and re-inserted. We do not feel that such replacement produced serious additional brain damage, since the electrodes were small. Figure 4 shows lateral and anterior-posterior ventriculograms with the electrodes in place.

The ends of the electrodes distal to the point of fixation to the skull were brought out of the scalp through individual needle tracts 3 cm. lateral to the scalp incision. This was accomplished by passing a 17-gauge needle through the scalp down to the open bone defect, threading the electrode out through the needle, and then withdrawing the needle. The scalp wound was then closed with two layers of interrupted quilting cotton sutures. A small sterile dressing was applied to the scalp wound. As mentioned above, the electrodes had individual exits from the scalp which were lateral to the dressing applied to the scalp incision. This allowed firm fixation of the electrodes to the scalp by adhesive tape, which was not disturbed when the operative wound dressing was changed for inspection of the scalp incision or removal of the sutures. A secondary dressing was then applied over the entire scalp and the exposed portions of the electrodes.

The patient was transferred to the recovery division for careful observation during the immediate postoperative period. Intravenous fluids were administered if necessary during this period, but sedation was avoided to minimize the danger of artifacts in the electrical recordings. Side rails and arm restraints were used until the patient had recovered from the anesthesia. While the patient was still under anesthesia, the secondary dressing was removed, so that the ends of the electrodes could be recovered and soldered to a special plug. This allowed for a rapid and repeated hook-up for recording and stimulating. The special plug was mounted on a plastic head piece, which in turn was firmly fixed to the patient's head when the secondary dressing was replaced.*

RESULTS

Subcortical electrode implantations by this method have been made in five patients to date. The number of electrodes placed in each patient varied from four to eight, depending on operative conditions present at the time of surgery. Attempts were made to place two electrodes 2 mm. apart in the rostral area of the basal part of the septal region, caudate nucleus, and septo-hypothalamic area, and also in the thalamus (see Chapter 9). Patient 21 tugged vigorously at his bandage and displaced the electrodes. These were then removed 5 days after the im-

*As in the open method, electrodes were removed by gentle pulling, after cutting any skin sutures that had been used to anchor them in place. They come out easily, like any surgical drain, and no hemorrhages or other undesirable consequences occurred relative to their removal.

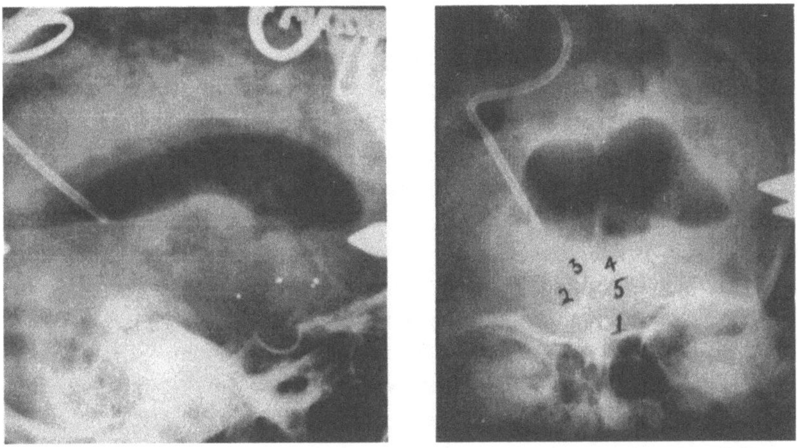

FIGURE X-4. Lateral and anterior-posterior ventrilograms showing electrodes in place in Patient 25

plantation. In two other patients the electrodes became displaced and were removed 48 hours after placement. All three of these patients were operated upon before we had adopted the cementing process for fixing the electrodes to the edge of the bone defect. In the fourth patient the electrodes remained in place 18 days without evidence of infection or other complications due to implantation.

No patient showed complications that could be attributed to the surgical procedure. Patient 21 died at another hospital 6 weeks following operation; this patient had far advanced pulmonary tuberculosis, but trauma incident to his attempting to remove his own electrodes might have contributed to his death. An autopsy was not obtained. Patient 25 died 18 days following surgery; the electrodes were still in place. An autopsy revealed gangrene of the bowel with intestinal obstruction and widespread metastases, including many to the brain in the region of the hypothalamus and pituitary (primary site breast). There were no intracranial complications secondary to implantation. In the other patients of this series there was no clinical evidence of surgical complications either during the time the electrodes remained in place or following their removal.

REFERENCES

1. Clarke, R. H., and V. Horsley. On a method of investigating the deep ganglia and tracts of the central nervous system (cerebellum), *Brit. M. J.*, 2:1799–1800 (1906).

2. Spiegel, E. A., H. T. Wycis, M. Marks, and A. J. Lee. Stereotaxic apparatus for operations on the human brain, *Science*, 106:349–350 (1947).
3. Wycis, H. T., and E. A. Spiegel. Symposium: psychosurgery; thalamotomy and mesencephalothalamotomy; neurosurgical aspects (including treatment of pain), *New York State J. Med.*, 49:2275–2277 (1949).
4. Hayne, R. A., and R. Meyers. An improved model of a human stereotaxic instrument, *J. Neurosurg.*, 7:463–466 (1950).
5. Talairach, J., H. Hecaen, M. David, M. Monnier, and J. de Ajuriaguerra. Recherches sur la coagulation thérapeutique des structures souscorticales chez l'homme, *Rev. neurol.*, 81:4–24 (1949).
6. Bailey, P., and S. N. Stein. A stereotaxic instrument for use on the human brain, *in Studies in Medicine: A Volume of Papers in Honor of Robert Wood Keeton*, pp. 40–49, Thomas, Springfield, 1951.
7. Jasper, H., and J. Hunter. A stereotaxic instrument for man, *Electroencephalog. & Clin. Neurophysiol.*, 1:263 (1949). Exhibited at the meetings of the American Electroencephalographic Society, June 11–12, 1949, Atlantic City.
8. Rémond, A. A stereotaxic instrument for man. Demonstrated at the meetings of American Neurological Association, May 8–10, 1952, Atlantic City.
9. Talairach, J., J. de Ajuriaguerra, and H. Hecaen. Étude topographique des images ventriculaires en fonction des noyaux gris centraux, *Ann. méd.*, 51:83–100 (1950).
10. Spiegel, E. A., and H. T. Wycis. Stereoencephalotomy (Thalamotomy and Related Procedures), Part I. Methods and Stereotaxic Atlas of the Human Brain, *in Monographs on Biology and Medicine*, vol. 1. Grune, New York, 1952.
11. Delgado, J. M. R. Permanent implantations of multilead electrodes in the brain. *Yale J. Biol. Med.*, 25:351–358 (1952).
12. Delgado, J. M. R., H. Hannibal, and W. P. Chapman. Technique of intracranial electrode implantation for recording and stimulation and its possible therapeutic value in psychotic patients. Read at the meeting of the Electroshock Research Association, May 10, 1952, Atlantic City.
13. Delgado, J. M. R. Some functions of the brain studied in waking animals with possible diagnostic and therapeutic applications to human patients. Demonstration presented at the meetings of the Federated Societies for Experimental Biology, April 6–10, 1953.

Physiological Data—Electrical Recordings

INTRODUCTION

ROBERT G. HEATH

The rationale for the specific procedure undertaken in our series of schizophrenic patients—namely, electrical stimulation of the septal region of the forebrain—was based on the assumption that a functional abnormality was present. Definite physiological data were not obtained on Patients 1 and 2, as the electrodes were not left in place long enough for recordings to be attempted. Recordings were taken from Patient 3, however, and from then on several variations in technique were made in order to secure better records of subcortical activity and also to determine whether abnormalities in the neural circuit were influencing the cortex. It was reasoned, on the basis of our accumulated data, that there might be a detectable physiological abnormality in this key region, reflecting the over-all alteration of dynamic brain activity that was associated with the clinically observed behavior disorder. The nature of the electrical abnormalities found consistently in patients in whom electrodes were satisfactorily placed will be discussed in detail and illustrated in Chapter 11.

As background information for this presentation, I shall briefly review reports in the literature concerning abnormalities detected in psychotic patients through electrical recordings. The most comprehensive review is that of Pond, Rey, and Hill.[1] Following a survey of 900 psychiatric patients, these workers reported abnormalities which they classify into three types on the basis of location. The first category includes diffuse bilateral fast waves (14 c/second plus) associated with slow waves (7 c/second and less) or slow wave activity only. The second category includes abnormal potentials lateralized and localized in the temporal region. The third category includes abnormal potentials localized by bipolar technique in the posterior and usually inferior areas of the temporal cortex. The first type of abnormality was widespread among psychotic patients, but the second and third were always correlated with shy, immature, inadequate, schizoid personalities. The investigators point out that abnormal slow wave activity was usually seen on the left and that there was apt to be a relation between sex and age, which is in accordance, they say with the later maturation of males. The abnormality encountered most frequently among the patients they surveyed was the temporal lobe spike—a finding that is in keeping with most of the other consistent reports in the literature. Pond and his group place great importance on the late ontogenetic development of the temporal lobe, to which they attribute the localization of spikes and other abnormalities.

Many workers in the field of electroencephalography tend to classify patients as psychomotor epileptics solely on the basis of spiking abnormality, even though their behavior disorders may be clinically that of schizophrenia. At the 1952 meetings of the American Neurological Association[2] some observers reported that the symptoms of patients whose EEG's show temporal lobe abnormalities are very similar to those seen in the endogenous psychoses; hence they inferred that those functions which are disturbed ictally during temporal lobe seizures may also be disturbed in a continuing, but not always recordable, fashion in the nonorganic psychoses.

One of the things we were continuously looking for in the subcortical records was a correlation between electrical patterns and emotional disturbances brought about by activation of painful memories. (There has never been a markedly consistent reflection of emotional disturbances on scalp recordings.) In a few cases we were able to make definite correlations between changes in the tracings from the subcortical leads and the patients' reports of emotionally charged thoughts. When this happened the change was usually detected through the septal, or facilitatory, circuit. Making such a correlation is extremely difficult, as it is impossible to know at all times the patient's thoughts and feelings. We succeeded best when we first noted a marked disturbance in the record and then questioned the patient on what he had been thinking and feeling.

On other occasions we attempted to disturb the patients by talking to them about emotionally charged topics. It was believed that changes reflecting emotional reactions frequently appeared in the records, but to be certain of this would require a much more extensive study. Definite material on this subject will be included in Chapter 11. Additional clear-cut data, gathered since the June 1952 meetings, are presented in Addendum E.

The question of the origin of clinical seizures has been discussed at some length in the literature on epilepsy. It was formerly held that idiopathic seizures begin largely at the cortical level. Recently, however, many persons have advocated the concept of a subcortical origin. In the course of taking deep recordings on patients, we were able to observe several seizures with both subcortical and scalp electrodes in place; inevitably, when clinical seizures occurred, abnormal electrical activity was noted first in the subcortical structures. In many instances the highly abnormal electrical activity noted in the subcortical recordings did not spread to the cortex. For further data see Addendum E.

It was apparent that, if many of our theoretical concepts were valid, there had to be some correlation between activity in the subcortical areas and various stages of awareness. Of particular interest, therefore, were the recordings obtained while a patient was in spontaneous sleep or when he passed from wakefulness into drowsiness and sleep and returned from sleep to a wakeful state. The patterns showed the manner of spread between the impulses in the subcortical electrodes and those placed on the scalp.

In the present series of patients we had only one who was clinically diagnosed as a depressive. He indeed showed many slow waves, as earlier reported (p. 49). In this connection it is interesting to note that there have been some reports in EEG literature of slow wave activity from scalp recordings obtained from depressed patients.

I have reviewed above some of the highlights from material to be presented in an attempt to correlate it with the over-all theoretical framework of the research and other aspects of the studies presented thus far. Chapters 11 and 14 will present in further detail some of the very extensive data that have been collected from recordings on our patients before and after stimulation. But even there we can only summarize the material in view of the fact that we literally have miles of recordings on each patient.

Important additional information has been gathered from human recordings since the meetings held in New Orleans in June, 1952, as the result of an improved technique of electrode implantation (see Addendum C). In Patient 26, whose case was demonstrated during the meetings, it was possible to leave electrodes in place for 21 days, so that recordings could be made at long intervals following stimulation. After stimulation the septal spikes flattened out but were replaced by slow wave activity. This suggested the possibility of damage from the stimulation procedure and led to further study of stimulation techniques (see Addendum D). As a result of these studies, the stimulation technique was altered, and it is our impression from long-term recordings following stimulation of subsequent patients that damage from stimulation has been eliminated or markedly reduced. With the new technique it is possible to follow stimulation effects without interference from the variable due to damage.

With the newer techniques of electrode implantation it has been possible to leave electrodes in place for prolonged periods (up to 11 months). Regular recordings from some patients have indicated a correlation between clinically observable psychotic behavior and subcortical spikes, with reduction of the spiking during periods of remission. Records to illustrate this finding are presented in Addendum E.

Variations in the types of electrode used and the techniques of implantation may present some difficulty in understanding recording and stimulating procedures.

In operations in which the open technique of implantation was used the electrodes were inserted in joined pairs (see Chapter 11, Figure 2). Since the two lead wires from such a pair were twisted together and brought through the skin as one, they were labeled as one lead. When attached to the electroencephalograph or stimulator, however, the distal ends of the intertwined wires were separated so that each pole became one EEG lead and similarly each pole of the pair could serve as one pole during stimulation. It must therefore be understood that the use of the term "lead" in conjunction with the description of *electrode place-*

ments means a joined pair, whereas use of the same term in conjunction with *recording or stimulation refers to only one pole of a joined pair.*

Virtually all recordings from the deep structures were bipolar (Chapter 11, Figure 1), that is, either between the two poles inserted as a joined pair or between one pole of a joined pair and one pole of another joined pair, or between one pole of a deep pair and a cortical or scalp electrode. Occasionally recordings were made from one deep pole of a joined pair and an indifferent, or noncephalic, electrode.

Stimulation in the series of patients described in this report was always bipolar; most commonly between two poles of a joined pair, but occasionally between a pole of one joined pair and a pole of another joined pair.

Less confusion will be encountered in regard to implantations by the stereotaxic, or closed, technique, where electrodes were implanted singly. Here each lead was brought through the skin individually and thus there was one EEG lead for each lead described in placement. Attempts were made to implant these single electrodes in pairs, since again all stimulations were bipolar and could be made between any combination of the leads. Similarly, recordings between any combination of leads were bipolar except when it is specified that the recording was from one specific lead to an indifferent, or noncephalic, electrode.

REFERENCES

1. Pond, D. A., J. H. Rey, and D. Hill. Biological correlates of constitutional EEG abnormalities of the temporal lobes, *Soc. Proc., 2nd Int. EEG Cong.*, 1:512 (1949), and *Electroencephalog. & Clin. Neurophysiol.*, 2:111 (1950).
2. Ostow, M. Psychodynamic disturbances in patients with disease of the temporal lobe, *Tr. Am. Neurol. A.*, 79–81, May 8, 1952.

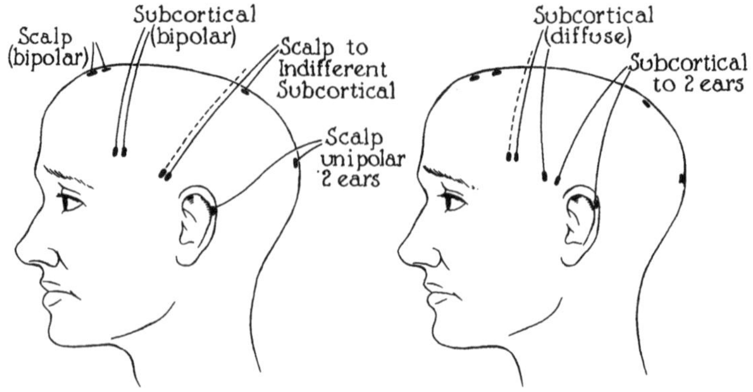

FIGURE XI-1. Diagram showing electrode connections

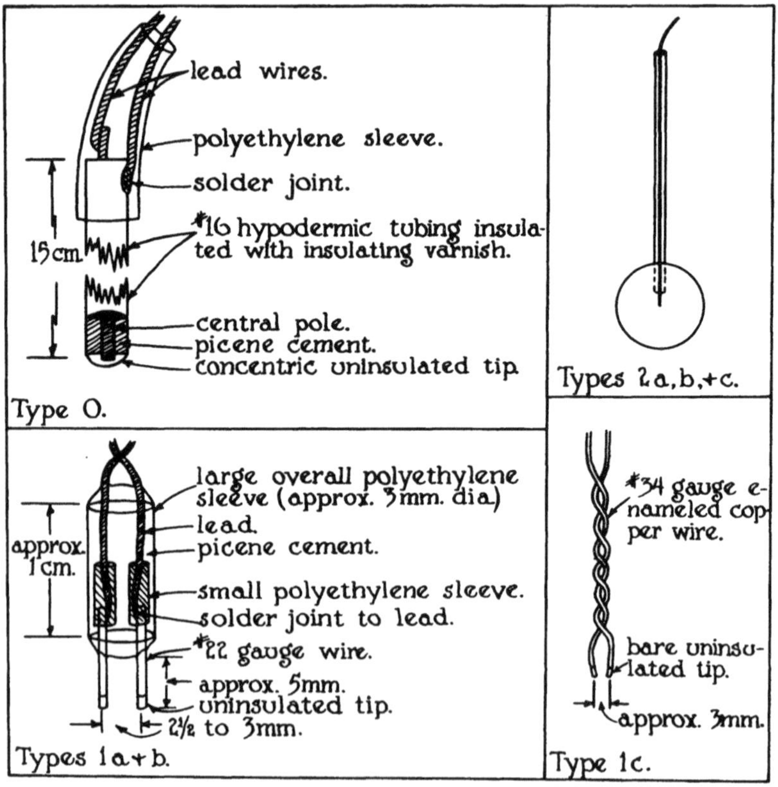

FIGURE XI-2. Details of electrode construction

CHAPTER 11

ELECTROENCEPHALOGRAMS AND SUBCORTICOGRAMS MADE BEFORE STIMULATION

ROBERT HODES
ROBERT G. HEATH
WILLIAM H. MILLER, JR.

ELECTROENCEPHALOGRAMS (SCALP RECORDINGS)

Prior to operation, from one to six scalp recordings were made in the routine electroencephalographic laboratory at Charity Hospital on all patients who were sufficiently cooperative.

The electrodes were small solder disks disposed in the usual fashion (see Figures 1 and 2). The scalp recordings were usually unipolar, but bipolar recordings were also made. The patient was studied in an air-conditioned, electrically shielded room, and the tracings were made on an eight-channel Grass electroencephalograph instrument, Model 3 C. Ordinarily from 1.5 to 3 grains of seconal sodium were given at the start of the procedure. The recordings usually lasted for at least 30 minutes. In all instances attempts were made to "activate" the EEG by hyperventilation and by sleep. This was not always successful with several of the psychotic patients. In some instances they either did not comprehend the request to hyperventilate or refused to do so. Some of them also actively resisted sleep.

Of the nineteen psychotic patients examined, thirteen had normal EEG's before operation. Of the six patients who presented at least one abnormal EEG prior to operation, three had been subjected to courses of electroshock, electronarcosis, or insulin therapy shortly before the records were taken. In two of these patients normal records had been obtained previously when the interval between the somatic therapy and the recording was approximately one year. The third patient of this group had been on the back ward for many years and had received large amounts of electroshock therapy. The grossly abnormal slow wave activity obtained from this patient could readily be ascribed to the effect of prolonged electroshock therapy. The fourth patient of this group showed a mild abnormality, one record being normal, the other two indicating questionable build-up on hyperventilation. The two remaining patients appeared to have abnormal brain waves unaccounted for by previous known therapy (Patient 6 and Patient 17). Patient 6 showed amplitude asymmetry, short bursts of fast negative spiking in the frontal and parietal leads, hypersynchronous 10 c/second waves, spiking in all leads, and occasional flat-topped 4 c/ and 6 c/second waves. Patient 17 on two occasions presented random spikes and hypersynchronous alpha in the occipital leads. Samples of abnormal records from these patients are shown in Figures 3 and 4. A summary of the EEG findings in all patients of this series is given in Table 1, at the end of this chapter.

In many cases the distinction between schizophrenic and psychomotor epilepsy cannot be made on clinical grounds alone.[1] This has been discussed previously (pp. 152–153). Nor is differentiation between these diseases simple on the basis of EEG findings, for although psychomotor epilepsy is often accompanied by temporal lobe spiking, it has also been shown that a relatively larger proportion of abnormal EEG's are presented by schizophrenic patients than by normal individuals. Thus recent studies by Hill and his coworkers[2] emphasize the nonspecific abnormalities of the EEG, as well as the small temporal spikes obtained from such patients. It is consequently of some importance to note that none of the patients in our series presented any electroencephalographic evidence of psychomotor epilepsy. Further, in view of the data to be given below on subcortical electrical activity, it is worthy of comment that most of the patients presented normal activity from the scalp derivations. Even those two patients whose abnormal EEG's could not be ascribed to EST did not show the electroencephalographic features which Pond, Rey, and Hill[2] described in some of the schizophrenic patients of their series.

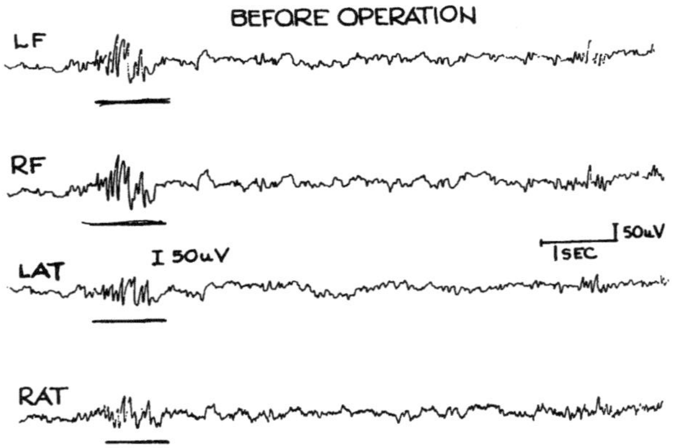

FIGURE XI–3. (right) Preoperative recording from Patient 6, showing abnormal activity

FIGURE XI–4. (below) Preoperative recording from Patient 17, showing abnormal activity

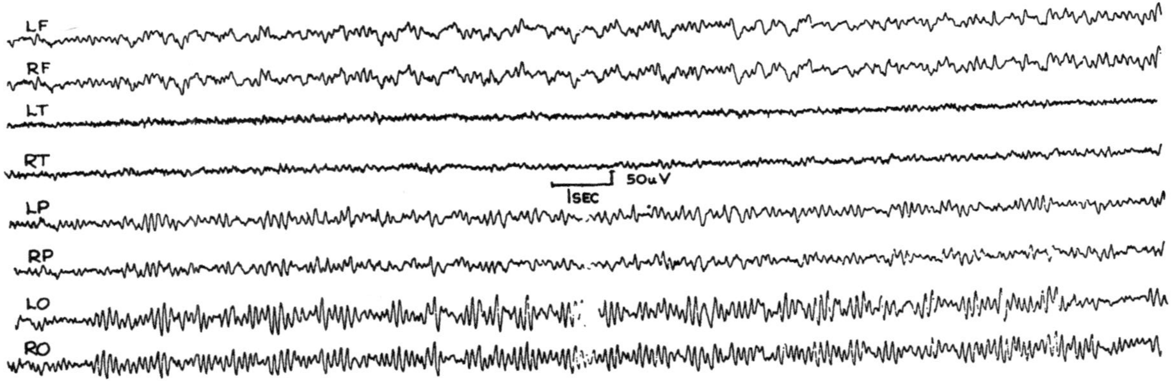

SUBCORTICOGRAMS (DEEP RECORDINGS)

METHODS

Subcortical recordings were usually begun within 6 to 12 hours after the operation at which the electrodes were implanted. The patient was placed on a cot in an electrically shielded room and recordings were taken almost continuously during the ensuing procedure, which usually lasted from 12 to 48 hours. After the stereotaxic technique for electrode implantation was developed (see Chapter 10), electrical activity could be followed for longer periods than when visual placement was employed. Patient 26 was followed in this way for 3 weeks after the insertion of the electrodes. This patient is not included in the present report, since the data were gathered after it was prepared (but see Addendum A).

Various types of electrodes were employed for recording, as shown in Figure 2. In one construction two 32-gauge enameled copper wires were bared for 2 to 3 mm. The uninsulated tips were separated from each other by 2 to 3 mm. and the lead-out wires were loosely twisted together and brought out to the surface. On a few occasions the bared copper tips of this electrode assembly were silver-plated. The plated electrodes appeared to offer no advantages over the bare copper, and the method was therefore abandoned. Because of the danger of insulation breaks in this type of electrode, heavy nylon-coated stranded copper wire was later used for the lead wires. Lengths of bare copper or silver wire measuring from 2 to 3 mm. were soldered to the ends of the heavy wire. The joint was covered with polyethylene tubing, and a polyethylene tube of larger diameter was then fitted around the two smaller pieces. Finally, the sheaths of polyethylene and the interelectrode spaces were filled with an insulating cement which had a low melting point and hardened quickly. De Khotinsky and picene were the materials most commonly employed for this filler. These electrodes were sterilized in aqueous zephiran chloride solution.

The silver or "silver solder" ball electrodes, with their lead-out wires made of stainless steel coated with quadruple teflon, are described in the section on stereotaxic placements (Chapter 10). The resistance between a pair of subcortical electrodes, measured with the electrodes inserted in the brain tissues, ranged from approximately 15,000 to 40,000 ohms.

The most common values were from 20,000 to 25,000 ohms. Neither the material used nor the type of construction of the electrodes appeared to have much influence on the resistance measured between the poles.

Scalp and subcortical recordings were taken simultaneously. Generally, from four to six channels of the eight-channel Grass instrument were used for subcortical recordings, the remainder being kept for scalp recordings. The various dispositions of scalp and subcortical electrodes are shown in Figure 1. As stated above, the scalp recordings were usually but not always unipolar. Opportunity for pick-up directly from the cortical surface was afforded by two patients in whom solder-disk electrodes had been placed on the pial surface at the same operation in which the deep electrodes were inserted. The recordings from the deep structures were almost always bipolar. Subcortical electrical activity was recorded routinely between the closely adjacent poles of an electrode pair. A more diffuse recording was also frequently employed, in which one pole of one electrode pair and one pole of a nearby pair of leads were taken to the grids of the amplifier. In such cases the poles from which the recordings were made were not more than 2 to 3 cm. apart. Sometimes, also, a deep electrode was coupled to two ear electrodes.

We frequently connected a scalp lead to a subcortical lead when the latter was picking up little electrical activity from the neural structures in its own vicinity. The effectiveness of this combination had been shown by Williams and Parsons-Smith[3] in recordings from two patients whose clinical status showed that they were having frank epileptic seizures. Whereas no electrical abnormalities could be obtained by the use of routine scalp leads, characteristic spikes appeared when a needle was inserted into the brain and recordings were taken between a scalp lead and a subcortical lead. Activity was thus uncovered which had presumably been obscured because it was distributed over a large expanse of cortex and hence "canceled out" by the usual recording techniques.

As will be discussed later, we sometimes used the scalp-subcortical derivation to sample the cortical activity when there was reason to suspect that the conventional scalp recordings were not registering significant information, as in the case of the epileptic patients of Williams and Parsons-Smith, noted above. Thus, when activity which we considered abnormal was obtained from subcortical leads but not from scalp electrodes, it became of considerable importance to be certain that the negative findings from the latter were not due to artifacts of recording. When no unusual activity from the cortex was obtained by using the method described above, the impression was indeed strengthened that the subcortical and the cortical electrical activity were not in fact congruent.

No subcortical recordings were attempted on the first two patients. Recordings from Patients 3 to 6 inclusive, were made on a four-channel Rahm EEG instrument. Because of the inadequate number of channels and for other reasons, this material is not considered technically satisfactory. Patient 5 was subjected to a second operation a little more than a year after the first. Adequate electrical recordings were obtained in this instance.

Subcortical and scalp recordings were generally taken for several hours before stimulation of the medio-basal and other regions was begun. During this time there was ample opportunity to observe the electrical patterns as they occurred spontaneously, in waking and in drowsy or sleeping states. One or more psychiatric interviews were conducted while recordings were being taken. The psychiatrist presented material which was presumed to have little significance to the patient as well as that which was thought to have emotional importance. Such a maneuver was performed in an attempt to determine whether any electrical correlates of emotional disturbance could be observed.

RESULTS

Spike Activity. Satisfactory recordings of subcortical electrical activity were taken from psychotic patients on sixteen occasions with the eight-channel Grass instrument. Spike activity, which varied considerably from patient to patient, frequently even in the same patient, was recorded for as long as several hours. It is difficult to give any simple description of this abnormal activity. Some of the outstanding features are noted below.

Frequently the spikes obtained were simple and sharply delineated; usually they were diaphasic and quite often followed by rather slow waves. A sample from the records of Patient 8 (15) is shown in Figure 5. The upper six channels represent responses from three bipolar electrodes.

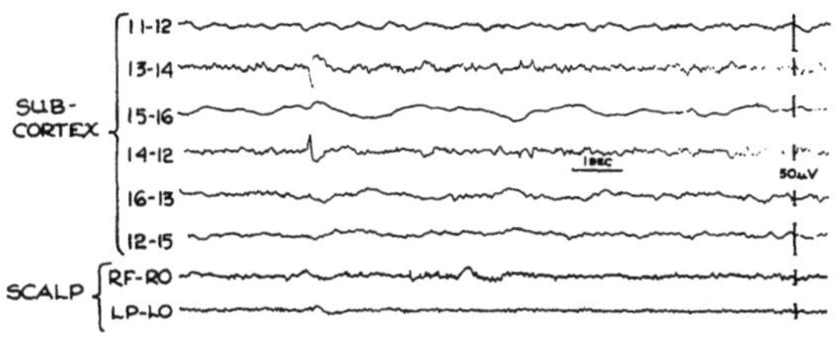

FIGURE XI-5. Recording from Patient 8(15)

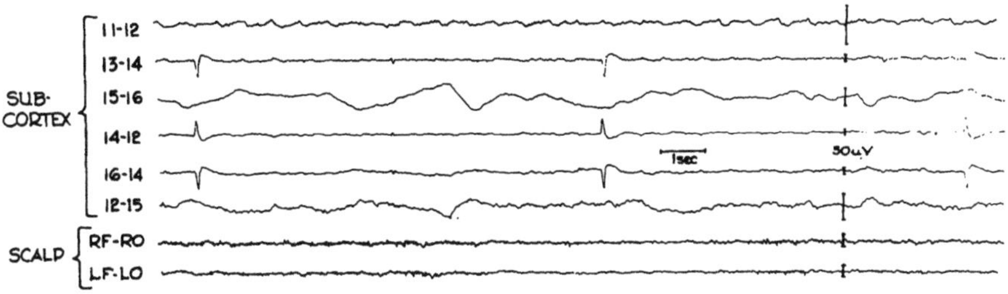

FIGURE XI-6. Recordings from Patient 8(15)

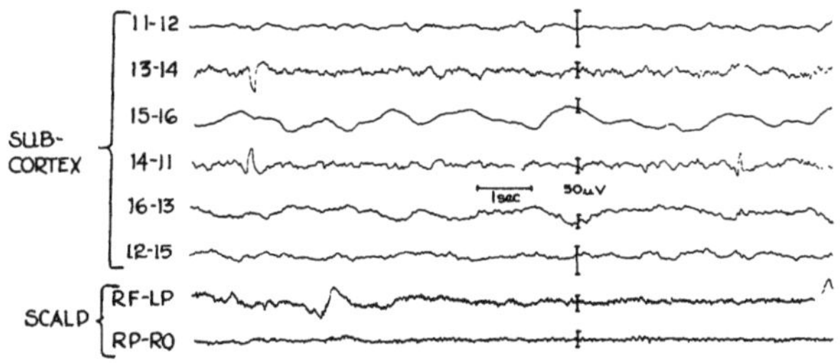

FIGURE XI-7. Recordings from Patient 8(15)

The first three channels are arranged for localized recording between the poles of a single electrode, while channels 4 to 6 represent diffuse recordings obtained by connecting elements of different electrode parts. The spike appears only on channels 2 and 4, both of which record lead 14. The locus of pick-up of this spike seems to be remarkably circumscribed, for no evidence of its occurrence was recorded in the two other pairs of leads, 11 and 12 or 15 and 16. Moreover, channel 5, in which the activity of lead 13 is also sampled, does not present the spike of channels 2 and 4. Thus the spike can be traced to lead 14 and excluded from lead 13, a few millimeters away. Although such sharp delimitation of the locus of a recordable spike was not common, it did occur in a few other instances. As will be noted throughout this report, the prominent spikes found in tracings from the subcortical leads were not found in those from the scalp leads.

Although we attach no special significance to the *magnitude* of spikes recorded, since the voltages were necessarily modified by the placement of electrodes and other technical variables, it nevertheless should be mentioned that amplitudes differed considerably from patient to patient as well as in the same patient during the course of the run. In bipolar recordings the amplitudes ranged from about 25 to about 200 microvolts.

Figure 6 is a record from the same patient as Figure 5. It is to be noted that amplitudes of the three large spikes localized in lead 14, are about twice as great as the spike response of Figure 5. In addition, a small spike (the second from the left in Figure 6) is shown mixed in with the other three spikes. The large spikes have more than three times the amplitude of the small one. In order to appreciate the variation in size of spikes obtained from different patients, Figures 5 and 6 should be compared with several succeeding figures.

Again as a matter of record, and without attempting to explain or attach particular importance to the observation, it was remarked on many occasions that spikes varied in *duration* as well as amplitude. This again held when comparing activity from one patient to another and also when observing various portions of the record from a single patient. The most common variation in duration of the sharp spikes ranged from about 60 to about 200 milliseconds. An example of such variation in two successive spikes in another record from Patient 8 (15) is shown in Figure 7. Here the duration of the large response on the left is about 150 milliseconds, whereas that of the one on the right is approximately 60 milliseconds.

Variation in spike size and fluctuation in spike duration in the records of Patient 16 are shown in Figure 8. These samples also illustrate the prominent slow wave associated with the spike and still another feature of the spike which has not yet been mentioned. On some occasions, instead of occurring singly, runs or trains of these large electrical impulses appeared together. Thus, in each of the first two records a single spike occurs with a particularly well-defined slow wave. In the third record two spikes run together without an intervening slow wave, and in the fourth record a series of three spikes in a row is followed by a

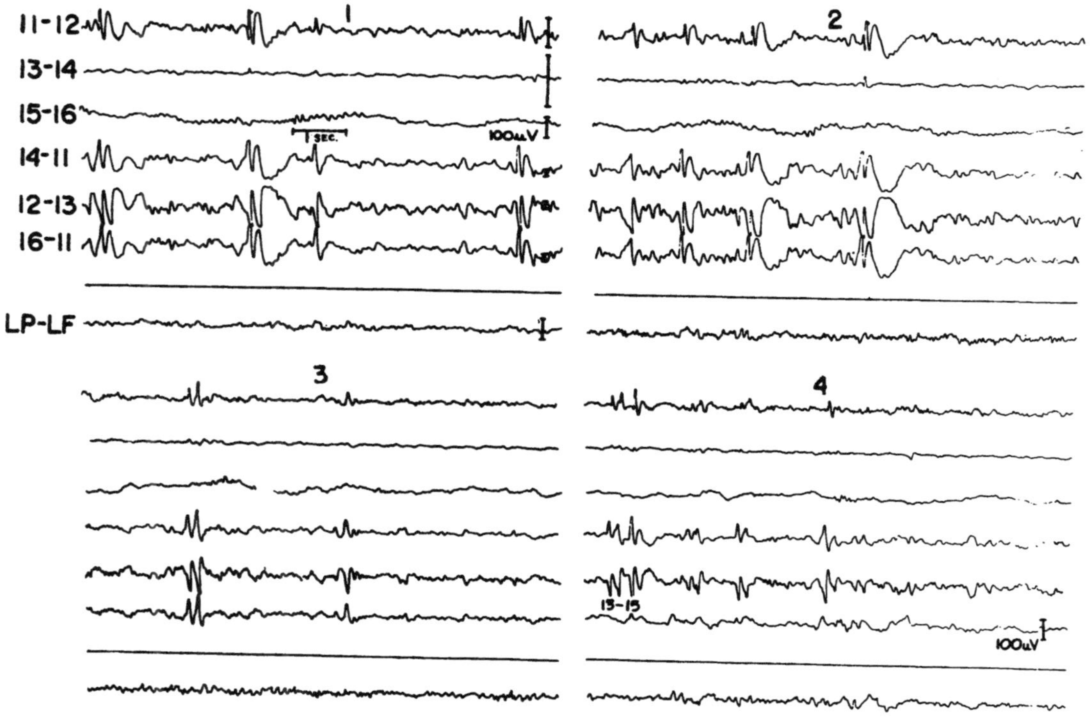

FIGURE XI–8. Recordings from Patient 16

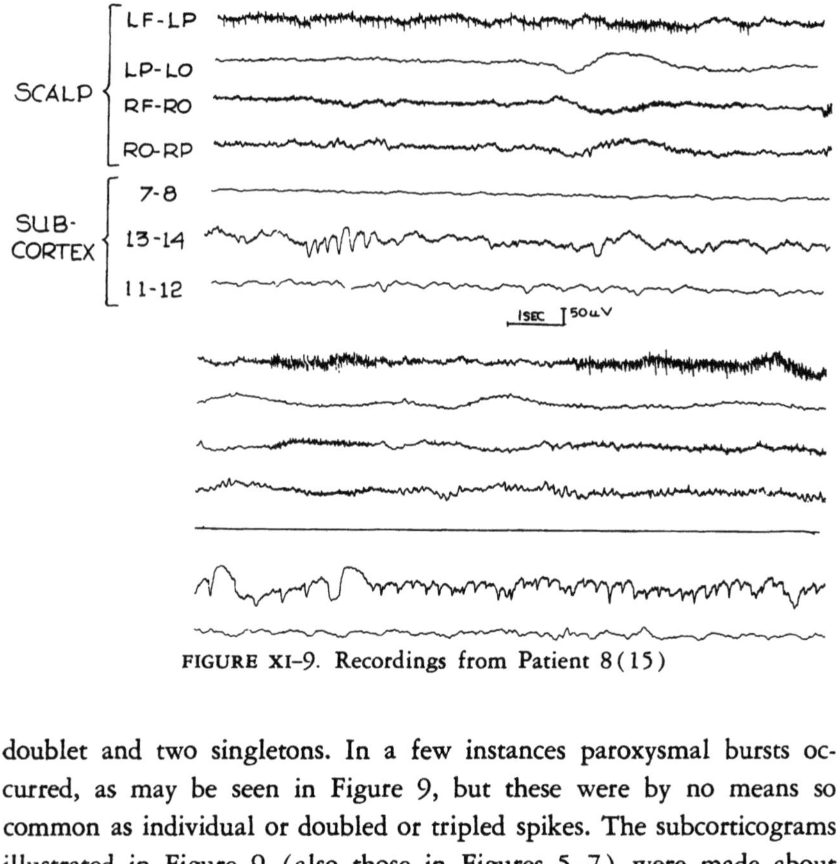

FIGURE XI–9. Recordings from Patient 8(15)

doublet and two singletons. In a few instances paroxysmal bursts occurred, as may be seen in Figure 9, but these were by no means so common as individual or doubled or tripled spikes. The subcorticograms illustrated in Figure 9 (also those in Figures 5–7) were made about seven months after the first implantation of electrodes in Patient 8 (15). The upper sample in Figure 9 presents a short burst of about 1.5 seconds' duration in channel 6, whereas the lower sample shows an extended train which seems to increase in frequency gradually. In the lower sample the spikes appear sharper than in the upper tracings, but the tops of the waves are less flat.

We have already pointed out that the spikes frequently appear to be limited to a single pair of subcortical leads separated from nonspiking leads by no more than a few millimeters. We have also mentioned that there is no evidence of abnormal spiking from the scalp leads. That unmistakable spike activity from subcortical regions need not be reflected on the cortex is demonstrated conclusively in Figures 10 and 11. These show recordings from a parieto-temporal scalp lead and from a scalp lead paired with a subcortical lead (Figure 10, channel 7, lead 15; Figure 11, channel 8, lead 14). In view of the previously mentioned suggestion by Williams and Parsons-Smith that scalp recordings may fail to pick up cortical activity for technical reasons, it should be noted that in the cases under discussion prominent spike activity was found in the subcortical lead but not in the scalp leads.

On many occasions the spikes obtained were not nearly so sharp as those just presented. As these are difficult to describe, a few are marked in Figure 12. A very complicated and rather smaller than usual disturbance is seen at the extreme left of the upper sample and at the right of the lower sample. The multiphasic character and slow wave components of these potentials are apparent. Again, no spikes were recorded from the cortex (channels 5 and 6).

In many patients slow wave activity was prominent in various subcortical leads. The reason why such high voltage slow waves were recorded is not known at present. One likely supposition is that they represent damage incident to placement of the electrodes or trauma resulting from the presence of a foreign body in the brain. Since knowledge of the electrical activity in the structures lying beneath the cortical mantle is fragmentary, it cannot be denied that the slow spontaneous rhythms noted in our patients may represent a particular phase of the normal response of certain deep-seated neural masses. But such an explanation appears less likely than the supposition that slow wave response indicates some damage to subcortical structures. This supposition is supported in principle by the findings of other workers. On the positive side, Williams[3] and his colleagues reported slow wave activity in recordings from patients with thalamic and other deep-lying tumors, and on the negative side various investigators (Meyers,[4] Gibbs,[5] and Spiegel[6]), whose techniques involved less interference than those employed for most of our patients, failed to observe slow wave activity in subcortical recordings. These negative findings further suggest that slow wave activity in the subcortex may be a concomitant of some impairment of function. At the moment, they contribute nothing new or significant to our understanding of the origin or origins of slow wave activity in the subcortex.

Fortunately for the main burden of the present report, this problem

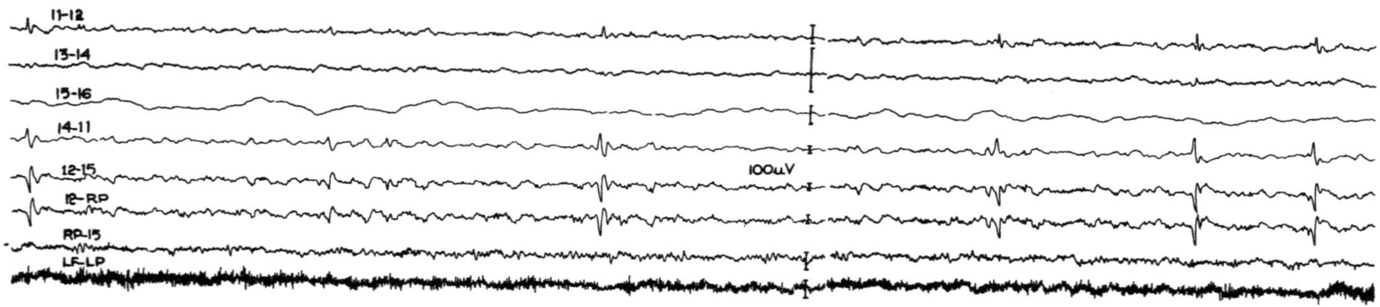

FIGURE XI-10. Recordings from Patient 16

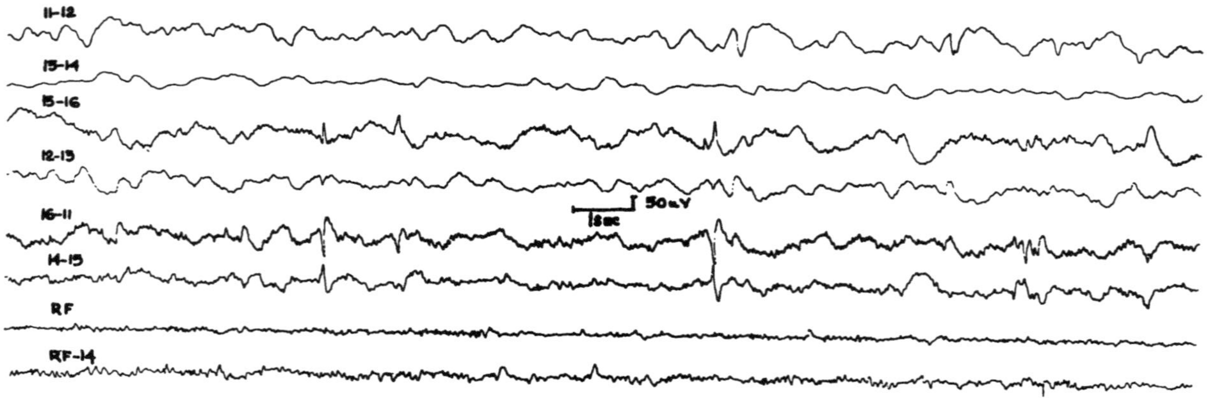

FIGURE XI-11. Recordings from Patient 18

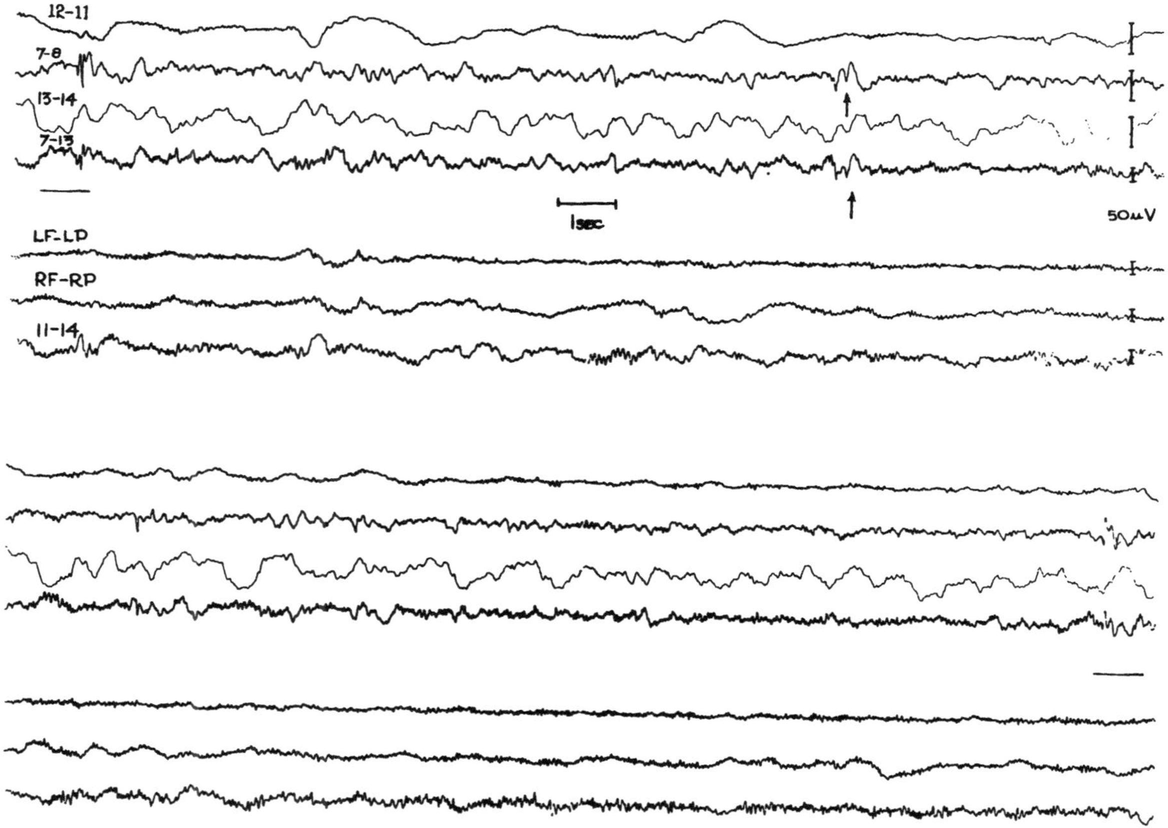

FIGURE XI-12. Recordings from Patient 10

is not germane to our interest in subcortical spike response. It should be noted, however, that slow waves added a significant technical difficulty to our major emphasis on spike characterization, for the rapid spikes were frequently overshadowed by the much greater amplitude of the slow waves. In one such record the almost continual occurrence of spikes was clearly brought out only when the slow waves had been filtered out; channel 1 in Figure 13 represents the unfiltered response and channel 4 the filtered response. These samples show how the spiking nature of the activity can be obscured by the method of recording. This patient's spikes are of an entirely different variety from those already presented; they resemble the activity observed in scalp recordings from a patient suffering from Jacksonian seizures.*

Clearly defined spikes occurred frequently in two pairs of leads in the case of Patient 13; these are seen to discharge independently in Figure 14. The spikes present in leads 15 and 16 are the sharpest (i.e., of the shortest duration) recorded from any patient in this series. Although their time course cannot be accurately resolved with the recording instrument used, it is clear that they were completed in less than the 60 milliseconds previously given (see p. 164) as the lower limit of the usual range of durations. The spikes present in leads 13 and 14 are of considerably longer duration than those present in leads 15 and 16 and resemble some of those shown in the preceding figures. Reference will be made later to the placement of electrodes of leads 15 and 16 (p. 175).

Figure 14 yields further support for the belief that the unusual subcortical discharge which has been called a spike is not present on the cortical surface. Electrodes had been placed on the pia of Patient 13, but the two large spike disturbances present in the subcortical recordings did not appear in the cortical or scalp recordings.

Discussion of Spike Activity. Thus far we have described various types of spike activity in the subcortex which are apparently not reflected in the cerebral hemispheres. No signs of such response can be detected by the use of scalp recordings or cortical recordings or by means of a

*This slow wave complication has been overcome by our new and improved procedure, in which stimulation is delayed from several days to a few weeks following implantation. It has become apparent that the slow wave activity formerly occurring was a temporary phenomenon present in diminishing degrees for two or three days after surgery.

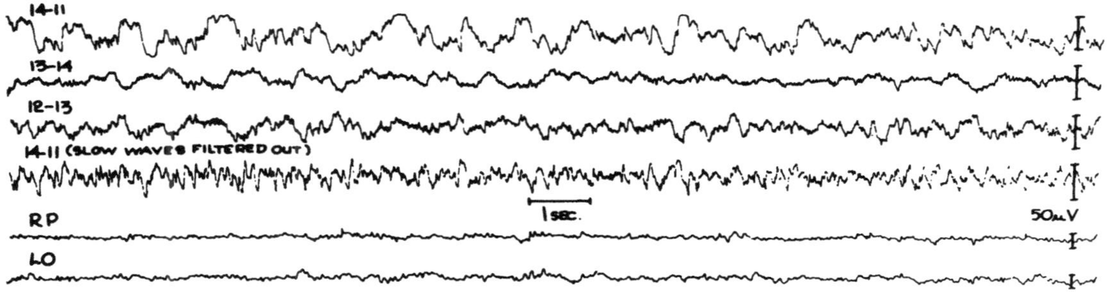

FIGURE XI–13. Recordings from Patient 20

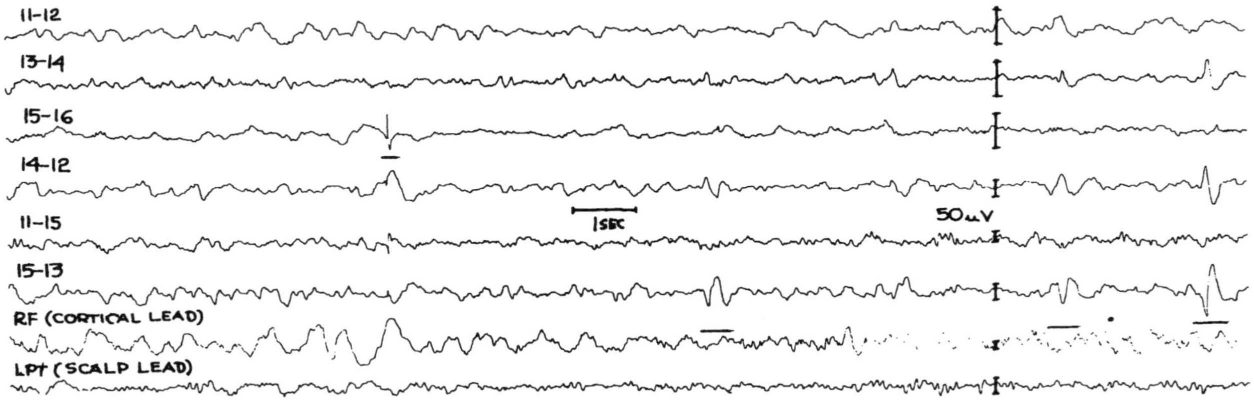

FIGURE XI–14. Recordings from Patient 13

special technique intended specifically to uncover such cortical activity as might be obscured by the artifacts of conventional recording. Furthermore, it has been suggested that the region of spiking is fairly limited in anatomical expanse, since it is usually restricted to a single bipolar electrode. The localization of activity that must be considered abnormal thus assumes considerable importance, for the correlation of morbid function with specific pathology is at once a time-honored method and a tempting lure of scientific medicine. Within the term "specific pathology," one must include not only the cellular and organic changes set forth by Virchow and his followers, but also physiological derangements and imbalances unaccompanied by demonstrable anatomic abnormalities. Thus, without prejudice as to the type or cause of the pathological process, we have sought at least one of its loci.

The quest for intracranial localization from extracranial landmarks has been long, arduous, and notoriously unsuccessful. Attempts have also been made to judge the position of one neural structure from certain prominent intracranial structures—for example, the ventricles, the pineal gland, the pituitary, and so forth. We have used the foramen of Monro and the lateral ventricles chiefly because some of the structures of major interest to us are in close proximity to these regions. But owing to the great variability in the size and shape of the human brain, all such attempts to place the position of one structure in the neuraxis by reference to a relatively constant intracranial landmark have not been entirely successful. Spiegel and Wycis[7] and Talairach, de Ajuriaguerra, and Hecaen,[8] spurred by the growing possibilities of human stereotaxy, have prepared atlases of the human brain. While these represent refinements in method, it is questionable whether they will completely overcome the basic difficulty of the human brain's inconstancy. Exact localization in most cases is impossible except at autopsy.

We thus approach the question of the localization of electrodes from which abnormal electrical impulses are recorded with a full realization of the inaccuracies inherent in our indirect methods. Only within the framework of these limitations can we speak of localization. To suggest more is to commit the unpardonable scientific blunder of ascribing more credibility to the abstraction devised to describe a physical system than to the physical system itself.

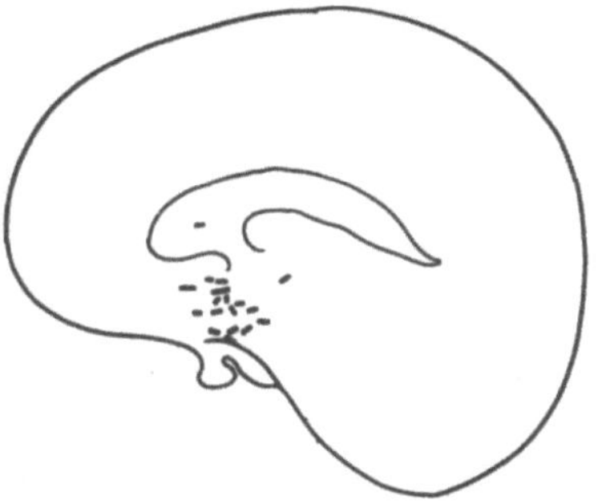

FIGURE XI–15. Locations of electrode points from which spiking was recorded. The anterior-posterior x-rays showed all points within 6 mm. of midline

Figure 15 shows a median sagittal section of the human brain, onto which has been projected the ventricular system. The composite was derived from study of the x-rays of several of the patients of this series. The markers represent the electrodes from which spikes were recorded. These markers were placed on the diagram roughly in accordance with the original position of the electrodes with respect to the foramen of Monro. Spikes were never recorded from what we considered to be the caudate nucleus, nor from any point more than 6 mm. from the midline. The most powerful region of spiking appears to extend rostro-caudally from the basal part of the septal region to the rostral reaches of the hypothalamus. Dorso-ventrally the area of abnormality extends in a continuous expanse from below the lateral ventricles to the base of the brain.

Figures 16–19 show the lateral and anterior-posterior roentgenograms of four of the six patients whose neurograms are detailed in Figures 5–14. X-rays from the fifth patient are shown in Chapter 9, Figure 3; none from the sixth patient are available. In Figure 19 two bipolar electrodes are marked in this fashion; the patient presented two distinct spikes, one sharp and fast, and the other of the more common slow variety. The more caudal and dorsal electrode in this figure gave the rapid spike. As nearly as could be judged from our indirect methods, it was the most caudally and dorsally placed of those from which spiking was secured. The films of Figure 19 also show electrodes in position on the pial surface.

Previous studies of the electrical activity of various parts of the subcortex have been made by other workers. Notable among these are Williams and Parsons-Smith,[3] Meyers,[4] Gibbs,[5] Spiegel and Wycis,[6] and Gastaut and Roger.[9] Although some of them have examined regions

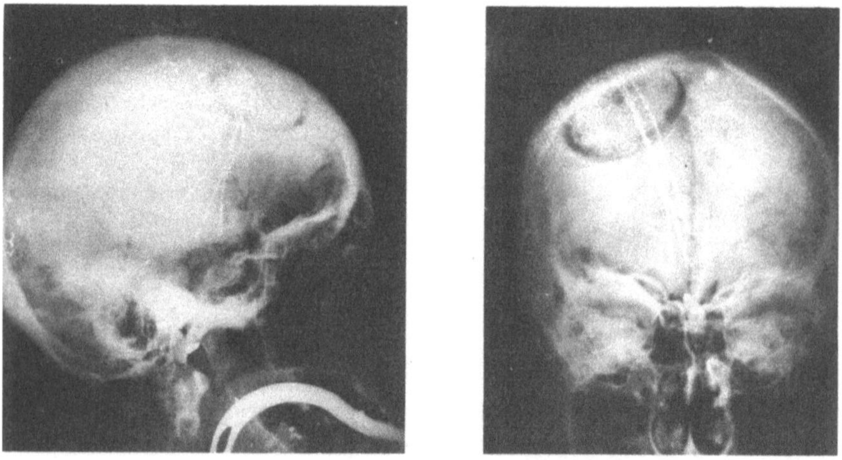

FIGURE XI–16. Lateral and anterior-posterior x-rays of Patient 16

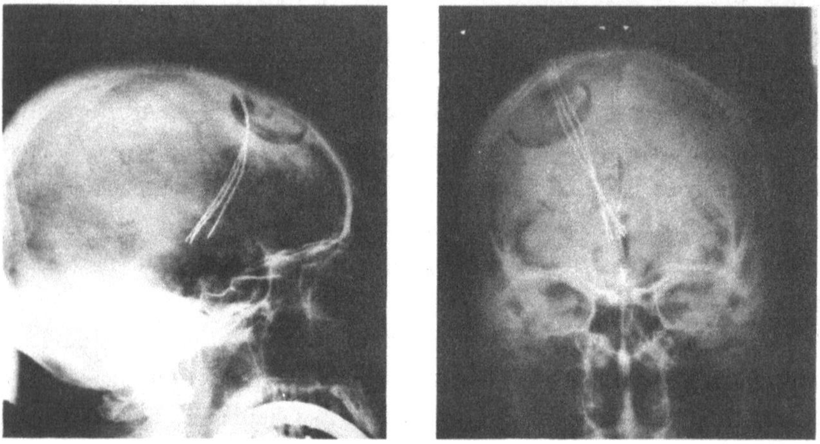

FIGURE XI–17. Lateral and anterior-posterior x-rays of Patient 18

in proximity to the areas described in this chapter, they report no significant spiking except in frank cases of epilepsy (Gibbs[1, 5]). Spiegel[6] mentions in a short note that he recorded subcortical spikes in two schizophrenic patients. However, his records are rather unconvincing. Further, Spiegel suggests in this same note that the spike activity may have been due to previous electroshock therapy which his schizophrenic patients had undergone. That our findings cannot be explained on this ground is evident from the fact that Patient 10 had never had EST and Patient 16 had received only three individual electroshock treatments before

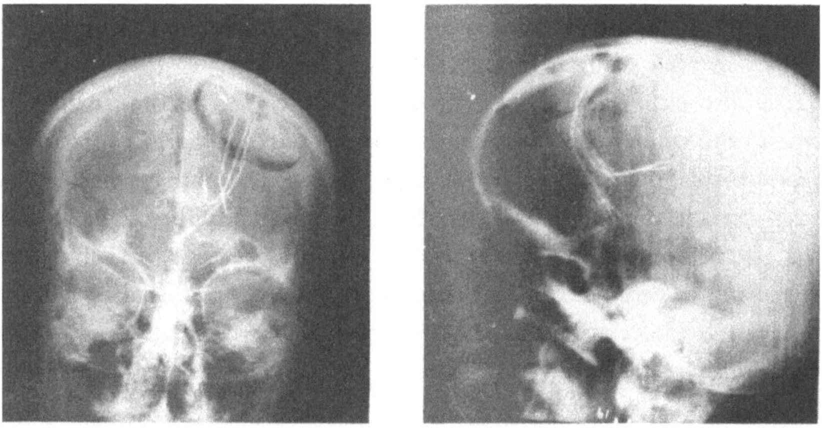

FIGURE XI–18. Lateral and anterior-posterior x-rays of Patient 10

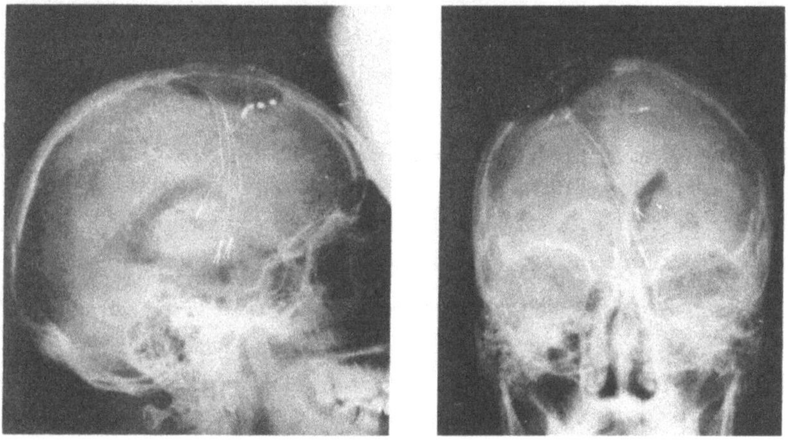

FIGURE XI–19. Lateral and anterior-posterior x-rays of Patient 13

subcortical recordings were taken. Yet both of them produced frequent and high voltage spikes (Figures 8, 10, and 12).

Additional indication that subcortical spiking may indeed be significant in schizophrenia is provided by electrical findings in three nonschizophrenic control patients. Two of these were cancer patients and the other a tuberculosis patient. All were in terminal stages of their disease, as has already been mentioned (p. 47). Several hours of recording, cortical and subcortical, were taken on these three patients, but no spikes were seen. This was especially important for our study in view of the fact that in all three patients there was evidence of some organic brain damage. Each of them showed some diffuse slow wave activity on scalp recordings, both before and after surgical intervention.

It is also clear that neither damage to the cortex nor destruction of some of the white matter was responsible for the recording of subcortical spikes in the schizophrenic patients, for the control patients suffered as much damage to the cerebral mantle as did the schizophrenics. Nor did there seem to be any difference in the amount of spiking, whether the operation was performed by a transcortical incision and visual placement or by the stereotaxic method, although it is obvious that the cortical damage suffered in the latter procedure was insignificant compared with that suffered in the former.

Spikes were apparently obtained equally well whether or not air had been injected into the ventricles. Further, if the irritation produced by air in the ventricles had any causal relation to the production of spikes, one would expect spiking in all leads rather than only from electrodes placed in a particular region.

We are thus left with the conclusion that subcortical spike activity is present in schizophrenic patients. Although we did not record cortical spikes, it is not impossible that both cortex and subcortex might on occasion be simultaneously involved in the production of aberrant electrical activity or that the cortex might be involved at one time and the subcortex at some other time. Such a situation would perhaps help to explain similarities in behavior and certain common features in the electroencephalograms found in psychomotor epilepsy and schizophrenia (p. 152). Further, from the physiological data of the Montreal group,[10] which describes corticifugal and corticipetal connections between the medio-basal septo-olfactory regions and the temporal lobe, it would not be difficult to imagine subcortical spike activity reaching this portion of the cortex or vice versa.

Although similarities between schizophrenia and psychomotor epilepsy have been mentioned frequently, it is important also to comment on the distinctions between the two diseases. Perhaps our results may help to explain some reasons for these distinctions, for it can perhaps be reasoned that the natural history of the two disease processes may differ precisely because of the regions of major pathological involvement—the temporal cortex in psychomotor epilepsy and the medio-basal septo-olfactory regions in schizophrenia. Although the end results of the depradations of these diseases may be amenable to physiological investigation, the etiological factors which lead to specific forms of pathology are beyond the scope of this paper.

The fact that the electrodes from which spikes were recorded were placed close to the midline appears to be of major significance. Dorsoventrally the spiking area extended from below the lateral ventricles to the base of the brain. Rostro-caudally the area of abnormal activity involved tissues located in the area we have described as the septal region and not extending caudally further than the most anterior reaches of the hypothalamus. Considering the extreme differences in anatomy between the cat brain and the human brain, such a localization agrees remarkably well with the regions in the carnivore which facilitated motor activity from the cortex exclusively (see Chapter 4), and in which destructive lesion led to the biochemical disturbances and bizarre behavioral patterns described in Chapter 3. The concepts that formed the bases for the current studies would therefore seem to have received some verification.

Spike Activity during Sleep. Because the electrodes were allowed to remain in our patients for comparatively long periods of time, we were able to utilize the opportunity, denied other workers, of observing subcortical activity during various stages of awareness—alertness, relaxation, drowsiness, and light or deep sleep. Of paramount concern to the electrophysiological analysis of schizophrenia is the effect of sleep on the subcortical spikes.

In every case drowsiness or sleep intensified either the amplitude of the spike or the frequency of its discharge. In fact, it was not always possible to observe spikes in some instances unless the patients were asleep. Strong or frequent "spikers" would show the synchronized discharge whether alert or asleep, but invariably the spiking was intensified with the occurrence of sleep. Relatively weak "spikers" often showed no spikes until the observers were out of the room, the light extinguished, and the noises from the outside reduced to a minimum. As the degree of awareness of the patient decreased from alertness, to relaxation, to sleep, the incidence of spikes progressively increased. This is shown clearly in Figure 20. The top record was obtained as Patient 10 slept. Spikes are seen in leads 7 and 8 and all combinations containing these leads. Sleep spindles are recorded from both deep and cortical leads, a finding similar to that previously noted in chronic experiments with monkeys (see Chapter 7). The middle record, in which only two spikes are seen, shows the patient semialert. The bottom record, taken when he had been fully aroused, presents no spike activity from the leads which yielded them frequently during drowsiness or light sleep.

Figure 21 also shows a rather striking difference in records taken during sleeping and waking states from the same patient. When the lower record was being registered, one minute after the upper tracing was made, a psychiatrist was questioning the patient on some material which was considered of a provocative nature to him. The disappearance of the spikes from this bottom record is quite evident.

Two similar records are seen in Figure 22. That Patient 10 was sleeping is apparent from the base line sway and small sleep spindles in the scalp leads of the upper record. Spikes are seen in leads 7 and 8 from the basal part of the septum. It should also be noted that slow waves are prominent in the deep recordings. When the patient wakened (lower record) there was a dramatic flattening in the subcortical records, and the spikes disappeared from leads 7 and 8. The abolition of high voltage slow waves on arousal has been reported in Chapter 7, which discusses the chronic experiments with monkeys.

Abolition of spikes and flattening of high voltage slow waves from deep electrodes is also apparent in a tracing from Patient 20. The upper record in Figure 23 shows the patient in the first stage of sleep. A few minutes later he presented premonitory symptoms of vomiting and began to wake up. This is evidenced by the alteration in the cortical activity. Eye blinks are reflected in the left frontal lead (channel 5), but, as usual, these movement artifacts are not recorded from the deep electrodes. The flattening of the slow waves and the abolition of the spikes from channels 1 and 3 of the lower record is immediately obvious.

Although always present, the sleep-dependency of the spikes was not always so complete as in the patients illustrated in Figures 20–23. In another patient, a frequent and strong "spiker," septal spikes were present during both the waking and the sleeping state but were markedly reduced in the former case. Such a situation is presented in Figure 24, in which

Patient 18 was drowsy while the upper record was being made and was interviewed by a psychiatrist while the lower record was being made. The spikes in the lower record are smaller, not so sharp, and less frequent than in the upper record.

Certain features of subcorticograms made during sleep have been noted. They are essentially similar to those characteristics described and illustrated in Chapter 7, which deals with chronic experiments with monkeys. The major points may be summarized:

1. Organized bursts of high voltage slow waves are commonplace in subcortical leads during drowsy or sleeping states. Sleep spindles and what appear to be "sleep humps" are often picked up from deep-seated electrodes.
2. These spontaneous outpourings frequently appear in some deep leads before they are noted in the scalp derivations. Whether this is due to gross recording artifacts, or whether these subcortical structures do in fact lead or drive the cortex it is not as yet clear.
3. In the transition from states of depressed consciousness to alertness, slow waves and spindle bursts are diminished or abolished in the subcortex. Tracings acquired in the waking state contain many low voltage fast waves, similar in many ways to those characteristic of scalp leads obtained during alertness or active cerebration.

Discussion of Spike Activity during Sleep. The major point demonstrated in this section is that sleep is a potent intensifier of abnormal subcortical spiking. Such a finding would appear to be quite reasonable, for sleep is among the most common "activators" of abnormal responses, routinely employed in most EEG laboratories. There is no *a priori* reason why sleep should not "activate" subcortical spikes as well as those from the cortical surface, for sleep is obviously a function of the total organism and not specifically localized to the cerebral hemispheres. In fact, evidence from human pathology as well as experimental neurophysiology have amply demonstrated the importance of subcortical influence on the production and maintenance of sleep. In earlier presentations (Chapter 7) we have demonstrated the participation of structures lying deep below the surface in the sleep process.

Thus, although association of sleep with abnormal activity should not be surprising, it appears to us to have special significance in this

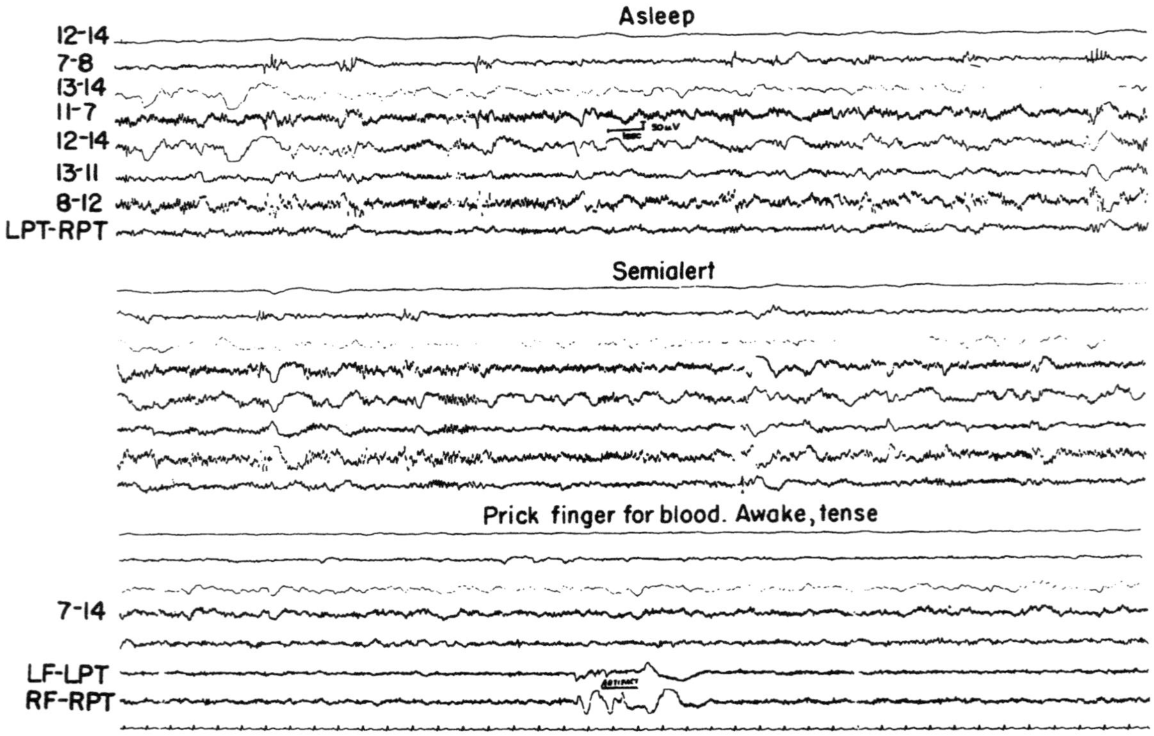

FIGURE XI–20. Recordings from Patient 10

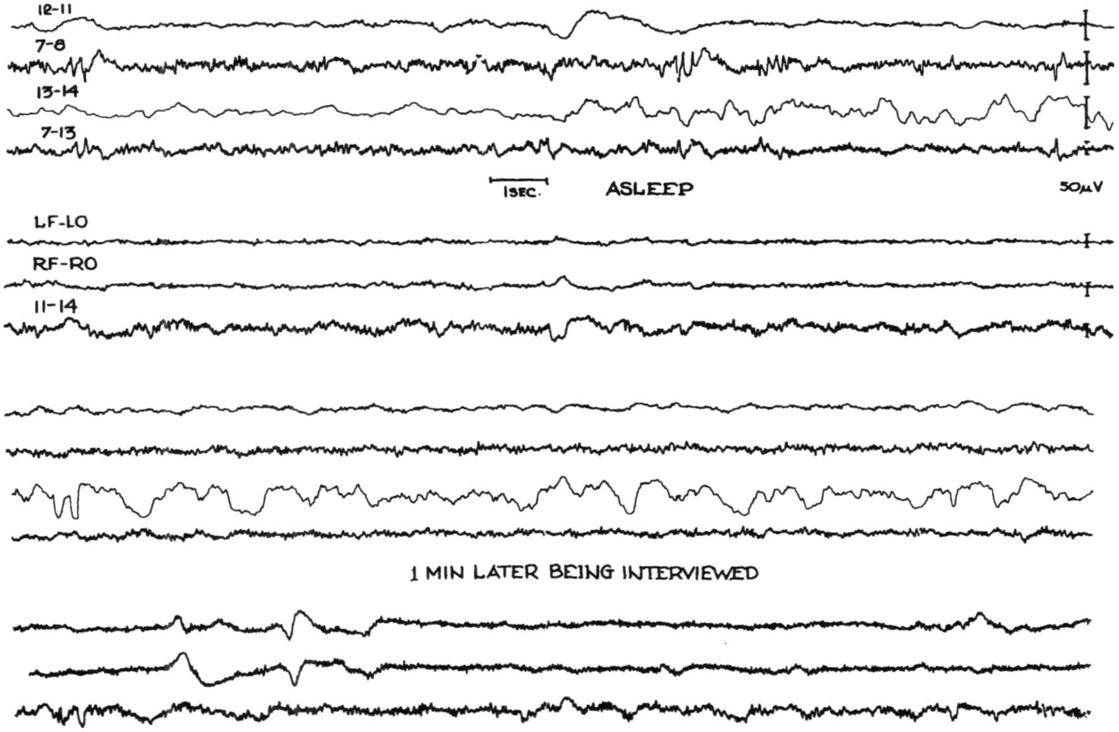

FIGURE XI-21. Recordings from Patient 10

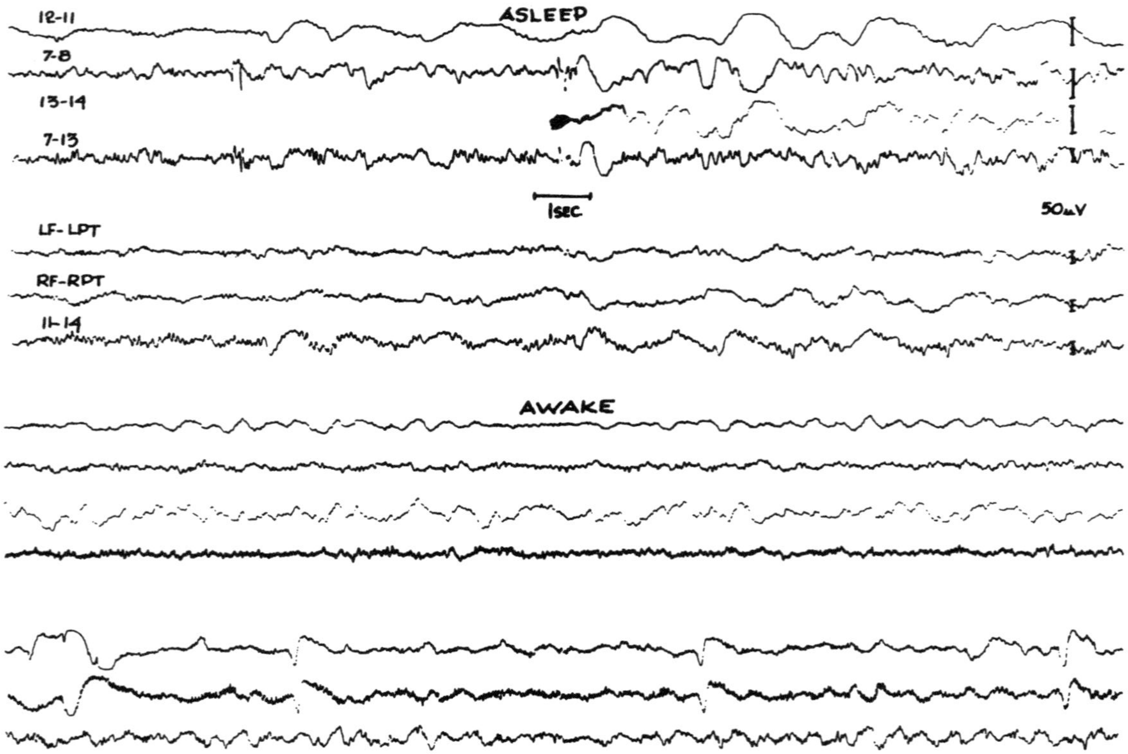

FIGURE XI–22. Recordings from Patient 10

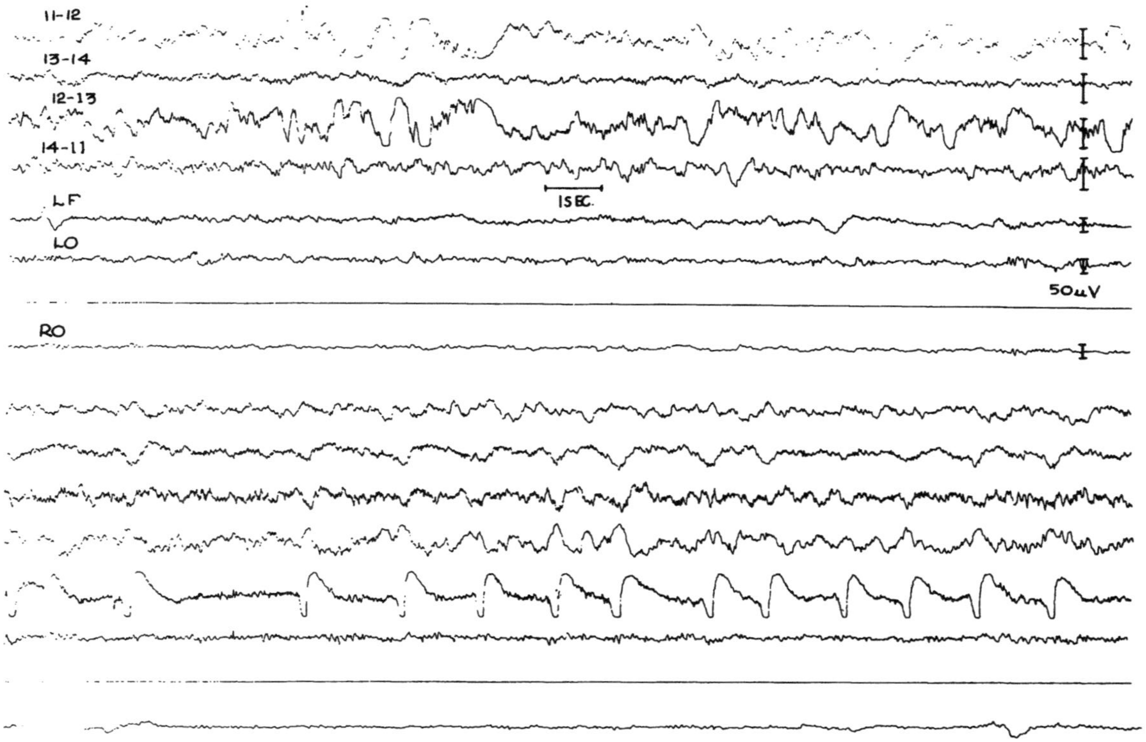

FIGURE XI–23. Recordings from Patient 20

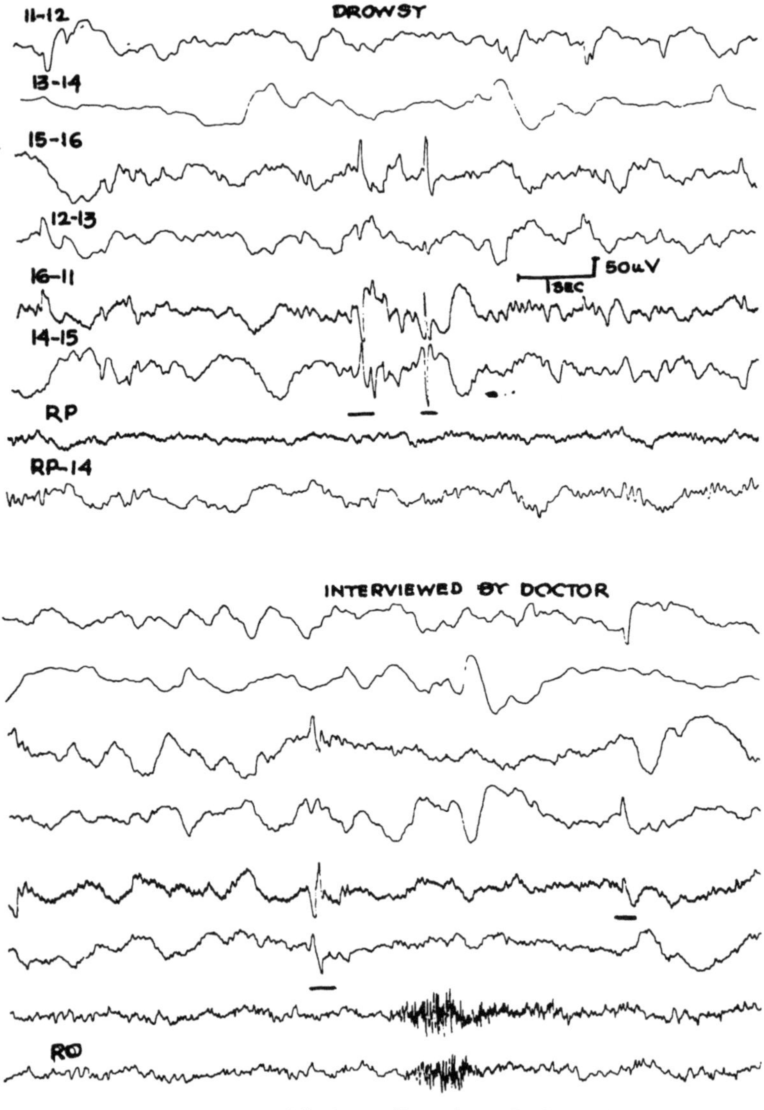

FIGURE XI–24. Recordings from Patient 18

instance, for similarities between schizophrenic behavior and psychomotor fits have been stressed by many workers and frequently discussed in this monograph. It therefore seems especially important in this connection to note that sleep is a more effective agent in uncovering the temporal lobe spikes of psychomotor epilepsy than metrazol, hyperventilation, or flicker. The latter agents, on the other hand, are more productive in other types of epilepsy, such as grand mal. Merlis[11] has found this to be true in a large series of epileptic patients of all types. Also of considerable significance in this connection are the findings of Dennis Hill, given at the May 1952 meetings of the American Electroencephalographic Society.[2] Hill analyzed with considerable care and great ingenuity the so-called nonspecific abnormalities frequently observed in patients with behavioral disorders. He showed that patients diagnosed as schizophrenics had small spikes localized particularly in the posterior temporal regions. These spikes were considerably more common in the schizophrenic patients than in individuals who were considered normal. Interestingly enough, these small spikes of the schizophrenic patients were markedly aggravated by sleep but were not intensified by hyperventilation.

Although we have now arrived at the point where we would be ready to accept the fact that sleep brings out the subcortical electrical defects in the schizophrenic, and although we have presented data from other sources which would tend to substantiate our findings, there appear to us no existing explanations of why such sleep dependence occurs. The following is a speculative attempt to explain this sleep-induced enhancement of abnormal activity.

Contrary to present-day fractionators of the central nervous system and current searchers after the seat of theoretical consciousness, we have assumed in our over-all concept that the cerebral cortex stands in intimate interrelationships with other portions of the nervous system and hence with the entire body. Further, we have assumed, as explained in Chapter 1, that the cerebral cortex is the dominant neural governor of the nervous system. For reasons as yet unknown, in schizophrenia this governor is defective. It therefore abdicates its prime function of control on lower centers. Either because of the reduced governing power of the cortex or for constitutional reasons, also still unknown, certain subcortical structures (facilitatory regions) respond to stimuli in an abnormal fashion (e.g., with spikes). In this view the severity of the disease process would be related to the degree to which the control of the lower centers by the cortex was lacking or inappropriate.

By almost universal consent, sleep is considered to be accompanied by a reduction of the cortical function. Pavlov,[12] Hess,[13] Moruzzi and

Magoun,[14] and others have offered material which could be interpreted as explaining sleep as an inhibition of cortical function. Hence it would be logical to suppose that abnormal activity noted during waking states would be even more apparent when the regulatory function of the cortex on subcortical structures is held in abeyance during sleep. The similarities between various states of reduced consciousness (sleep, dreams, hypnosis, fugue states, etc.) and schizophrenic behavior are everyday observations and would seem to us to have at least one common causative factor—diminished control by the phylogenetically new cerebral cortex.

The hypothesis advanced above is illustrated in the schema of Figure 25.

Emotional Stimulation and Subcortical Recordings. The original hypothesis on which the present work on schizophrenic patients was based suggested that abnormal cortical activity might be reflected in the so-called facilitatory region of the subcortex. It was of considerable interest therefore to determine whether emotional material could in any way be related to the electrical response from these same regions. Consequently, frequent discussions between patients and members of the psychiatric staff were conducted while electrical activity was continuously recorded. The results of this procedure are unquestionably the least certain of any of the findings obtained from subcortical and cortical recordings. In many ways, however, they are among the most interesting. We therefore present a few suggestive results from this type of study. It cannot be too strongly emphasized that the material is given with full knowledge of its incompleteness and its highly speculative character.

Large paroxysmal outbursts of high voltage slow waves as well as frequent occurrence of spiking in the septal leads are shown on channels 1, 3, 4, and 8 of Figure 26. This record is a 1-minute sample taken during a psychiatric interview, in which the discussion related to the patient's thoughts about death. Such a record must be interpreted with extreme caution, for it should be noted that paroxysmal bursts evident in the figure did not occur at the beginning of the psychiatric interview with Patient 20, but approximately 20 minutes later. No similar activity was seen during several hours of recording—but on the other hand several other discussions with the patient, on material apparently as noxious as this, did not result in similar electrical activity.

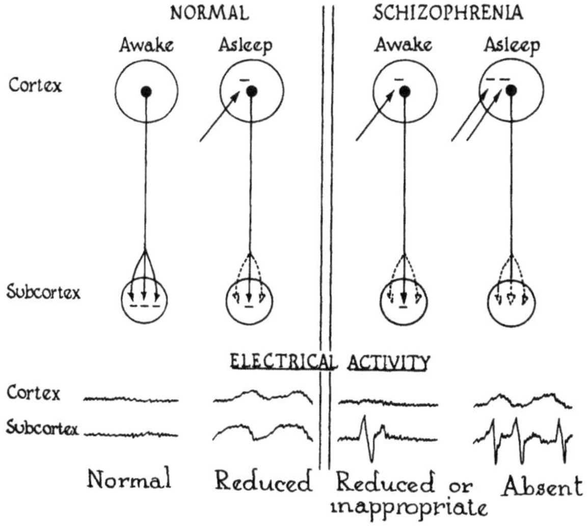

FIGURE XI–25. Diagram showing hypothetical control of subcortex by cortex

Another example of a similar but less dramatic outburst from the septal leads is shown in Figure 27, taken from a different patient. The upper left record shows the relatively flat, featureless recordings obtained before the psychiatric interview. Leads 13 and 14 begin to show slow wave response in the upper right record, taken 3 minutes after the discussion of emotionally charged material had begun. In the lower left record, taken a little more than 5 minutes after the discussion had started, there is a great increase in high voltage slow wave response. Three and a half minutes after termination of this interview (lower right record), subcortical activity returned approximately to its state before the discussion with the patient began. This figure illustrates the more common type of activity seen during positive interviews—that is, those in which changes in subcortical recordings were noted during emotional excitation. The most common type of such activity was an upsurge of high voltage slow waves.

In order to restore the note of caution with which this section was introduced, for comparison with Figure 27 we present in Figure 28 excerpts taken from the same patient's recordings. Here are shown three samples obtained within 15 to 20 minutes of each other, during which time no psychiatric interview took place. Notice here, as in Figure 27,

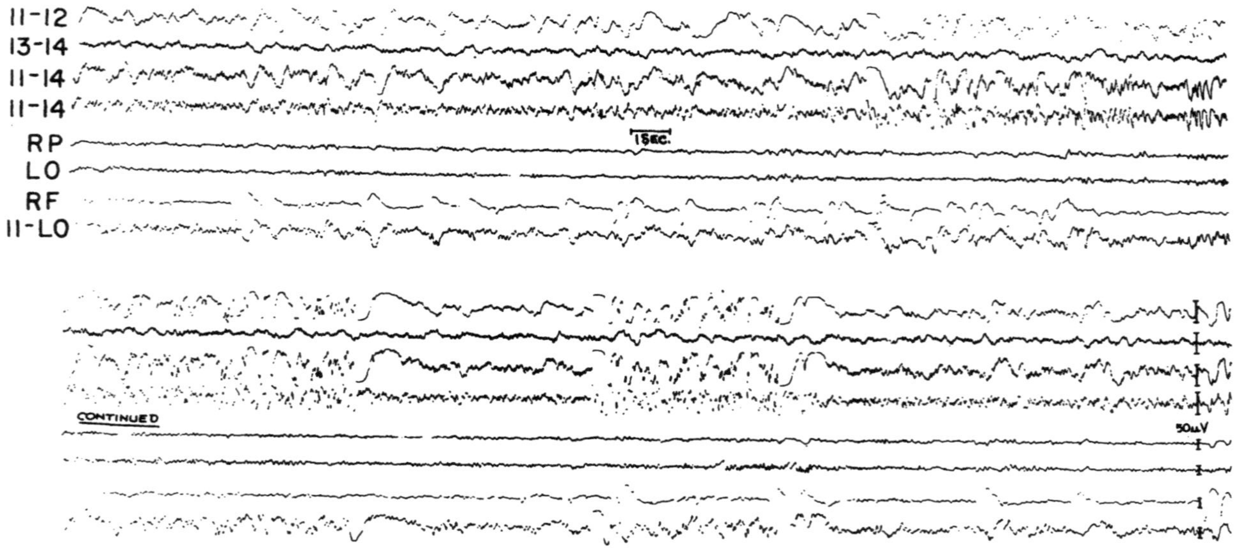

FIGURE XI-26. Recordings from Patient 20. In leads 11-12 the slow waves have been filtered out

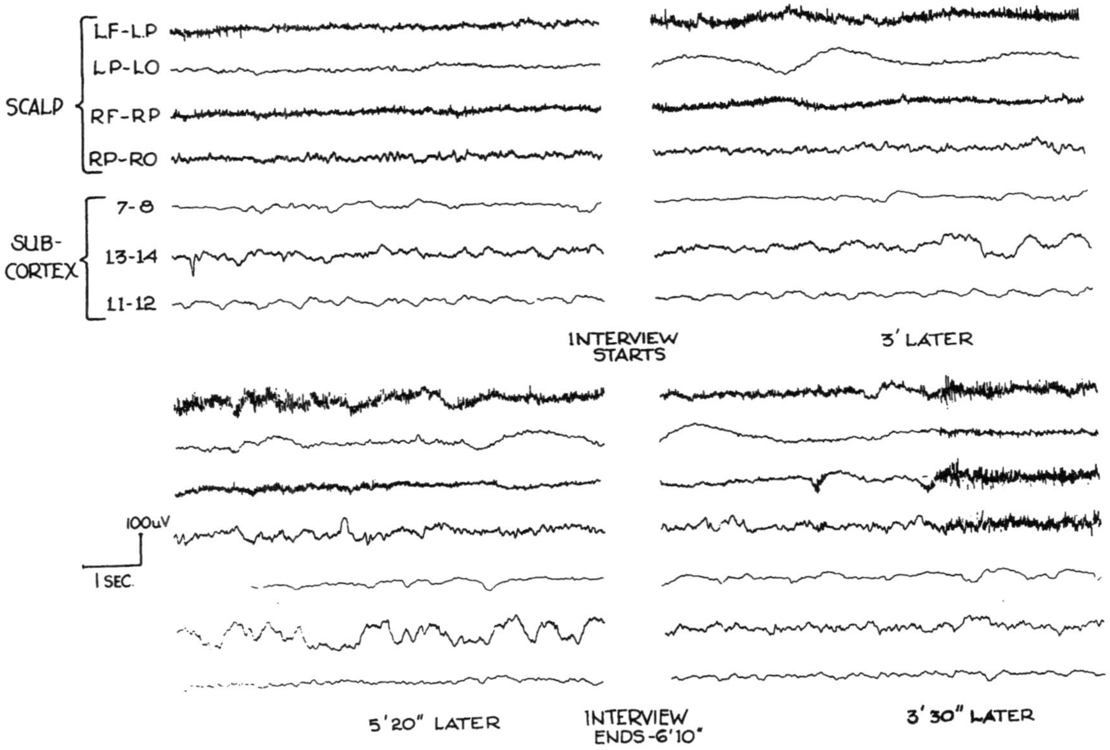

FIGURE XI–27. Recordings from Patient 8(15)

that record 1 shows flat activity from leads 13 and 14, but records 2 and 3 show considerable high voltage response from the same leads.

Discussion of Emotional Stimulation and Deep Recordings. The objection may be made, and with good justification, that the psychologically harmful stimulus responsible for the unusual subcortical activity of Figure 27 was not necessarily applied to the psychotic patient from without but might have originated as a result of his own painful memories or fantasies. This objection cannot be summarily dismissed; further work will decide between the alternative explanations.*

Although it appeared to us that the activity which seemed to be aroused by psychiatric examination most frequently occurred in those leads from which the spiking was also obtained, such activity was also seen from time to time in leads which gave no such evidence of abnormality. Again such negative evidence can be countered by many and varied speculations which at the moment it appears fruitless to discuss. More explicit data than are now available are needed to determine the meaning, if any, of these results.

The findings discussed above may be explained if the thesis is accepted that emotional stimulation may precipitate abnormal reactions which are reflected as changes in subcortical electrical activity. The explanation to be offered is in keeping both with our over-all theoretical concept and with the results concerning the intensification of abnormal activity during sleep, as given in this report; for one would simply have to assume that certain stimuli are sufficiently painful to depress cortical function—whether they are delivered from the outside or are recalled by means of the psychiatric interview or arise spontaneously from memories of life experiences. The end result is lack of control, or inappropriate control, of the subcortical masses (see Figure 28).

SUMMARY

Two of the psychotic patients of this series had abnormal electroencephalograms which could not be readily ascribed to the effects of prior electroshock therapy. The findings in these records were not suggestive of psychomotor epilepsy, nor were they similar to the positive findings sometimes noted in the EEG's of schizophrenics.

*For results obtained since this writing see Addendum E.

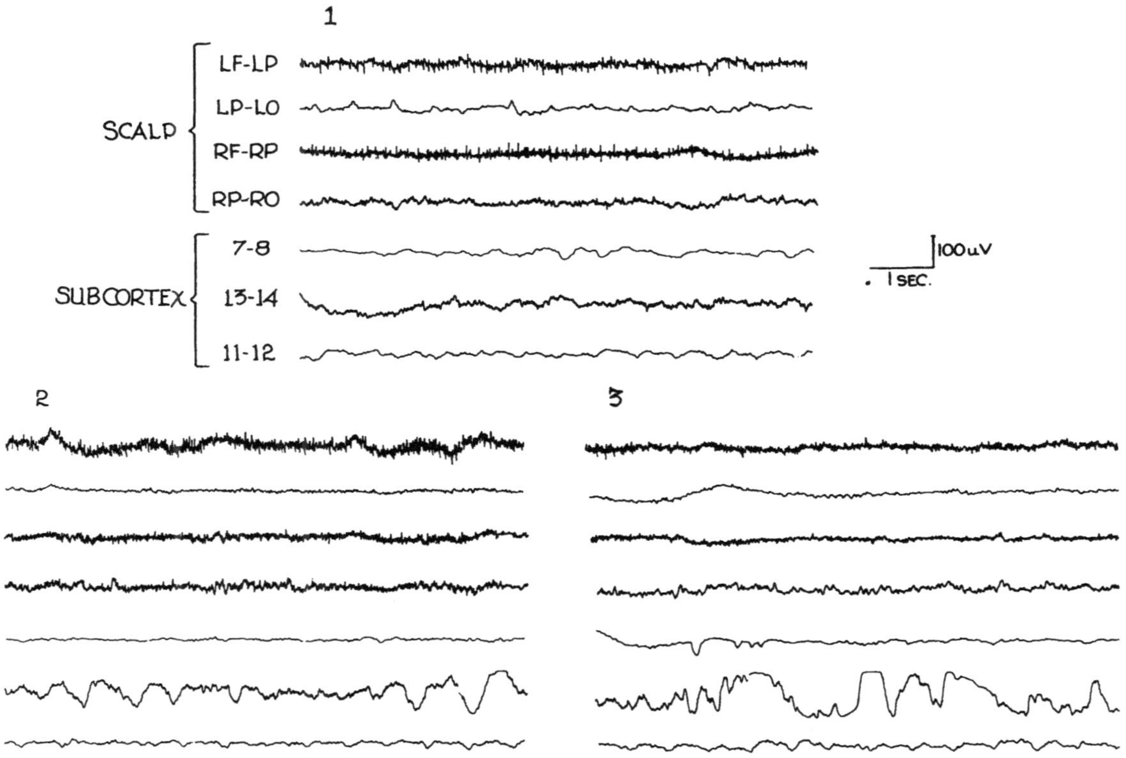

FIGURE XI–28. Recordings from Patient 8(15)

TABLE XI–1. Electroencephalographic findings in nineteen schizophrenic patients. No electroencephalographic data were obtained from Patient 1. The operation-stimulation procedure was repeated in the cases of Patients 5 and 8.

Patient	2	3	4	5(24)	6	7	8(15)	9
Age	17	20	26	22	28	35	41	39
No. of recordings before EST, ENT, or insulin (all normal)	1	—	—	—	—	1	—	—
Shortest time between DX and recordings (in months)	0.5	12	3.5	0.8	8	3.2	8	2
PRE-STIMULATION EEG's								
No. of recordings after EST, ENT, or insulin	2	1	1	3	4	1	2	2
Normal recordings	0	1	1	3	2	1	2	0
*Type of abnormality**	RSp S_3	—	—	—	SpF AA HS RSp	—	—	GPS_2 GPS_3
Time between end of EST, ENT, or insulin and stimulation (in months)	5.5	24	2.4	3.1	24	6.4	14	2
POST-STIMULATION EEG's								
No. of recordings	6	2	2	3		3	3	5
Normal recordings	0	0	0	3		1	2	0
Type of abnormality	S_2F SpF	S_3F SSF	S_3F	—		S_3F	S_3F	S_3F SSF
Duration of abnormality after stimulation (in months)	12	4	2	—		10	1	3

*KEY

RSp	Random spikes
S_3	Extremely slow (delta)
BU on HV	Build up on hyperventilation
SpF	Spike focus
AA	Amplitude asymmetry
HS	Hypersynchrony
GPS_2	Generalized paroxysmal moderately slow (theta)
GPS_3	Generalized paroxysmal extremely slow (delta)

(TABLE 1—continued)

10	11	12	13	14	15(8)	16	17	18	19	20	22	24(5)
56	19	23	35	22	41	47	26	39	32	37	21	22
2	—	—	—	—	—	—	—	—	—	—	—	—
—	12	Con-cur-rent	36	15	8	18	12	30	35	96	Con-cur-rent	0.8
PRE-STIMULATION EEG's												
—	1	6	2	2	2	3	2	3	3	1	3	3
—	1	6	2	2	2	3	0	1	3	1	1	3
—	—	—	—	—	—	—	HS RSp	±BU on HV	—	—	GS_2 S_2F	—
No EST	12	1.2	36	17	21	19	14	31	37	96	Con-cur-rent	16.5
POST-STIMULATION EEG's												
3	6	4	2	1	1		1	1	0	1	1	2
2	1	2	0	0	1		0	0	—	1	0	2
RSp	S_3F SSF RSp St	RSp	S_3F RSp	S_2F SS Dep	—		S_2F S_3F HS	GS_2	—	—	GS_3	—
2.5	1	2.5	7	4.5	—		5	4.5	—	—	0.3	—

GS_2 Generalized moderately slow (theta)
S_2F Moderately slow focus (theta)
S_3F Extremely slow focus (delta)
SSF Sleep spindle focus
SS Dep Sleep spindle depression
St Stupor
GS_3 Generalized extremely slow (delta)

Abnormal activity in the form of spikes of various shapes, sizes, frequencies, and durations was noted in subcorticograms obtained from schizophrenic patients. These spikes were not recorded from the cortical surface either in scalp leads, direct cortical leads, or scalp leads combined with indifferent subcortical leads. Significantly increased spiking occurred during drowsiness or light sleep. Emotional influences may sometimes be reflected in the activity of those subcortical structures from which abnormal spike activity is recorded, but considerably more data are required before any positive correlation can be made.

The possible relevance of these results to an understanding of the pathophysiology of schizophrenia has been discussed.

REFERENCES

1. Gibbs, F. A., and E. L. Gibbs. *Atlas of Electroencephalography*, vol. 2: *Epilepsy*. Addison-Wesley, Cambridge, 1952.
2. Hill, D. EEG in episodic psychotic and psychopathic behavior, *Electroencephalog. & Clin. Neurophysiol.*, 4:419–442, 1952. See also Pond, D. A., J. H. Rey, and D. Hill. Biological correlates of constitutional EEG abnormalities of the temporal lobe, *Soc. Proc., 2nd Int. EEG Cong.*, 1:512 (1949), and *Electroencephalog. & Clin. Neurophysiol.*, 2:111 (1950).
3. Williams, D., and G. Parsons-Smith. Spontaneous electrical activity of the human thalamus, *Brain*, 72:450–482 (1949).
4. Meyers, R., J. R. Knott, R. A. Hayne, and D. B. Sweeney. The surgery of epilepsy, *J. Neurosurg.*, 7:337–346 (1950).
5. Gibbs, E. L., and F. A. Gibbs. EEG evidence of thalamic and hypothalamic epilepsy, *Neurology*, 1:136–144 (1951).
6. Spiegel, E. A., and H. T. Wycis. Thalamic recordings in man with special reference to seizure discharges, *Electroencephalog. & Clin. Neurophysiol.*, 2:23–27 (1950).
7. Spiegel, E. A., and H. T. Wycis. *Stereoencephalotomy*, part 1: *Methods and Stereotaxic Atlas of the Human Brain* (*Monographs in Biology and Medicine, vol. 1*). Grune, New York, 1952.
8. Talairach, J., J. de Ajuriaguerra, and H. Hecaen. Étude topographique des images ventriculaires en fonction des noyaux gris centraux, *Ann. méd.*, 51:83–100 (1950).
9. Gastaut, H., and J. Roger. Les Preuves électro-encéphalographiques d'une importante participation thalamique dans les syndromes myocloniques, *in Communications au IVe Congrès Neurologique International*, vol. II, p. 19. Masson, Paris, 1949.

10. Stoll, J., Jr., C. Ajmone-Marsan, and H. Jasper. Electrophysiological studies of subcortical connections of the anterior temporal region in the cat, *J. Neurophysiol.*, 14:305–316 (1951).
11. Merlis, J. K., C. Grossman, and G. F. Henriksen. Comparative effectiveness of sleep and metrazol-activated electroencephalography, *Electroencephalog. & Clin. Neurophysiol.*, 3:71–78 (1951).
12. Pavlov, I. P. *Conditioned Reflexes: An Investigation of the Physiological Activity of the Cerebral Cortex*, Oxford Univ. Press, London, 1927. See also Pavlov, I. P. *Lectures on Conditioned Reflexes, II: Conditioned Reflexes and Psychiatry*, Int. Pubs., New York, 1941.
13. Hess, W. R. *Das Zwischenhirn; Syndrome, Lokalizationen, Functionen.* Schwabe, Basle, 1949.
14. Moruzzi, G., and H. W. Magoun. Brain-stem reticular formation and activation of the EEG, *Electroencephalog. & Clin. Neurophysiol.*, 1:455–473 (1949).

Physiological Data—Electrical Stimulation

INTRODUCTION

ROBERT G. HEATH

As our studies progressed, we felt that the accumulating data were filling in many of the theoretical gaps in our over-all theoretical concept. The electrical recordings reported in Chapter 11 not only appeared to offer some confirmation of our basic hypothesis—that is, that schizophrenia is associated with abnormalities in the septal region of the forebrain—but also suggested that spiking in the septal leads of the subcorticograms might constitute physiological evidence of abnormalities observed in schizophrenic patients by other techniques. Our next and most important problem, then, appeared to be the development of satisfactory techniques for correcting these abnormalities. Chapter 12 will describe our attempts to alter the pathological mechanisms of the disease process by introducing stimuli into the facilitatory circuit of the septal region. The above statements do not imply a localization for schizophrenia in the septal region, but rather that this region is a key area, in which the dynamic process is reflected.

Before the electrical recordings had been completed, stimulation had in fact been used as a therapeutic procedure, but with the finding that spikes consistently occurred in the records of all schizophrenics in whom electrodes were satisfactorily placed, though not in the records of three nonschizophrenic controls, elimination of spikes from the record was regarded as a therapeutic gauge. Spiking was subsequently reduced in varying degrees from the records of different patients. As might be expected, many variables were encountered.

The stimulation procedure itself was of course dependent primarily on the success with which the electrodes were placed. The difficulties inherent in the open method of implantation have been described in detail in Chapter 9. Not only was it impossible to place the electrodes in exactly the same way in the brains of any two persons, but in the interest of the patient it was necessary to remove them soon after the operation. It was therefore impossible to determine over an extended period the degree to which the supposed abnormalities had been eliminated or reduced by electrical stimulation. Although the situation was considerably improved through utilization of the stereotaxic apparatus, we continued to encounter many technical difficulties. As reported in Chapter 10, in the first case in which the closed, or stereotaxic, method was employed the electrodes were moved out of position during closure of the scalp. In the second case the electrodes were not firmly fixed, and so the patient managed to dislodge them before the end of the intended period of observation. The third patient operated upon by the closed method was not schizophrenic; in this case the recordings were so complicated by organic brain disease that the data referable to the changes following stimulation could not be applied to the schizophrenic group.

At the outset it was decided to use the type of stimulus that was most effective in facilitating induced background motor activity in the animals—that is, a frequency of 100 cycles per second, 1 millisecond square wave pulse. We have consistently adhered to this stimulus throughout the patient series thus far, although after the first two stimulations the method of administration was altered. The later changes consisted largely in setting up better safeguards. These will be described in Chapter 12. We are by no means certain that the stimulation used by us is the most effective type that can be administered. Likewise, we are not certain that the most effective way of altering abnormalities in the septal region is by applying a stimulus directly to that site. In the present series of schizophrenic patients, a complication in operative technique made it necessary to stimulate one of the patients in the caudate nucleus, the hypothetical location of the inhibitory circuit. Following this stimulation the patient temporarily improved. It may well be that the most effective way of altering pathological mechanisms in the septal region would be to stimulate elsewhere—in structures which play into the septal region. Since spikes supposedly represent asynchronous massive discharge of cells, it would not be illogical to assume, for example, that a massive inhibitory effect might establish a more normal rhythm. It is possible, too, that introducing a stimulus into an already abnormally firing region would accentuate the abnormality.

Several technical advances have been made in stimulation technique since the meetings held in New Orleans in June, 1952, and a description will therefore be included in Addendum C. Patient 26 (the demonstration patient, see Addendum A) was the first patient without complicating brain disease in whom it was possible to follow recordings for an extended period following stimulation. Although septal spiking was reduced in this patient, persistent slow wave activity appeared after stimulation, indicating the possibility that damage was being done. The whole stimulation procedure was therefore reviewed. It was found that a stimulus of the type used in the last 23 operations resulted in release of gas and changes in pH of the area surrounding the electrode. This had not been so with the type of stimulus given in the first two patients. Accordingly, the stimulation technique was modified.

Following the observation that the one patient in the series who was given caudate stimulation markedly improved, we have, in two patients operated upon since the meetings, again stimulated the caudate region. Insufficient time has elapsed to permit a therapeutic evaluation. In only one of the two cases were septal recordings satisfactory; these indicated that caudate stimulation was temporarily effective in reducing spikes in the records (see Addendum E). In several recent patients following stimulation to the septal region we have recorded persisting high amplitude paroxysmal activity in the septal region. Such activity has not persisted following stimulation to other subcortical structures (see Addendum E).

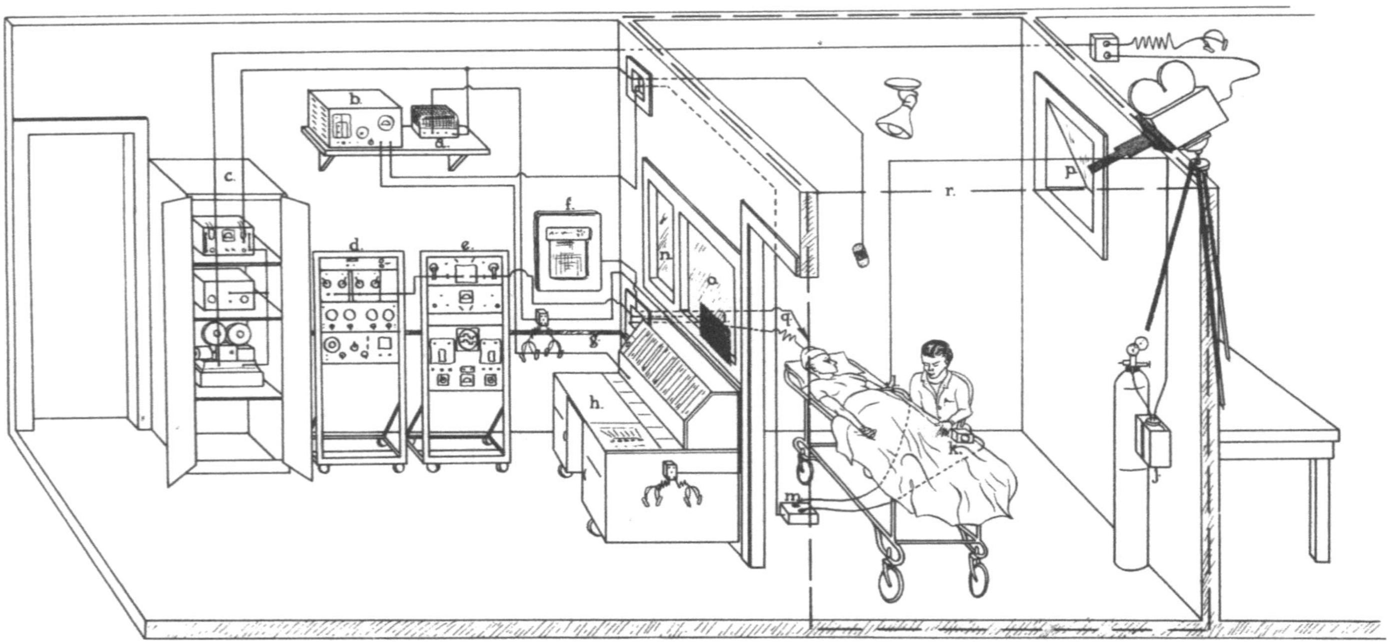

FIGURE XII–1. Cross-section of shielded room and instrument room. (a) Audio amplifier fed by microphone in shielded room, the output being connected to headphones for personnel in instrument room, and fed to motion picture sound-recording equipment. (b) Electronic equipment for recording intra-arterial blood pressure on EEG. (c) Motion picture sound-recording equipment. (d) Electrical stimulating equipment. (e) Stimulus monitor and calibrating equipment. (f) Skin temperature recorder. (g) Electrical ground bus. (h) Electroencephalograph. (i) Stimulate-record panel (in shielded room). (j) Saline reservoir and pressure tank with regulator. (k) Utility blood pressure indicating meter. (l) Blood pressure transducer. (m) Blood pressure junction box. (n) and (o) Semi-transparent mirrors. (p) Motion picture camera port. (q) Thermocouples to eight points on the body. (r) Electrostatic shield. The shielded room is paneled with acoustic tile

CHAPTER 12

SUBCORTICAL STIMULATION TECHNIQUES

HAL C. BECKER
SAMUEL M. PEACOCK, JR.

In research projects like ours, there always arises a conflict between the ideal methodological approach to the various phases of the program and the physical time available in which to make the program productive. In the particular problem of delivering an effective electrical stimulus to specific subcortical structures in man, a compromise is forced among the following requisites: sufficient stimulus to excite the desired neural elements; safeguards against brain damage in the patients; and time and personnel available to develop and construct the special electronic equipment necessary to achieve these ends.

Such equipment not only must be capable of producing such a stimulus but also must have built-in facilities for quantitatively monitoring those parameters necessary to assure reproducibility of the stimulus. The stimulus parameters currently in use in our laboratory represent what we feel to be the best compromise among the factors mentioned above. Addendum D describes these parameters and explains the reasons for their adoption. The present chapter covers the chronological development of the electrical stimulation techniques in use in our laboratory up to the meetings held in New Orleans in June, 1952.

The sketch in Figure 1 shows the physical layout of the various types of electronic and photographic apparatus which were required to produce sound motion pictures of the patient during stimulation and to gather the other data here presented.

Patients 1 and 2 of our series were stimulated in the neurosurgical operating room immediately following electrode placement. The rest of the patients were stimulated in the shielded room shown at the right in Figure 1—Patient 3 having been previously stimulated in the operating room under general anesthesia.

METHODS

Four general methods of electrical stimulation were used in the present series of patients. These methods and the electronic equipment used in them are shown in block diagram in Figure 2. In each method the electrical stimulation routinely consisted of the application of a rectangular voltage pulse of 1 millisecond duration, with a repetition frequency of 100 cycles per second, to the stimulating electrode. The few cases in which other pulse durations and repetition frequencies were used are specified on the Stimulation Data Sheet of the individual patient. The four methods of stimulation came into use in the following order:

A. Grass Model 3C stimulator connected to the stimulating electrode through a General Radio No. 578-A isolation transformer.

B. Model 3C Stimulator connected to the stimulating electrode through Grass Stimulus Isolation Unit, Type SIU-3.

C 1. Same as B, except for the addition of a dual channel D.C. coupled oscilloscope connected between the stimulus isolation unit and the stimulating electrode to provide means for monitoring[1] and measuring the peak amplitudes of the current and voltage of the stimulus pulse. MRP* not used.

C 2. Same as C 1, except that MRP was used.

C 3. Same as C 2, with the addition of another stimulus isolation unit in series with the first to provide the higher stimulus voltages required to maintain the desired stimulus current levels.

D. Same as C 2, except that ERP† was used. This symmetrical stimulus probably tends to reduce brain damage resulting from ion transport[2] instead of MRP to reduce polarization.[3]

The other parameters of stimulation—temporal duration of stimulus, peak current§ of stimulus pulse in milliamperes, peak voltage of stimulus pulse in volts, pulse duration in milliseconds, pulse repetition frequency in cycles per second, type of stimulating electrodes, and location of electrodes—are given in the Stimulation Data Sheet of each patient.

*MRP refers to manual reversal of the polarity of the stimulus pulse at a rate of about 1 per second in order to reduce the effects of electrode polarization at the higher current levels.

†ERP refers to electronic reversal of stimulus pulse polarity.

§The current pulse amplitudes employed in these stimulations were governed by the intensity and type of psychological response obtainable within the limits of immediate physiological safety.

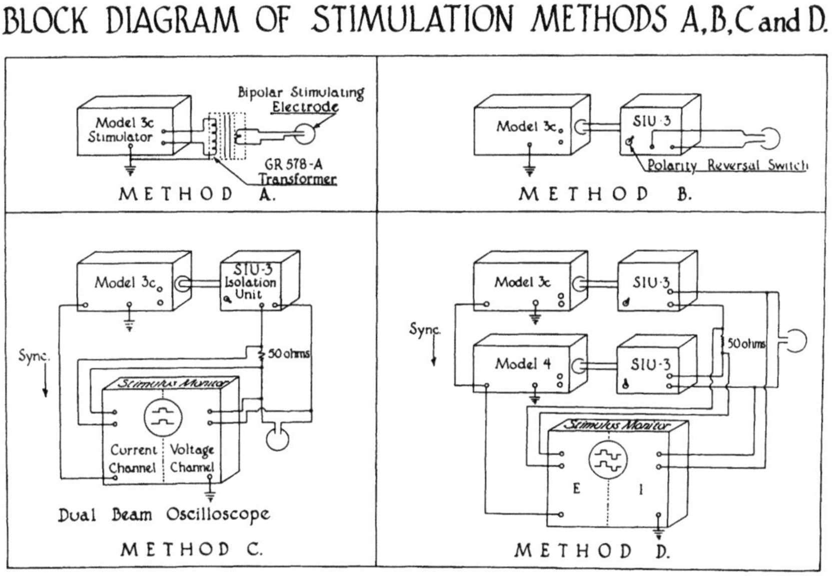

FIGURE XII–2. Block diagram of stimulation methods A, B, C, and D. Method C was used in the majority of the cases reported. See description in text

METHOD A

In Method A, which was used for stimulating Patients 1 to 5, a rectangular stimulus pulse of known voltage, pulse duration, and repetition frequency was applied to the stimulating electrode through a General Radio 578-A isolation transformer, voltage stepdown connected. Since current was not measured in this system, estimates of peak pulse current were made subsequently on the basis of data obtained from animal experiments, in which peak currents were measured with the stimulus monitor, using this same method of stimulation.

METHOD B

In Method B, which was used for stimulating Patients 6 to 8, the Grass Stimulus Isolation Unit was substituted for the G-R isolation transformer. In the majority of the stimulations in which this method was used, and in which the patient had responses that were clinically detectable, it was observed that the most striking and dramatic phase of the response began during the first few seconds of stimulation, and then rapidly decreased in intensity during the next 10 to 20 seconds.

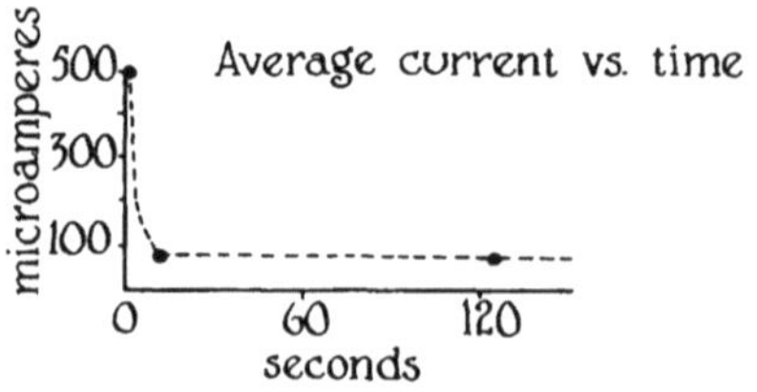

FIGURE XII-3. Polarization, Method B, used in case of Patient 8(15). This shows decrease of average current as a function of time. Repetition freq. = 100 c/sec.; pulse duration = 1 msec.; peak voltage = 16 volts; unidirectional rectangular pulse

The possibility that this effect might be at least partially due to polarization of the stimulating electrode was investigated by inserting a milliammeter in series with the electrode. A typical curve of average current flowing through the tissue in which the electrode was placed versus duration of stimulation is shown in Figure 3. Curves of this sort clearly demonstrated that polarization was taking place in the cases in which such measurements were made.

These undesirable effects (decrease of stimulus current and decrease of intensity of psychological response as a function of time), apparently the result of electrode polarization, were reduced by manually reversing the polarity of the stimulus pulse at a rate of about 1 per second (MRP). In those cases in which it was necessary to go to the higher current levels to produce the various responses the MRP technique served to extend the duration of the responses.

The degree of polarization[4] in each case was, of course, a complicated function of many parameters such as intensity of current, repetition frequency, duration of pulses, electrode surface area, electrode material, total duration of stimulus, and immediate environment of the stimulating electrode.

METHOD C

In order to get quantitative data on the instantaneous current and voltage of the stimulus pulse, reverse voltage and current resulting from the polarization phenomenon, a two-channel dual-beam D.C. coupled oscilloscope was connected to the stimulator-electrode circuit in such a way that two pulses were displayed on the oscilloscope. The amplitude of one of these pulses was made proportional to the intensity of the instantaneous current which flowed between the poles of the bipolar electrode by measuring the voltage drop across a 50 ohm resistor in series with the electrode. The amplitude of the other pulse was made proportional to the instantaneous voltage which appeared across these poles. This system comprised Method C, which was used in the rest of the cases reported. Thus, the addition of the two-channel oscilloscope in its role of stimulus monitor provided quantitative dynamic measurements of instantaneous currents and voltages, respectively flowing between and existing across the poles of the bipolar stimulating electrode. By virtue of these data quantitative determinations could be made of instantaneous current density at the electrode surface, and instantaneous and average power delivered to the electrode.

METHOD D

This method represents a more complicated, but a more satisfactory way of reducing the effects of polarization (that is, decrease of stimulus current with time for a given voltage, production of gas bubbles, alteration of pH, etc.). It differs from the foregoing method in that the potential of alternate pulses is reversed electronically, that is, successive stimulus voltage pulses and, of course, current pulses, are reversed in sign. This method was used in only one case, and adequately served to reduce the polarization to a negligible degree at a current of 11 ma. (peak level).

Figures 4a and 4b demonstrate reduction of polarization with MRP, and further reduction of polarization with ERP. Figures 4c–4j illustrate some other interesting observations made with the Stimulus Monitor, which are described in the captions.

STIMULUS MONITORS

The particular stimulus monitor described above in Methods C and D was inadequate when the peak voltage of the stimulus pulse exceeded 40 to 50 volts. This resulted from the poor common mode rejection characteristic of the two differential oscilloscope input amplifiers at these high voltages. However, this monitor could be used at these voltage levels if the inputs to both current and voltage amplifiers were made single-ended, with one grid of each grounded, and the corresponding pole of the bipolar stimulating electrode grounded. With this connection it was necessary to remove all other grounds from the patient to prevent

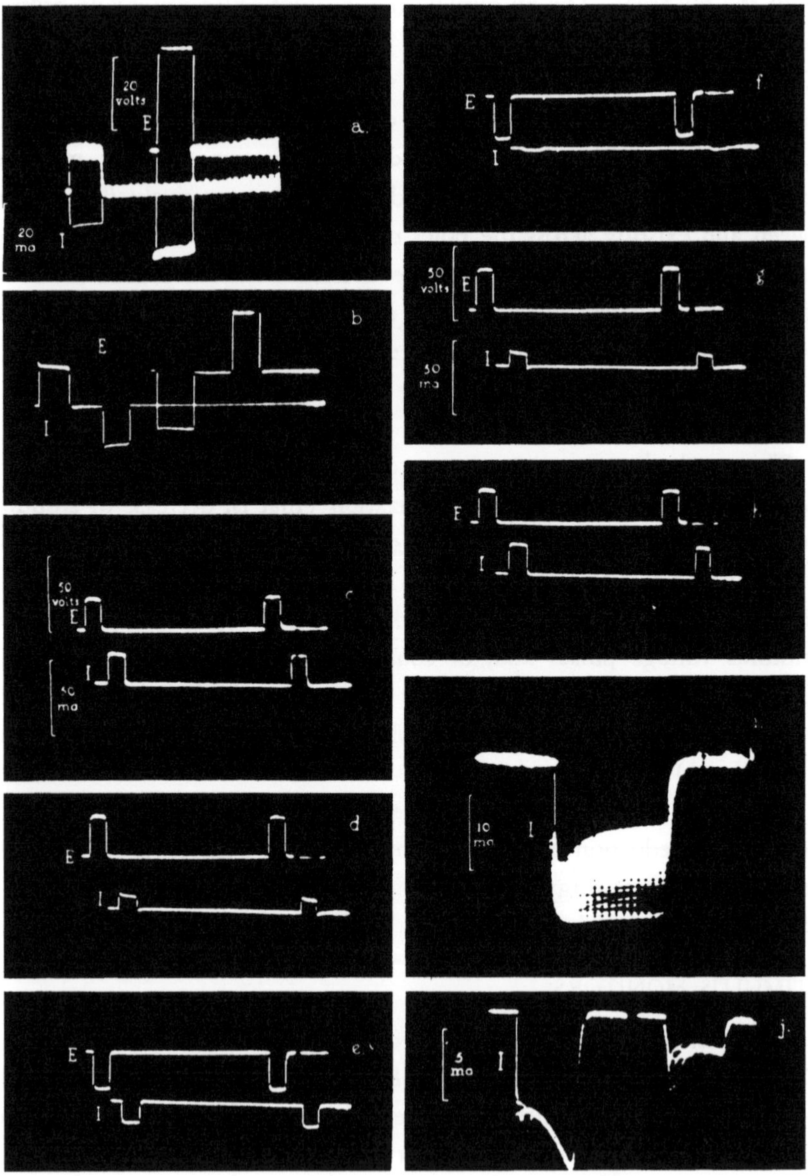
20 volts
E
a.
20 ma
I
b
E
I
50 volts
E
I
50 ma
d
E
I
E
e.
I
f
E
I
50 volts
E
g
50 ma
I
E
I
10 ma
I
5 ma
I
j.

FIGURE XII–4. Photographs of stimulus monitor oscilloscope. (Pulse repetition frequencies are 100 per second. Pulse durations are 1 millisecond. The very fast phases of the CRT trace have been drawn in for clarity.) (a) Time exposure of current and voltage pulses just before and just after reversal of stimulus polarity using MRP. Patient 23. Electrode type 1b. Stimulation Method C. (b) Current and voltage pulses using ERP, demonstrating smaller voltage to current ratio (lower effective resistance) than that in (a) above. Same patient, same electrodes. (c) 5:39 P.M. Stimulus had been on for 7 minutes.

Figures 4c through 4h were photographed serially over a period of 16 minutes. Stimulation method C, electrodes type 2c (bipolar silver spherical electrodes approximately 3/4 mm. in diameter) placed 4 mm. apart in brainstem of Cat No. D1. These figures demonstrate the wide range of currents obtainable (with constant voltage) as a function of electrode history and stimulus polarity. (d) 5:43 P.M. Four minutes later. Note decreased amplitude of current pulse. (e) 5:43:30 P.M. Stimulus polarity was reversed at this time. (f) 5:46:30 P.M. Three minutes later. Note decreased amplitude of current pulse. (g) 5:50 P.M. Stimulus polarity was reversed at 5:49, causing amplitude of current pulse to build up to value shown during the minute from 5:49 to 5:50. Stimulus turned off at 5:50. (h) 5:55 P.M. Five minutes later. Stimulus turned on at this time. Note larger current pulse than in (g), demonstrating depolarization of electrodes while stimulus was off. (i) Time exposure (3 seconds) showing decrease of current pulse amplitude (and contour change) with each successive stimulus pulse from the time when stimulus was turned on. Voltage pulse not shown but was constant at 30 volts during exposure. Electrode type 0. (j) Two time exposures showing erratic current variation resulting from electrode lead fracture at its point of entry into silver ball electrode. Voltage pulse (not shown) was constant during time exposures. Presumably erratic current changes are caused primarily by changes in electrode impedance resulting from formation of gas bubbles on conducting surface of broken wire diffuse spread of current. Figure 5 shows a quantitative determination of diffuse stimulating current resulting from a simulated extraneous ground when "one side grounded" stimulus source is used.

A new dual channel stimulus monitor[5] having good common mode rejection for large common mode input voltages has been designed and is currently in use in this laboratory.

CONNECTION OF ELECTRODES

The stimulating electrodes constitute an integral and obviously critical part of the electrical stimulation system. Ideally they should be treated in this section. However, data on the various types of electrodes used in our series of patients are presented in another section (p. 160), since the authors of the present chapter had virtually no part in the selection of electrode material or in the basic electrode design.

The spherical electrodes used in this series of patients, although "unipolar" from the physical point of view, were always stimulated bipolarly, and in at least this respect they were electrically equivalent to those of the latter type. That is, the spherical electrodes were always stimulated in pairs.

The early method of connecting the electrode leads to the "Stimulate-Record" panel (Figure 6) was simply to solder additional lengths of light, flexible wire to the short leads which emerged from the dressing, and to fit these wires with pin plugs which were inserted into the appropriate pin jacks of the S-R panel. Later, the plug-in arrangement consisting of a plastic headpiece fitted with a special connector,* shown in Figures 7 and 8, was developed by the authors. This was used on the last patient reported.

The electrical connections of the S-R panel were such that operation of the S-R switch allowed the electrode or electrodes plugged into the two S-R jacks to be connected either to the stimulating equipment for stimulation, or to the EEG jack box for recording.

INTRA-ARTERIAL BLOOD PRESSURE MEASUREMENTS

Intra-arterial blood pressure was determined by means of a brachial artery puncture using a special large-bore hypodermic needle (No. 18).

*Cannon Electric Company, No. DA-15.

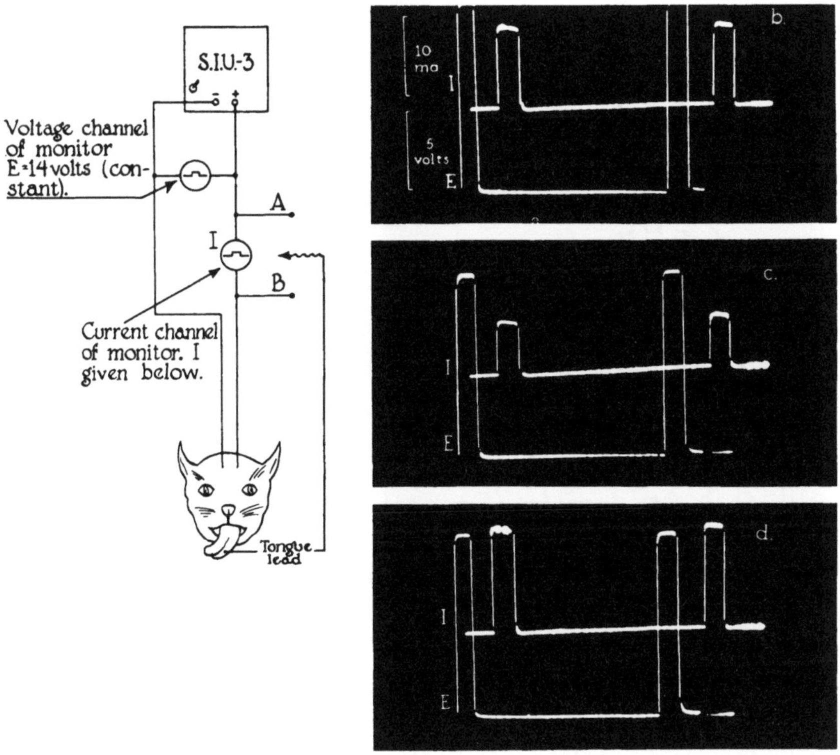

FIGURE XII-5. Quantitative determination of diffuse stimulating current to extraneous ground. (The very fast phases of the CRT trace have been drawn in for clarity.) (a) Diagram of circuit connections to stimulator, stimulus monitor, and animal. Stimulus voltage constant at 14 volts throughout (b), (c), and (d). Pulse repetition frequency, 100 cycles per second. Pulse duration, 1 millisecond. Tongue lead simulates an extraneous ground. Data below provide determination of the diffuse stimulating current which would flow to such a ground if a "one side grounded" stimulus source were used. (b) Photograph of stimulus voltage and current pulses to two type 2c (silver spherical) electrodes spaced approximately 3 mm. apart in white matter. Tongue lead connected to neither A nor B. Current pulse amplitude = 10 ma. (c) Same conditions as (b) except tongue lead connected to point A. Current pulse amplitude = 7 ma. (d) Same conditions as (b) except tongue lead connected to point B. Current pulse amplitude = 14.5 ma. Note that with tongue lead connected to either A or B, the stimulus voltage (14 volts) is applied not only between the two electrodes in the white matter, but also between tongue electrode (alligator clip) and the electrode in the white matter on the left. The voltage drop beween points A and B (monitor current channel input terminals) is negligible in this case. The difference between current pulse amplitudes in (c) and (d) represents the amplitude of the diffuse current flowing from tongue electrode through the brain to the electrode in the white matter on the left

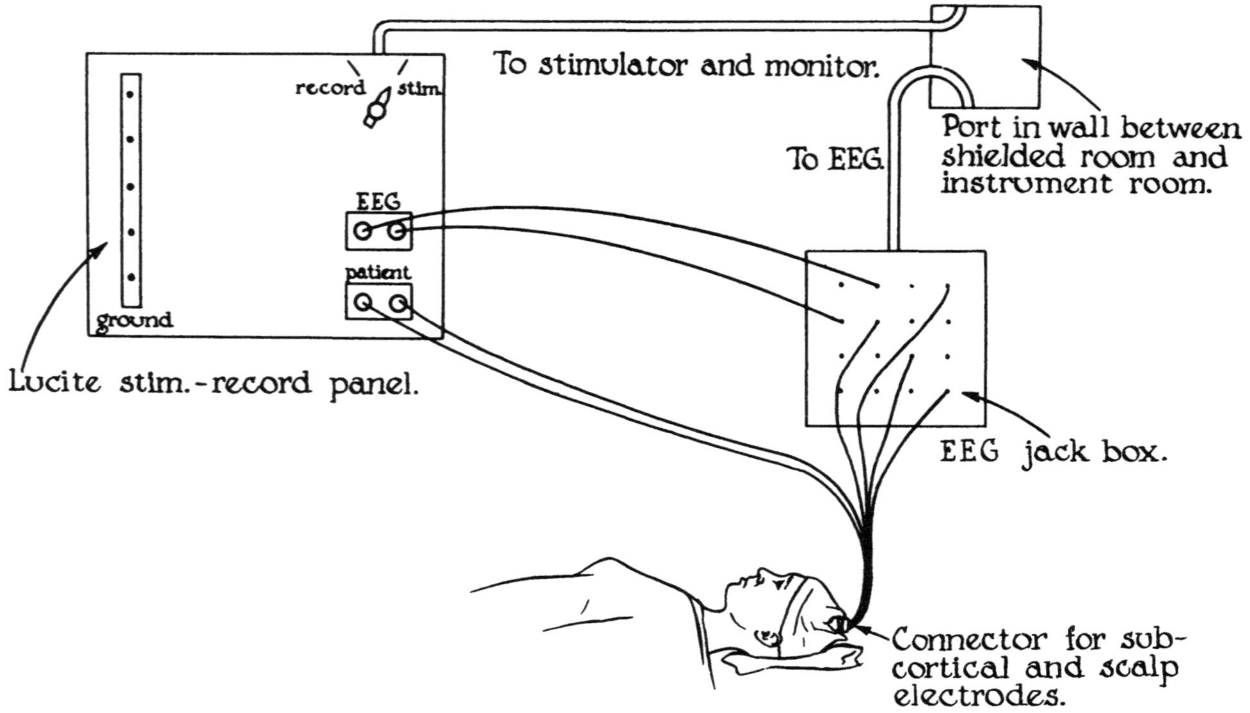

FIGURE XII–6. Electrical connections to patient in shielded room. Detailed sketch of stimulate-record panel (also shown in Figure 1) and its connections to patient, stimulating, equipment, and recording equipment

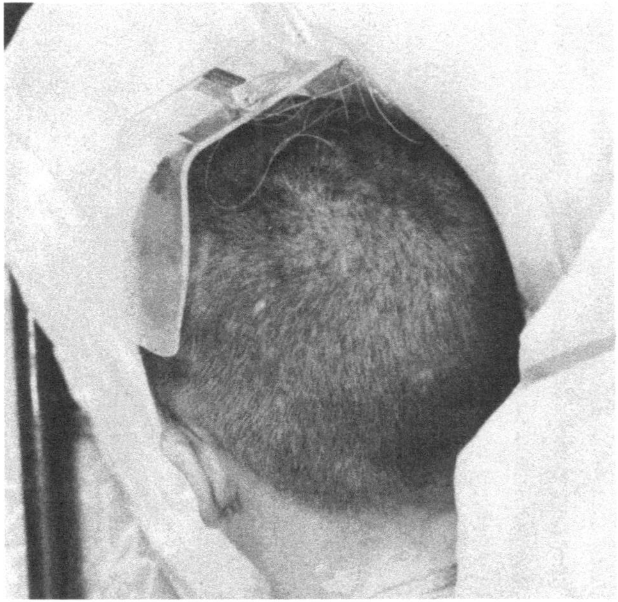

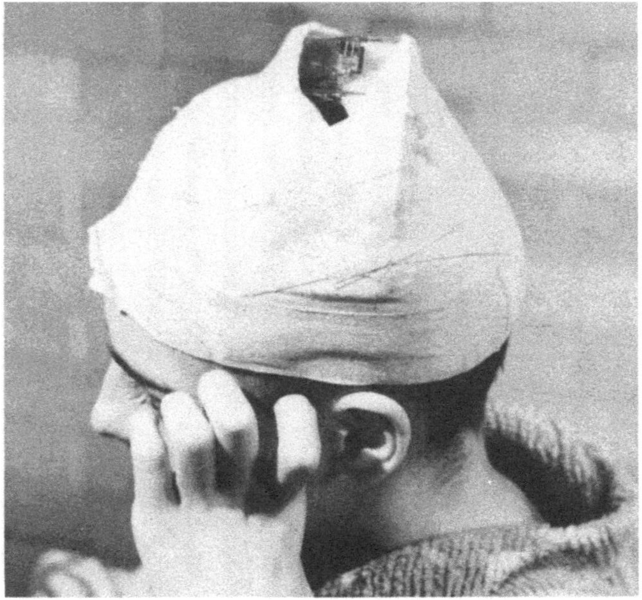

FIGURE XII–7 (left). Plastic headpiece and plug-in electrical connector, with electrode lead wires soldered to connector pins

FIGURE XII–8 (right). Plastic headpiece taped in place

This was connected to a three-way stopcock fitted with a needle valve (Figure 9), which introduced a carefully metered small rate of flow of physiological saline through the needle into the artery to prevent clotting. The saline supply was held under about 15 pounds of pressure. The stopcock was connected to a Hathaway PS–8A pressure-sensing element. The PS–8A element is essentially a differential transformer having for its core a movable ferromagnetic slug connected to a thin corrugated stainless steel diaphragm. This diaphragm was exposed to the instantaneous arterial pressure in the hypodermic syringe. It had a frequency response (0 to 100 cycles per second) such that the arterial pressure pulses were portrayed accurately by the use of appropriate electronic circuits connected to one channel of a Grass electroencephalograph. This channel of the EEG was equipped with a special wide angle pen, so that a pressure range of approximately 40 to 300 millimeters of mercury was spread over a distance of 3 1/2 cm. Since the EEG recorder was in another room, a remote milliammeter calibrated in terms of blood pressure was used as a guide to accomplish the arterial puncture. The "constant flush" method which was used here to prevent clotting is a modification of that described by Peterson and Dripps in 1949.[6] It should be pointed out here that near the upper and lower limits of the blood pressure range, the pen deflection versus pressure was somewhat nonlinear, so that some distortion of pulse contour occurred in those patients in which great BP changes were recorded (see Figure 10).

SKIN TEMPERATURE MEASUREMENTS

Skin temperatures were measured by means of eight iron-constantan thermocouples secured with small pieces of scotch tape to various points of the patient's body. The temperature recording unit was a Leeds and Northrup Speedomax Recording Potentiometer arranged to sample and record the output of each of the eight thermocouples in a cyclic manner once every 32 seconds.

REFERENCES

1. Lane, C. T., W. S. McCulloch, C. H. Prescott, and J. G. Dusser de Barenne. A new method for the investigation of the electrical properties of living tissues, *Am. J. Physiol.*, 113:85–86 (1935).

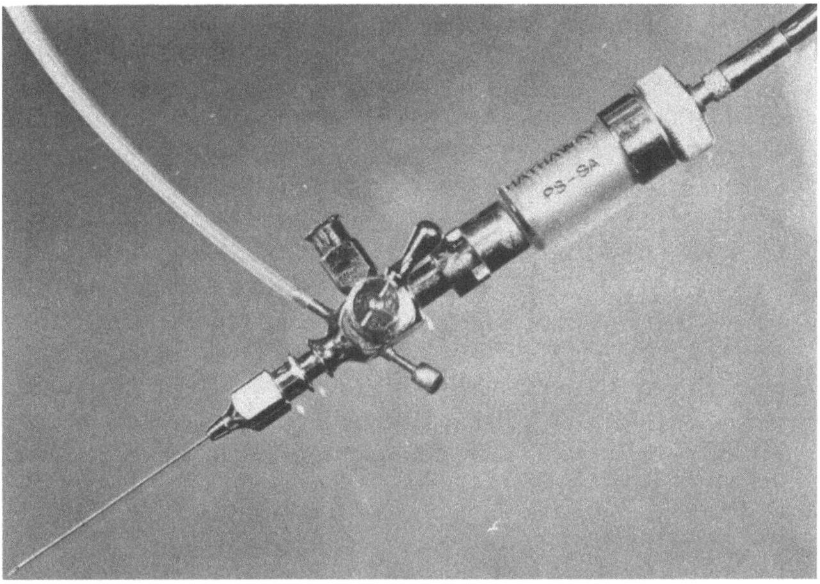

FIGURE XII–9. Special needle valve built into three-way stopcock shown attached to blood pressure transducer and thin wall no. 18 hypodermic needle. Threaded needle valve stem extending toward lower right controls rate of flow of physiological saline

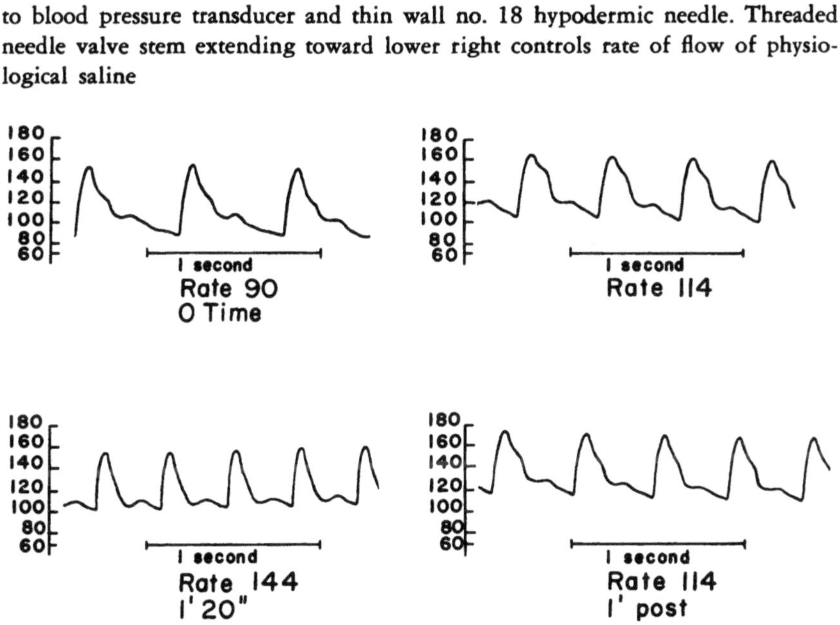

FIGURE XII–10. Samples of pulse contour changes encountered during electrical stimulations. These records show intra-arterial blood pressure and pulse contour wave forms as recorded on one channel of the EEG, using the equipment described in the text

2. Lilly, J. C. Personal communication.
3. Wyss, O. A. M., and S. Obrador. Adequate shape and rate of stimuli in electrical stimulation of the cerebral motor cortex, *Am. J. Physiol.*, 120:42–51 (1937).
4. Jones, G., and S. M. Christian. Galvanic polarization by alternating current, *J. Am. Chem. Soc.*, 57:272–284 (1935).
5. Becker, H. C. A dual channel stimulus monitor ("stimonitor") for electrophysiology (in preparation).
6. Peterson, L. H., R. D. Dripps, and G. C. Risman. A method for recording the arterial pressure pulse and blood pressure in man, *Am. Heart J.*, 37:771 (1949).
7. Lilly, J. C., G. M. Austin, and W. W. Chambers. Threshold movements produced by excitation of the cerebral cortex and efferent fibers with some parametric regions of rectangular current pulses in cats and monkeys, *J. Neurophysiol.*, 15:319–341 (1952).

STIMULATION DATA SHEETS OF PATIENTS 1 TO 25

In each case these data sheets have been "cut" because of space limitations. Only three parametric points are given for each separate stimulation period—one at the beginning, the second at approximately half of the total period, and the third at the end of the period.

The sheets are self-explanatory except for the following points.

Under "Electrode(s)" the numbers and letters in the right column refer to the types of electrodes illustrated in Chapter 11, Figure 3.

Under "Stimulation(s)" the letters in the right column refer to the methods of stimulation described in the present chapter (see Figure 2).

Peak current is given in milliamperes. In cases where the drop was more than approximately 20 per cent during the duration of the current pulse, two figures are given, one over the other. The upper figure represents peak current; the lower figure represents the amplitude of the current pulse at its trailing edge.

Under "Peak voltage" the figures represent the peak voltage of each pulse, as determined by the stimulus monitor.

STIMULATION DATA SHEETS

PATIENT & DATE	SURG. TECH.	ELECTRODE(S) NO.	& TYPE	LOCATION	STIMULATION(S) NO.	& TECH.	DURATION (MIN.–SEC.)	PEAK CUR. (MA.)	PEAK VOLT. (VOLTS)	COMMENTS
1 (4/18/50)	open	1	0	ant. thal.	1st	A			8	No physiological or psychological response
2 (10/18/50)	open	1	0	septal	1st	A	0– 0	1	2	
							0–30	1	2	
					2nd	A	0– 0	1	2	
							0–30	1	2	
					3rd	A	0– 0	3	6	
							0–30	3	6	
					4th	A	0– 0	3	6	
							0–30	3	6	
					5th	A	0– 0	4	8	
							0–20	4	8	Multiple generalized seizures
3 (1/18/51)	open	1	1a	septal						As a result of a shorted electrode patient probably received no current
4 (2/8/51)	open	2	0	septal	1st	A	0– 0	2	4	1st stimulation given in operating room. X-ray revealed broken lead on electrode. Patient probably received no current from 5 later stimulations. No apparent physiological response
			1a				1–00	2	4	

PATIENT & DATE	SURG. TECH.	ELECTRODE (S) NO. & TYPE	LOCATION	STIMULATION (S) NO. & TECH.		DURATION (MIN.–SEC.)	PEAK CUR. (MA.)	PEAK VOLT. (VOLTS)	COMMENTS
5	open		septal	1st	A	0– 0	2	6	
(2/23/51)						1–00	2	6	
See also				2nd	A	0– 0	2	6	No appreciable physiological
Patient 24						1–00	2	6	response
6	open	3 pr. 1a	septal	1st	B	0– 0	2	6	
(3/15/51)						1–00	1	6	
						2–00	0.7	6	
			caudate &	2nd	B	0– 0	3	10	
			thalamus			1–00	1	10	Minimal physiological effects of
						2–00	0	10	diffuse sympathetic type
7	open	3 pr. 1a	high in	1st	B	0– 0	3	10	
(4/25/51)			septal			1–00	1	10	
						2–00	1	10	
				2nd	B	0– 0	6	17	
						0–15	2	17	No apparent physiological
						1–00	1.5	17	response
8	open	3 pr. 1a	septal	1st	B	0– 0	5	14	
(5/2/51)						1–00	1	14	
See also						2–00	1	14	No apparent physiological
Patient 15									response
9	open	3 pr. 1a	septal	1st	C2	0– 0	4	10	
(5/24/51)						1–10	4.8	10	
						2–00	4.8	10	Stimulation produced blood pres-
				2nd	C2	0– 0	8		sure rise from 120/86 to 150/
						1–30	8		106. No other apparent physio-
						2–00	8		logical effect

10	open	3 pr.	1a	septal	1st	C2	0– 0	10	30	
(6/7/51)							0–15	8	22	
							2–00	8	22	
				corp. cal.	2nd	C2	0– 0	4	6	
							2–00	4	6	
				septal	3rd	C2	0– 0	10	30	Stimulation of septal electrode
							3–00	10	30	produced blood pressure rise from
				septal	4th	C2	0– 0	10	20	116/82 to 186/124 with no
							5–00	10	20	other apparent physiological effect.
				septal	5th	C2	0– 0	10	30	Stimulation of corpus callosum
							9–00	10	30	electrode produced no apparent
							11–20	10	30	physiological effect
11	open	3 pr.	1b	septal	1st	C(1)(2)*	0– 0	8	10	Stimulation of septal electrode
(9/20/51)							2–00	8	8	produced mild blood pressure rise
				high in	2nd	C(1)(2)	0– 0	8	4	from 124/80 to 148/100 with
				caud. or			1–00	8	4	no other apparent physiological
				corp. cal. (3)						effect. Stimulation of high cau-
				septal	3rd	C(1)(2)	0– 0	12	8	date electrode produced no ap-
							7–00	14	14	parent physiological effect
							15–00	14	15	*The notation C(1)(2) denotes
										very slow MRP at rate of about
										1/30 sec. This technique was used
										because silverplated electrodes did
										not polarize as rapidly as copper

PATIENT & DATE	SURG. TECH.	ELECTRODE (S) NO. & TYPE	LOCATION LEAD & TIME	STIMULATION (S) NO. & TECH.		DURATION (MIN.–SEC.)	PEAK CUR. (MA.)	PEAK VOLT. (VOLTS)	COMMENTS
12 (10/11/51) (10/12/51)	open	3 pr. 1a							Since the locations of the electrodes were questionable, stimulations at low frequencies were given to determine whether leads 2 and 3 were in internal capsule. Lead 2 was subsequently localized in the caudate, near the capsule. Stimulations 8–22 were given at pulse repetition frequencies of 1–5/sec.; pulse duration of 5 msec., with peak currents up to 20 ma. Total stimulation time was less than 4 min. After stimulation 26 the internal capsule electrode was pulled out about 2 mm., and after stimulation 27 it was withdrawn 2 more mm. Physiological response summary: Stimulation of internal capsule electrode (labeled septum) produced autonomic effects including flushing, sweating, dilatation of
			caudate (near int. cap.) (2) 3:10A	1st	C1	0– 0 0–06	12 12		
			caudate (near int. cap.) (2) 3:19A	2nd	C1	0– 0 0–04	6 6		
			caudate (near int. cap.) (2) 3:27A	3rd	C1	0– 0 2–00	2 2	4 5	
			int. cap. (3) 3:38A	4th	C1	0– 0 2–00	4 4	7 6	
			bas. caud. (1) 3:50A	5th	C1	0– 0 2–00	4 4	5 6	
			caudate (near int. cap.) (2) 4:07A	6th	C1	0– 0 2–17	4 4	9 9	

caudate						pupils, and increased respiration.
(near						The most pronounced effects were
int. cap.) (2)	7th	C1	0– 0	1	3	tonic movements of right arm and
4:50A			2–00	1	2	leg, turning of body to right, and
bas. caud. (1)	23rd	C1	0– 0	4	6	rolling of eyes outward and up-
3:23P			2–45	4	6	ward to right. This was followed
bas. caud. (1)	24th	C1	0– 0	8	10	by a period of stupor. Stimulation
3:33P		C2	2–00	8	12	of the other capsular electrode
bas. caud. (1)	25th	C2	0– 0	12	18	(labeled thalamus) produced sim-
3:50P			2–00	12	26	ilar effects. There were fewer au-
bas. caud. (1)	26th	C2	0– 0	4	6	tonomic responses. Mild sweating,
3:57P			3–00	4	6	dilatation of the pupils, and an
bas. caud. (1)	27th	C2	0– 0	4	6	increased rate in respiration, to-
4:09P			1–00	8	12	gether with the tonic movements
			2–00	8	16	of arm and leg and turning to
caudate						right. Stimulation of basal cau-
(near						date electrode (labeled caudate)
int. cap.) (2)	28th	C2	0– 0	8	12	produced dilatation of pupils and
4:20P			2–00	12	26	at first generalized increase in
			4–00	12	30	motor activity, which gradually
						blended into a decreased state of
						awareness indistinguishable from
						sleep

PATIENT & DATE	SURG. TECH.	ELECTRODE(S) NO. & TYPE	LOCATION LEAD & TIME	STIMULATION(S) NO. & TECH.		DURATION (MIN.–SEC.)	PEAK CUR. (MA.)	PEAK VOLT. (VOLTS)	COMMENTS
13	open	3 pr. 1b	septo-hypothal.	1st	C1	0– 0	2	1	
(10/22/51)			(2)			0–30	2	1	
			septo-hypothal.	2nd	C1	0– 0	4	2.5	
			(2)			2–00	4	2.5	
			left	3rd	C1	0– 0	4	7	
			mid-thal.			0–33	4	7	
			(3)						Stimulation of hypothalamic elec-
			hypothal. (1)	4th	C1	0– 0	2	1.9	trode at 2 ma. produced an initial
						0–36	2	1.9	blood pressure rise from 148/92
			hypothal. (1)	5th	C1	0– 0	4	4	to 175/115, together with dif-
						11–00	6	10	fuse sympathetic discharge, clonic
					C2	16–50	4	6	movement of right arm and leg,
			septo-hypothal.	6th	C2	0– 0	4	3	left internal strabismus, followed
			(2)			1–54	4	3	by convergence as current was in-
			hypothal. (1)	7th	C2	0– 0	4	3	creased. Patient complained of
						23–40	4	3	nervousness, urinary urgency, and
						40–00	4	3	chills. Stimulation of septo-hypo-
			septo-hypothal.	8th	C2	0– 0	6	4	thalamic electrode produced no
			(2)			1–30	8	6	immediate blood pressure response
						4–00	8	6	but as current was increased pres-
			left	9th	C2	0– 0	4	4	sure rose from 140/70 to 190/
			mid-thal.			2–30	4	5	108. Tachycardia of 180, flushing,
			(3)			6–00	6	8	sweating, and dilatation of the

			hypothal. (1)	10th	C2	0– 0	10	10	pupils were noted; and as stimu-
							10	9	lation was continued there devel-
			hypothal. (1)	11th	C2	0– 0	12	12	oped clonic 3/sec. movement of
						1–30	12	10	right thumb with what appeared
			hypothal. (1)	12th	C2	0– 0	2	2	to be a petit mal variant seizure.
						2–00	2	2	Stimulation of left midthalamic
			hypothal. (1)	13th	C2	0– 0	6	5	electrode produced apnea, asso-
						12–00	6	5	ciated with a decreased sense of
						16–00	6	5	awareness
14	open	3 pr. 1b							Stimulation of septo-hypothalamic
(11/21/51)									electrode at 2 ma. produced initial
(11/22/51)			septo-hypothal.	1st	C2	0– 0	4	4	blood pressure rise from 120/86
			(2)			2–00	4	4	to 210/160. This response was
			8:42A						a maximal one, pressure dropping
				2nd	C2	0– 0	8	6	as stimulation was continued to
			9.03A			4–40	8	6	160/90. Tachycardia of 174,
						6–20	8	6	flushing, sweating, dilatation of
				3rd	C2	0– 0	2	1	pupils, tremor, and increased rate
			11:28A			5–10	6	4	of respiration were noted and pa-
						10–55	8	4	tient expressed great fear, which
				4th	C2	0– 0	8	6	lasted for some minutes following
			1:09P			3–00	8	6	stimulation

PATIENT & DATE	SURG. TECH.	ELECTRODE (S) NO. & TYPE	LOCATION LEAD & TIME	STIMULATION (S) NO. & TECH.		DURATION (MIN.–SEC.)	PEAK CUR. (MA.)	PEAK VOLT. (VOLTS)	COMMENTS
15	open	3 pr. 1b	septal (2)	1st	C2	0– 0	4	3	Stimulation of septal electrode pro-
(12/6/51)			10:49P			3–00	4	3	duced blood pressure rise from
See also				2nd	C1	0– 0	6	3	140/80 to 160/86. Heart rate
Patient 8			11:26P			2–10	8	6	increased slightly, and patient
						3–00	8	6	gradually became cyanotic and
				3rd	C2	0– 0	10	8	then apneic. There were tonic
			11:33P			1–00	10	8	movements of right arm and leg
						1–57	6	4	and patient became disoriented
(12/7/51)				4th	C2	0– 0	4	3	after stimulation but said he felt
			12:54A			3–50	6	4	more relaxed. Several minutes
						10–17	6	4	after stimulation he went into
									generalized convulsion
16	open	3 pr. 1b	septal (1)	1st	C2	0– 0	2	1	
(12/11/51)			11:13P			1–07	2	1	
			septal (1)	2nd	C2	0– 0	6	2	
			11:23P			1–15	6	2	
						2–01	6	2	
			septal (1)	3rd	C2	0– 0	10	4	
			11:49P			0–45	10	5	
						2–02	10	5	
(12/12/51)			septo-hypothal.	4th	C2	0– 0	4	1	
			(2)			1–10	4	1	
			12:10A			2–07	4	1	

				septo-hypothal.	5th	C2	0– 0	10	2	
				(2)			4–10	14	4	
				12:41A			8–00	14	4	
				septo-hypothal.	6th	C2	0– 0	12	4	
				(2)			4–25	16	5	
				2:11A			10–00	16	5	
				septal(1)	7th	C2	0– 0	12	10	
				2:42A			2–38	16	14	
							5–01	16	14	Stimulation of septal electrode produced blood pressure rise from 120/87 to 130/98. Stimulation of septo-hypothalamic electrode produced blood pressure rise from 118/80 to 178/110. Patient complained of agitation
				septo-hypothal.	8th	C2	0– 0	6	2	
				(2)			1–25	6	2	
				3:05A			2–00	6	2	
				septal(1)	9th	C2	0– 0	6	5	
				3:25A			1–45	6	5	
							2–30	6	5	
17	open	3 pr.	1b							
(12/19/51)										
(12/20/51)				septal(2)	1st	C2	0– 0	4	5	
				2:58A			3–35	4	6	
							4–00	4	6	
				vent. hypothal.	2nd	C2	0– 0	2	2	
				(1)			3–05	6	7	
				3:23A			4–00	6	7	
				vent. hypothal.	3rd	C2	0– 0	8	9	
				(1)			5–00	8	9	
				3:50A						

17 (continued on next page)

PATIENT & DATE	SURG. TECH.	ELECTRODE (S) NO. & TYPE	LOCATION LEAD & TIME	STIMULATION (S) NO. & TECH.		DURATION (MIN.–SEC.)	PEAK CUR. (MA.)	PEAK VOLT. (VOLTS)	COMMENTS
17 (continued)									Stimulation of septal electrode
(12/20/51)			vent. hypothal.	4th	C2	0– 0	6	6	produced blood pressure rise from
			(1)			2–00	6	6	110/70 to 180/100. The sus-
			4:56A						tained effect was erratic; tachy-
			septal (2)	5th	C2	0– 0	8	9	cardia of 162 and a startle reac-
			4:59A			3–00	10	13	tion were noted, both eyes opened,
						6–00	12	17	and patient expressed fear. Stimu-
			vent. hypothal.	6th	C2	0– 0	4	4	lation of ventral hypothalamic
			(1)			3–00	4	4	electrode produced blood pressure
			5:35A						rise from 140/80 to 200/120.
			vent. hypothal.	7th	C2	0– 0	12	13	Again maintenance of this pres-
			(1)			2–00	14	16	sure was erratic; marked tachy-
			6:15A			5–00	14	17	cardia, startle reaction, and open-
			thalamic (3)	8th	C2	0– 0	2	5	ing of the eyes were noted, as well
			6:39A			1–25	6	12	as right external strabismus. The
						1–45	6	12	patient again complained of fear.
			septal (2)	9th	C2	0– 0	4	4	Stimulation of thalamic electrode
			6:45A			0–40	8	8	had no apparent physiological
						2–00	8	8	effect

18	open	3 pr.	1b						
(1/8/52)									
(1/9/52)				septal (3)	1st	C2	0– 0	4	5
				12:11A			1–00	4	5
							2–00	4	5
				septal (3)	2nd	C2	0– 0	8	10
				12:27A			3–50	12	20
							5–45	14	25
				septo-hypothal.	3rd	C2	0– 0	4	7
				(1)			0–20	4	7
				12:57A					
				septal (3)	4th	C2	0– 0	6	8
				1:32A			2–00	6	7
				septo-hypothal.	5th	C2	0– 0	2	4
				(1)			1–35	2	3
				2:01A			4–50	2	3
				septo-hypothal.	6th	C2	0– 0	2	3
				(1)			4–48	3	4
				2:20A					
				septal (3)	7th	C2	0– 0	6	5
				2:31A			2–00		
							6–25		
				septal (3)	8th	C2	0– 0	6	6
				3:31A			2–30	10	10
							3–00	10	10
				septo-hypothal.	9th	C2	0– 0	2	3
				(1)			10–01	2	3
				3:40A					

18 (continued on next page)

PATIENT & DATE	SURG. TECH.	ELECTRODE (S) NO. & TYPE	LOCATION LEAD & TIME	STIMULATION (S) NO. & TECH.	DURATION (MIN.–SEC.)	PEAK CUR. (MA.)	PEAK VOLT. (VOLTS)	COMMENTS
18 (continued)								
(1/9/52)			septal (3)	10th C2	0– 0	12	11	
			4:11A		2–05	17	22	
					5–00	17	22	
			septal (3)	11th C2	0– 0	14	18	
			4:30A		5–40	20	22	
					15–00	16	17	Stimulation of septal electrode
			septal (3)	12th C2	0– 0	14	14	produced initial rise in blood
			5:14A		3–00	16	16	pressure from 116/76 to 142/96.
					32–07	16	16	This response was maintained.
			septo-hypothal.	13th C2	0– 0	2	2	There was tachycardia; patient be-
			(1)		2–00	2	3	came pale and sweaty and both
			6:19A					pupils were seen to dilate. Stimu-
			septo-hypothal.	14th C2	0– 0	3	3	lation of septo-hypothalamic elec-
			(1)		3–00	4	4	trode produced blood pressure
			6:33A					response of 180/120, and there
			septal (3)	15th C2	0– 0	14	13	was tachycardia of 192. Patient
			6:36A		1–30	16	15	flushed, sweated, and complained
					10–00	16	15	of feeling faint. Dilatation of the
			leads 1 to 3	16th C2	0– 0	1	2	pupils was noted first on right
			7:07A		1–15	4	4	side and then on both sides.
					4–00	6	7	Stimulation between these two
			septal (3)	17th C2	0– 0	14	14	leads produced sweating, and pa-
			7:30A		30–00	19	24	tient was seen to make a tonic fist

19	open	3 pr.	1b							
(1/22/52)										
(1/23/52)				thalamic (2)	1st	C2	0– 0	0.5	1	
				4:23A			2–15	2.2	4	
							5–00	4.8	7	
				rost. hypothal.	2nd	C2	0– 0	0.6	3	
				(1)			2–40	4	22	
				4:33A			3–30	4	22	
				thalamic (2)	3rd	C2	0– 0	4	7	
				4:53A			1–30	12	21	Stimulation of rostral hypothalamic electrode (lead 1) produced marked slowing and deepening in respiration. Stimulation of rostral hypothalamic electrode (lead 3) had no apparent physiological effect except a marked internal strabismus. Stimulation of thalamic electrode (lead 2) had no apparent effect. This patient developed acute cardiac failure immediately after operation and was digitalized rapidly. He was exhibiting a pulsus alternans at time of stimulation. Blood pressure was 250/150; pulse rate was 168; respiration was 32
							2–20	12	21	
				rost. hypothal.	4th	C2	0– 0	2	2	
				(3)			1–25	12	12	
				5:00A			2–35	14	16	
				rost. hypothal.	5th	C2	0– 0	6	20	
				(1)			1–35	8	30	
				5:11A			2–05	8	30	
				rost. hypothal.	6th	C2	0– 0	40	20	
				(3)			2–10	10	10	
				5:19A			10–00	10	8	
				thalamic (2)	7th	C2	0– 0	15	23	
				5:58A			4–15	9	34	
							10–00	9	32	
				rost. hypothal.	8th	C2	0– 0	15	12	
				(3)			11–45	10	10	
				7:16A			33–03	4	4	

PATIENT & DATE	SURG. TECH.	ELECTRODE(S) NO. & TYPE		LOCATION LEAD & TIME	STIMULATION(S) NO. & TECH.		DURATION (MIN.–SEC.)	PEAK CUR. (MA.)	PEAK VOLT. (VOLTS)	COMMENTS
20 (1/31/52) (2/1/52)	open	2 pr.	1b							Stimulation of septal electrode produced initial rise in blood pressure from 130/80 to 200/120. There was generalized sympathetic discharge. Patient said she felt warm and faint. Stimulation of septo-hypothalamic electrode produced marked blood pressure rise. Current was kept on for 4 sec. During this time there was diffuse sympathetic discharge, and patient said she felt pins and needles all over. Blood pressure continued elevated for some time
				septal(2) 12:44A	1st	C2	0– 0	4	10	
							1–30	4	11	
							3–10	4	13	
				septal(2) 1:03A	2nd	C2	0– 0	6	14	
							2–25	8	22	
							6–00	8	20	
				septo-hypothal. (1) 2:13A	3rd	C1	0– 0	4	6	
							0–08	4	6	
				septal(2) 3:54A	4th	C2	0– 0	2	3	
							5–10	2	4	
							10–00	2	4	
21 (3/6/52) (3/8/52)	stereo-taxic	3	2a							
				rost. sept. (11–12) 12:06A	1st	C2	0– 0	2	2	
							1–30	2	2	
				rost. sept. (11–12) 12:10A	2nd	C2	0– 0	4	3	
							1–30	4	3	

				rost. sept.	3rd	C2	0– 0	8	5	
				(11–12)			2–01	8	5	
				12:12A						Stimulation of rostral septal elec-
				rost. sept.	4th	C2	0– 0	12	6	trode produced blood pressure rise
				(11–12)			1–55	14	8	from 118/68 to 170/110. In-
				12:22A			2–30	14	8	creased pulse rate, dilatation of
				septal	5th	C2	0– 0	2	2	pupils, and generalized tremor
				(12–13)			2–45	15	4	were noted. Stimulation of septal
				1:45A			5–30	20	6	electrode produced no blood pres-
				septal	6th	C2	0– 0	12	4	sure response. However, there
				(12–13)			1–35	24	10	were increases in pulse rate and
				1:58A			4–00	30	12	flushing. *Isolation unit was not
				rost. sept.	7th	C2	0– 0	40	14	used here. The output of the
				(11–12)			5–00	20	12	Model 3C stimulator was con-
				2:06A			10–00	30	16	nected to electrodes through the
				rost. sept.	8th*		0– 0	20	8	monitor and patient was complete-
				(11–12)			6–00	40	18	ly ungrounded elsewhere. MRP
				3:32A			12–00	40	36	throughout stimulation no. 8
22 (3/25/52)	stereo-taxic	8	2b		This patient received a total of 12 stimulations to 5 combinations of 8 subcortical electrodes which appeared on x-ray to be pulled up into the subcortical white matter. Current pulse amplitudes ranged from 2 to 20 ma.; durations ranged from 1–50 to 12–36					Stimulation produced motor responses characteristic of stimulation of area 6 and/or area 8, which involved complex movements of eyes and of left and sometimes of right side of the face, arms and legs. Associated with this was generalized autonomic discharge

PATIENT & DATE	SURG. TECH.	ELECTRODE(S) NO. & TYPE	LOCATION LEAD & TIME	STIMULATION(S) NO. & TECH.		DURATION (MIN.–SEC.)	PEAK CUR. (MA.)	PEAK VOLT. (VOLTS)	COMMENTS
23	open	3 pr. 1b	septal	1st	C1	0– 0	2		Stimulation of septal electrode pro-
(3/27/52)			(13–14)		C2	4–20	11	30	duced initial blood pressure rise
(3/28/52)			12:28A		C2	10–00	11	30	from 134/76 to 160/105. Tachy-
			septo-hypothal.	2nd	D	0– 0	2	2	cardia and flushing were noted,
			(15–16)			7–45	2	2	and pre-existing tremor was seen
			1:20A						to stop. Patient became euphoric.
			septal	3rd	D	0– 0	4 to 8		Stimulation of septo-hypothalamic
			(13–14)			1–15	12	16	electrode with current pulse of 2
			2:16A			10–00	11	16	ma. produced initial blood pres-
			septal	4th	C2	0– 0	10		sure rise from 140/80 to 180/
			(13–14)			3–30	18		135, associated with tachycardia
			2:31A			20–10	10	26	of 172, flushing and sweating.
									Patient experienced brief episode
									of auricular fibrillation, pupils
									dilated, and eyes converged. Re-
									peated stimulation of the septal
									electrode threw patient into gen-
									eralized convulsion and status
									epilepticus

24 (4/11/52) See also Patient 5 (4/12/52)	stereo-taxic	7	2b							Stimulation of septal electrode (leads 12–13) produced rise in blood pressure from 110/76 to 144/110. This was associated with marked tachycardia, flushing, and sweating. Stimulation of septal electrode (leads 11–13) produced blood pressure response of 150/100. There was marked tachycardia, and alternating movements of both hands with MRP were noted
				septal (12–13) 7:53A	1st	C1	0– 0	2		
						C2	5–20	12	12	
						C2	10–00	18		
				septal (12–13) 8:18A	2nd	C2	0– 0	8		
							4–30	28	20	
							10–00	32	22	
				septal (11–13) 5:32P	3rd	C1	0– 0	4		
						C2	4–20	18	16	
						C3	13–40	34	22	
25 (5/1/52)	stereo-taxic	5	2b	septal (2–3) 11:56P	1st	C2	0– 0	2	0	
							4–10	10	9	
							8–10	20	18	
(5/2/52)				septal (3–4) 12:28A	2nd	C2	0– 0	6		
							1– 0	6		
				septal (3–4) 12:33A	3rd	C2	0– 0	8	9	
							5–15	16	14	
							12–15	20	17	
				hypothal. (4–5) 12:59A	4th	C2	0– 0	4		
							1–45	12	15	
							3–15	20	20	

25 (continued on next page)

PATIENT & DATE	SURG. TECH.	ELECTRODE(S) NO. & TYPE	LOCATION LEAD & TIME	STIMULATION(S) NO. & TECH.		DURATION (MIN.–SEC.)	PEAK CUR. (MA.)	PEAK VOLT. (VOLTS)	COMMENTS
25 (continued)									
(5/2/52)			septal(2–3)	5th	C2	0– 0	8		
			1:15A			0–20	12		
						1–35	22	20	
			septal(2–3)	6th	C2	0– 0	6	6	
			12:09P			10–00	24	32	
						20–15	24*		
			leads 2–4	7th	C2	0– 0	8	7	
			3:26P			4–00	20	16	
						10–30	20	16	
			hypothal.	8th	C2	0– 0	6		
			(4–5)			1–35	14	15	
			4:34P			3–40	20	17	
			septal(2–3)	9th	C2	0– 0	2*	20	
			5:08P			0–58	2		
			septal(2–3)	10th	C2	0– 0	4		
			5:13P			0–12	?		
(5/6/52)			leads 2–4	11th	C2	0– 0	8	8	
			3:18P			10–00	22	16	
						22–10	22	22	
			leads 1–2	12th	C2	0– 0	2		
			3:55P			3–15	18	16	
						6–20	18	16	

	septal (2–3) 4:14P	13th	C2	0– 0	?		Stimulation of septal electrode (leads 2–3) produced initial blood pressure rise from 135/80 to 140/90. Pressure rose to 190/100 as current was increased. There was marked tachycardia. Stimulation of the septal electrode (leads 3–4) produced initial blood pressure response of 160/100 and as current was increased the pressure rose to 200/115, accompanied by marked tachycardia. Stimulation of hypothalamic electrode produced an initial blood pressure response of 200/110; again there was marked tachycardia, and in this case internal strabismus was noted. Patient said she felt tense. Stimulation on subsequent days was less effective, and 7 days postoperatively there was a reversal in effect—patient showing slower pulse rate and drop in blood pressure on septal stimulation. *Current erratic as a result of a defect in lead 3
				0–50	8*		
	leads 1–4 4:25P	14th	C2	0– 0	4	5	
				2–15	20	17	
				4–45	26	20	
(5/9/52)	leads 2–4 3:40P	15th	C1	0– 0	4	5	
			C2	5–00	10		
			C2	10–00	24	18	
	leads 1–4 4:07P	16th	C2	0– 0	4	4	
				2–40	12	9	
				5–25	12	9	

CHAPTER 13

PHYSIOLOGICAL RESPONSES TO SUBCORTICAL STIMULATION

SAMUEL M. PEACOCK, JR.

The data to be described in this particular report will deal with the physiological effects observed at the time of electrical stimulation of our series of patients. It has been pointed out from time to time in the preceding chapters that many variables were unavoidable throughout the project and that this fact has necessitated discussions of the patients individually rather than classifications in groups according to some common factor or factors.

The major factors confounding the physiological data are primarily the localization of electrodes within the brain, the dearth of quantitative information on the spread of current flux in the subcortical structures of variable homogeneity for various electrode configurations, and the almost complete lack of information on current thresholds (as opposed to voltage thresholds) in a parametric line in the various neural structures involved.

In the parametric sets used throughout this project, only pulse duration and pulse repetition frequency were maintained as fixed parameters from patient to patient, while train duration, train repetition frequency, pulse amplitude, and electrode design and locale varied widely from one stimulation to the next in each patient, and from patient to patient. Frequently there were no appreciable effects until current pulse amplitude was increased to fairly high levels, and yet, on the other hand, there were occasional electrode positions which produced vigorous physiological responses at very low current pulse amplitudes. When this occurred, however, psychological responses were usually unfavorable. It should be emphasized that the psychological response governed the intensity of the stimulus within the obvious limits of physiological safety and that the parameters used to produce the desired psychological response varied greatly. It is probable that this variability in "threshold" was primarily a function of electrode position and, to a lesser extent, electrode design. In a majority of the patients, despite the many variables, a certain uniformity in physiological response was seen, but because of the difficulties in electrode localization and the high current pulse amplitudes used, only the most guarded localization of function should be made from this physiological data.

The observations reported were made by at least three members of the team. The observation room routinely contained one member at the patient's side, one to conduct the psychiatric interview, another to handle the intra-arterial blood pressure apparatus, and another to assist in the event of any untoward effects from electrical stimulation. Physiological responses were noted by all observers, and a report was dictated immediately after stimulation. Since there was an element of the unknown in each stimulation, all responses, regardless of type or timing were noted. These seemed to be restricted primarily to the various autonomic and somatic motor responses of various types and in various distributions.

The recording of intra-arterial blood pressure as a continuous record became desirable as the project progressed.* It was found that, during the course of the stimulations early in the project, when patients were appearing to "brighten" during stimulation, they were also showing moderate rises in blood pressure and other vasomotor phenomena. It was therefore decided to abandon the use of the clinical sphygmomanometer in favor of a continuous intra-arterial recording of blood pressure in those patients cooperative enough to permit arterial puncture. The continuous record of blood pressure during the course of stimulation gave some indication of the physiological effectiveness of stimulation, although this was not always correlated with psychological changes. It also served as a warning in those cases in which blood pressure and pulse rates showed very brisk rises at low stimulus intensities.

It is important to remember that the experimental technique evolved gradually as the project progressed. For example, the first two patients were stimulated in the operating room under direct vision via a long bipolar concentric electrode. Patients 1 to 7 had very low current pulse

*Although in many cases excellent pulse contours were obtained, no attempt has been made to analyze the records for the possible significance of the changes in contour recorded. Such an analysis awaits more complete data.

amplitudes and stimulations of relatively short duration, and hence there was a minimal physiological response. As time went on, however, it became customary to increase pulse amplitude gradually in 2 or 3 ma. steps over the course of the stimulation period, which varied from a few seconds to over 30 minutes, depending upon the magnitude and nature of the psychological and physiological responses observed. Some patients received several stimulations of this type from each of three bipolar electrodes. Intra-arterial blood pressure recording was started on Patient 13, for the reasons given above, and has since been used routinely up to the present time when possible. The intra-arterial cannula was usually left in place long enough to obtain records from the stimulation of each electrode position in each patient. This resulted in a minimum continuous recording over a 2-hour period and in some cases much longer.

OBSERVATIONS

As it is felt to be unwise to group these patients either with respect to their responses or to electrode placement, for the reasons discussed above, they will be taken up here individually. A summary of these results is seen in Table 1. The first seven patients are omitted from this chart, since with one exception they showed minimal physiological responses.

Of the first seven patients, only Patient 2 had an appreciable response. As mentioned above, she was stimulated in the operating room under local anesthesia. A bipolar concentric electrode was implanted in the septal region under direct vision. As the pulse amplitude was increased slightly, the patient went into a generalized convulsion and continued to have a series of such seizures during the first postoperative day. She remained in stupor or semi-stupor for several days, and it was even deemed necessary at this time to perform a tracheotomy. After the first few days her recovery was rapid and uneventful.

The remaining five patients had electrodes implanted in the septal region by the open technique. Stimulation was delayed in these patients until they had reacted from the anesthesia, except in the case of Patient 3, who was also stimulated in the operating room under anesthesia without any effects.

Patients 8, 9, and 10 all underwent stimulations of the septal region and showed only moderate blood pressure rises. There was no other apparent physiological response in these patients, but it is believed that in some of them psychological responses were quite profound (see Chapter 17).

Patient 10 also had a single anterior thalamic stimulation, again without observable effect. The pulse amplitude of all stimulations in the first ten patients was of 10 ma. or less, at a repetition frequency of 100 pulses per second, with a pulse duration of 1 msec. However, on this first group, stimulus was not monitored, so that these parameters insofar as pulse amplitude and wave form are concerned are only approximate.

With Patient 11, an extremely important modification in technique was made in the introduction of a stimulus monitor into the stimulating circuit (Chapter 12). In this case peak current to the septal electrodes was taken to 14 ma. This produced a moderate rise in blood pressure from 124/80 to 148/100, and with the maintenance of a relatively constant *current* pulse amplitude, the response was maintained for the duration of stimulation. Prior to this, each response had been primarily an "on" effect, gradually decreasing as the current pulse decayed with polarization. Stimulation to a second pair of electrodes in the region of the caudate nucleus was ineffective in this patient. Localization on the early group of patients was relatively inaccurate, however, so that there is a possibility that this electrode was elsewhere.

Patient 12 inadvertently had two bipolar electrodes placed in the region of the internal capsule on the side opposite to that of entry into the brain, and one in the basal portion of the caudate nucleus on that side. Stimulation to the capsular region evoked tonic high frequency responses of the right arm and leg, with turning of the head and trunk toward the right side and conjugate movement of the eyes in this direction. This response was accompanied by flushing, sweating, pupillary dilatation, and an increase in respiratory rate. Single pulse stimulation of these structures, or stimulation carried out at 2 pulses per second, produced phasic movements of these same contralateral extremities. High frequency stimulation was followed in each case by semi-stupor, which lasted for several minutes. Stimulation to the electrode in the basal part of the

TABLE XIII–1. Autonomic and motor responses following stimulation of Patients 8–25. Patient 5 received a second stimulation (see Patient 24), as did Patient 8 (see Patient 15)

NOTE: Some shifts in localization were made after the data in this chart were compiled. In Patient 10 the electrode intended for the anterior thalamus was localized in the corpus callosum. In Patient 11 it was thought that the "high caudate" electrode might also have involved the corpus callosum. In Patient 12 lead 2 was localized in the caudate *near* the internal capsule. In Patient 19 lead 2 was localized in the thalamus rather than the caudate

			AUTONOMIC EFFECTS — BLOOD PRESSURE			PULSE						MOTOR			
	ELECTRODE LOCALIZATION	STIM. CURRENT Ma	PRE-STIM.	IMMEDIATE	MAX.	PRE-STIM.	MAX.	VASO-MOTOR	SWEAT	PUPIL	RESP.	RIGHT	LEFT	EOM	REMARKS
8	Septal	5-1	154/86	—	160/96	86	90	O	O	O	O	O	O	O	O
9	Septal	4-8	120/86	—	150/106	90	110	O	O	O	O	O	O	O	O
10	Septal	10	116/82	—	186/124	80	—	O	O	O	O	O	O	O	O
	Ant. Thalamus	4	116/82	—	116/82	80	—	O	O	O	O	O	O	O	O
11	Septal	8-14	124/80	—	148/100	64	84	O	O	O	O	O	O	O	O
	High Caudate	8	124/80	—	124/80	68	66	O	O	O	O	O	O	O	O
12	Capsule-Caudate	4-12	128/76	—	128/76	84	96	flush	↑	dilate	↑	arm, leg tonic	O	conjugate to right	alert.→stupor
	Int. Capsule	4	130/78	—	130/78	86	90	O	↑	"	↑	"	O	"	"
	Caudate	1-12	126/72	—	126/72	80	90	O	O	"	O	increased activity		O	sleep-like
13	Hypothalamic	2-12	148/92	175/115	200/135	84	156	O	O	"	↓	arm leg clonic	O	Lt. int. strabis. convergence	urin. urgency agitated chills
	Septo-hypothal.	2-8	140/70	140/70	190/108	90	180	flush	↑	"	O	clonic thumb	O	O	alert.→pmv
	Lt. Mid-thalamic	2-8	140/70	140/70	140/70	86	88	O	O	O	apnea	O	O	O	stupor
14	Septo-hypothal.	2-8	120/86	210/160	210/160	96	174	flush	↑	dilate	↑	tremor		O	fear
15	Septal	4-10	140/80	160/86	160/86	84	90	O	O	—	apnea	arm leg tonic	O	O	disoriented → gm
16	Septal	2-16	120/87	120/87	130/98	—	—	O	O	—	O	O	O	O	agitation
	Septo-hypothal.	4-16	118/80	118/80	178/110	—	—	—	—	—	O	O	O	O	
17	Septal	4-12	110/70	110/70	180/100	96	162	—	—	—	—	startle		O	fear
	Vent. Hypothal.	2-14	140/80	180/100	200/120	96	144	O	O	O	O	startle		right ext. strabismus	fear
	Thalamic	6	130/76	130/76	130/76	96	96	O	O	O	O	O	O	O	O
18	Septal	4-20	116/76	142/96	142/96	120	144	pale	↑	dilate	O	O	O	O	O
	Septo-hypothal.	2-4	118/76	180/120	180/120	108	192	flush	↑	dilate (R first)	↑	O	O	O	faint
	Between above	6	118/76	118/76	118/76	110	110	O	↑	O	O	O	tonic fist	O	O
19	Rostral Hypothal.	0.6-8	250/150	O	O	168	O	O	O	O	O	O	O	O	O
	Caudate	0.5-15	"	O	O	"	O	O	O	O	O	O	O	O	O
	Rostral Hypothal.	2-40	"	O	O	"	O	O	O	O	O	O	O	int. strabis.→ convergence	O
20	Septal	2-8	130/80	200/120	220/130	114	132	—	—	O	O	O	O	O	warm, faint
	Septo-hypothal.	4	146/82	250/–	off**	"	↑	flush	—	dilate	↑	startle		O	paresthesias
21	Septal	2-40	118/68	—	170/110	80	↑	—	—	dilate	—	tremor		O	—
	Septal	2-20	120/70	—	118/78	"	112	flush	—	O	O	O	O	O	—
22	5 Combinations in subcortical white matter.	2-20	108/70	108/70	144/80	78	↑	"	↑	dilate constriction	↑	turns head, trunk bilateral tonic movement		conjugate to right convergence	fear
23	Septal	2-18	134/76	134/76	160/105	108	120	"	O	O	O	stopped tremor		O	euphoric gm
	Septo-hypothal.	2	140/80	180/135	180/135	fibrillating 108	172	"	↑	dilate	—	"		convergence	—
24	Septal	2-32	110/76	—	144/110	100	160	"	↑	O	O	O	O	O	O
	Septal	4-34	"	—	150/100	98	144	O	O	O	O	alternating head movement c̄ smp		O	O
25	*Septal	2-24	136/80	140/90	190/110	126	162	O	—	—	O	O	O	—	euphoric
	*Septal	6-20	140/98	160/100	200/115	141	165	flush	—	dilate	O	O	O	—	euphoric
	Hypothalamic	4-20	140/100	200/110	200/110	138	160	"	—	dilate	O	O	O	int. strabis	tense

*Reversal of effects on 7th postoperative day. **Stimulation terminated in 4 seconds.

caudate, as previously described, produced only dilatation of the pupils and a change in his state of awareness, somewhat resembling deep sleep, from which he could not be aroused for several minutes after stimulation. Finally, on arousal, when the patient was questioned about this episode, he stated that he had just felt sleepy and therefore had gone to sleep (see x-ray of skull, Chapter 19, Figure 7).

Patient 13 had one bipolar electrode placed in the hypothalamus, one in the septo-hypothalamic area, and one in the mid-portion of the thalamus (see Figure 1). The effect of stimulation to the hypothalamic lead at an initial pulse amplitude of 2 ma. was that of a rise in blood pressure from 148/92 to 175/115. When pulse amplitude was increased to 8 ma., blood pressure rose to 200/135. Pulse rate increased from 84 prestimulation to 156 during stimulation, and this was associated with dilatation of the pupils, slow deep respiration; eventually there was a tonic, right-sided seizure during stimulation to this electrode.

The septo-hypothalamic response was similar. It consisted of a maximum blood pressure rise at 8 ma. to 190/108 and an increase in pulse rate to 180, along with flushing, sweating, and dilatation of the pupils. During stimulation to this electrode what appeared to be a petit mal seizure with alternating movements of the right thumb was noted. Initially, there was a left internal strabismus, which gave way to convergence as peak current was increased. The patient complained of nervousness, urinary urgency, and chills.

Patient 14 was stimulated several times in the septo-hypothalamic area. The response was similar to that of Patient 13. A maximum blood pressure rise of 210/160 from a prestimulation level of 120/86 was associated with tachycardia of 174, flushing, sweating, dilatation of the pupils, and increased respiratory rate. During the course of stimulation the patient also developed a generalized tremor, which appeared to be associated with his extreme apprehension and fear and which persisted for several minutes after stimulation. Figure 2 shows the anatomical position of the electrodes.

Patient 8(15) received several septal stimulations at a maximum pulse amplitude of 10 ma. A moderate blood pressure response associated with mild tachycardia was observed. Toward the end of one of these stimulations, the patient developed a tonic response of the right arm

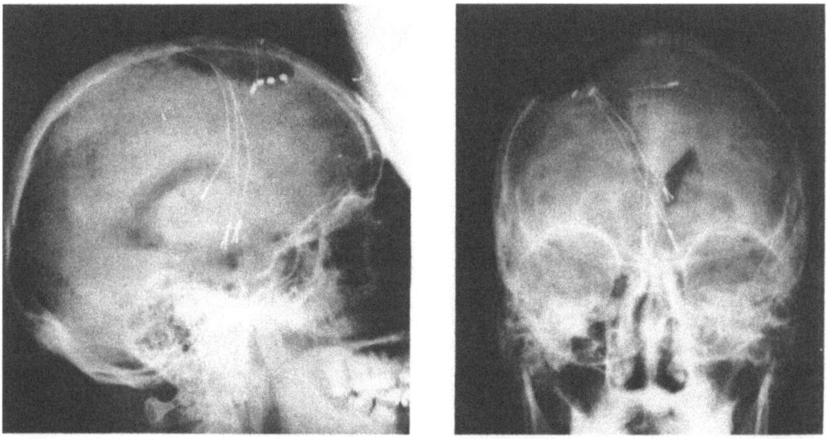

FIGURE XIII–1. Patient 13. Lateral and anterior-posterior views showing position of subcortical electrodes at base of the diencephalon

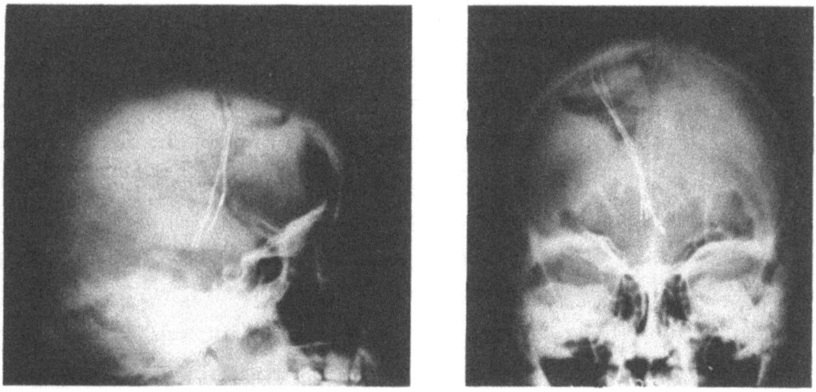

FIGURE XIII–2. Patient 14. Lateral and anterior-posterior views showing position of subcortical electrodes

and leg, and shortly after this became apneic and cyanotic, at which point stimulation was stopped. Respiration was immediately resumed, and the patient appeared to be quite normal. Several minutes after this, he went into a generalized seizure from which he recovered in the usual manner.

Patient 16 received several ineffective septal stimulations with pulse amplitudes of 16 ma. One bipolar electrode was located in the septo-hypothalamic region, and from this point a blood pressure rise from 118/80 to 178/110 was recorded. The patient became quite agitated during this stimulation.

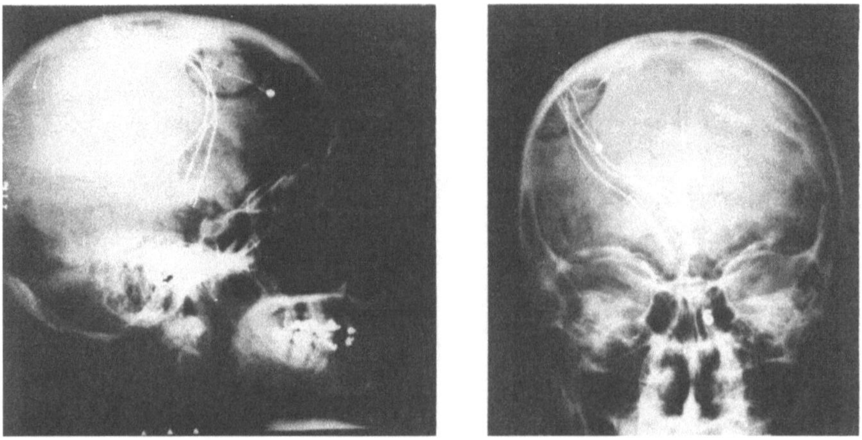

FIGURE XIII–3. Patient 17. Lateral and anterior-posterior views showing position of subcortical electrodes. Stimulation of the deepest of these resulted in post-stimulation arrhythmia

Patient 17 had one bipolar electrode in the septal region, one in the thalamus, and one in the ventral part of the hypothalamic area (Figure 3). Stimulation of the latter produced a blood pressure rise to 200/120 (Figure 4) and tachycardia of 144, and this was associated with a generalized startle reaction. A right external strabismus was noted, and the patient expressed subjective feelings of fear and anxiety. Following stimulation there was a marked cardiac arrhythmia (Figure 5), which is believed to have been the result of transient unopposed vagal activity initiated by way of the carotid sinus reflex in the presence of increased ventricular irritability as a result of circulating epinephrine. It is unfortunate that EKG leads were not available, for it would then have been possible to demonstrate the probable ectopic origin of the isolated pulses seen in the record. Such a situation was found to be present in cats, as shown in the other portions of Figure 5. These effects are believed to be due to vagal activity, since they were abolished following vagotomy.

Stimulation of the septal region had much the same effect, but the blood pressure response reached only 180/100. No vagal effect was evident here. In both stimulations, the patient's eyes were seen to open widely, and she said she was afraid. Stimulation of the thalamus was ineffective at the same pulse amplitude that was used in the other stimulations.

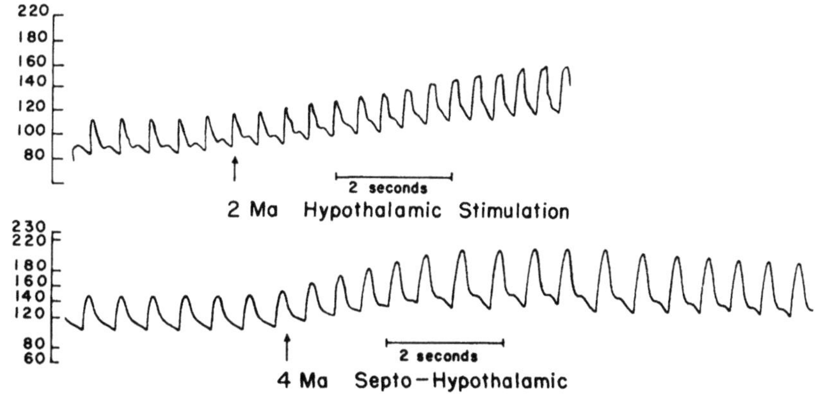

FIGURE XIII-4. Patient 17. Blood pressure rises in response to stimulation to two deep leads. Intra-arterial blood pressure recorded from brachial artery

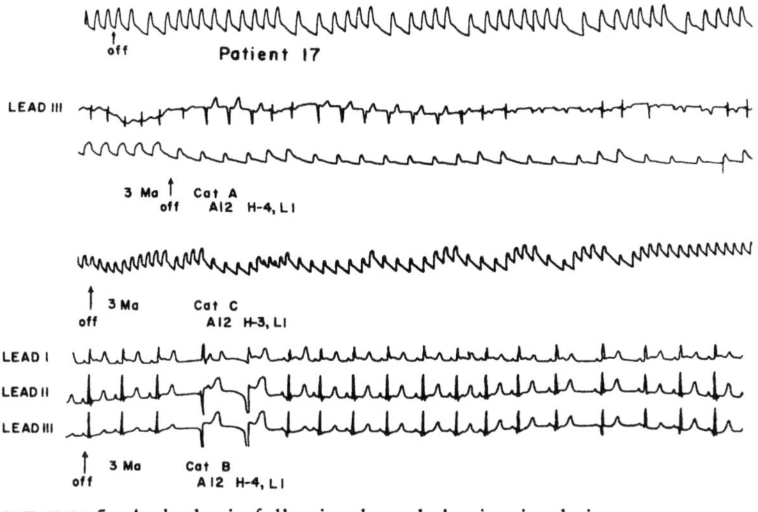

FIGURE XIII-5. Arrhythmia following hypothalamic stimulation

Patient 17: record of intra-arterial blood pressure, showing poststimulation arrhythmia. See further discussion in the text

Cat A: Simultaneous EKG lead III and femoral pulse and blood pressure record. Note the marked irregularity of the pulse record and the small pulse pressures at the time of the numerous multifocal ectopic ventricular beats.

Cat C: Femoral pulse and blood pressure record taken immediately after hypothalamic stimulation. Note similarity between this and the patient's record.

Cat B: Simultaneous EKG leads showing two ectopic ventricular beats of different origins followed by return to RSR. Ectopic beats occurred after the sudden onset of relative bradycardia. Toward the end of the record the slowing was more marked, but RSR was maintained. This arrhythmia was not obtained following bilateral vagotomy

Patient 18 was stimulated in the septal region and in the septo-hypothalamic region. The responses were essentially the same, but much more intense in the septo-hypothalamic region. Blood pressure rose from 118/76 to 180/120. There was tachycardia of 192, flushing, sweating, pupillary dilatation, which persisted for several minutes following stimulation, and the patient also complained of feelings of faintness. Stimulation was then carried out between one pole of the septal electrode and one pole of the septo-hypothalamic electrode at 6 ma. The only responses that were noted here were sweating and tonic movement of the left hand, consisting primarily of clenching and unclenching the fingers.

Patient 19 had a bipolar electrode in the caudate nucleus and two in the hypothalamus. He showed no response to stimulation except a slowing and deepening of respiration elicited from the caudate lead and an internal strabismus from a hypothalamic lead. This patient, however, was an unusual one, for he went into operation with malignant hypertension and a history of several episodes of cardiac failure. Immediately after operation, he had an acute episode of cardiac failure and was rapidly digitalized. His cardiac status seemed to improve enough to warrant stimulation, but at this time he was running a pressure of 250/150, a pulse rate of 168, and a respiratory rate of 32. There was a pulsus alternans, due apparently to over-digitalization. It is apparent that his vasomotor responses were somewhat restricted by the extent of the blood pressure, tachycardia, and acute decompensation which he was already showing, and which probably accounted for the ineffectiveness of these stimulations.

Patient 20 had one bipolar electrode implanted in the septal region and one in the septo-hypothalamic region. Stimulation to the former produced tachycardia and a rise in blood pressure from 130/80 to 220/130. The patient stated that she felt warm and faint but that the "feeling was good." Stimulation to the hypothalamic electrode, with a pulse amplitude of 4 ma. for several seconds, produced an immediate rise in blood pressure to 250/—. (The intra-arterial cannula was not used in this patient, and therefore the blood pressure recording depended upon the use of the sphygmomanometer, which of course has its well-known inaccuracies.) Her pressure remained up for several minutes after stimulation, her diastolic then being picked up at 120. She flushed, her pupils dilated, and she complained of generalized "pins and needles."

Patient 21 was the first one operated upon by the so-called closed, or stereotaxic, technique. He had three unipolar electrodes placed in the septal region. Blood pressure responses from stimulation between pairs of these electrodes ranged from 118/68 to 170/110 with pulse amplitudes up to 40 ma. This technique involves the use of relatively large spherical electrodes about 1 1/2 mm. in diameter, thus increasing the surface area considerably.

Patient 22 was also operated upon by the stereotaxic technique. In the immediate postoperative period the electrodes were inadvertently pulled up, so that they lay in subcortical white matter, probably in the radiations from areas 8 and 6. Stimulation between pairs of these unipolar electrodes produced generalized autonomic responses without blood pressure rises —mainly increases in pulse rate, flushing, and sweating. In addition there were tonic movements of the face, left arm, and left leg and complicated eye movements, consisting of conjugate movements, external strabismus, internal strabismus, and vertical nystagmus. During stimulation the patient expressed great fear, and at one point it took four or five people to restrain her.

Patient 23 was operated upon by the old open technique, and bipolar electrodes were placed in the septal and septo-hypothalamic regions. At pulse amplitudes of 18 ma. on the septal lead, the blood pressure was seen to rise from 134/76 to 160/105. The patient developed tachycardia and flushing and became quite euphoric. Stimulation to the septo-hypothalamic lead at 2 ma. evoked a blood pressure rise to 180/135, tachycardia of 172, flushing, sweating, and dilatation of the pupils, along with convergence. At this point the patient had a transient episode of auricular fibrillation. A prolonged stimulation of the septal region was terminated when a generalized seizure developed.

Patient 24 was a repeat from the earliest group. This time she was operated upon by the stereotaxic technique, and electrodes were placed in the septal region only. Stimulation at high current pulse amplitude (34 ma.) produced a blood pressure rise from 110/76 to 150/110. Tachycardia, flushing, and sweating were associated with the rise in blood pressure. One stimulation was also seen to evoke a tonic clenching of the fists on manual polarity reversal.

Patient 25 had two pairs of electrodes in the septal region and one in the hypothalamic region. Implantation was again done by the stereotaxic technique. The responses were much the same. Blood pressure rose from 136/80 to 190/110 on septal stimulation, and to 200/110 on hypothalamic stimulation. There was an internal strabismus on the hypothalamic stimulation, and tachycardia was associated with all stimulations.

DISCUSSION

In evaluating and discussing the physiological data, it is apparent that the septal and especially the septo-hypothalamic and hypothalamic areas are potent in producing brisk autonomic responses, primarily sympathetic, consisting of marked rises in blood pressure, tachycardia, sweating, pupillary dilatation, and an increase in respiratory rate. These physiological responses probably represent a diffuse sympathetic discharge, centrally initiated, and would be predicted on the basis of much well-known animal work. Most of our patients almost at the onset showed an alerting response, with widening of the palpebral fissures, and an increase in responsivity. Again, this effect would be predicted from animal experiment, especially from Magoun's work on the rostral extension of the activating system which extends through this basal portion of the diencephalon.[1] However, the pseudo-affective responses seen in animals were not present. Rage was never shown and only rarely an inappropriate amount of fear or anxiety, in spite of the vigorous physiological responses with the concurrent subjective feelings which must have been experienced.

In addition to the usual autonomic responses, deep stimulation in the hypothalamic region sometimes produced extra-ocular movements, which consisted of either internal strabismus, external strabismus, or convergence. These extra-ocular movements are difficult to explain on the basis of stimulation to tissues immediately surrounding the electrodes. In the two patients which showed convergence, both leads were quite deep, and it is apparent that the eye movements were the result of spread of stimulus current to the midbrain producing threshold current densities there. In the case of internal and/or external strabismus, it is believed that the electrodes, again, were quite deep, and that these movements resulted either from stimulation of the nerves along their course at the base of the brain or from spread of stimulus current to the medial longitudinal fasciculus or oculo-motor nuclei of the mesencephalon. The latter hypothesis seems to be borne out to a certain extent in one patient who, on deep stimulation at low current pulse amplitude, showed a left internal strabismus which was then converted to convergence as the current pulse amplitude was increased.

In the summary shown here (Table 1), it can be noted that Patients 9, 10, 13, 14, 16, 17, 18, 20, 21, 22, 23, 24, and 25 all showed large blood pressure changes along with other responses usually associated with generalized sympathetic discharge. It is interesting to note that we did not encounter parasympathetic effects of any magnitude. The last patient of the series, on stimulation 7 days after operation, did show a slight response in this direction. But she is the only patient in whom these effects were seen, and there is some question as to the validity of the observations in her case, since at autopsy she was found to have had a metastatic lesion involving the hypothalamus. It will also be noted that Patients 12, 13, 14, 15, 18, 21, 22, and 24 showed some somatic motor activity. Of this group, two showed only tremor, which can be interpreted as the result of diffuse sympathetic discharge, two others were patients having electrodes either in the internal capsule proper or in the subcortical white matter. The rest, that is, Patients 13, 15, 18, and 24, showed somatic motor activity which can best be explained on the basis of current flux in corticifugal fibers in the diencephalon or mesencephalon. Since the current densities at the site of stimulation must have been very high, it seems quite probable that they were of movement threshold strength for some distance from the electrodes. Indeed, this factor is a major variable yet to be evaluated. Patients 15 and 23 both had generalized seizures immediately following stimulation or during stimulation. These seizures in all probability were the result of a combination of many factors and not attributable to electrical stimulation per se. Although a number of patients did show paroxysmal electrical activity during the course of the procedure, only these two spilled over into generalized activity.

SUMMARY

In summarizing these observations, it can be said that a series of 23 patients* have received multiple subcortical stimulations to various structures. Thirteen of these patients showed a definite diffuse sympathetic

*The series of 25 operations included two repeats.

discharge. The electrodes to which stimulation was applied were located in the basal portion of the brain, the majority localized in the region of the septum and extending back into the hypothalamus. Pressor vasomotor responses tended to be greater when stimulation was applied to electrodes placed in the region of the basal diencephalic nuclei, that is, the more caudal electrodes. The emotional responses observed in those patients with more caudal electrode placements were in keeping with but less intense than those which would be predicted on the basis of animal work. Stimulations to the more rostral leads produced a favorable psychological response, but physiological effects were relatively minor until high current pulse amplitudes were used. Eight patients showed somatic motor activity of a type which is believed to be characteristic of stimulation of the motor corticifugal radiations, or, in the case of extra-ocular movements, the midbrain. Indeed, in two of these patients the electrodes were found to lie in the subcortical white matter of the internal capsule or radiations. In the remaining patients who exhibited somatic motor activity other than seizures, electrode positions were deep, and it was believed that the movements observed were due to spread to the corticifugal fibers in the midbrain or to the medial longitudinal fasciculus and/or oculo-motor nuclei at this level. Two patients who showed somatic motor activity in response to stimulation also had generalized seizures during the course of the procedure. The actual localization of the precise anatomical structures stimulated is extremely difficult because of the variability of anatomical structures and the difficulty in placing of electrodes within these variable structures. Moreover, the current flux set up during stimulation may have resulted in current densities of threshold strength in tissue other than that in the immediate vicinity of the electrodes.

No discussion of the electrical activity recorded in these patients has been made here, for that appears in a different section of this book.

REFERENCE

1. Magoun, H. W. An ascending reticular activating system in the brain stem. *Arch. Neurol. & Psychiat.*, 67:145–154 (1952).

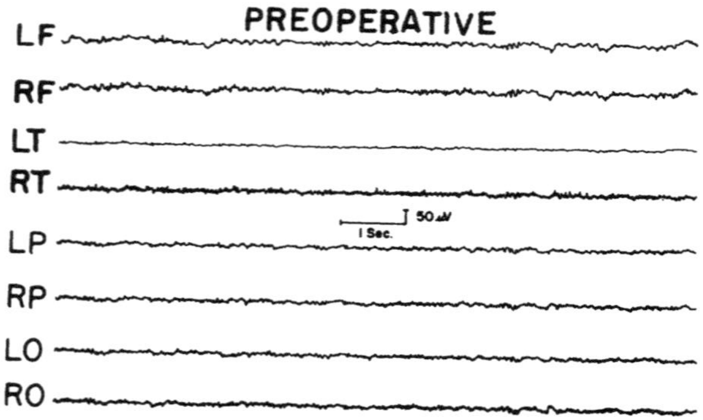

FIGURE XIV–1. Recordings from Patient 10

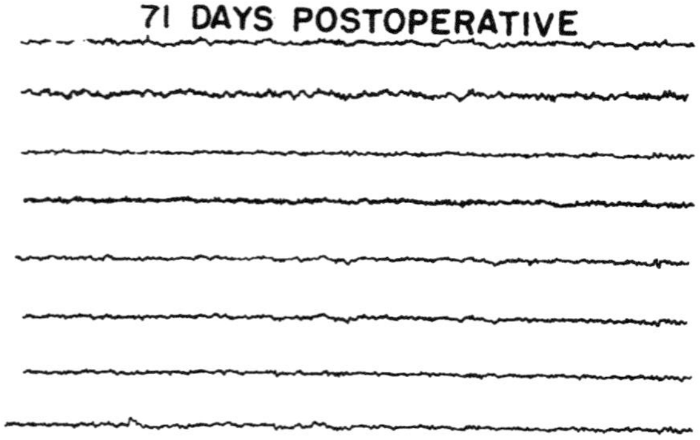

FIGURE XIV–1 (continued)

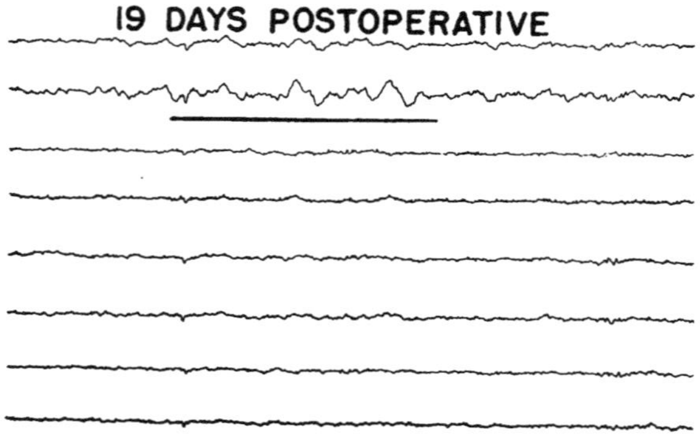

FIGURE XIV–1 (continued)

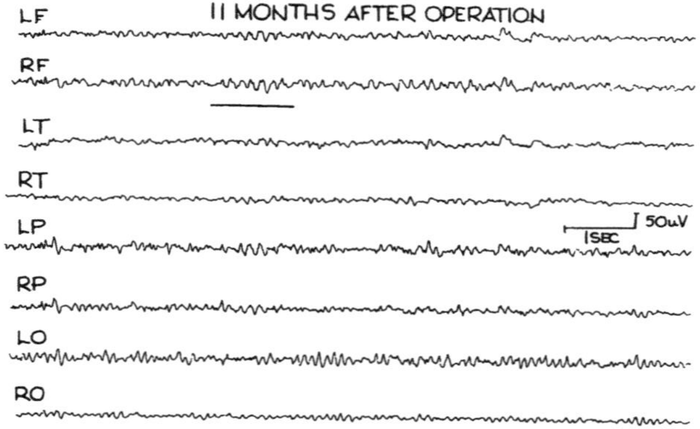

FIGURE XIV–2. Recordings from Patient 7

CHAPTER 14

ELECTROENCEPHALOGRAMS AND SUBCORTICOGRAMS FOLLOWING STIMULATION OF SUBCORTICAL STRUCTURES

ROBERT HODES
ROBERT G. HEATH
WILLIAM H. MILLER, JR.

ELECTROENCEPHALOGRAMS (SCALP RECORDINGS)

Electroencephalographic records were made on 18 of the 21 psychotic patients in this series (see Table 1) for varying periods after subcortical stimulation. One patient became uncooperative and could not be persuaded to subject herself to recording after the stimulation procedure. For other reasons, no postoperative EEG's were secured from two additional patients. As a rule, EEG's were taken a few days postoperatively, during the next few months of recovery, and as shortly before this report was written as was feasible. The longest period between the first EEG and the last follow-up EEG was more than 1 year (Patient 2). The intervals following stimulation at which EEG's were made, as well as the number of recordings obtained, are given in Chapter 11, Table 1.

Most of the patients presented abnormal EEG's for a few months after stimulation. The major abnormality noted during this period was slow wave frontal activity, greatest on the operated side (Figure 1, upper right record); this sometimes tended to disappear with time, to be replaced by a normal pattern. Evidence of pathological changes in the brain are not apparent in the lower record of Figure 1, taken 71 days after surgical intervention. This record is indistinguishable from those obtained from the patient preoperatively (Figure 1, upper left). Often there was spread from one frontal focus to the opposite frontal region as shown in Figure 2, or to more posterior areas of the homolateral hemisphere.

Of the 18 patients from whom postoperative EEG's were obtained, eleven presented definitely abnormal brain waves more than 2 months after surgery and subcortical stimulation. Included in these eleven patients are the five described in Chapter 11, whose preoperative records were abnormal. As infectious processes of the encephalon developed in two other patients, the pathological electrical activity shown in their records may well have been related to this cause. There remained, however, four patients whose records showed consistent abnormalities more than 2 months after surgery. The anomalous EEG's cannot be characterized by any single description, for there was no constant abnormal feature common to the tracings from the different patients.

Slow wave foci, in bursts of 4–6 c/second, or generalized slow activity dominated the records of some patients, random spikes persisted in others, and spike foci were observed in several of the records. Figure 2, taken from a patient subjected to surgery 11 months previously, shows bursts of slow wave activity in all leads. The 4–5 c/second patterns are most prominent in the right frontal lead. The trains of 6 c/second waves in the occipitals are noticeably asymmetrical. This patient experienced a "spell" and is discussed further below.

In Figure 3 sharp spikes are clearly apparent in the right frontal lead; in all probability there was conduction spread to homolateral temporal and parietal regions and to contralateral frontal regions. This record was taken 7 months after operation. The patient, like some of the others, had had symptomatic seizures between the time of operation and the time at which the records in Figure 21 were made. Such attacks are consistent with the EEG findings.

No epileptiform episodes were reported by the patient whose abnormal EEG's 1 year after operation are shown in Figure 4. The 5 c/second bursts underlined in the figure are prominent bilaterally in parietal and occipital leads. This activity is not so apparent in the right and left temporal leads and does not seem to be present in the frontal leads. In addition to the slow wave activity, fast spike-like responses of about the same frequency as normal alpha appear in both occipital derivations. This activity, present throughout the record, is especially clear in the two bursts at the middle and left side of the figure.

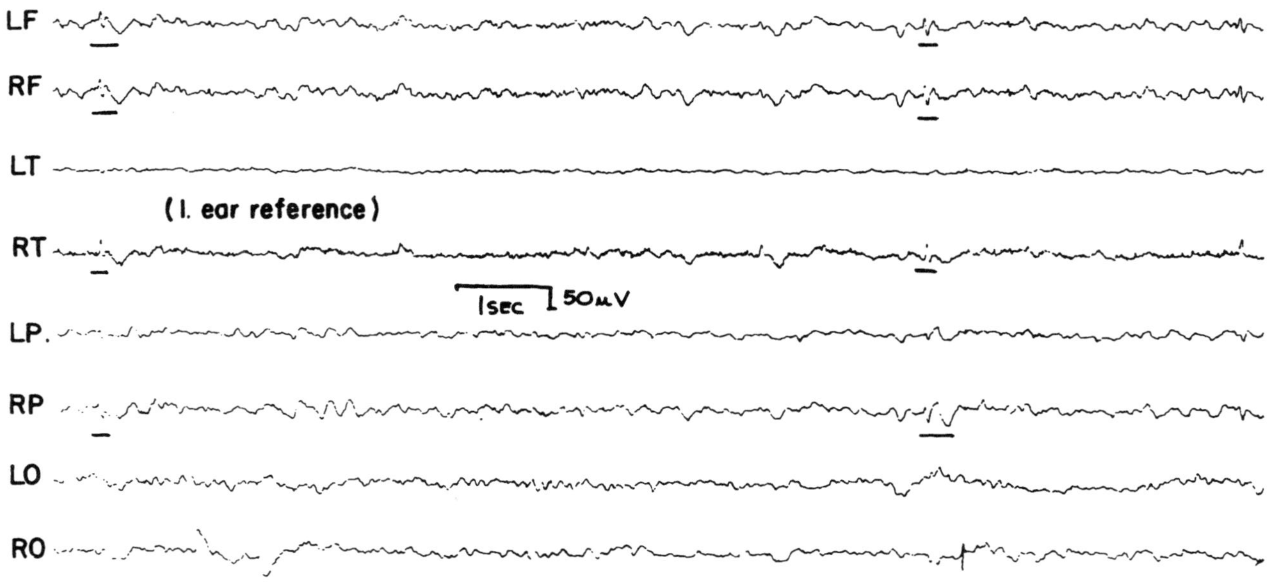

FIGURE XIV–3. Recordings from Patient 13

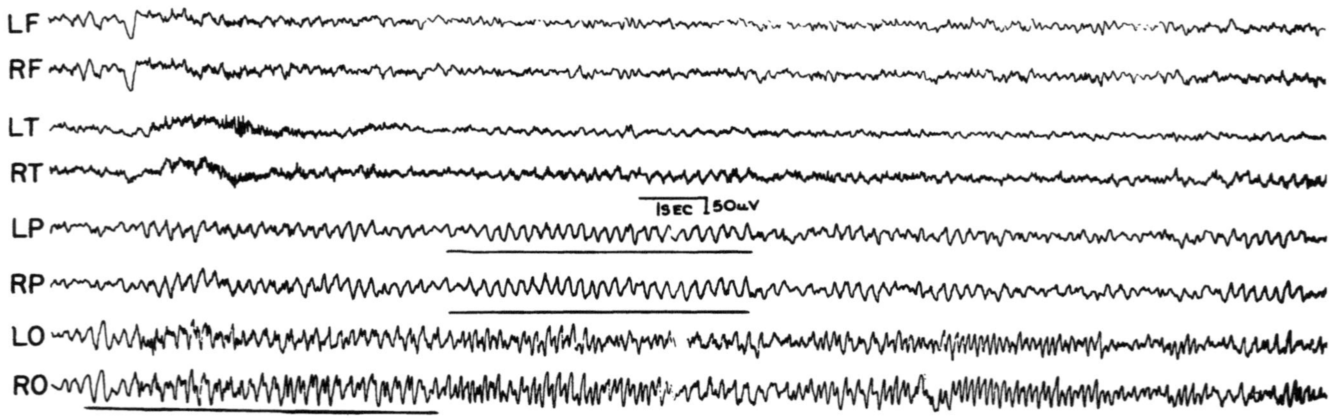

FIGURE XIV–4. Recordings from Patient 2

TABLE XIV-1. Summary of EEG findings in psychotic patients

	21 Patients		18 Patients			
	BEFORE OPERATION		AFTER OPERATION AND STIMULATION			
All EEG's normal	15		4			
All EEG's abnormal	6		14			
Abnormalities due to	EST	Other causes	Previous abnorm.	Infection	Effects of surg.?*	Effects of stim.
	3	3	5	2	3	4

*Postoperative period was less than 2 months.

In the summary given in Table 1 it should be noted that at this writing three of the nine patients with normal preoperative EEG's but abnormal postoperative EEG's had been followed for less than 2 months. Whether their electrical abnormalities would continue was of course an open question. In any event, it is clear that, whereas only four patients presented normal brain waves within a few months after operation, at least four patients who had normal EEG's prior to surgery showed evidence of gross abnormality. No other cause than some effect of the procedure can be held responsible for the apparently permanent change in the character of the recordings. At the present time it is not possible to state whether these effects were the consequences of stimulation, or of cortical or subcortical trauma or other damage incident to surgery, or of both of these major procedures. Some indication that stimulation per se was at least partially responsible for the enduring abnormalities in the EEG's is given later.

SUMMARY

Normal EEG's were consistently observed in four of the eighteen psychotic patients who were followed electroencephalographically for several months after surgery. On the other hand, four patients whose patterns had been normal prior to operation showed diverse abnormal activity on at least some of the postoperative recordings. Of the remaining ten patients examined, five had abnormal activity before operation, two suffered from infectious processes that may have been responsible for the abnormal activity that appeared after operation, and three were not studied for a sufficiently long period to determine whether their postoperative EEG deviants would disappear or become permanently entrenched.

SUBCORTICOGRAMS

Our original intent in implanting subcortical electrodes in schizophrenic patients was to alter the course of the disease by stimulation of the facilitatory region—that is, the rostral, medial, and basal areas of the forebrain. When consistent and localized spike activity (see Chapter 11) was discovered in the region on which our attention had been focused —for the theoretical considerations given in earlier chapters—the assumption was entertained that perhaps the abnormal electrical activity and the disease process were related. From this followed the hopeful corollary that alteration of the spike activity would constitute evidence of alteration in the course of the disease.

It was reasoned that the imposition of an external force (electrical stimulation) might change the abnormal rhythms which had been postulated before the research was begun and which actually had been found during the progress of the work. The hope was held that the effect of such a stimulus would be similar to that of the stimulus applied to a heart exhibiting "circus movements." In the latter instance abnormality may disappear permanently after temporary interruption of the rhythm. Another analogy from pathophysiology is that of the "trigger point" in a painful muscle. Here, a locus of irritation sets up afferent impulses which, kept in continuous activity by self-reexciting circuits, produce sensations of pain. A single injection of a local anesthetic such as novocaine may abolish the pain permanently. Presumably in this case manifestations of the disorder cease after disruption of abnormal neural activity.

Most of the stimulations were delivered to those electrodes from which subcortical spikes were recorded. In a few instances, other electrodes were activated for other reasons. Results obtained in later cases are beyond the scope of this report and will be given elsewhere (Addendum E). Bipolar stimulation was employed, 100 square waves of 1 millisecond duration and of variable intensity being delivered from a Grass Model 3C stimulator and isolation unit. Because of the stimulation artifacts, recording was not possible during the period of stimulation, which varied from a few seconds to 30 minutes.

The following account will be divided into two main parts. The first will describe the occasional bouts of paroxysmal electrical activity which followed shortly after termination of the stimulus. This activity was sometimes confined to the specific subcortical regions through which the current was delivered and sometimes spread to the cerebral mantle. For the sake of convenience, these responses will be referred to as subcortical and cortical "fits," respectively. The second part will describe immediate and long-term effects of stimulation on subcortical spikes.

SUBCORTICAL FITS

Abnormal high voltage, rhythmic spike and wave patterns were obtained from the electrodes through which the stimulation was applied. This activity was observed in almost every instance as soon as the stimulus was ended and the amplifiers were turned on.

Typical prestimulation recordings are illustrated in the upper record of Figure 5. The spikes from lead 13 appear in channels 2 and 5, as described in Chapter 11, under spontaneous activity before stimulation. Outbursts of large spikes and waves at a frequency of about 1 c/second appear exclusively in the stimulated leads. It is of interest to note that within 20 seconds of the cessation of stimulation the electrode of lead 14 became a site of seizure activity, whereas before stimulation the spontaneously produced spikes were recorded only in lead 13. Thus, in this case, the neural elements in the vicinity of the electrode of lead 14 were either thrown into synchronous discharge by the applied stimulus or involved by conduction spread from the neighboring tissues around the electrode of lead 13. If the paroxysms of abnormal spikes and waves were conducted, the spread must have been quite limited in extent, for it is obvious that subcortical structures only a few centimeters away were not involved. No seizure activity is noted from leads 11 and 12 or leads 15 and 16, in channels 1 and 3, respectively. Moreover, the two bottom channels give no indication that the scalp electrodes were involved. All this would suggest circumscribed activation and remarkably small spread for a disturbance of such magnitude. The dramatic activity evoked by stimulation began to subside about 1 minute after cessation of the exciting current, became irregular 1 minute 40 seconds after stimulation (Figure 5, lower left record), and disappeared at 2 minutes 5 seconds. The synchronized outburst did not return, as shown by the lower right tracings of Figure 5, recorded 14 minutes after the stimulation was terminated. The patient was conscious during the subcortical outburst.

A short outburst of high voltage spike and wave response, evoked by high frequency activation of leads 7 and 8 to the basal part of the septum is illustrated in the lower record of Figure 6. The upper record was made shortly before stimulation was begun. Spikes had been obtained in leads 7 and 8 during several hours of prestimulation recording. After 11 minutes of stimulation an immediate burst of seizure activity appeared in the leads from the stimulated electrodes but not in the scalp leads sampling the electrical activity of the hemispheres. This burst decelerated rapidly and disappeared in about 20 seconds. The large downward deflections seen in the scalp recordings (channels 5 and 6) are eye-blink artifacts and have no relation to the seizure response seen in the subcortical leads. Such movement artifacts are practically never noted in subcortical leads.

Sharp waves or spikes of long duration are seen in the records in which lead 15 or lead 16 was involved (Figure 7). When these leads were recorded together (channel 3) the potentials were somewhat greater than 100 microvolts. This pronounced activity, which occurred about once every second, subsided quickly and disappeared about 45 seconds after stimulation was terminated. As before, no cortical spikes were noted. The few marked disturbances recorded from leads 11 and 12 (channels 1 and 4 were not related to the activity aroused in the tissues in proximity with the stimulating electrodes. Whether they were induced by stimulus spread and activation, or by the firing of connections linking the neural elements around the stimulating electrodes (leads 15 and 16) to neural tissue in propinquity to leads 11 and 12, cannot be determined from these data.

Figure 8, recorded after 10 minutes' stimulation to spiking leads 12 and 13 from the electrode located in the rostral part of the septal region, exhibits a paroxysmal outburst which lasted approximately 1 minute. The discharge frequency decelerated rather smoothly from about 1.5 c/second to approximately .5 c/second. Spikes and waves of approximately 100 microvolts peak-to-peak amplitude declined to about 50 microvolts (middle right record) before disappearing. The pattern resembles in form the productions of petit mal epilepsy. However, no

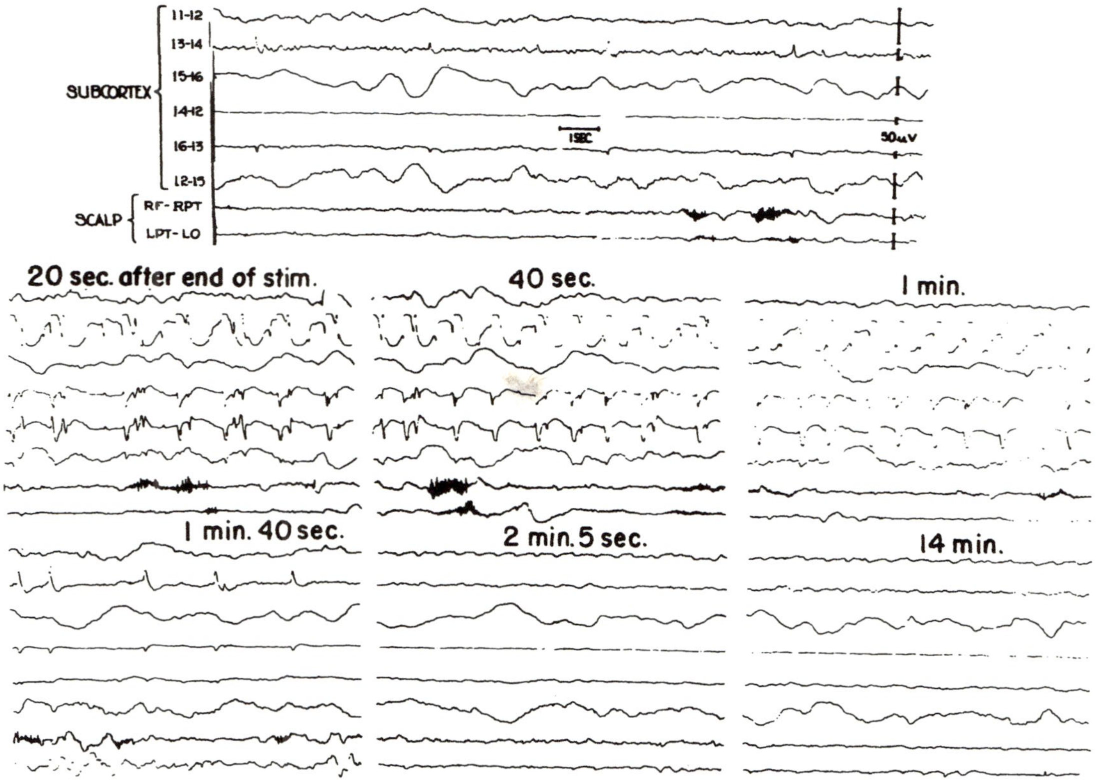

FIGURE XIV–5. Recordings from Patient 8(15)

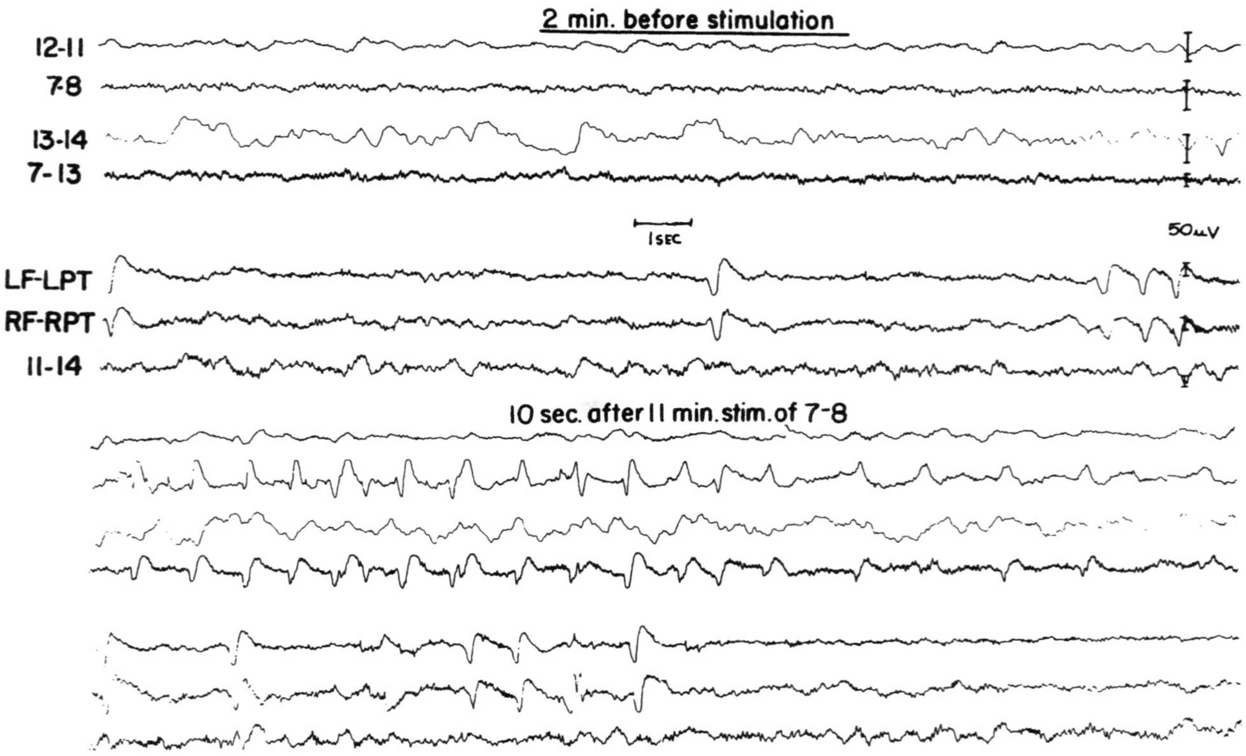
2 min. before stimulation
12-11
7-8
13-14
7-13
1 SEC
50 µV
LF-LPT
RF-RPT
11-14
10 sec. after 11 min. stim. of 7-8

FIGURE XIV–6 (above). Recordings from Patient 10

FIGURE XIV–7 (below). Recordings from Patient 18

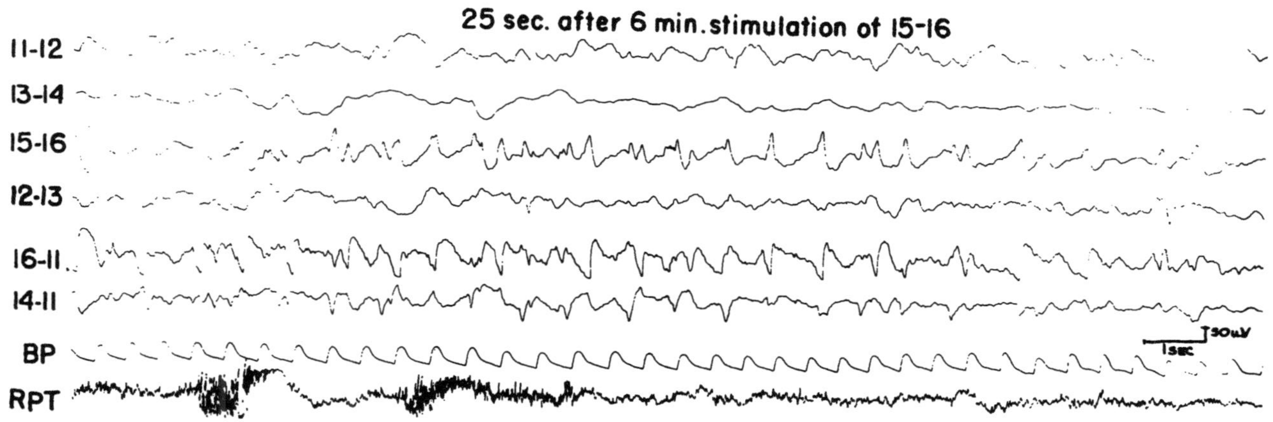

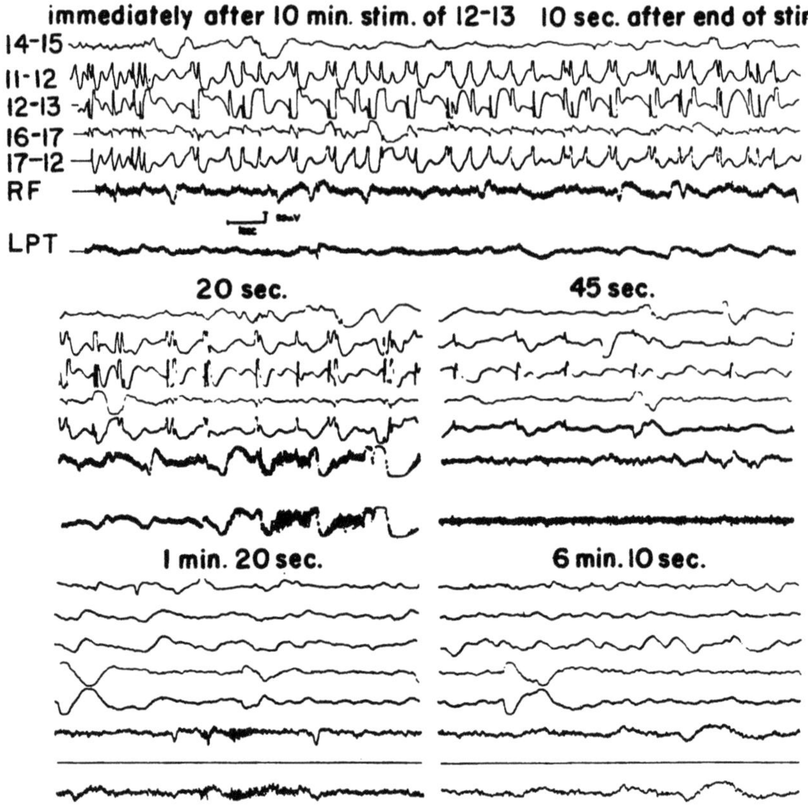

FIGURE XIV–8. Recordings from Patient 5 (24)

spike and wave activity was recorded from the cortex, and the patient gave no evidence of loss of consciousness during this subcortical turbulence. There is no evidence that the electrodes placed in the caudate nucleus (leads 14–15) were involved. However, a minor degree of spiking appeared in lead 16 (channel 4). This electrode was about 1.5 cm. caudal to those stimulated. The placements had been made in this patient by the stereotaxic technique (see Chapter 10).

Figures 9, 10, and 11 illustrate an interesting type of response to subcortical stimulation which is intermediate between the grossly abnormal but highly circumscribed activity discussed above and that which also involved the cortex. The patient who provided these tracings presented spikes in two pairs of leads—a slow disturbance in leads 11 and 12, and a rapid potential in leads 15 and 16, as marked in the upper

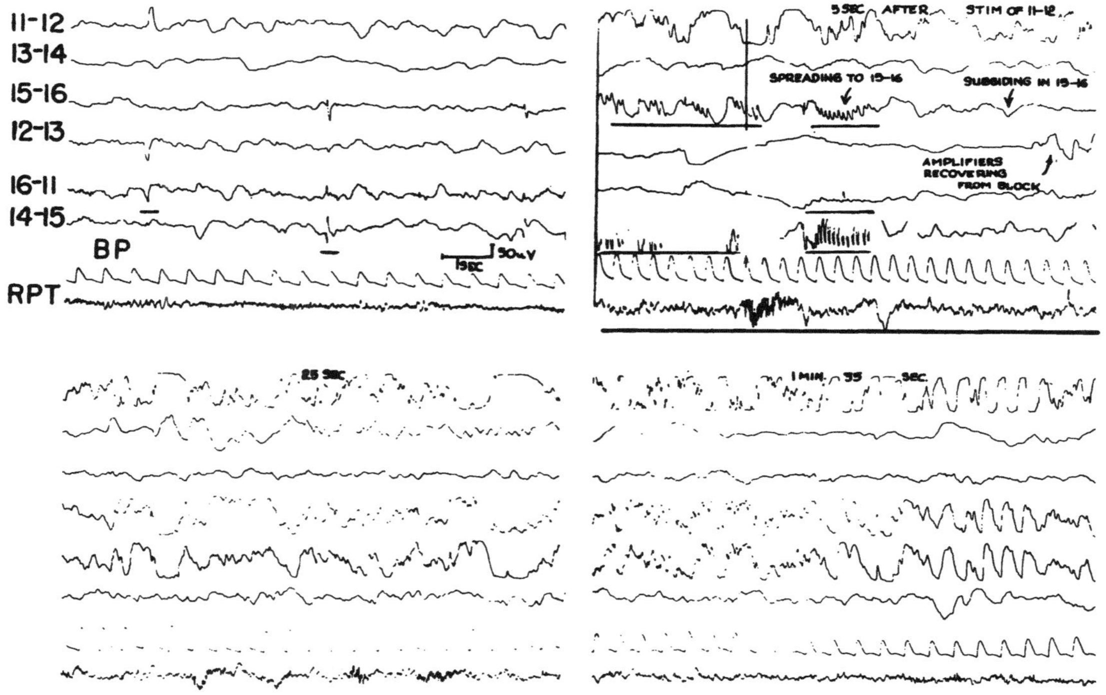

FIGURE XIV–9. Recordings from Patient 18

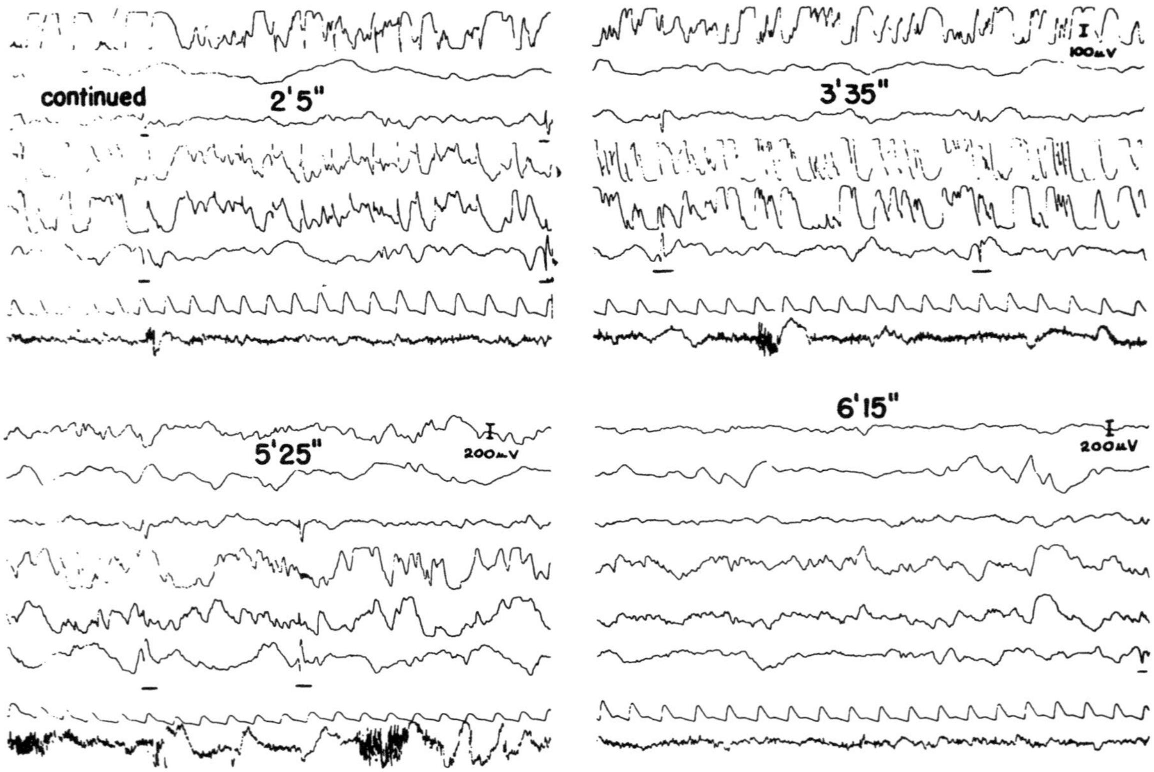

FIGURE XIV–10. Recordings from Patient 18

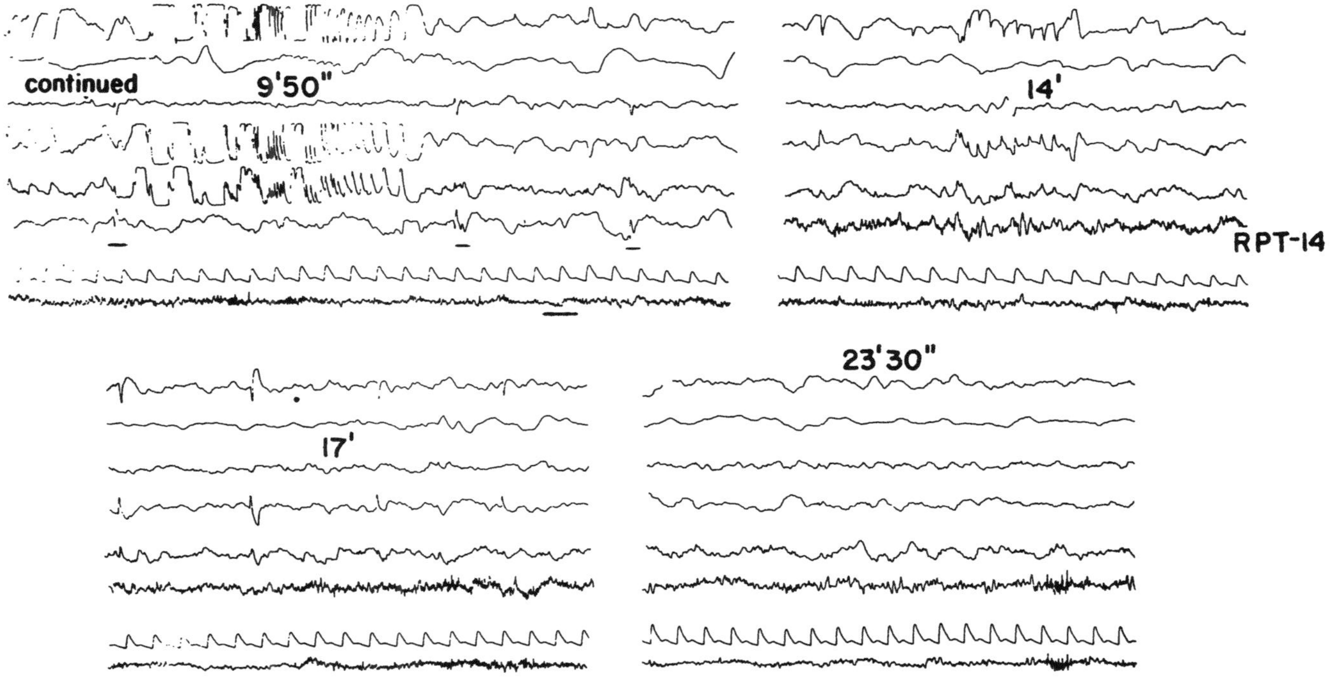

FIGURE XIV–11. Recordings from Patient 18

left record of Figure 9. Violent electrical disturbances were seen to begin in leads 11 and 12 as soon as the recording instrument was turned on. Abnormal response was also present in a neighboring pair, leads 15 and 16. Within 10 seconds after cessation of stimulation, the high voltage, 10–11 c/second runs of sharp spikes subsided in leads 15 and 16, as indicated in the upper right tracing. Evidence that the third pair of deep leads (13 and 14) was also involved, but to a lesser degree than leads 15 and 16, is seen in the upper right and lower left records. That the involvement was also very brief is indicated by the disappearance of unusual electrical activity from leads 15 and 16 after 1 minute. (Figure 9, lower right-hand record.) Frequent spikes, commingled with very large slow waves, continued to be prominent from the activated tissue even while the abnormal potentials from the adjacent leads were subsiding. Indeed, such explosive synchronous discharges continued for the ensuing 5 minutes (Figure 10), and then appeared sporadically during the final abatement of the fit (Figure 11). Scalp recordings failed to suggest significant invasion of the hemispheres by the tempest below. Even when scalp leads were connected to an indifferent subcortical lead (Figure 11, lower left record), cortical activity did not parallel the distinctive aberrations observed in the deep leads. On rare occasions, with the scalp-subcortical leading method, there were suggestions of cortical abnormality related to the subcortical events. Such an instance is illustrated in the upper right record of Figure 11. Approximately 25 minutes elapsed between the end of stimulation and the subsidence of this subcortical fit. Its severity and duration were the greatest of all of those which did not involve the cerebral cortex to any major extent.

CORTICAL FITS

In a few instances stimulation of subcortical regions of the forebrain resulted in frank convulsions and loss of consciousness. The electrical signs of a cortical seizure were apparent in these cases. The most dramatic convulsion occurred in Patient 23, a control patient whose records are given in Figures 12, 13, and 14. The electrodes of leads 13 and 14 were activated for 20 minutes. Immediately after the termination of the exciting current a cataclysmic outburst was recorded. The peak-to-peak voltages measured in Figure 12 were of the order of 200 microvolts, but

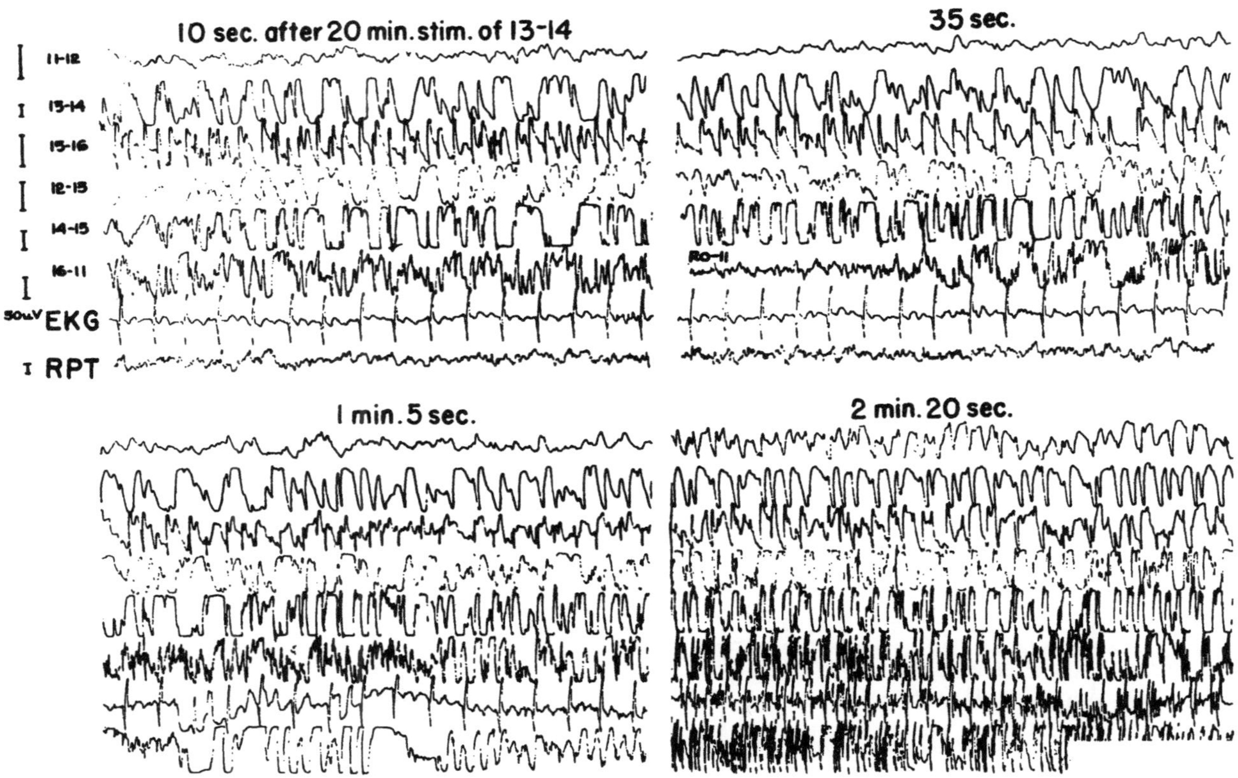

FIGURE XIV-12. Recordings from Patient 23

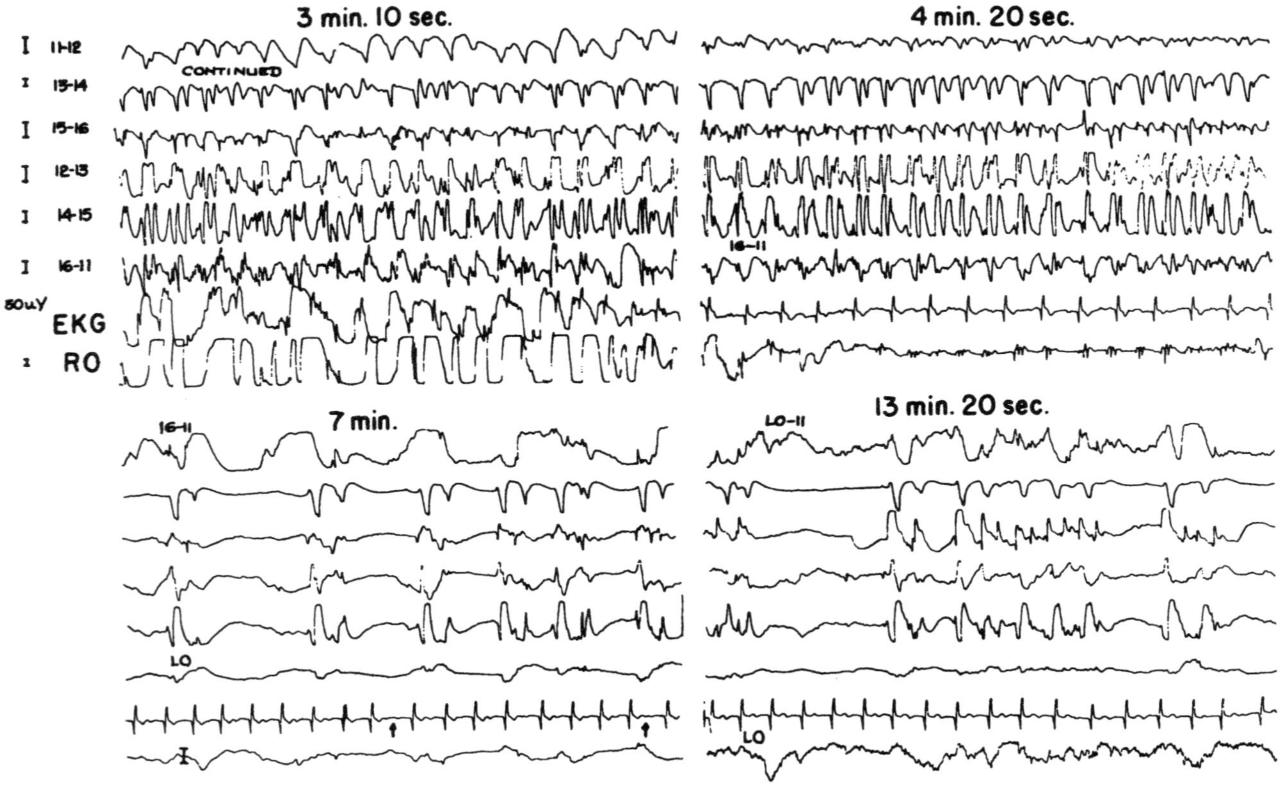

FIGURE XIV–13. Recordings from Patient 23

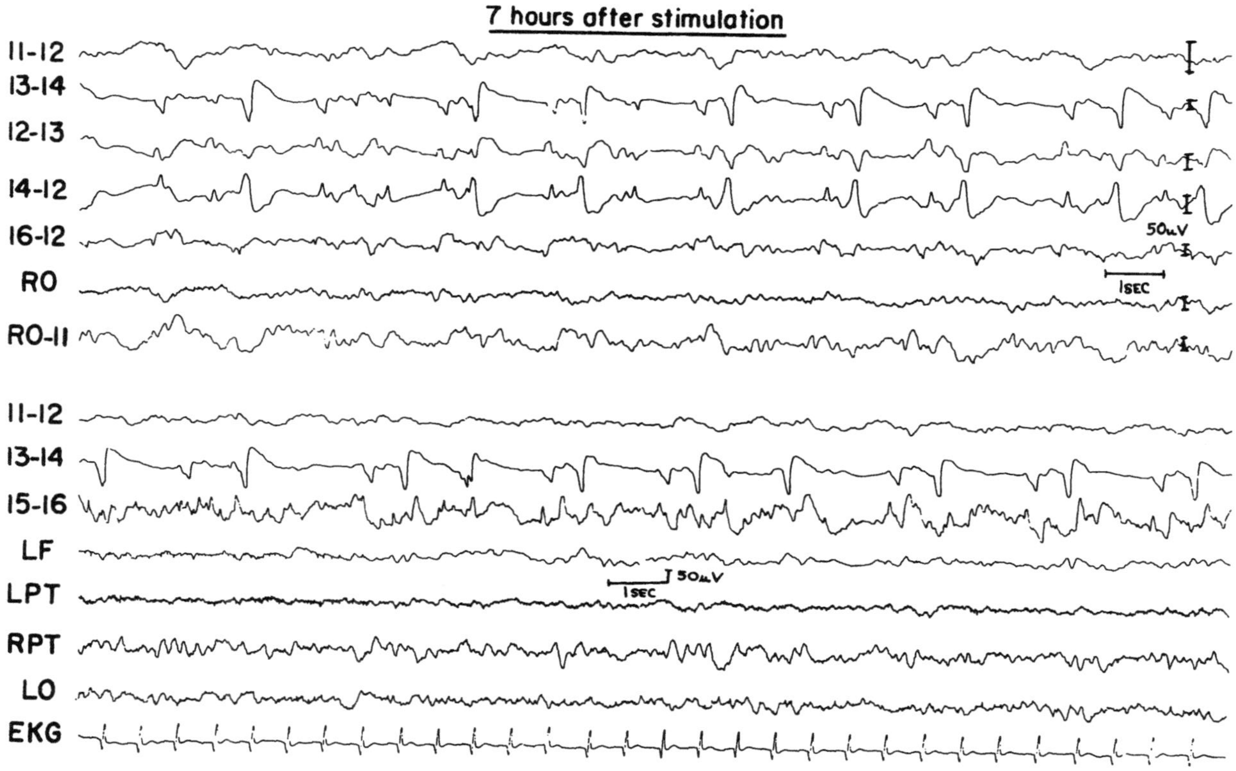

FIGURE XIV–14. Recordings from Patient 23

some waves must have been of even greater magnitude, since rounding and squaring of the tops showed that the amplifiers were blocked and so could not record true maximal values. Whereas convulsive electrical activity is obvious in the subcortical leads, the scalp leads (bottom channel) show only slow waves for about 1 minute following the end of the stimulation. At about this time an abrupt alteration in the character of the cortical activity occurred and bursts of large slow waves preempted the lower left record. This activity continued to build up in frequency and intensity until unmistakable electrical evidence of a convulsive seizure appeared (lower right record). Clinical signs of convulsion were also present, both the involuntary spasms of the musculature and the loss of consciousness being obvious. There seems little reason to doubt that the cortical fit was initiated by the spread of this subcortical paroxysm to the hemispheres. Seizure patterns did not appear on the surface until about 1 minute after they were well established in the subcortex. It is also unlikely that such synchronized bursts were present but not recordable on the hemispheres, for scalp-subcortical leads were employed 25 seconds after the stimulation was finished. The development may be seen in channel 6 of the upper right record and in the following traces of Figure 12. In the first half of the upper right record only the abnormal slow, low voltage patterns appear, as in the scalp derivations of channel 8; then the dramatic shift from slow wave response to seizure type of outburst occurs. Seizure spikes and waves of large amplitude progressively dominate channel 6; the lower right tracing is practically identical with the convulsive patterns obtained from the scalp recordings of channel 8. The essential duplication, especially in the lower right-hand record of the electrical entries in the two channels containing cortical leads indicates that the cortical activity is dominant; otherwise the potential fluctuations of lead 11 would also be chronicled in channel 6.

The sequence of a subcortical outburst gradually invading the hemisphere thus seems clear from examination of Figure 12. In view of the discussion in the preceding paragraph, the late appearance of the cortical fit cannot logically be ascribed to artifacts of recording. Further, the fact that seizure activity does eventually appear on the cortex also argues against its presence (but nonrecordability) at an earlier time. The sequelae of the stimulation described above took place with such rapidity that it was not possible to determine the point in time at which consciousness was lost. From the failure of limited subcortical outpourings to produce unconsciousness (Addendum E) and from the well-known reduction of consciousness which accompanies convulsive disorders, one would be inclined to suggest that the involvement of the cortex in the electrical rampage of Figure 12 coincided with the failure of the patient to remain in touch with her surroundings. It is of some interest that this loss of awareness did not occur *during* stimulation but only after its termination. The neural mechanisms that were responsible for preventing the postulated overwhelming of the cortex in this instance are unexplainable at present.

Continuation of the profound involvement of the entire nervous system in the patient just described is shown in Figures 13 and 14. The abnormalities need not be described in detail. The highly synchronized spikes and waves, both cortical and subcortical, are obvious in Figure 13, as are the rhythmic subcortical bursts and cortical patterns characteristic of stupor and poststuporous states in Figures 13 and 14. Cardiac irregularities are marked by arrows in the lower left record of Figure 13. For this patient's history and postoperative course, see Section IV.

DISCUSSION

Two major types of paroxysmal high voltage spike and wave activity were observed. One type of fit, appearing in the subcortical leads through which the electrical pulses are delivered, failed to involve significant expanses of adjacent neural masses and was not recordable from the cerebral hemispheres. The other kind of fit originated in the region stimulated, expanded to activate other subcortical structures, and then spread to the cortical surface. An intermediate type of response to subcortical stimulation was also observed, in which the excitation of contiguous subcortical regions subsided quickly and did not invade the hemispheres. Subcortical fits were not accompanied by loss of consciousness, whereas those which reached the cortex were attended by motor and sensorial manifestations of the clinically familiar convulsion.

That seizure response of the magnitude seen in several of the illustrative examples remained quite circumscribed is not without parallel in routine electroencephalographic experience. Electrical manifestations of Jacksonian fits are frequently localized in the fronto-parieto-temporal cortex and fail to spread caudally or involve the contralateral hemisphere. Likewise, the spreading fits that we have observed in some of our patients subjected to artificial subcortical activation have their counterparts in petit mal and grand mal epileptic attacks. Almost invariably electrical anomalies characterizing these maladies are observed over the entire cerebral mantle.

The localization of seizure outpourings to a small area of the brain-stem provides additional support for the validity of the results obtained in an earlier section dealing with the presence of spontaneous spikes from the subcortex (see Chapter 11); for it seems quite logical to assume that, if the dramatic electrical productions of the subcortical fit can be confined to its area of origin, the much smaller outbursts may be similarly confined. (For later data see Addendum E.)

Most of the stimulations which caused paroxysmal outbursts were from the midline rostro-basal structures of the septal region. To our knowledge, such effects have not been reported previously. Whether these outbursts were related to the activity resembling petit mal seizures obtained by Hunter and Jasper[1] from stimulation of midline diencephalic structures remains a subject for further study. Likewise, future work must determine the relationship of our data to the seizure patterns evoked on the cortex from stimulation of the septal and other regions in animals (Stoll, Ajmone-Marsan, and Jasper;[2] Ajmone-Marsan and Stoll[3]).

Our data may be of some importance for the eagerly sought understanding of the neural substrata of consciousness. That the cerebral cortex is likely to be an important region whose deranged function leads to loss or reduction of awareness is suggested by the fact that frank unconsciousness supervened, in our experience, when considerable and grossly obvious abnormal activity involved the hemispheres, but did not occur when similarly dramatic disturbances were confined to one of the various subcorticai areas sampled in these studies. Such a finding may well serve to add a note of caution to the interpretation of some studies which implicitly appear to minimize the importance of cortical damage for the production of diminished states of awareness. Thus, Penfield[4] remarks that "highest level seizures" may emanate from a region designated by him as the "centrencephalon." Although Penfield's suggestions are based on sound pathological and physiological observation, it is also well to emphasize that the effect of various lesions described by him on cerebral *function* should not be overlooked. And since, in our present state of knowledge, the absence of demonstrable cellular pathology or electrical abnormality is in no sense proof of the vitality of the neuraxis, the temptation to emphasize subcortical phenomena and to disregard cortical effects, or vice versa, should be avoided. Such caution is in the interests of a central nervous system physiology based on the synthesis of integrated and mutually interacting systems, rather than one suggesting the compartmentalization and isolation of more or less independent anatomical entities. In this connection also, it is perhaps worthy of comment that the findings of abnormal activity in certain subcortical regions of schizophrenic patients (see Chapter 11) should help not only to concentrate attention to these regions, but should also serve as a stimulus to further objective study into the failure of that cortical-subcortical harmony which must lie at the basis of consciousness and appropriate behavior. When such information becomes available, the neurophysiological concomitants of schizophrenia and other states of altered awareness may be described —along with the known behavioral phenomena attendant upon these states.

EFFECT OF STIMULATION ON SUBCORTICAL SPIKES

Diminution in frequency, reduction in amplitude, or disruption in form—singly or in combination—were the effects most frequently recorded after stimulation through the leads from which spikes were recorded. The period of altered spike-firing obtained after stimulation varied from patient to patient. Because of the frequent changes in technique (electrode materials, methods and sites of electrode implantation, surgical innovations, etc.) that are inevitably introduced in a preliminary investigation of this kind, we are unable at the present time to quantify the spike-depressing efficiency of the various intensities, durations, or other characteristics of the stimulation employed. Such a relation between stimulation features and effect is highly desirable and may become applicable when the technical details have become fixed. Even in the latter event, however, it is not unlikely that the complications and variations introduced by the subtle fluctuations of the conscious human brain may well forestall fulfillment of this highly desirable correlation.

An example of stimulation that was effective for only a short period of time is given in Figure 15. Frequent, well-defined spikes from the septal lead 14 were appearing when the top record was made. Spiking then decreased until 4 minutes after stimulation (middle record), when only one spike appeared. Following this the tendency was reversed; but 11 minutes after stimulation (bottom record) the frequency of the spikes was still somewhat less than before stimulation and their amplitude was somewhat reduced. It is interesting that whereas the spikes in the top record are seen in combinations involving lead 14, in the middle and lower records they are seen in combinations involving lead 13. This situation continued throughout the entire ensuing several hours of recording. Although the spiking in lead 14 seemed to have been abolished, for the practical purposes of our procedure the electrical abnormality was considered to be essentially unchanged at the termination of this record.

A more prolonged reduction in spiking is seen in the next two figures, taken from a different patient. The first of these, Figure 16, shows 1/2 minute of continuous recording of Patient 18, with the usual prominent subcortical spike. Figure 17 shows 1 consecutive minute of recording about 1 hour and 15 minutes after a 30-minute stimulation of the previously "spiking" lead. This record is typical of the last hour of recording on this patient—only a few, extremely small spikes occurred even when the patient was asleep.

In one of the most prolific "spikers" of this series (Patient 16) the pathological activity was essentially abolished for at least two hours after a series of stimulations applied chiefly to the "spiking" leads. Figure 18 shows 40 seconds of recording during a fairly typical prestimulation period. Figure 19 shows the last minute of recording on the evening and morning of the stimulation. The spikes are gone, and only slow waves are present throughout the record. No sharp, high voltage activity in any way resembling that in the prestimulation records had been observed for the 2 hours preceding the final stimulation. The appearance of slow waves was not an infrequent sequel to stimulation. Since it was felt that this activity was not desirable, attempts were always made to stimulate

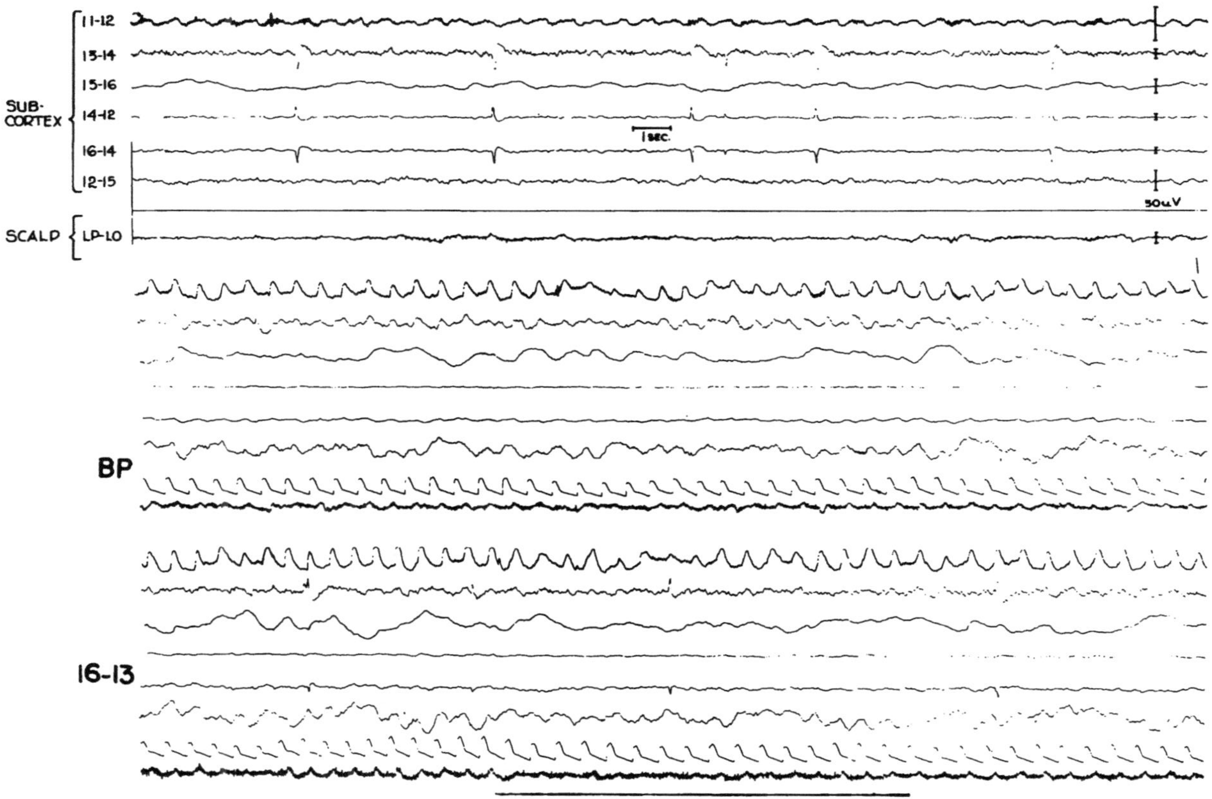

FIGURE XIV–15. Recordings from Patient 8(15)

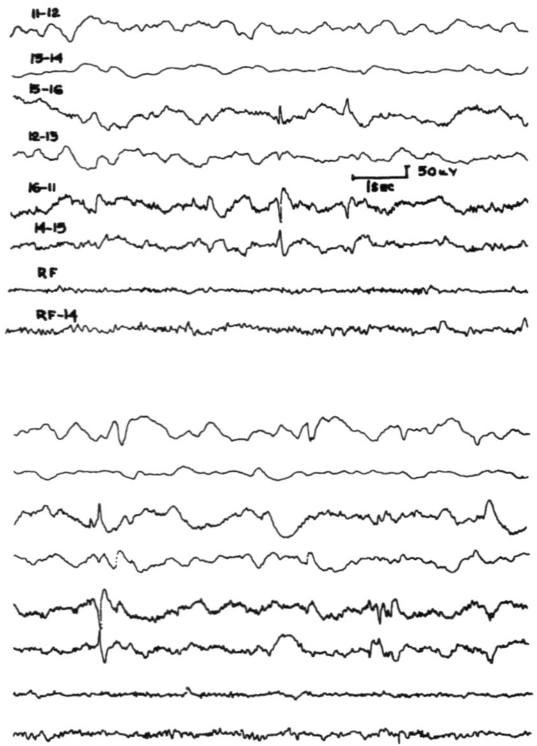

FIGURE XIV-16. Recordings from Patient 18

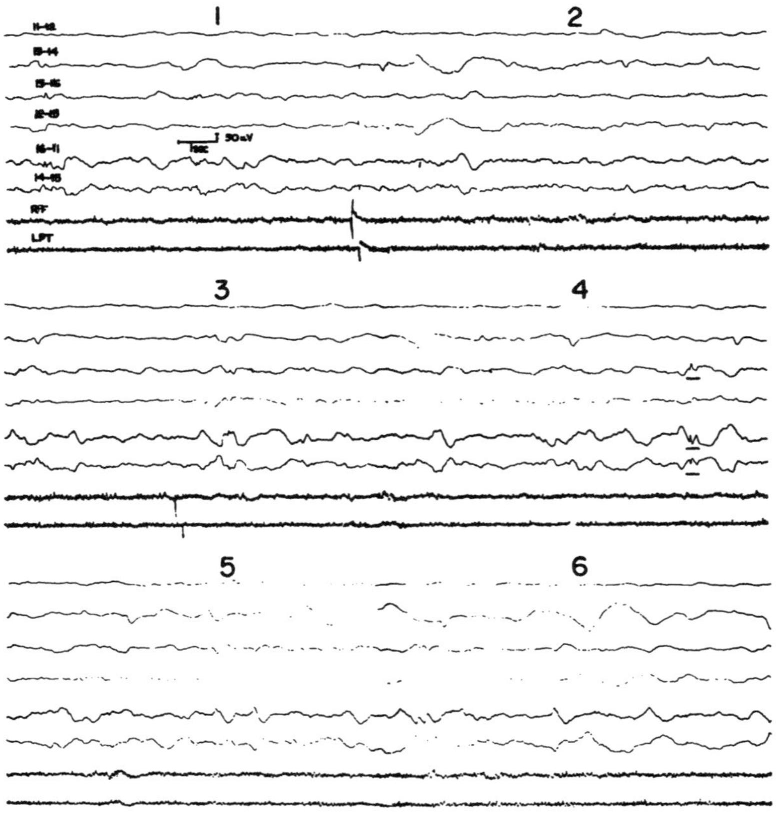

FIGURE XIV-17. Recordings from Patient 18

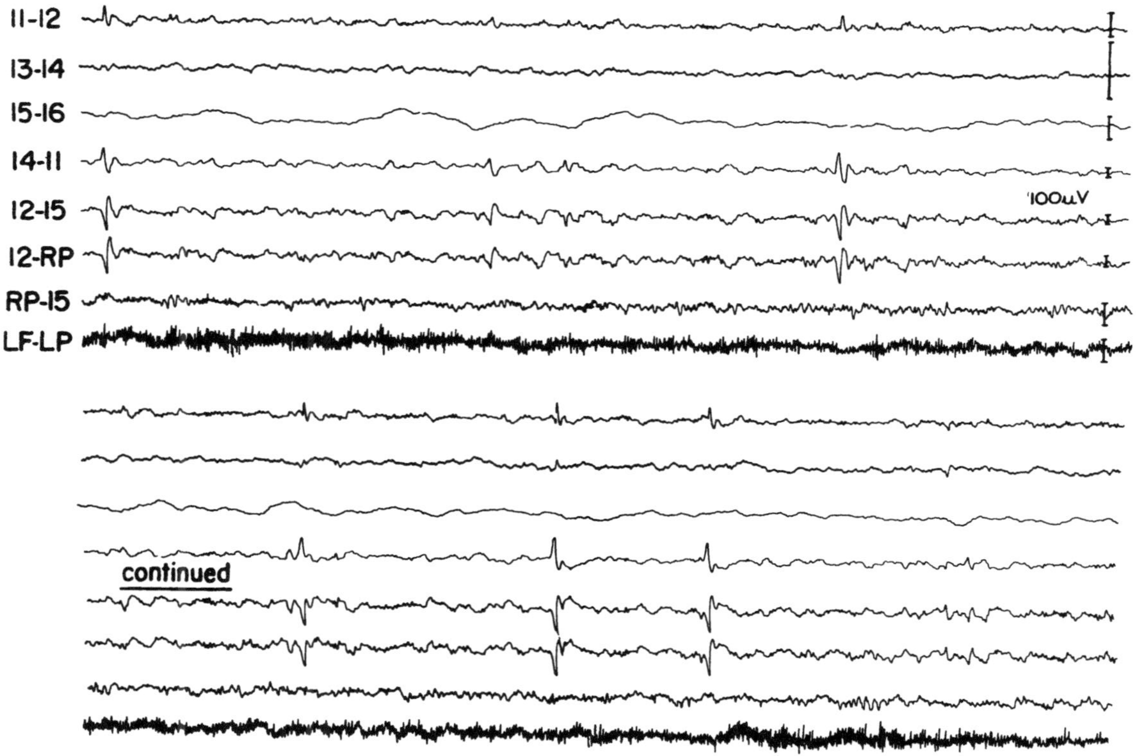

FIGURE XIV–18. Recordings from Patient 16

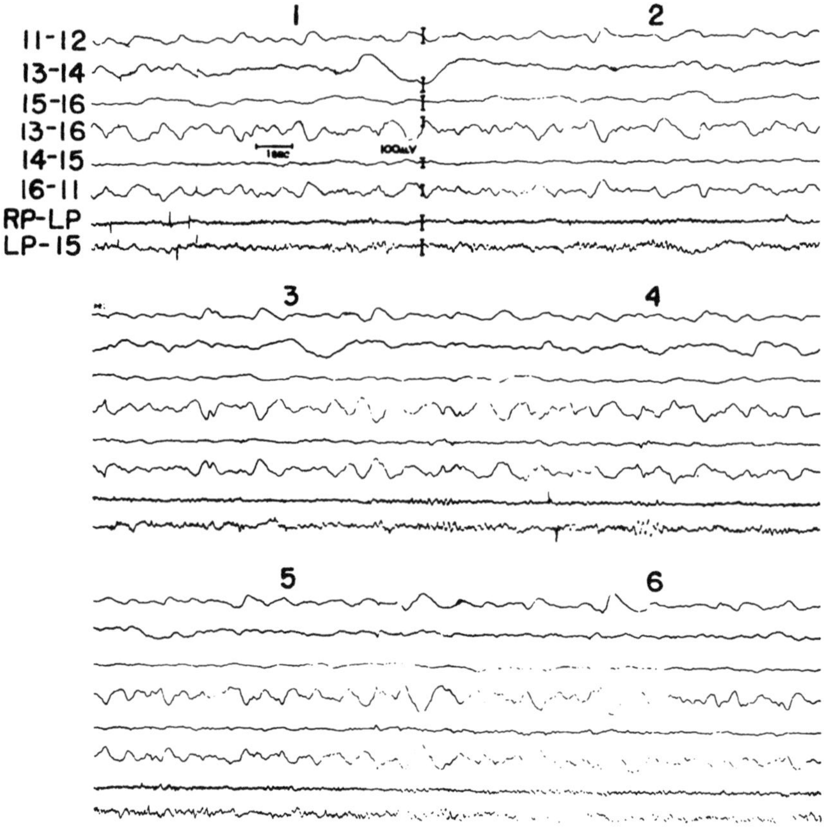

FIGURE XIV–19. Recordings from Patient 16

in such a manner as to eliminate or reduce them. This was, however, not completely successful in any case. Figure 19 illustrates the persisting slow wave activity. The meaning of the residual slow activity is not yet clear.*

In the top record of Figure 20, powerful spike discharge is noted at the extreme left and right of channel 3 (containing leads 15 and 16), as well as channels 5 and 6 (containing lead 16). The prominent, long-lasting disturbances in channel 2 (leads 13 and 14) are not germane to the present discussion. Seven and a half minutes after a 4-minute stimulation applied to the brain through leads 15 and 16 (middle record) slow wave activity was derived from these leads, but the sharp spikes

*For later information see Addendum E.

characteristically recorded from them prior to stimulation are not seen. Throughout the ensuing 2 1/2 hours no spike activity was ever noted from these same leads. This is clear from the bottom record, taken at the end of the observations on the day of operation. The patient was returned to the ward and another tracing made 3 hours later. The extremely disappointing result of this final recording is seen in Figure 21. Spikes have reappeared in leads 15 and 16 (channel 3) at this time. In spite of the resurgence of abnormal synchronized activity proper surgical care of the patient made it essential to proceed with the removal of the electrodes as planned.

COMPLICATIONS OF SUBCORTICAL STIMULATION

In addition to the occasional subcortical or cortical seizures described earlier we also found random spikes in the scalp leads of two patients. These appeared within an hour after stimulation and were occasionally synchronized with the subcortical spikes (Figure 11). With the passage of time, they disappeared from the cerebral hemisphere.

In the case of Patient 7 cortex and subcortex showed synchronized spikes and/or slow wave activity for at least 7 hours after the final stimulation. The striking synchrony of scalp and septal leads is apparent in Figure 22. The upper record was taken about 30 minutes after the final stimulation of the septal region (leads 11 and 12) and is relatively featureless when compared with the lower record, which was taken nearly 7 hours later. The latter shows the tremendous surge of high voltage spikes and slow waves which occasionally burst through to the cortex.

The fact that in a few cases subcortical stimulation was followed by a condition in which the subcortex and cortex fired together in an abnormal fashion may have some bearing on the clinical status of those patients in whom symptomatic seizures later occurred. Patient 7, whose record (Figure 22) provided the most outstanding example of synchronized discharge, had a routine electroencephalographic examination 1 month after operation. The outstanding finding at that time was a slow wave focus in the frontal regions. Two months after operation the waking record was normal. No further EEG's were obtained until about 11 months after the operation. During this interval the patient had a

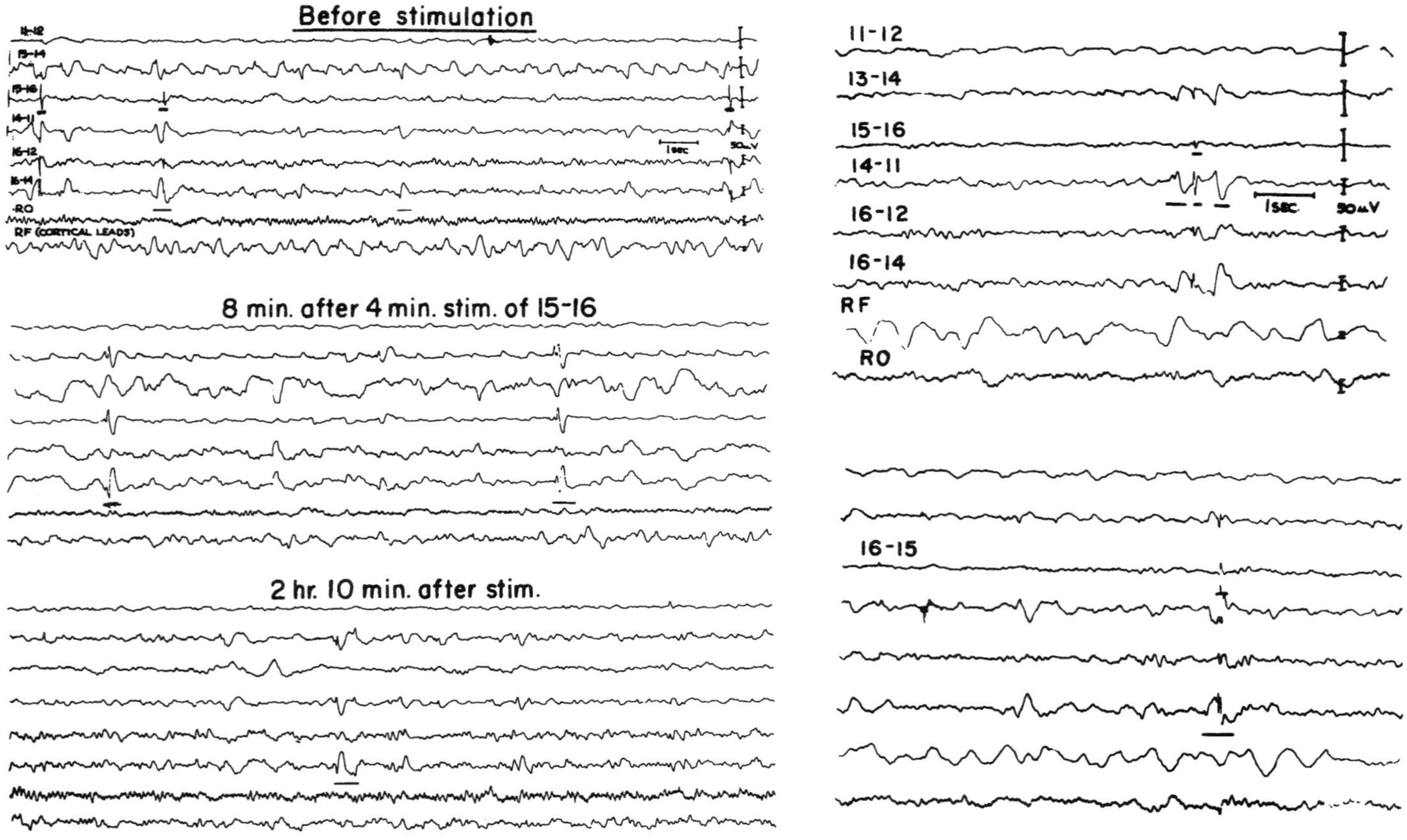

Before stimulation
11-12
13-14
15-16
14-11
16-12
16-14
RO
RF (CORTICAL LEADS)
1sec
50µV
8 min. after 4 min. stim. of 15-16
2 hr. 10 min. after stim.
11-12
13-14
15-16
14-11
1SEC
50µV
16-12
16-14
RF
RO
16-15

FIGURE XIV–20 (above, left). Recordings from Patient 13

FIGURE XIV–21 (above, right). Recordings from Patient 13

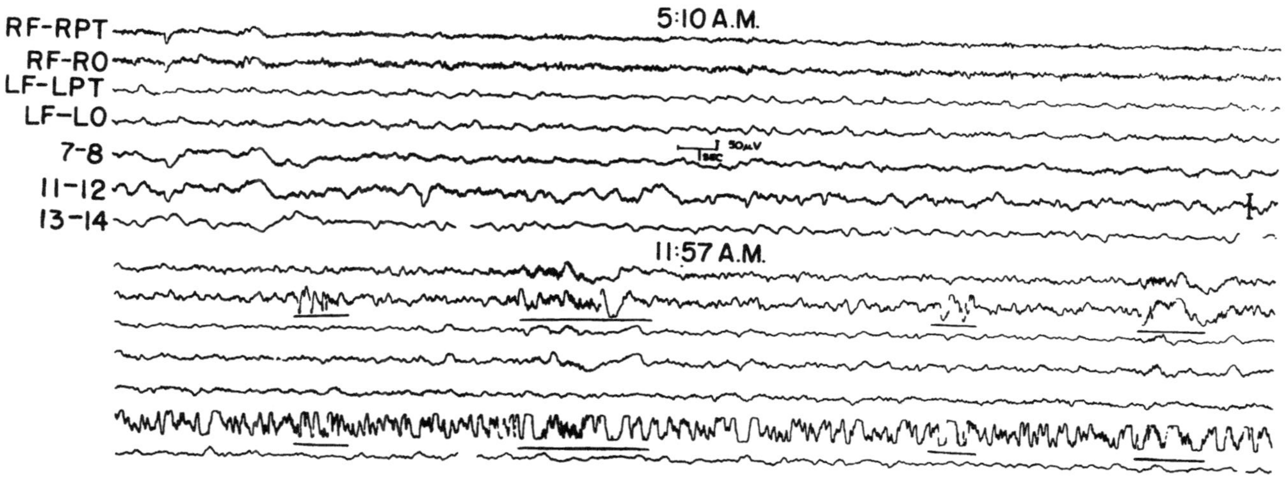

FIGURE XIV–22. Recordings from Patient 7

fit, or fainting spell, whose exact features cannot be determined from the subjective account. Another EEG was made a few days after the "spell," and this record showed, in addition to the frontal focus, an amplitude asymmetry in the occipitals. It is not inconceivable, therefore, that the prolonged tonic-clonic convulsions or impairments of consciousness which some of the patients experienced were due to the effects of subcortical stimulation.

DISCUSSION

Although we had no definite correlation between the presence of subcortical electrical abnormality and the status of the disease process, we tended to concentrate our thinking along these lines because of the striking character of the patterns obtained from the medio-basal areas discussed at length elsewhere in this report (Chapter 11). We had hoped that we should be able to disrupt the spike activity by electrical intervention, with the implicit assumption that the schizophrenic state would be concomitantly altered for the better. It was therefore a source of considerable discouragement that we were not able to abolish this activity for longer than a few hours in some patients and even less in others. Even in those cases in which spiking was abolished up to the end of the recordings, it appears unlikely that we succeeded in extinguishing it permanently. This conclusion is supported by the fact that in several cases in which this activity was eradicated for a time it reappeared in recordings made a few hours later. Moreover, there were two patients in our series who had two operations and courses of stimulation. The first, Patient 5(24), presented evidence of septal spiking during the first subcortical exploration. For a few months after stimulation her clinical status was somewhat improved. Then she gradually returned to a psychotic condition similar to that existing before the intervention. Thirteen and a half months later she was operated on again, preparatory to a second, more intense stimulation. Several hours of prestimulation recordings from the subcortex produced ample evidence of spike response in the same regions from which such activity had been obtained after the first procedure. Patient 8, who showed potent and frequent spikes, was stimulated with minimal current after his first operation. He subsequently followed approximately the same course as Patient 5. Seven months later he was operated upon again, and again responded in the usual fashion. The spikes were recorded in the same general area in which they had been localized on the previous trial.

Although we believe that spikes were abolished in few, if any, cases, it is impossible from the present data to be certain that they were not affected by the stimulation in other respects. Indeed, from the character of the records obtained we are inclined to suggest that in some cases the spikes may have been altered in frequency, size, and sharpness for considerable periods of time. It may be, even, that the degree of clinical improvement was related to the degree and duration of the modification of the abnormal response. But because of the methodological and biological variants previously discussed in these pages, the above suggestion should be recognized merely as a working hypothesis, cautiously made, and open to future validation or disavowal.*

The possibility exists, however, that subcortical spikes are not directly related to the schizophrenic state. In this view the spike and the aberrant mental attitudes may be separate products of a fundamental disorder. Conceivably, electrical intervention might produce clinical improvement without changes in the subcortical potentials and vice versa. Analogies drawn from electroencephalographic experience make such a postulate seem easily credible. Following a blow on the head, for example, slow wave cortical activity may be obtained during the period of unconsciousness produced by the accident and may persist long after the patient has apparently regained his normal clinical status.

Yet the appeal of a simple hypothesis, that the electrical and behavioral disorders are causally related remains, in spite of the rationalization given above and many others which might be put forward. Although the discussion thus far has emphasized the discouraging aspects of our failure to eliminate the subcortical spike, certain real satisfaction may be derived, on the other hand, from some of our results. For the idea that bizarre electrical patterns can be either altered or abolished has been confirmed, even if in a very limited sense. There can be no question that in many instances such activity was either abolished or reduced for a period long outlasting the stimulation. If spike and disease process are indeed related, we have

*Long-term correlations between recordings and behavior are reported in Addendum E.

then uncovered a tool for further work. The bright possibility is then open that intermittent stimulation over a long period, continuous stimulation over a longer period, or entirely different types of stimulation or other means of intervention (e.g., drugs) would be effective in abolishing this activity.* With the recent introduction into our technical armamentarium of the human stereotaxic apparatus for the implantation of subcortical electrodes, the stimulating of and recording from subcortical structures over a period of weeks has been achieved.

With advances in technique which allow prolonged physiological studies in conscious patients, the relationships between neurophysiological, biochemical, psychological, and psychiatric concomitants of schizophrenia may become more apparent than heretofore.

REFERENCES

1. Hunter, J., and H. Jasper. Effects of thalamic stimulation in unanesthetized animals; arrest reaction and petit mal-like seizures, activation patterns and generalized convulsions, *Electroencephalog. & Clin. Neurophysiol.*, 1:305–324 (1949).
2. Stoll, J., Jr., C. Ajmone-Marsan, and H. Jasper. Electrophysiological studies of subcortical connections of the anterior temporal region in the cat, *J. Neurophysiol.*, 14:305–316 (1951).
3. Ajmone-Marsan, C., and J. Stoll, Jr. Subcortical connections of the temporal pole in relation to temporal lobe seizures, *Arch. Neurol. & Psychiat.*, 66:669–686 (1951).
4. Penfield, W. Memory mechanisms, *Arch. Neurol. & Psychiat.*, 67:178–198 (1952).

*Further studies are reported in Addendum E.

CHAPTER 15

BIOCHEMICAL STUDIES ON THE PATIENT GROUP

ROBERT G. HEATH
T. DUANE PRICE
FLORENCE B. STROHMEYER

The humeral changes that accompany schizophrenia and their relationship to the humeral changes associated with the mechanism of stress have been summarized in the introductory chapter on the theoretical framework of our research program. They will be briefly touched on here by way of introducing the biochemical deviations from the normal of our series of schizophrenic patients.

The idea, often reported, that the adrenal cortex is underactive in schizophrenia is based on the resemblance of schizophrenics to Addisonians (a) in chronic metabolic status, as evidenced by low oxygen consumption, anemia, and similar aberrations in sugar metabolism,[1] and (b) in diminished response to stress. The changes reported as significant in the latter category include decreased retention of administered sodium[2] and smaller drops in circulating eosinophils[3] and lymphocytes.[4, 5]

There is much evidence to indicate that the alterations suggesting adrenocortical underactivity do not result solely from actual deficiency in the adrenal cortex. The most important evidence in this regard is the consistent finding that administration of adrenocortical substances or ACTH does not change the clinical course of schizophrenia.[6, 7, 8] Another important consideration, which is somewhat debated in the literature, is that schizophrenics respond normally, or almost normally, to ACTH.[3, 9, 10]

In our over-all theoretical concept we advanced the hypothesis that even though many schizophrenic patients display symptoms resembling those seen in persons with underactive adrenals, and even though the biochemical findings which have been briefly reviewed are correct, such deviations from the normal need not be due to a pathological condition, either functional or histological, in the adrenal cortex. We held that the primary defect was in the neural circuit—the decompensated schizophrenic reaction in most instances being triggered off by stressful situations associated with painful memories. This contention was based on the adaptational theory of behavior, on psychiatric observations, and on observations following frontal lobe surgery and other methods of therapy in schizophrenia. We further hypothesized that suppression of function in a specific area of the brain might be responsible for humeral changes similar to those effected by adrenalectomy. If this should be true, then activation of the area might provide a method of treating schizophrenic patients.

For the above reasons, and others that are less pertinent here, experimental studies were undertaken with animals. These are reported in Chapters 2–7. Chapter 2, which is the most relevant to the present discussion, demonstrates that damage to specific subcortical structures in the septal region of the forebrain can produce a picture similar to that produced by removal of the adrenals. Subsequent chapters discuss the interconnections between the septal region and the cerebral cortex and the integration of cortical and subcortical function.

On the strength of these animal studies, we then attempted to determine whether chemical changes similar to those produced by activation of the adrenal cortex could be observed in schizophrenic patients following electrical stimulation of the septal region of the forebrain.

The chemical data are incomplete on the first few patients, since we lacked facilities for setting up an efficient routine during the first year. During the second year, however, our methods were gradually developed and improved, and the amount of meaningful data increased as the series grew. By the time that adequate chemical evidence was in hand, it had been already established that there was a physiological abnormality in the septal region, the nature of which has been described in Chapter 11. Also by this time, it seemed probable from the marked increase in blood pressure following septal stimulation that the humeral mechanism was being activated.

In our attempts to gather meaningful chemical data many obstacles were recognized, and some we overcame as our technique improved. One of the principal obstacles was referable to the technique of electrode placement and stimulation. When the open method was used, the electrodes could be kept in place only 24, or at most, 54 hours. This meant that the first stimulation had to be given within 8 to 12 hours after the completion of surgery. Since the eosinophils drop markedly, or completely disappear for a period of 2 to 3 days following major surgery,[11] it was very difficult to separate the metabolic consequences of electrical stimulations from those of the surgical operation. Therefore, the eosinophil count, as well as many other measurements, could not be utilized in this connection. The lymphocyte count, likewise a valuable indicator of stress,[12, 13] returns to a preoperative level much sooner. In our series, the lymphocytes were usually approaching the preoperative level by the time the stimulation was administered. However, this was not always the case. In a few instances, they were still climbing rapidly, but the result was interpreted as minimizing rather than exaggerating the lymphopenic effect of stimulation. With this criterion it was clearly possible to separate the effects of stimulation from those of surgery plus stimulation. In the present report we have emphasized the findings which appear to be independent effects of the two procedures.

There were, throughout the series, some unavoidable minor variations in operative technique—particularly in the placement of the electrodes. This lack of uniformity made it useless to attempt an over-all statistical survey. By and large, each patient had to be studied individually, and the analytical values determined with exceptional accuracy, since checking values by subsequent collection of another sample was not possible.

We wish to express our appreciation to Philip M. Manson and Beryl O'Reardon, for their important part in testing and developing methods, as well as for making most of the measurements.

RESULTS

TESTS OF PITUITARY AND ADRENOCORTICAL FUNCTION

Tests of the Thorn type—that is, the 4-hour epinephrine test and the 4-hour ACTH test[14]—have been widely used to compare the anterior pituitary and adrenocortical responses of different individuals and groups. These tests involve measuring the concentration of eosinophils in the circulating blood before and after administering .3 mg. of epinephrine hydrochloride or 25 mg. of ACTH.[11, 14] The "normal," or "adequate," response is considered to be one in which a drop of 50 per cent or more is obtained in the eosinophil count; an inadequate response is indicated by a decrease of *less* than 50 per cent. We extended these tests to include control measurements of the individual diurnal variation of each patient in order to ascertain whether the measured change might reasonably be considered to reflect only the patient's *normal eosinophil variation* during the experimental period. Such normal variations, in tests covering a similar period, have been reported by Rud[15] and subsequently by Swanson, Bauer, and Ropes,[16] who describe them as occasionally interfering with the Thorn test. We further included in our battery of tests a procedure involving the administration of two 100-mg. doses of cortisone at zero and 24 hours, eosinophil concentrations being measured at zero and 48 hours.[17] This last test was designed to assure us that the patient could respond by a 50 per cent drop in eosinophils if the eosinophil-removing tissues were supplied with a high concentration of 11-17-oxy-corticosteroids. As regards determination of the concentration of the circulating eosinophils, we tried the Thorn-Dunger procedure[11] but found it to be too unreliable for routine use, since the eosinophil granules break up spontaneously, if the blood is allowed to stand in contact with the eosin-acetone mixture for longer than 3 minutes and the stained granules break up into many small particles unless a rigidly standard pipet-shaking technique is applied. We then tried the Randolph procedure.[18] Although it proved to be accurate—the results being comparable to those obtained on the same samples rapidly counted by the Thorn-Dunger technique—this method was found to have disadvantages from the standpoint of routine use because it is not only very time-consuming, but hard on the eyes of technicians required to do a large number of samples. Moreover, carelessness in the use of this technique was found to give high results due to the registering, under low power, of reticulocytes as eosinophils. We then observed that if heparin were added to the Thorn-Dunger diluting fluid the eosinophils would be much more stable. This method possesses all the advantages of the Thorn-Dunger technique as regards speed and ease of manipulation, and the additional virtue that a sample can be allowed to stand in contact with diluting fluid for about 4 hours before damage to the eosinophils becomes significant. However, by the time we were prepared to embark on the studies covered in this report, we had tested Pilot's method[19] and found it to be nearly as rapid as the acetone-heparin method and better suited to our purpose in that samples could be allowed to stand for as long as 8 hours before being counted. The findings on Patient 12 and all that followed were obtained by measurements with Pilot's method[19] alone or Pilot's method plus the eosin-acetone-heparin method. The results by the two methods agreed well.

Initially, we used the epinephrine and ACTH tests and the cortisone test as prognoses of the operative procedure, since the literature[14] indicated that consistent non-responders to either type of test were poor surgical risks. This theory rests on the assumption that non-responders will fail to elaborate the adrenocortical hormones considered necessary for recovery and so run the danger of irreversible shock. In order to ascertain whether stimulation would produce a change in reaction in schizophrenic patients, we also performed follow-up tests on preoperative non-responders.

Figure 1 shows the results obtained in the case of Patient 12. Although this patient consistently failed to respond to epinephrine or ACTH, cortisone produced an appropriate eosinopenic reaction. Moreover, the circulating eosinophils decreased to a negligible value after implantation of the electrodes and indeed not one eosinophil could be found in the sample taken only a few hours later than that represented by the last bar of the figure. Yet the patient showed no evidence of shock and recovered from the combined implantation and stimulation procedure without untoward incident. In a series of eight Thorn tests performed over the course of 7 months following stimulation, he continued as a characteristic non-responder, only one of the tests producing a 50 per cent decrease in eosinophil concentration. The findings on several other patients showed no change in response to epinephrine in the poststimulation period. However, Patient 14 showed an improved response, and Patient 18, a preoperative responder, appeared to have been converted to a non-responder. When extensive studies by Steele and Stratton[20] of the Tulane Medical School Department of Surgery indicated that about 33 per cent of the Thorn tests performed on various types of patients show inadequate response, it became clear that this reaction had no specificity relatable to schizophrenia. Since the Thorn test had

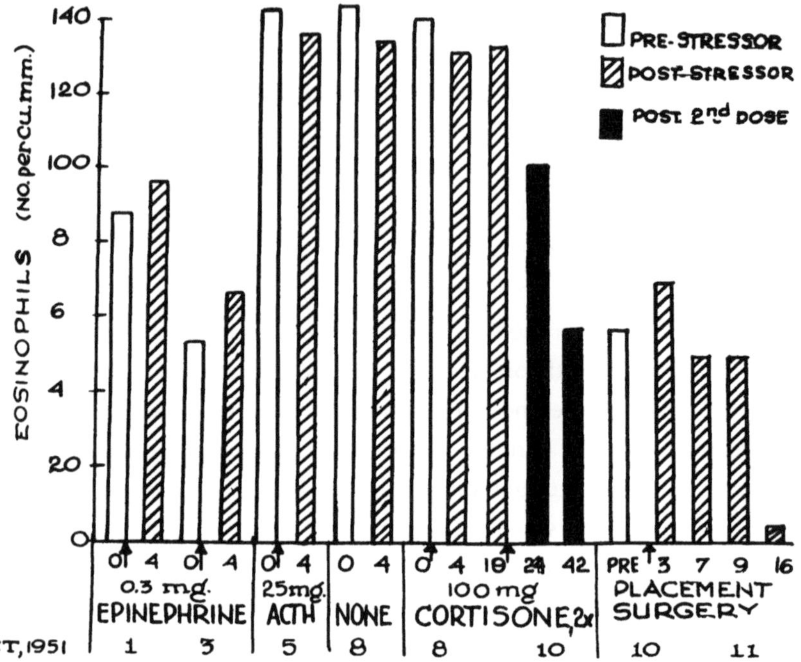

FIGURE XV–1. Responses of Patient 12 to epinephrine, ACTH, and cortisone tests

also proved unreliable in the prognosis of surgery, it was used routinely for the last time in the case of Patient 18.

EOSINOPENIC AND LYMPHOPENIC RESPONSES TO ELECTRODE IMPLANTATION

Our findings indicate that the brain surgery involved in electrode implantation constitutes a very great stress. With the open method of placement, the eosinophils decreased continuously for approximately 12 hours, in most cases reaching a value of zero shortly before or after this period; the highest concentration observed within 12 to 24 hours was 10 cells per cu. mm.* Although usually on the ascending grade at the time stimulation was applied, the lymphocyte concentrations had sometimes decreased as much as 90 per cent and rarely less than 60 per

*Inasmuch as we counted the total number of eosinophils in 1.2 or 2.4 cu. mm. of blood, much larger volumes than are usually examined, our figures may be considered exceptionally reliable.

cent—in fact, the leukopenic reaction was frequently prolonged into the stimulation period. Thus, both the eosinophil count and the magnitude and duration of the lymphopenic reaction testify to the stress imposed by electrode implantation as compared with other types of operation as recorded in the literature.

LYMPHOPENIC RESPONSES TO STIMULATION

The lymphopenic response is the most transitory of the stress reactions and proved to be the only one which could be consistently used as a criterion of the stress elicited by stimulation alone in contrast to the additive effects of the surgery and stimulation, which together are reflected by many other measures of adrenocortical activity. Of the twelve patients in whom the lymphopenic response was followed in detail during and after stimulation, eight showed marked decreases in poststimulation concentrations as compared with prestimulation concentrations. This is considered particularly noteworthy in view of the fact that in each case the lymphocyte concentration had reached its lowest point and was ascending to the normal level at the time of stimulation. In these studies the lymphocyte count was determined from the total concentration of white cells obtained from duplicate samples, four chambers being counted, and from differential concentrations in which from 400 to 1,000 cells were counted instead of the usual 100, the smears being made at least in duplicate and frequently in quadruplicate.[21]

Table 1 shows the results obtained on twelve patients. The breakdown of this table was motivated by the findings of Hume[22] and McGoon,[23] who produced an eosinopenic response in dogs and cats by hypothalamic stimulation, and those of Harris,[13] who elicited lymphopenia in rabbits by the same means. However, it must be pointed out that our analysis of the data was based on presumptive evidence that the stimulation was applied to the hypothalamus in the case of each of the twelve patients in Table 1. Such a breakdown may be probably unjustified at the present time because of inadequate criteria for localizing the stimuli. The MLR column shows the decrease in lymphocyte concentration as compared with the prestimulation value, the lowest point being chosen and the decrease expressed in percentage. It will be noted that in two of the three cases in which the MLR value was nil (Patients 16 and 24) a

TABLE XV–1. Lymphopenic responses in relation to electrode location

Patient	*Time of stim. (hrs. post no. 1)* Septal	*S–H*	*Time of L.R. (hrs. post no. 1)*	*L.R. (%)*	*M.L.R. (%)*	*Comments*
I. PATIENTS WITH AT LEAST ONE ELECTRODE NEAR HYPOTHALAMUS						
14		0.1	3.75		80	
		0.35				Steady fall
		2.77				from pre-stim.
		4.45				
		0.0	1.0		70	15 min. rise, then steady fall
16	0.0	0.95	1.4	53	0	Never below
	0.17	1.47	to 1.9	(1700		pre-stim.
	0.60	2.97		to 800)		
	3.48	3.87				
	4.20					
17			2.54		32	
19			4.6		54	Rise to 1.2 hrs., then steady fall
20	0.0	1.48	2.1		16	Seemed held
	0.32					down. Rise
	3.17					from 6.3 et seq.
22	Subcort. white matter		2.2		0	
23	0.0	0.87	3.54		76	Initial rise,
	1.80					stayed low
	2.05					after 3.5
25			1.8		24	Rose later. Deemed nil
II. PATIENTS RECEIVING SEPTAL STIMULATION BUT WITH ALL ELECTRODES REMOVED FROM HYPOTHALAMUS						
15					73	
18					38	
21					56	
24			0.65 to 1.65	38 (1850 to 1150)	0	

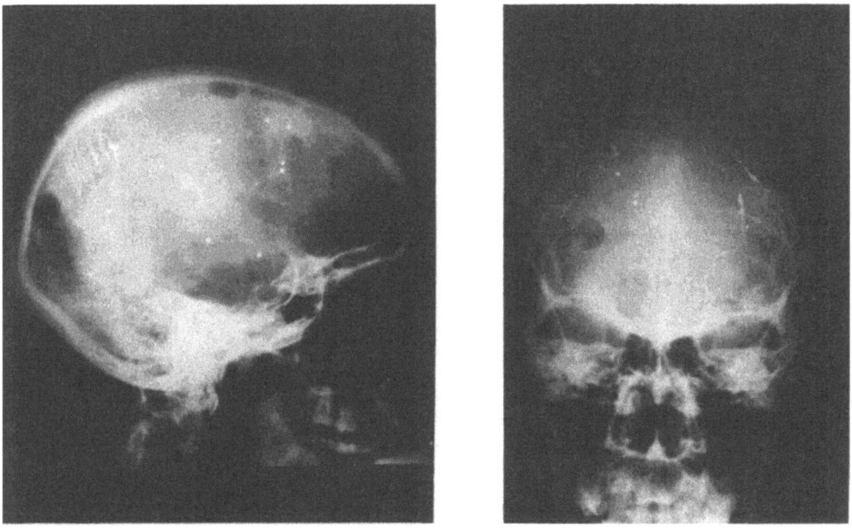

FIGURE XV–2. Location of electrodes in Patient 22

marked lymphopenic reaction occurred during or immediately after stimulation. However, the lowest poststimulation value did not fall below the prestimulation value. These two cases are considered significant, inasmuch as the initial values were still very low in consequence of surgery and the curves would ordinarily have been ascending continuously within experimental error unless a stress had been applied. In the case of Patient 22, who at no time showed a lymphopenic reaction, x-rays revealed that the electrodes were inadvertently dislodged during closure of the scalp, with the result that the conducting ends were pulled up into the white matter near the cortex (Figure 2). When the stimuli were applied, the patient had tonic seizures, which, if anything, should have increased the stress. This case, therefore, turned out to be a control on the specificity of electrode location and the stress of minor seizures.

Although thorough studies of lymphopenic response were worked up for all twelve of the patients represented in Table 1, only six cases are illustrated here in detail (Figures 3–9). Each of these examples was selected on the basis of the type of lymphopenic response obtained and the presumed location of the stimulating electrode. Eosinophil changes are also shown, though somewhat less dramatically, in Figures 3–9.

Figure 3 illustrates the findings in the case of Patient 25, who was

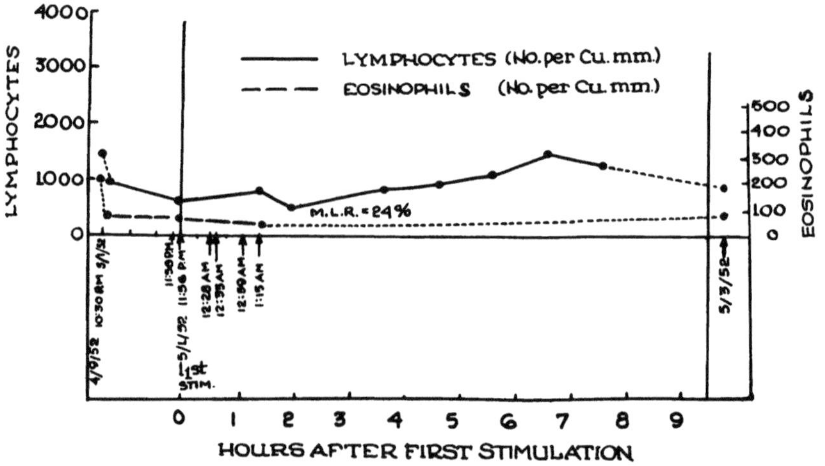

FIGURE XV–3. Lymphocyte and eosinophil changes in Patient 25

known to be in the terminal stage of cancer at the time of operation. Post mortem examination showed that widespread metastases had invaded both the hypothalamus and the pituitary from the primary site in the breast. As previously mentioned, the location of the nearest stimulating electrode to the hypothalamus was inadequately established.

Figures 4 and 5 demonstrate the profound lymphopenic response of Patient 14 to stimulation in the septo-hypothalamic region. When the stimuli were applied, nearly 20 hours had elapsed since surgery, and the lymphocyte concentration had regained its normal level. We recall from the literature no other type of stressor which has been shown to decrease the lymphocyte count so sharply or extensively; however, it will be shown in other cases in our series that the stress of electrode placement often produced an equally profound effect. In this particular patient the electrodes remained *in situ* for 2 days. Figure 4 illustrates the effect of surgery and stimulation on the first day, Figure 5 the effect of stimulation for 3 minutes at 8 ma. on the second day. In this study 1,000 cells were counted for each point. The preliminary short-lived lymphophilia previously reported as an immediate consequence of various stresses, appeared in this case at 15 minutes; the maximum lymphopenic response was observed at 1 hour—the value being 70 per cent. No further samples were taken until 3.5 hours—at which time the customary rise had occurred. The spacing of these samples is attributed to the fact

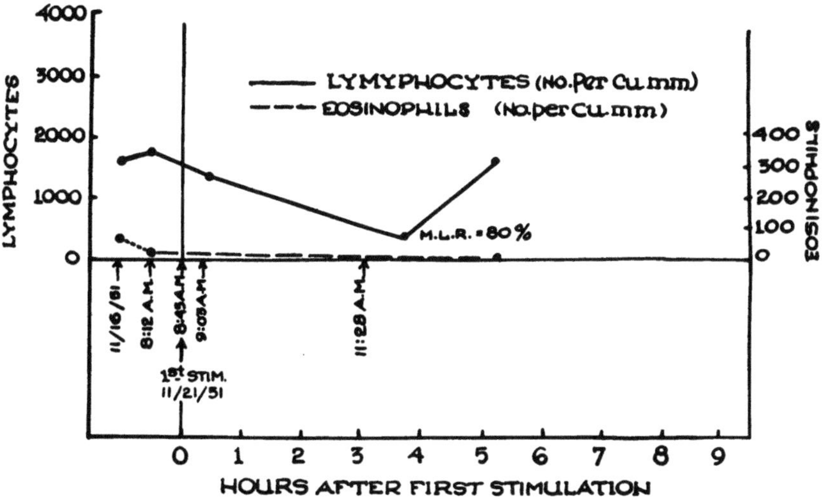

FIGURE XV–4. Lymphocyte and eosinophil changes in Patient 14, November 21, 1951

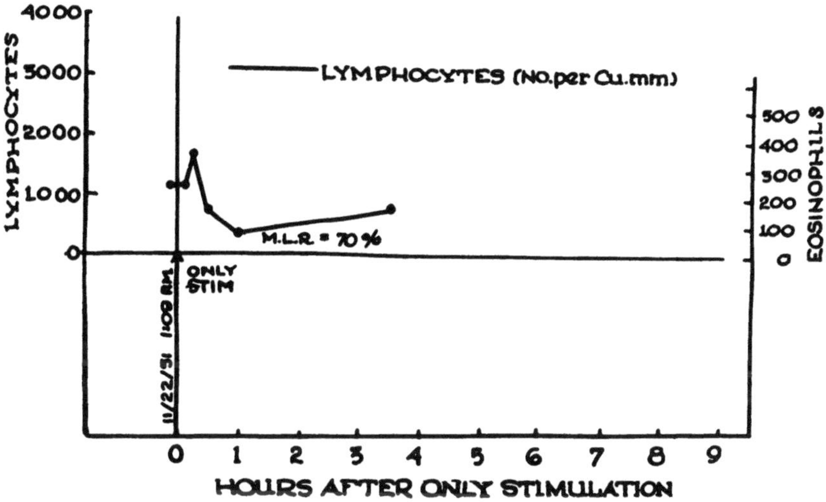

FIGURE XV–5. Lymphocyte changes in Patient 14, November 22, 1951

that the last interval represents the time which elapsed between the hours of 2 and 4:30 on Thanksgiving Day.

The eosinopenic reaction of Patient 14 to surgery is also shown in Figure 4. Immediately after operation the rather low initial count of 50 was diminished to 10 and shortly thereafter the value decreased to zero. It is not obvious but likely that the disappearance of the eosinophils

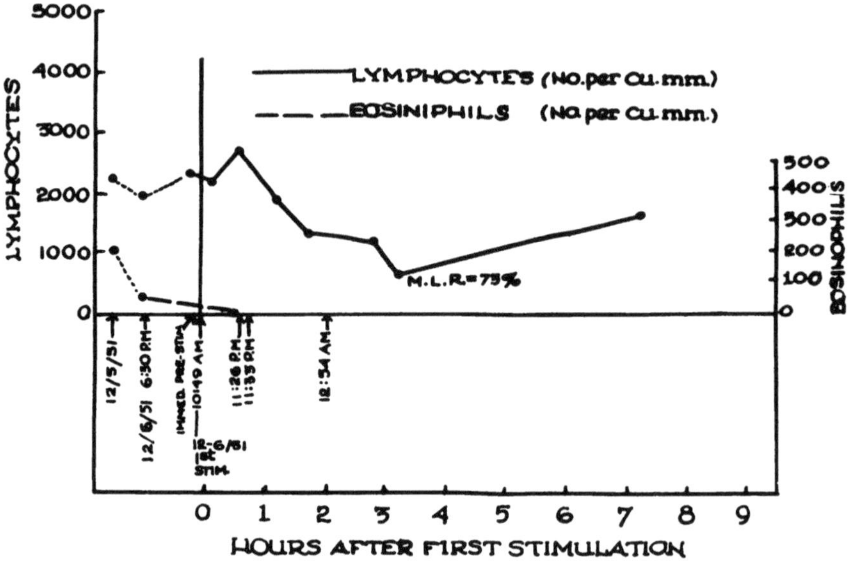

FIGURE XV–6. Lymphocyte and eosinophil changes in Patient 15, December 6, 1951

was due to stimulation. As a rule, the eosinophil concentrations of our patients followed the usual pattern of response to major stress in remaining low for 2 days (at less than 10 per cu. mm.) and then mounting on the third—this increase being known as the "third day rise" or "third day eosinophilia." Seven days after the first stimulation they reached 150 per cu. mm.

Figure 6 shows the lymphopenic response obtained from Patient 8 (15) by multiple stimulations. All of these were septal, and none was regarded as being near the hypothalamus. The magnitude of the lymphocyte drop is 73 per cent, which is comparable to that obtained from Patient 14 with the electrodes adjacent to, but not clearly in, the hypothalamus.

Figure 7 shows the lymphopenic response obtained from Patient 19 after stimulations to several points which could not be isolated. It further shows the drastic eosinopenic effect of surgery on an epinephrine nonresponder. The rise which occurred 4 hours after administration of epinephrine on 1/14/52 is plotted at the left. The relatively low prestimulation value of 70 eosinophils per cu. mm. was due to the patient's having responded normally to a Thorn-type ACTH test. Patient 19 subsequently

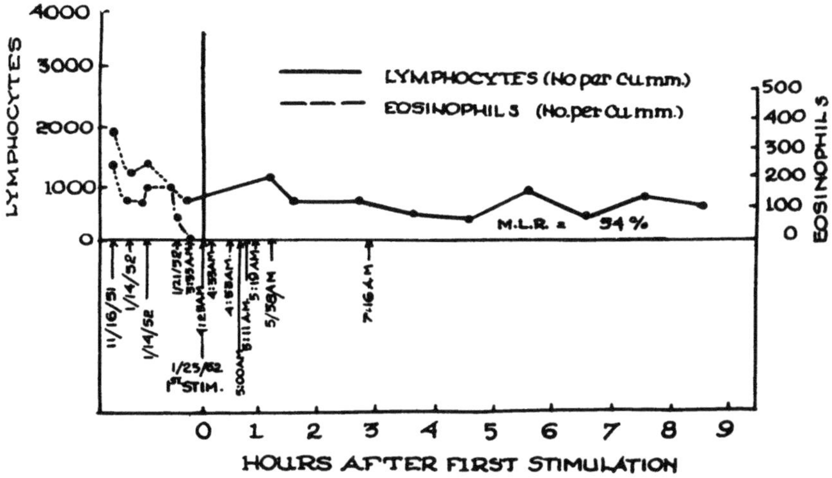

FIGURE XV–7. Lymphocyte and eosinophil changes in Patient 19, January 23, 1952

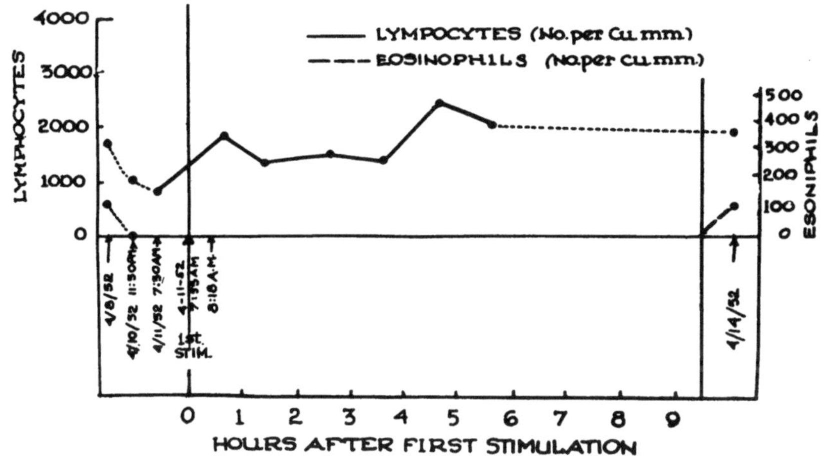

FIGURE XV–8. Lymphopenic curve on Patient 24, who failed to respond with lymphopenia to stimulation, April 11, 1952

developed an abscess involving the septum, the consequences of which will be discussed in relation to the electrolyte findings.

Figure 8 shows the findings on Patient 5 (24)—one of the three from whom no MLR value was obtained. At no point did the lymphocyte concentration fall below the initial value of approximately 800. However, when it is considered that the samples were taken from a patient

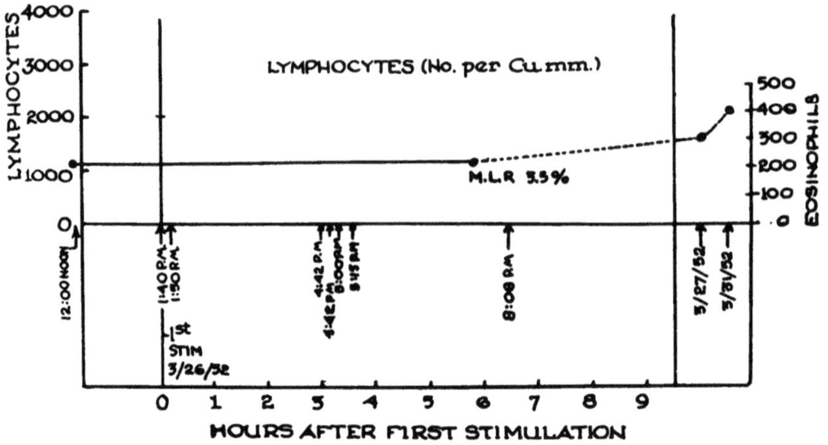

FIGURE XV–9. Effect on circulating lymphocytes of stimulation of the subcortical white matter in Patient 22, March 26, 1952

whose lymphocyte concentration was initially low as a consequence of surgery, the values in Figure 8 also indicate a transitory lymphophilia followed by a lymphopenic reaction, which amounted to 38 per cent.

Figure 9 shows a curve plotted from stimulation to the higher regions of the brain (see Figure 2). As previously explained, Patient 22 should be considered a control for demonstrating the specificity of initiating lymphopenic response to electrode placement in the septo-hypothalamic region. In this patient neither the stimulation procedure nor the tonic seizures developed during stimulation induced lymphopenia. The lymphocyte concentration remained unperturbed following surgery.

CHANGES OF ELECTROLYTE CONCENTRATION IN PLASMA AND URINE

As reported in Chapter 2, our experiments with cats indicated that destructive lesions in the basal part of the septum and the orbital region of the cortex produce drastic depletion of plasma sodium. The cells of this region may control sodium retention by hormonal processes or by regulation of nerve stimulation to endocrine glands, or may act directly upon functional tissues. Regardless of the mechanism, it would seem probable that electrical stimulation of this region would produce the reverse effect of ablation—namely, retention of sodium, which would be manifested by an increased plasma concentration. We have obtained evidence that septal stimulation does indeed produce sodium retention in man. Such effects of septal stimulation and the surgery which preceded it were, however, short-lived. Patients followed before and after stimulation, on a long-term basis, showed no greater variation than do normal individuals in concentrations of plasma sodium and potassium except in the immediate poststimulation period. Perhaps greater refinement of technique, with excretion studies conducted while patients are on controlled diets, may show changes to parallel the psychiatric and psychological effects. Our electrolyte findings are not incompatible with the observations of alterations in psychiatric and psychological status following stimulation on a normal *ad libitum* diet.

The routine long-range study of Patient 19 proved, in retrospect, to be of exceptional interest. The analytical findings are reported in Table 2.

This patient, being a hypertensive, was maintained on a low-salt diet while a patient at Charity Hospital. Preoperatively the plasma sodium concentration remained within normal limits on this regimen. The potassium was on the lower border of the normal range. The first plasma sample taken after operation showed the sodium, potassium, and chloride exceptionally low. An immediate attempt was made to rectify this condition by placing the patient on a normal diet, somewhat high in carbohydrates and proteins, and by supplying extra sodium and potassium chlorides as indicated. The administered potassium was adequately retained, as demonstrated by plasma analysis performed 2 weeks later in two different laboratories. The low concentration of sodium showed that a profound change had occurred subsequent to, or as a result of, the operation. The patient died shortly afterward, and autopsy showed that an abscess involving the septal region had developed. Although more extensive, the brain lesion was comparable to those placed artificially in the cats. The effect of such a lesion on the retention of sodium was thus extended from cats to humans. Brain sections of this patient showing invasion of the septal region by the abscess are shown in Figure 10.

Most of our short-term studies on changes in plasma and urine sodium and potassium demonstrate only that there is marked retention of sodium following the combined procedures of electrode placement and stimulation. Table 3, which shows the results obtained from Patient 22, is pre-

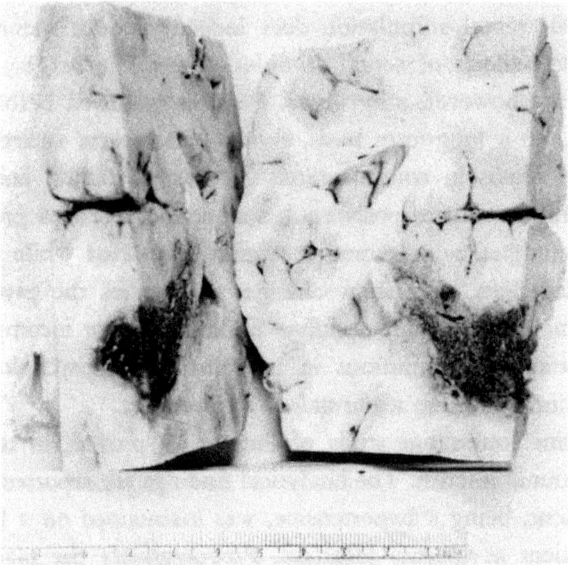

FIGURE XV–10. Section of brain of Patient 19. The abscess was a complication of the operative procedure

sented as an example of the marked sodium retention that may occur in consequence of the combined influences of electrode placement and stimulation. Although the results are inconclusive as regards the specific effect of stimulation on this process, the rise in plasma sodium and the decrease in plasma potassium show a very definite trend, considering the conditions of the study. Routinely we do not claim that the determination of sodium can be made closer than plus or minus 1 meq. per liter, and potassium to plus or minus .1 meq. per liter. However, when all of the determinations of a single experiment are made in one series, and the readings of the standards do not fluctuate throughout the course of flame photometric analysis, such differences as are shown in this table are definite and reliable.

Table 3 also illustrates dramatically the superiority of electrolyte measurements on urine instead of plasma for determining the consequences of a process in which increased potassium excretion and decreased sodium excretion both occur. The body pools of sodium and potassium are large, and drastic changes in excretory pattern can occur without an appreciable alteration of the plasma concentration. Expression of urinaly-

TABLE XV-2. Plasma electrolyte changes on development of brain abscess in hypertensive patient (Patient 19)

Date	*Na-K Intake*	*Plasma*		
		Na	*K*	*Cl*
11/15/51	Low salt	145	3.0	
1/14/52	Low salt	135	2.8	
1/23/52	*Operation*			
2/5/52*	Low salt	119	2.2	68
2/18/52	Normal, also infusions of NaCl, oral KCl*	123.5 (124)	4.8 (4.8)	

*Started normal diet. Infusions 154 meq. NaCl 3 times per week; oral KCl.

TABLE XV-3. Short-term changes of plasma sodium and potassium concentrations and of urinary potassium-sodium ratios in response to surgery and stimulation in Patient 22

Time		*Plasma*		
Date	*Hour*	*Na* (*meq/l*)	*K* (*meq/l*)	*Urinary K-Na ratio*
2/18/52				0.43
3/21/52		136.7	5.0	
3/25/52	AM.	*Surgery*		
3/25/52–3/26/52	12 N–1 A.M.			0.72
3/26/52	12:30 A.M.	135.9	4.3	
3/26/52	1:13–2:54 A.M.	*Cortical stimulation*		
3/26/52	3:30 A.M.	136.3	5.0	
3/26/52	12 N	137.4	5.2	
3/26/52	1:40–8:08 P.M.	*Subcortical stimulation*		
3/26/52	6:30 P.M.	138.1	4.2	
3/26/52	7:30 P.M.	140.0	4.4	
3/27/52	10:45 A.M.	140.0	4.3	
3/27/52				3.6

sis results as potassium-sodium ratios instead of concentrations of the individual elements in urine merely simplifies presentation of the results, since the actual concentrations are so markedly influenced by variations in water intake. The range in magnitude of potassium-sodium ratios is between 0.3 and 0.8 in normal subjects on normal diets. The values which we actually obtained on all except one of the patients from whom urine was collected preoperatively and between 2 and 5 days postopera-

TABLE XV–4. Preliminary report on the influence of surgery and stimulation on urinary excretion of potassium and sodium

	Prestimulation			Poststimulation	
Patient	*Date of sample*	*K-Na ratio*	*Stim. dates*	*Date of sample*	*K-Na ratio*
11	pre-	0.67	9/20	9/24	1.18
12	10/12	0.85	10/12	10/17	2.8
13	10/23	0.56	10/23	10/25	0.78
18	1/4	0.39			
	1/7	0.44			
	1/8	0.67	1/9 12:11 A.M.	1/9 2 P.M.	1.08
22	2/18	0.43	3/26	3/27	3.6
25*	5/9	0.64	5/9*	5/10	0.69
				5/11	2.43
				5/12	1.56

*Stimulated 8 days after surgery.

tively are listed in Table 4. Whereas, preoperatively, the work-up values were always within the normal range when schizophrenic patients remained on the hospital diet, most of the postoperative ratios shown here from patients on the same diet are above normal. In each case, it will be noted that the ratio increased postoperatively.

Findings obtained after an isolated septal stimulation of Patient 25, the only subject in whom the electrodes remained in place for a sufficient time to allow recovery from the metabolic consequences of surgery, are shown in the last rows of Table 4. On the first day after the isolated stimulation there was a negligible increase in the potassium-sodium ratio, which was accompanied by polyuria, on the second day there was an appreciable increase, and on the third day a decrease, but the third-day value remained well above the first day value. During this period Patient 25's electrolyte excretion pattern following the isolated septal stimulation was essentially the same as that of patients subjected simultaneously to the effects of surgery and stimulation. Unfortunately, this study could not be continued because infusions of physiological saline were required for therapeutic reasons. Further details on the electrolyte balance of Patient 25 consequent to combined surgery-stimulation and to isolated septal stimulation are presented in Tables 5 and 6. Normal values for plasma and urine over the 3-day period before surgery are shown in the upper section of Table 5. Plasma and urine concentrations of potassium and sodium are expressed in meq. per liter—the potassium-sodium ratio being entered under the urinary heading. The volume of urine excreted during the period covered by the test is entered in the third from the last column (all samples having been collected by catheter); and the milliequivalents of potassium and sodium excreted during the 24-hour period are totaled in the last two columns. There was an increase in the potassium-sodium ratio on the first postoperative day; and this continued until 7 o'clock on the morning of the second postoperative day, which included the first stimulation. The resulting high ratio was due primarily to sodium retention, as shown in the last column. Sodium retention by this subject, and on this occasion only, did not persist beyond the first day after stimulation.

Table 6 shows the effects on electrolyte balance of the isolated stimulation of Patient 25. The metabolic trend following the stimulation, uncomplicated by surgery or infusions, is most dramatic. We hesitate to say, however, on the basis of this one study, that such changes are characteristic results of septal stimulation. Although the subject was a terminal cancer patient and although the metabolic changes recorded for the period of 13 or 14 days prior to stimulation are not given here, it will be noted that the latest prestimulation values of both constituents had returned approximately to normal, and that the stimulation was followed by a profound diuresis without significant increase in sodium retention or in the potassium-sodium ratio. The diuresis was characterized by excretion of 3.7 liters of urine by this very small patient (who weighed only 70 pounds); the results of the water loss were manifested in concentrations of both potassium and sodium in the blood and also showed up in the erythrocyte counts (not listed here).

On the second day following stimulation marked sodium retention was accompanied by increased potassium excretion, resulting in a potassium-sodium ratio of 2.43. On the third day the urine was divided into two portions, showing potassium-sodium ratios of 1.54 and 1.74, respectively. For once the therapeutic regimen served to simplify rather than complicate interpretation of our chemical findings. Twelve hours after administration of the saline infusion an enormous sodium retention was demonstrated by the concentrations in the blood (156 and 160

TABLE XV–5. Effects of surgery and stimulation on the electrolyte balance of Patient 25

	Time			Plasma		Urinary Excretion					
										Total meq. per 24 hours	
Treatment	*Date*	*Hour*	*Status*	K (meq/1)	Na (meq/1)	K (meq/1)	Na (meq/1)	K–Na ratio	Vol. in liters	K	Na
None	4/28–4/29	11–11 A.M.	Pre-			17.2	25.3	0.68	—	—	—
	4/29	——		3.6	133						
	4/29–4/30					21.7	30.0	0.72	2.35	50.9	70.4
	4/30–5/1	4 P.M.–7 A.M.				19.8	50.4	0.39	1.60	31.7	80.7
Surgery	5/1	10 A.M.–2 P.M.									
	5/1	10:30 P.M.	Post-surg. & pre-stim. no. 1	4.5	144						
	5/1–5/2	7–7 A.M.	Through stim. no. 1			35.0	26.3	1.33	1.55	54.3	40.8
Stimulation no. 1	5/2	1–3 A.M.									
	5/2	7:30 A.M.	Post-	3.6	139						
	5/2–5/3	7–7 A.M.				24.9	38.2	0.65	1.98	49.3	75.7
	5/3	1:30 P.M.		4.0	133						
	5/3–5/4	7–7 A.M.				21.8	34.3	0.64	1.80	39.3	61.7

TABLE XV–6. Effects of isolated septal stimulation on the electrolyte balance of Patient 25

	Time			Plasma		Urinary excretion					
Treatment	*Date*	*Hour*	*Status*	*K (meq/1)*	*Na (meq/1)*	*K (meq/1)*	*Na (meq/1)*	*K–Na ratio*	*Vol. in liters*	*Total meq. per 24 hours K*	*Total meq. per 24 hours Na*
None	5/8–5/9	1–1 P.M.	Pre no. 4			25.8	41.4	0.62	2.05	52.9	85.0
	5/9	3 P.M.		4.0	128						
	5/9	1–3 P.M.				24.7	32.4	0.76	—	—	—
Stimulation no. 4	5/9	3–4 P.M.									
	5/9	4–9:30 P.M.	Post no. 4			17.6	26.5	0.66	0.59	10.4	15.6
									3.70	49.3	71.9
	5/9–5/10	9:30–4 P.M.				12.5	18.1	0.69	3.11	38.9	56.3
	5/9	7:40 P.M.		4.1	130						
	5/10	7 P.M.		5.3	149						
	5/10–5/11	4–4 P.M.	Post no. 4			43.3	17.8	2.43	1.95	84.5	34.7
	5/12	2 P.M.		5.2	149						
	5/11–5/12	4–1 P.M.				34.6	22.4	1.54	1.64	53.3	34.5
									1.79	59.3	37.9
	5/12	1–4 P.M.				40.0	23.0	1.74	0.15	6.0	3.4
Infusion regimen —water, glucose, NaCl	5/12–5/17	4 P.M.–3 P.M.									
154 meq. NaCl 2000 ml.	5/14	12 N		4.2	156						
5% glucose daily	5/14	3 P.M. (spot sample)				11.4	62.2	0.18	—	—	—
1500 ml. 5% glucose	5/16	11 A.M.		4.7	160						
4 P.M. 5/16, to 11 A.M., 5/17	5/17	11:30 A.M.		3.6	140						

meq./L). It was not reflected in the urinary potassium-sodium ratio because the amount of sodium administered was so large. To restore the normal balance, aqueous glucose was administered alone the following day.

SUMMARY

1. Studies of biochemical and hematological changes resulting from mild electrical stimulation applied to the septal and septo-hypothalamic regions of the human brain have been reviewed. Stimulations in this general region elicited a marked lymphopenic reaction, the decreases in blood lymphocyte concentration frequently being as large as 60 to 80 per cent.
2. In a single case, a terminal cancer patient with metastases to the pituitary and hypothalamus, septal stimulation evoked a 24-hour diuresis resulting in marked dehydration. On the second and third days following stimulation, marked retention of sodium occurred. None of the stimulations applied to this patient elicited significant eosinopenic or lymphopenic responses; these findings suggest that the brain can regulate, by separate mechanisms, two categories of the functions generally ascribed to the adrenal cortex and believed to be mediated by the single hormone, ACTH.
3. Another patient developed a brain abscess in the septal region; the consequent irreversible loss of plasma sodium proceeded as previously described for cats with lesions in the septal region of the forebrain and the orbital cortex (see Chapter 2).
4. Studies of the response to electrode placement show that such surgery often constituted an exceptionally great stress.
5. In general, responses of schizophrenic patients to epinephrine were found to be normal. Response to tests of the Thorn type contributed nothing to surgical prognosis that was not shown by ordinary evaluation of pituitary and adrenal function. Those patients who failed to respond preoperatively to epinephrine or ACTH responded normally with a profound eosinopenia and lymphopenia to the surgery of electrode placement, and their recovery was not marked by shock.
6. Changes in urinary potassium-sodium ratios, used in measuring electrolyte response to stressors, were found to be more sensitive for this purpose than were changes in plasma electrolyte concentrations.

REFERENCES

1. Hoskins, R. G. *The Biology of Schizophrenia,* p. 105. Norton, New York, 1946.
2. Pincus, G., and Hoagland, H. Adrenal cortical responses to stress in normal men and in those with personality disorders; some stress responses in normal and psychotic subjects, *Am. J. Psychiat.,* 106:641–650 (1950).
3. Lee, R. E., L. Babcock, R. Reilly, L. Schlann, and C. G. Pfeiffer. Thorn test on institutionalized schizophrenic patients, *Fed. Proc.,* 10:318 (1951).
4. Pincus, G., and F. Elmadjian. The lymphocyte response to heat stress in normal and psychotic subjects, *J. Clin. Endocrinol.,* 6:295–300 (1946).
5. Hoagland, H., F. Elmadjian, and G. Pincus. Stressful psychomotor performance and adrenal cortical function as indicated by the lymphocyte response, *J. Clin. Endocrinol.,* 6:301–311 (1946).
6. Freeman, H., and F. Elmadjian. Carbohydrate and lymphoid studies in schizophrenia, *Am. J. Psychiat.,* 106:660–667 (1950).
7. Hoagland, H., and G. Pincus. Pituitary-adrenocortical function in patients with severe personality disorders, *in Proceedings of the First Clinical ACTH Conference.* Blakiston, Philadelphia, 1950.
8. Cleghorn, R. A., B. F. Graham, M. Saffran, and D. E. Cameron. A study of the effect of the pituitary ACTH in depressed patients, *Canad. M. A. J.,* 63:329–331 (1950).
9. Parsons, E. H., E. F. Gildea, E. Ronzoni, and S. Z. Hulbert. Comparative lymphocytes and biochemical responses of patients with schizophrenia and affective disorders to electroshock, insulin shock and epinephrine, *Am. J. Psychiat.,* 105:573 (1949).
10. Pincus, G., and H. Hoagland. Adrenal cortical responses to stress in normal men and in those with personality disorders; analysis of the pituitary-adrenal mechanism in man, *Am. J. Psychiat.,* 106:651–659 (1950).
11. Roche, M., G. W. Thorn, and A. G. Hills. The levels of circulating eosinophils and their response to ACTH in surgery; their use as an index of adrenocortical function, *New England J. Med.,* 242:307–314 (1950).
12. Michael, S. T. Adaptation to brief stress; the blood level of leucocytes and adrenal function in epilepsy, electrically induced convulsions, and after injection of epinephrine, *Yale J. Biol. & Med.,* 22:71–92 (1949).
13. Harris, G. W. Hypothalamus and endocrine glands, *Brit. M. Bull.,* 6:345–350 (1950).
14. Roche, M., A. G. Hills, and G. W. Thorn. The levels of circulating eosinophils and their response to ACTH in surgery; their use as an index

of adrenal cortical function, *in Proceedings of the First Clinical ACTH Conference.* Blakiston, Philadelphia, 1950.
15. Rud, F. *The Eosinophil Count in Health and in Mental Disease.* Tanum, Oslo, 1947.
16. Swanson, J. N., W. Bauer, and M. Ropes. Evaluation of eosinophil counts, *Lancet,* 262:129 (1952).
17. Rosenthal, R. L., *et al.* Effects of cortisone and ACTH therapy on eosinophils of the bone marrow and blood, *Proc. Soc. Exper. Biol. & Med.,* 75:740–741 (1950).
18. Henneman, P. H., H. Wexler, and M. M. Westenhaver. A comparison of eosin-acetone and phloxine-propylene glycol diluents in eosinophil counts, *J. Lab. & Clin. Med.,* 34:1017–1020 (1949).
19. Pilot, M. L. Use of base in fluids for counting eosinophils, *Am. J. Clin. Path.,* 20:870–871 (1950).
20. Steele, H. G., and A. F. Stratton. The epinephrine test; its use on pre-operative patients, *New England J. Med.* (in press).
21. Bray, W. E. *Synopsis of Clinical Laboratory Methods,* 2nd ed. Mosby, St. Louis, 1938.
22. Hume, D. M., L. Recant, P. H. Forsham, and G. W. Thorn. Studies on the effect of epinephrine on the pituitary-adrenocortical system, *J. Clin. Endocrinol.,* 10:187–229 (1950).
23. McGoon, D. C., A. R. Rich, and T. H. Cochran. Marked lipemia resulting from the administration of cortisone, *Bull. Johns Hopkins Hosp.,* 88:101–109 (1951).

CHAPTER 16

PSYCHOLOGICAL OBSERVATIONS BEFORE AND AFTER STIMULATION

H. E. KING
KATHLEEN M. YOUNG
ROBERT CORRIGAN
LEONA BERSADSKY

Previous chapters have indicated that certain formulations from psychology were in the minds of the research group when working out the over-all theoretical framework for the present cooperative study. In addition, the psychologists of the group have attempted to aid in the appraisal of the effects of electrophysiologic stimulation of the septal region of the brain by examining each case prior to and following the stimulation procedure by the application of psychological test methods. No attempt will be made in this chapter to describe the stimulus variable employed; that complexity has been left to the physiological discipline. We shall attempt to describe how, using psychological techniques, we have undertaken long range studies of the patients concerned in an effort to plot the course of their response to stimulation, if any, and to aid in the group effort to identify the life processes involved.

To begin, it will be necessary to describe briefly our view of the problem before us and the selection of the battery of psychological tests to be used in the study of this patient group. In recent years experience with partial ablation of the human frontal cortex has modified our ideas considerably about the sort of thing which it is important for psychologists to investigate when attempting to study brain function in the wake of surgical or physiological procedures.[1,2,3] The results of such studies, plus the weight of the evidence arising from trauma, tumors, and many other organic conditions, have made it amply clear that most of the behavioral changes which can be seen to follow brain alteration lie in the general sphere of motivational and affective changes in the personality and that few, if any, clear changes occur in the individual's use of such aspects of his mental machinery as intelligence, memory, learning,

TABLE XVI–1. The psychological tests employed

APHASIA—Eisenson tests

INTELLIGENCE—Wechsler-Bellevue Adult Intelligence Scale (short form: Comprehension, Vocabulary, Picture Completion, Block Design)
Porteus Maze Test

MEMORY-LEARNING—selected items from the Wechsler Memory Scale (a, b, c); Benton Visual Retention Test (d);

a. Rote	c. Associative
b. Logical	d. Memory for designs

RORSCHACH TEST

THEMATIC APPERCEPTION TEST—Cards: (female) # 1, 2, 4, 9GF, 10
(male) # 1, 4, 6BM, 7BM, 14

PSYCHOMOTOR TESTS
Reaction time (RT)
Response, or jump reaction time (RspT)
Tapping speed (T)
Finger dexterity (in simple movements, RLB)
" " (in more complex movements, Am)

BEHAVIOR RATINGS—Tulane scale

sensation, perception, and so on. This does not, of course, deny that changes in these abilities may occur, but it is to state that such changes are overshadowed by the personality changes when they occur. In our earlier studies of cortical function this sort of inquiry had been deliberately avoided as the subject of psychological investigation because it appeared that this might best be covered by the psychiatrists' clinical reports, and that any work we might undertake would only be a duplication. In some ways the outcome of these studies made us regret this decision, for the principal changes in patient status following prefrontal topectomy were found to be alterations in the affective life of the patient. We therefore planned to include much more investigative work in this sphere in future experimentation. This was, unfortunately, more easily said than done, owing to the almost complete absence of valid test methods to sample the affective elements of the personality. There followed a period of attempting to devise new techniques and instruments which would prove applicable, first reports on which have recently been published.[2] The experience gained by this experimentation with methods gave some notion of what we might find profitable to include in the present investigation.

We faced, then, the task of trying to measure changes which subcortical stimulation might produce in the status of the individual with regard to his over-all adaptation to the environment. In our earlier studies of cortical ablation we had sought to find a relationship between a cortical area and a psychological function. The situation faced in the present stimulation studies was, however, a quite different one. In this instance we were attempting, instead, to help identify by psychological techniques any changes in the status of the patient that might occur as a result of stimulation, with particular attention to possible changes of an affective nature. For this purpose we needed a relatively small battery of tests which could be applied to our patients before and after stimulation in order to appraise any alterations in the psychological functions tested. The group of tests finally selected is shown in Table 1.

METHODS

The tests group broadly into two categories: *intellective* and *personality*. Naturally, each receives some of its components from the other, and so the distinction is not a hard and fast one. Brief descriptions of the tests and the reasons for their inclusion are given below.

DESCRIPTION OF THE BATTERY OF TESTS

Aphasia. The possibility of producing aphasic or related disturbances concerns anyone who attempts a new operative procedure on the brain. We therefore made careful examinations of such functions, using the Eisenson tests[4] for the detection of receptive and expressive disturbances.

Intelligence. To answer the primary question of whether the intelligence of the patient was in any way affected by stimulation procedures, we employed two tests, the Wechsler-Bellevue (a shortened form) and the Porteus Mazes. These two tests were used as a pair because, although both are called tests of intelligence, the Wechsler-Bellevue is representative of a type of test validated against academic achievement (i.e., age-progress, grades, etc.), whereas the Porteus Maze Test is validated against social achievement (i.e., self-sufficiency, social adaptability, planfulness, etc.). The tests yield similar but not identical scores, since they differ fundamentally in their concept of intelligence. (See Chapter 14 of the Columbia-Greystone report[1] for further discussion of this point.) These tests are too well known to require further elaboration here. We used both with an eye to appraising intelligence from a more universal point of view. The Wechsler-Bellevue Test was administered in shortened form (see Table 1) and scored in the standard manner.[5] The Porteus Maze Test was administered and scored in standard form, complete.[6]

Memory-Learning. Since electroshock therapy and organic damage to the brain often produce disturbances in memory-learning, we included representative tests of rote, logical, and associative memory in our test series. Three of the tests employ auditory stimulus material, and one uses visually presented material. The three auditory memory tests are from the Wechsler Memory Scale, Form 1, Tests IV, V, and VII, administered and scored in the standard manner.[7] The visual memory test used was the Benton Visual Retention Test, Form A, given and scored in the standard manner.[8]

Personality. To attempt the appraisal of the effect of physiological stimulation on the personality as a whole, we employed two tests, both of a projective nature, the Rorschach Test and the Thematic Apperception Test. The Rorschach Test was administered in standard form and evaluated according to the Beck scoring system.[9] The TAT[10] was shortened to a five-card series (see Table 1), and protocols were inspected for an estimate of:

1. Length of story
2. Type of ending
3. Quality of description
4. Hero characterization
5. Occurrence of consistent themes
6. Environmental presses

Both of these are well known tests and require no further description here, except, perhaps, to emphasize that the Beck scoring system rests primarily on elements in the production (movement, color, etc.) rather than an extensive analysis of content (i.e., *what* is seen), and that our scoring on the TAT is perhaps minimal, but is of a less interpretive quality than the usual scoring methods.

Psychomotor. The psychomotor measurement methods employed were drawn from a new technique about which little has been published to date.[2, 3, 11, 12] Briefly, we have found that fine psychomotor measurement methods are sensitive to the presence of behavioral disorder and to a considerable extent reflect the degree to which behavior is disturbed. A full description of the tests employed and the strength of the relationship existing between psychomotor performance and behavioral disorder is now being prepared for publication.[13] In applying the techniques to the present group of stimulation patients, data obtained from groups of normal subjects and from groups of psychotic, neurotic, and pseudoneurotic schizophrenic patients were used for comparison. Three essential factors involving speed in simple psychomotor performance were studied: measures of the speed with which an individual may initiate a movement, the speed of continued movement, and movement dexterity while working at high speed. The scores reported are simple raw time scores, or are expressed as percentages of normal performance.

Systematic Behavior Ratings. In the course of psychological experimentation with psychotic subjects in a variety of past studies it became necessary for us to make some on-the-spot evaluations of the quality of performance on our tests, if we were to have any confidence in the scores as adequate representations of the patients' abilities (e.g., CFF or auditory thresholds) when the time came for data analysis. This notation was originally undertaken exclusively for the benefit of the experimenters in helping to evaluate the meaningfulness of their results. However, it soon became apparent that we could rate such aspects of behavior on graphic scales, along a continuum for some item of behavior from zero expression to complete expression, with a very high degree of correspondence between raters. Becoming interested in this as a method of obtaining behavioral data on psychotic patients, we undertook to build a systematic scale for such use. Turning to the literature, we found very few attempts at scales for the observation of the behavior of psychotic patients. That of Malamud and Sands[14] was perhaps the most ambitious but was primarily intended to represent the patient in his ward and interpersonal relationships. What we wanted, and constructed, was a scale which would indicate the activities of the patient as seen at the time of taking psychological tests. The scaling was to be made after the patient had completed a test interview and had performed on several types of psychological tests—intelligence, Rorschach, brightness discrimination, and so forth. Table 2 shows the several items on which we made judgments immediately upon the conclusion of a test session, usually while the patient was still present. The rater was provided with definitions of

TABLE XVI–2. The Systematic Behavior Rating Scale

1. Cooperation	5. Grasp of instructions	9. Self-criticism	13. Confusion
2. Relevant verbalization	6. Effort on test	10. Self-confidence	14. Personal concern with the examiner
3. Apparent memory	7. Willingness	11. Rapport	*15. Over-all evaluation of the data
4. Expressive play	8. Attention to test	12. Intrusion of psychotic influence	*16. Testing conditions

Sample item: COOPERATION

0	10	20	30	40
No performance	Much urging and many repetitions required to obtain performance	Adequate but minimal compliance with instructions, some urging required to obtain performance	Fair compliance with instructions, little urging required to obtain performance	Complete compliance with instructions, no urging required to obtain performance

*Items for the use of the examiner and are not included in the analysis of results.

TABLE XVI–3. Average ratings obtained by several groups of patients using the Systematic Behavior Rating scales

	n	*M*
Chronic schizophrenic	100	25.9
Hospitalized PNS* and neurotic	14	30.8
OPD† PNS* and neurotic	28	30.0
Normals	50	39.1
This series (preoperative)	10	24.8

* Pseudoneurotic schizophrenic
† Outpatient Department

each category, and each item was anchored at five points along the continuum. The sample at the bottom of Table 2 shows the anchoring of the judgment at various points along the scale from one extreme to the other. Checks might be placed anywhere on the line and later assigned numerical values depending on their distance from the end of the scale.

Inter-rater reliability was found to be satisfactorily high when the tasks performed were remotely similar. On a study of patients receiving electronarcosis therapy, the correlation between two raters—one using the scale after intelligence testing, the other after memory testing—was +.87. When the tasks were very different (same raters as above), as in the solitary carrying out of one set of instructions on a paper-and-pencil task and psychomotor testing, the correlation fell to +.66, which was still not bad considering the diversity of activity observed. In the present study the preoperative inter-rater reliability (same two raters) was +.90. Table 3 shows some average ratings obtained by various patient groups on the basis of this scale. Each patient was rated by three different examiners at each interview period. In scoring, the ratings are given numerical value from 0 to 40, with 0, 10, 20, 30, and 40 opposite the five stated anchor points. Scores for both individual items and a total were obtained.

This, then, was the battery of tests used in making the psychological evaluation, and with these tools we set to work.

The patient series was selected, as explained in Chapter 8, from a severely disturbed, "hopeless" group on an acute psychiatric ward. This took the expected toll of our psychological data, because the presence of strong symptoms such as negativism, mutism, and so forth, made the testing of some patients impossible. Moreover, experience had taught us that postoperative testing is of no value whatsoever without a preoperative comparison point, and so unless we were able to gather data from a patient preoperatively, we made no attempt to follow him postoperatively. Complete psychological records were obtained for 10 of the 25 stimulation procedures, comprising nine patients, one of whom received a second stimulation after a lapse of time.

Our time schedule on the first year's cases was: preoperative testing about two weeks before operation and postoperative testing three months after operation. The psychomotor tests and systematic behavior ratings were used one month, as well as three months postoperatively. We found that this did not provide sufficient data and therefore planned to follow succeeding cases preoperatively and at one month, four months, and eight months postoperatively with all tests. This course has been followed and to date all patients are past their four months' testing, and none has reached his eight months' postoperative testing yet.

RESULTS

It is not possible to discuss the patients of this series as a group, for each case is highly individual and has been subject to a different experimental procedure. The only recourse is to the clinical method, with a description of each case, supported by the objective scores available, as seen at each testing interval. Brief sketches are given below of the course of each patient studied, and sample graphs of the psychomotor and systematic behavior rating scores will be presented for an improved patient, one who did not change, and one who became worse, to help illustrate our attempt to plot the postoperative course of such patients.

Incidentally, having just explained what procedures and schedule would be followed, we are forced to begin with the description of a case which does not exactly conform. This exception is a result of the patient's having been the first case we studied; all the rest do adhere to the schedule described.

Patient 2

Aphasia. No disturbances were noted at any test period.

Intelligence. Wechsler-Bellevue: A low level of performance was given by the patient preoperatively. On postoperative testing there were slight and consistent increases in score.

The Porteus Maze Test was not administered.

Memory-Learning. On preoperative testing all scores were quite low. On postoperative testing all scores remained at the same level except for a marked gain in associative memory.

Personality. Rorschach: On preoperative testing a severe schizophrenic process was seen in the patient's rejection of six cards and in her evasive responses to the others. One month postoperatively the patient was more productive (R 29) and showed considerable anxiety (4 FY, 4 FV). Schizophrenia was plainly reflected in the following areas: poor reality contact (F+% 18), disturbance in thought processes (A% 24), somatic preoccupation, and primitive emotional reactions (3 C, 1 CF). Two months postoperatively there was an improvement in reality grasp, although the rating still fell within the pathological range (F+% 58). Somatic preoccupation was still marked, but there was an attempt at handling the emotions in a more adequate manner (1 CF, 3 FC). The anxiety noted one month postoperatively had dropped out. Five months postoperatively somatic preoccupation was still present and reality grasp was at the same level, but there were gains in other areas. There were signs of increased awareness of people (6 H) and inner resources (2 M), and the patient's attempt to handle her emotions in a more suitable manner continued but was less successful than at the former postoperative testing (CF 4).

The TAT was not administered.

Psychomotor. The preoperative performance of the patient was in the low portion of the schizophrenic range. One month after operation there was decided and consistent improvement in scores; by two months there was a reduction of this improved level of performance but it was not so great as to constitute a return to the preoperative level. Five months postoperatively there were unmistakable and consistent gains in all scores except *Assembly,* which is in keeping with a marked improvement in clinical appearance. The nature, pattern, and extent of change indicate that the patient remained schizophrenic but showed a much better level of psychomotor performance within the schizophrenic range.

Systematic Behavior Rating. A marked psychotic interference in test performance was seen preoperatively. One month postoperatively there was a reduction of such interference; by two months this had abated somewhat, but by five months a very marked reduction was visible in the degree of psychotic interference in the test situation. In over-all view, postoperatively there was a clear alteration in a positive direction on all items of behavior rated (14+, 0–). The average change in item value from pre- to postoperative was +27.8. The largest increases (2 steps, or 20 points) were in expressive play, relevant verbalization, and willingness to perform, and in personal concern with the examiners. There were also some changes (1 step, or 10 points) in other aspects of rated behavior, such as: (in descending order of rank) increased self-criticism, increased effort on tests, increased rapport, lessened psychotic intrusion, increased attention to tests, better cooperation, better grasp of instructions, and reduction in confusion.

Summary. On preoperative testing this patient scored low in her performance on intelligence and memory-learning tasks. Personality measures indicated a severely disturbed, schizophrenic individual, and psychomotor scores placed her at the low end of the schizophrenic range. Behavior ratings reflected a marked psychotic interference in test performance. One month postoperatively, she showed a slight increase in intelligence scores, with memory-learning scores remaining at the preoperative level except for a marked gain in associative memory. Personality measures showed little change except that the patient was more productive than on preoperative testing. Psychomotor scores showed a marked and consistent improvement. Less psychotic interference was seen in behavior ratings at this test period. Two months postoperatively personality measures showed a considerable decrease in the degree of psychosis (no intelligence or memory-learning scores available).

Psychomotor scores were at approximately the same level as one month postoperatively, although somewhat reduced. Behavior ratings again showed marked psychotic interference but not a full return to the preoperative level. Five months postoperatively personality measures showed a still further decrease in the degree of psychosis. Psychomotor scores increased markedly and consistently with the exception of *Assembly*. Behavior ratings at this period showed a very marked lessening of psychotic interference in test performance. The over-all picture is one

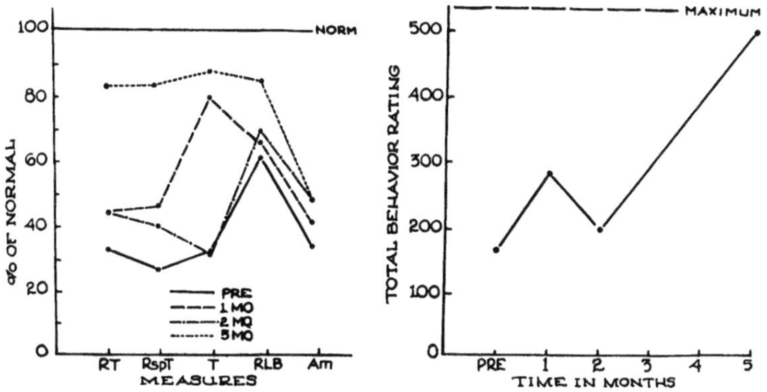

FIGURE XVI–1. Psychomotor performance (left) and total Systematic Behavior Rating (right) for Patient 2 at each test. NOTE: For abbreviations used in Figures 1–3 see Table 1. The curve points have been joined to simplify inspection and do not imply continuity.

of a very marked improvement in the degree of psychosis in this patient. A graphic illustration of the changes in psychomotor and systematic behavior rating scores is given in Figure 1.

PATIENT 6

Aphasia. No disturbances were noted at any test period.

Intelligence. Wechsler-Bellevue: The patient performed at an average level on preoperative testing. The postoperative scores were nearly identical with the preoperative.

Porteus Mazes: A low level of performance was given preoperatively, with no change in score postoperatively.

Memory-Learning. On preoperative testing the patient showed superior performance on rote, associative, and memory for designs subtests, while logical memory was below average. Postoperative scores remained at about the same level.

Personality. Rorschach: The preoperative record reflected a severe schizophrenic process. This patient showed poor reality grasp (F+% 33), lack of conformity in thinking (A% low, P 2), and impulsive, primitive emotional reactions (2 C). The postoperative record showed some increase in productivity (R 19), which allowed for an increase in bizarreness of percepts (jelly, bile, etc.). Reality grasp was still poor (F+% 33), and thought processes were disrupted (A% 31). He did respond more rapidly and showed more awareness of his emotional disturbances (T col: 14″; T unc:8″). Essentially there was little change in the schizophrenic process from pre- to postoperative testing.

TAT: The preoperative stories were fairly well developed and fairly cohesive. Most of them had happy endings, and people always did the "right thing" in the end. The postoperative stories, while similar in content, showed much less cohesiveness. The patient digressed a number of times in telling the story and was sidetracked by his own discussions.

Psychomotor. Preoperative scores placed the patient in the middle of the schizophrenic range. One month postoperatively he showed some improvement, although this was not completely consistent. By three months after operation he had lost some of these gains and retained others. The general pattern of changes was suggestive of a highly variable patient with a very slight improvement.

Systematic Behavior Rating. The patient's preoperative scores showed relatively little psychotic interference in test performance. One month postoperatively no remarkable change was seen in rated behavior; by three months a very slight lessening of psychotic interference could be noted. In over-all view, there was no gross alteration in rated behavior, with extremely slight but consistent gains noted (11+, 2−). The average change in item value from pre- to postoperative was +1.0. The largest change (2 steps) was an increase in expressive play, and there was also a change of 1 step in the reduction of psychotic intrusion into the test situation and an increase in personal concern with the examiners.

Summary. At the preoperative testing this patient showed fair performance on intellective and memory-learning tasks. Personality measures indicated a severe schizophrenic process, and psychomotor performance placed him in the middle of the schizophrenic range. Behavior ratings showed relatively little psychotic interference in test performance. On postoperative testing there was no change in intellective scores. Personality measures showed little change in the schizophrenic process. Psychomotor performance showed no marked changes but reflected some inconsistent improvement. The over-all picture was one of little change in status from pre- to postoperative testing.

Patient 7

Aphasia. No disturbances were noted at any test period.

Intelligence. Wechsler-Bellevue: On preoperative testing the patient performed at an average level. Postoperative testing showed a marked loss in comprehension and vocabulary tests, a slight gain in picture completion, and the same score on block design.

Porteus Mazes: The patient gave a poor performance preoperatively but showed a slight gain postoperatively.

Memory-Learning. The patient showed poor performance preoperatively, particularly on logical memory. Postoperatively most scores remained at the same level except for a further loss in logical memory.

Personality. Rorschach: The preoperative record was that of a severely disturbed individual, with four cards rejected and only five responses given. The meager record contained perseveration and color-naming, both pathognomonic of schizophrenia. The postoperative protocol was practically identical, with four cards rejected and six responses given, the latter having the same content as the preoperative responses.

TAT: At the preoperative testing the patient produced no stories but after much urging would describe the cards. His only spontaneous production concerned a mother and a son, with the mother being disappointed in the son because he had done something wrong. The postoperative record was identical with the preoperative one in all respects, including the spontaneous production.

Psychomotor. The patient's preoperative score placed him at the low end of the schizophrenic range. One month postoperatively a slight improvement was noted, although this was not fully consistent. The results obtained three months postoperatively were almost identical with those obtained one month postoperatively. The gains and losses indicate no particular change in psychopathology.

Systematic Behavior Rating. Marked psychotic interference in performance was seen at the preoperative test period. One month after operation there was a slight reduction of this interference, but by three months the preoperative level had been reached again. In over-all view, there was no gross alteration in rated behavior postoperatively, only very slight gains and losses (9+, 4–). The average change in item value from pre- to postoperative was +2.1. The largest change (1 step) was an increase in self-criticism.

Summary. On preoperative testing this patient scored low in his performance on intelligence and memory-learning tasks. The personality

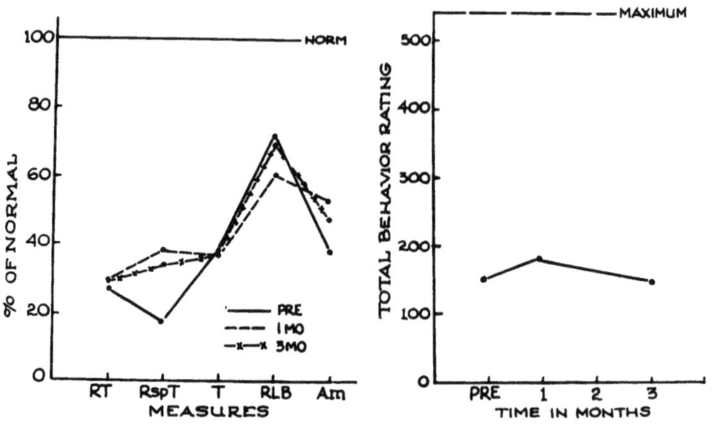

FIGURE XVI–2. Psychomotor performance (left) and total Systematic Behavior Rating (right) for Patient 7 at each test

measures indicated a severely disturbed schizophrenic individual, and psychomotor scores placed him at the low end of the schizophrenic range. Behavior ratings reflected a marked interference of psychosis in test performance. On postoperative testing there was no significant change in intelligence or memory-learning scores. Personality measures were nearly identical pre- and postoperatively. Psychomotor scores showed very slight and not fully consistent improvement. Also, a very slight improvement, which did not continue, was noted in behavior ratings. The over-all picture is one of essentially unchanged status from pre- to postoperative testing. A graphic illustration of the changes in psychomotor and behavior rating scores is given in Figure 2.

Patient 8 (15)

Aphasia. No disturbances were noted at any test period.

Intelligence. Wechsler-Bellevue: On preoperative testing the patient was slightly above average on all items except block design, which was very low. Postoperatively there were no changes in his scores.

Porteus Mazes: The patient gave a low level of performance preoperatively, which remained the same on postoperative testing.

Memory-Learning. The patient's preoperative performance was average on all tests except logical memory, which was very low. Postoperatively there was no change in scores except for a slight increase in logical memory.

Personality. Rorschach: The preoperative record revealed an individual who displayed good reality grasp (F+% 87) but who was severely constricted (high F%, R 13) and showed little emotional reactivity (no color). Thought processes tended to be stereotyped (high A%) and to show conformity (P 8). The postoperative record was very similar in content to the preoperative record, but it did show some impulsive emotional reaction which had not been present before (1 C) and indications of increased anxiety (T unc:35″; T col:19″). The patient stated that he found the task harder to do.

TAT: All the stories produced were fairly well developed. There was no dominant theme throughout. The preoperative stories had happy endings preceded by quarrels or failures of some sort. The postoperative stories were similar in content and structure to the preoperative stories but were much shorter, and more urging was required from the examiner to elicit production.

Psychomotor. The patient's preoperative performance was quite good and in the upper portion of the schizophrenic range. One month after operation there was a marked and consistent drop in scores; at three months there were further losses on two scores and slight gains on two. The pattern and direction of change would tend to indicate a more hebephrenic-catatonic type of reaction than was observable preoperatively.

Systematic Behavior Rating. Preoperatively this patient showed very little psychotic interference in test performance. One month after operation there was increased psychotic disruption in performance, but by two months the preoperative level was again approximated. In over-all view, there were no gross alterations in rated behavior, only very slight gains and losses (7+, 6−). The average change in item value from pre- to postoperative was +1.1. The largest change (1 step) was an increase in self-criticism.

Summary. On preoperative testing this patient made average scores on intellective tasks, with the exception of low scores on block design, Porteus Mazes, and logical memory. Personality measures indicated a mild degree of schizophrenia characterized by constriction and little emotional reactivity. Psychomotor performance placed the patient in the upper portion of the schizophrenic range. Behavior ratings revealed very little psychotic interference in test performance. Postoperatively there was no change in his intellective scores. Personality measures showed greater difficulty in production and some increase in the degree of psychosis. Psychomotor performance showed marked and consistent loss one month postoperatively and inconsistent gains and losses at about the same level three months postoperatively. No gross alteration in rated behavior was noted. The over-all picture is one of increased psychosis for this patient in the postoperative period.

Patient 12

Aphasia. There was some difficulty in executing items on the aphasia test preoperatively, specifically in object-naming from pictures and in spelling. One month postoperatively these same difficulties were exaggerated; specifically, spelling became more bizarre. By four months after operation object-naming was normal and only spelling remained poor.

Intelligence. Wechsler-Bellevue: On preoperative performance scores were exceedingly low and the patient appeared pathologically retarded. By one month after operation a definite increase had occurred in vocabulary score and in picture completion; other tests were at zero performance. Four months postoperatively clear positive changes in all tests were seen, with the greatest gains in block design and comprehension.

Porteus Mazes: The preoperative performance was exceedingly low. One month postoperatively zero performance was obtained, although the patient made an attempt throughout the test; at four months marked improvement was seen.

Memory-Learning. Prior to surgery this patient was in such poor contact with his environment that he was unable to carry out the instructions of the examiner adequately. His preoperative memory-learning performance was very low. One month after operation performance was actually at zero throughout; at four months there were clear positive gains on the test as a whole, especially in associative memory-learning.

Personality. Rorschach: The preoperative record showed a severe schizophrenic process in that only three responses were given and seven cards were rejected despite continual urging by the examiner. The three responses given were frequently seen percepts, all with good form, and suggested that the patient had good potentialities, but was unable to cooperate at the time. One month postoperatively he was more cooperative; eight responses were given and three cards rejected. Of the eight responses, two were color-naming (invariably pathognomonic of schizophrenia) and the remainder suggested poor reality contact. There was some increase in responsiveness, but the protocol was still extremely limited and reflected little basic change from the preoperative protocol. Four months postoperatively a somewhat clearer picture was obtained of this patient's personality structure, since no cards were rejected and thirteen responses were given. Although no cards were rejected outright, a number of responses were given in the vague, evasive manner which is usually considered a more sophisticated form of rejection. This record showed the patient to be highly constricted (high F%), with stereotyped thought processes (A% 69). His reality grasp was impaired, but he made an attempt to maintain his contact with reality, poor though it might be, and he succeeded to some extent (F+% 72, P 3). There was some evidence of inner life (M 1) but no attempt to utilize emotional feelings in reacting to various situations (no color responses).

TAT: Preoperatively no stories were produced despite much urging. Only a few words of description were elicited on each picture—a meager and unproductive protocol. One month postoperatively stories were elicited, and the descriptions given then were more spontaneous than before. All characters seen in the cards were described as "quiet." Four months postoperatively no complete stories were elicited, but after urging by the examiner a few hints were given about the attitudes of the people in two of the pictures.

Psychomotor. The patient's preoperative performance was in the lower part of the schizophrenic range and rather variable. Tests made one month postoperatively showed dramatic gain in *Reaction Time*, with losses in *Tapping*, and no change in *Dexterity*. Tests made four months postoperatively showed a return of *Reaction Time* to the preoperative level, with some consistent gain in all other scores. The pattern of scores and changes indicated that the patient had made a definite quantitative improvement in degree of psychosis but clearly remained in the schizophrenic range (about the middle of the range).

Systematic Behavior Rating. Severe psychotic interference in test performance was shown preoperatively. One month after operation this was reduced but still strong; by four months it had lessened dramatically. In over-all view, there was a clear alteration in a positive direction, all gains and no losses (13+, 0–). The average change in item value from pre- to postoperative was +30.1. The largest changes (2 steps) were increases in cooperation, relevant verbalization, expressive play, grasp of instructions, effort on tests, attention to tests, self-criticism, and rapport; reduction in confusion; and an increase in personal concern with the examiners. There were also changes, but not to so marked a degree (1 step), in the patient's willingness to perform and the lessened intrusion of psychotic influence.

Summary. Preoperatively this patient demonstrated retarded performance on all tests. His cooperation and willingness to attempt the tests were always adequate, but his very poor contact with his environment severely influenced his performance. For this reason scores on intelligence tests and memory-learning were probably pathologically low. His meager production on the personality tests reflected a severe schizophrenic disturbance. His psychomotor performance placed him in the lower portion of the schizophrenic range, and behavior ratings showed an extremely retarded, unproductive patient. One month postoperatively his performance on intelligence and memory-learning tests was at the zero point. Personality measures indicated some increased responsiveness, but with the schizophrenic disturbance still severe. Psychomotor performance showed slight improvement, as did behavior ratings. By four months after operation the patient had improved to a marked degree. His performance was definitely improved on intelligence, memory-learning, and psychomotor tasks and in rated behavior. The productions on all personality-behavior tests still remained within the schizophrenic range but demonstrated a quantitative improvement in status. The over-all picture is one of marked improvement in the degree of psychosis in this patient.

Patient 13

Aphasia. No disturbances were noted at any test period.

Intelligence. Wechsler-Bellevue: The preoperative performance indicated that the patient was below average on all tests and particularly defective in comprehension. Marked improvement in comprehension and vocabulary appeared one month postoperatively, and continued gains in comprehension and picture completion appeared four months postoperatively. Scores on other tests remained at the preoperative level.

Porteus Mazes: A low level of performance was given preoperatively, which was unchanged after operation.

Memory-Learning. Low scores were obtained preoperatively, and by one month after operation there was no change in rote or logical memory, but a marked decrease in associative memory and memory for designs was apparent. By four months after operation there were general gains, chiefly in associative and logical memory.

Personality. Rorschach: The preoperative record showed a disorganized personality, with impairment in reality contact (F+% 60) and little conformity in thought processes (A% 17, P 2, 1 Hdx). Signs of negativism were present (s 3). The patient was attempting to maintain himself in strict control (high F%) but showed few inner resources (1 M–), and when he reacted emotionally it was in an uncontrolled manner (2 CF). There was evidence of deep, all-pervasive anxiety which the patient could not control (FV, FY, midline anxiety, content of canyons and caves). One month postoperatively he refused to be tested. In the record obtained four months postoperatively the patient still showed impairment in reality contact (F+% 63) but exhibited more conformity in thinking (A% 53, P 3), and his negativism had lessened from its preoperative level (s 1). Although his personality was quite constricted (F% high), the signs of marked anxiety and impulsive emotional response had disappeared (only 1 FV, 1 FC). The patient was more controlled, and hence more organized than he had been prior to operation, but the basic schizophrenic pattern was still in evidence.

TAT: At preoperative testing the stories given contained a good deal of extraneous verbal material in the form of digressions but emerged, nevertheless, as units. They usually ended happily, because the heroes were "good, strong men," characterized as intelligent, having exceptional talent, and always doing the "right thing." In one case, where the hero was in a state of tension, the patient remarked, "he will recover because he is good." No performance was elicited one month postoperatively, but the stories produced four months postoperatively were short and to the point. There was no longer any emphasis on the sterling qualities of the hero—in fact, in two stories the hero wound up in difficulty. The material on the whole was more neutral, and in at least two stories the patient produced a more realistic situation. He appeared to show less concern with self, or himself as he wanted to be, and better reality grasp than he had preoperatively.

Psychomotor. The patient's preoperative performance indicated schizophrenia in an individual with relatively good organization. One month postoperatively the tests showed a "leveling" of scores, with a slight general improvement but a loss in organizational aspects. By four months after operation the record showed further gains, with an inconsistent return to preoperative level in *Tapping* score. In over-all view, there was a slight improvement in the psychosis, although its schizophrenic character remained.

Systematic Behavior Rating. The preoperative record showed only moderate psychotic interference in test performance. One month after operation the disturbance was markedly increased but at four months the scores had again approximated the preoperative level. In over-all view, there was no gross alteration in rated behavior. Both gains and losses were shown (5+, 8–). The average change in item value from pre- to postoperative was –0.3. The largest changes (1 step) were increases in attention to tests and willingness to perform and decreases in self-confidence, rapport, and personal concern with the examiners.

Summary. This was a very cooperative patient, whose performance was colored by the bizarre aspects of his behavior. Below-average scores were obtained on intelligence and memory-learning tests. Personality tests showed schizophrenia with uncontrolled anxiety. The psychomotor pattern was schizophrenic with good organization. Behavior ratings showed the clear intrusion of psychosis in the patient's behavior. One month postoperatively some improvement was noted in the Wechsler-Bellevue score, no change in the Porteus Maze score, and some loss in memory-learning. No performance could be obtained on either the Rorschach or the TAT. Psychomotor performance was slightly improved, but there was greater psychotic intrusion in rated behavior. By four months after operation some continued improvement in the Wechsler-Bellevue score and some gains in memory-learning were visible, but there was no change in the Porteus Maze score. Personality measures showed basic schizophrenia still in evidence but with anxiety dropped out and better organization. Psychomotor performance remained much the same, and there was a return to the preoperative level of rated behavior. The over-all picture of this patient indicated some improvement in personality with accompanying gains in intellectual work following operation.

Patient 14

Aphasia. No disturbances were noted at any test period.

Intelligence. Wechsler-Bellevue: The patient performed at a high level preoperatively. One month after operation there was some shifting of scores among the subtests, but by four months there was a return to preoperative levels in all subtests.

Porteus Mazes: Superior performance was given preoperatively; this was followed by a marked loss one month postoperatively, but there was a return to the preoperative level at the end of the four months' test interval.

Memory-Learning. The patient gave a very superior performance on all subtests preoperatively. An appreciable loss on all items was noted one month after operation; by four months there was a full return to the preoperative level.

Personality. Rorschach: The preoperative record was that of a severely disturbed individual who retained adequate reality contact (F+% 75), with adequate conformity in thinking (A% 38, P 6). At this time the patient's inner resources were meager (1 M), as most of the emotional energy he possessed went into primitive, uncontrolled reactions (1 C, 2 CF; M/C: 1/4). His need to express himself intellectually was strong (emphasis on W, R 55), although at times this revealed bizarreness in percepts (such as numbers 3 and 4, the letter A). Severe, constricting anxiety was a dominant feature of this record (5 VF, 2 FV, 1 FY), and it appeared to be expressed in the patient's marked oppositional trend directed toward the environment (s 6, M/C: 1/4). Some of his disturbance was reflected in the content of his percepts (i.e., explosion, fire, and a single human form). One month postoperatively the record was marked by diminution of the patient's need to express himself (R 29, W normal). He showed considerably less opposition to his environment (s 2) and his marked anxiety had practically disappeared (1 FY, 1 YF). His grasp of reality had increased (F+% 84), but his thinking was more stereotyped (A% 51). There was no bizarreness in percepts as in the preoperative record. The patient's emotional life was still strongly outgoing (M/C:2/5), for the most part expressed in reactions of a primitive type (2 C, 2 CF). At four months the record showed some of the features of the two previous tests. He was impelled to express himself intellectually (R 57), but succeeded in doing this in a more organized manner (W normal). His reality grasp was within normal limits (F+% 89), as were his thought processes (A% 38, P 7). There was an increase in inner resources (M 3), and even more emphasis on outgoingness (M/C:3/10.5)—the reaction type still being one of strongly primitive, uncontrolled emotional responses (C 4, CF 3). There was a return of opposition to his environment stronger than ever (s 9, M/C:3/10.5), and along with this a return of anxiety (4 FY, 1 YF, 3 FV), which now contained some depressive elements that had not been present before. In over-all view, this patient made some gains in reality grasp and general organization of thought processes, but the pattern of his emotional life remained similar in structure to that seen in the preoperative record and his anxiety returned after a brief disappearance.

TAT: On preoperative testing the patient's stories were told with much verbalization, many side comments, and frequent changing of plots. They all ended happily, as a rule with resolution of a moral conflict. This dominant theme included little material on interpersonal relationships. The resolution of the conflict usually found the hero on the "right" side. The record suggested that the patient was much concerned with morality and displayed much intellectualization. Two of the stories produced one month postoperatively were identical with the preoperative stories, but most of them were much shorter and more cohesive. There was less emphasis on moral issues and less effort to resolve all conflicts happily. More interest was shown in interpersonal relationships, and, when these were involved, much satisfaction was derived from them. At the four months' test period the protocol was much more similar in its formal elements to the preoperative record than to that given one month postoperatively. The plots were changed and the stories lengthened, with side comments and long discussions of particular points not necessarily relevant to the narrative. There was an interesting inconsistency in presentation, in that the patient said that he was going to make up happy stories but proceeded in four of the five stories to present a "gruesome" circumstance with a violent ending (a nervous breakdown, death by a plane crash, poisoning, etc.). For the first time he mentioned his own particular symptom of fear of germs as part of a story. It appeared that he had returned to his preoperative status, with increased concern about self and personal reference.

Psychomotor. Preoperatively the patient's performance was near normal, with only a minor tendency toward a schizophrenic type of performance. One month postoperatively his record showed a dramatic and consistent loss on all scores. Four months postoperatively it showed a marked improvement in the direction of the preoperative level, but despite a general recovery of the immediate postoperative losses some impairment in *Reaction Time* was still present. There was no doubt that this patient's psychosis had been temporarily exacerbated by stimulation. His status four months after operation was very much like his preoperative status.

Systematic Behavior Rating. The preoperative scores showed only moderate psychotic interference in test performance. One month after operation there was a slight increase in such disturbance, but by four months a marked reduction had occurred. In over-all view, there was a clear alteration in a positive direction (12+, 1–). The average change in item value from pre- to postoperative was +9.4. The largest changes (1 step) were increases in cooperation, expressive play, willingness to perform, self-criticism and self-confidence and a reduction of confusion.

Summary. Preoperatively this patient rendered superior performance on most tasks set for him. His scores on intelligence and memory-learning tasks were high. Personality tests reflected a disturbed individual, anxious, constricted, intellectualizing, and in opposition to his environment. His psychomotor performance was high and borderline with normal. Behavior ratings indicated considerable psychotic intrusion. One month after operation he showed marked impairment on intellectual and memory-learning tasks. Personality tests showed less need for intellectualization, less opposition to environment, and the disappearance of anxiety, but more stereotypy in thinking. Psychomotor performance showed a dramatic and consistent loss on all scores. Behavior ratings showed a tendency to increased psychotic intrusion. At the four months' testing period the patient demonstrated a clear return to the preoperative level on intelligence and memory-learning tasks. Personality measures showed a closer resemblance to those of the preoperative level, with a return of intellectualization, anxiety, and opposition to the environment but also with improved reality contact and thought organization. Some depressive elements appeared which had not been present before. His psychomotor performance returned approximately to the preoperative level. Behavior ratings showed a clear alteration in a positive direction, indicating lessened psychotic intrusion in test performance.

The over-all picture is that of a patient with a high preoperative level of performance on psychological tests, a clear loss on all tests except the Rorschach and TAT one month postoperatively, followed by a reinstatement of his preoperative level on all tests in the four months' test period.

PATIENT 15 (8)*

Aphasia. No disturbances were noted at any test period.

Intelligence. Wechsler-Bellevue: Preoperative testing showed average scores on all tests except block design, which was very low. Four months postoperatively there was a slight but general improvement in intelligence scores.

Porteus Mazes: A low level of performance was given preoperatively, followed by a significant drop at the four months' test period.

Memory-Learning. Preoperative scores were all below average. Four months postoperatively there was a general increase in memory-learning scores, with a marked increase in associative and logical memory.

Personality. Rorschach: The preoperative protocol showed an individual who was clearly schizophrenic (M/C: 1/6.5; three color-naming responses). He showed little control over his emotional responses and had regressed to a primitive mode of expressing his emotions. Despite this he showed good reality contact (F+% 84), and his thought processes

*This patient had a previous stimulation, and so the testing at one month following the second operation was omitted in order to reduce transfer effects from repeated testing.

were reasonably intact (A% 55, P 5). He showed some awareness of his struggles (color shock: T unc:20″; T col:42″) but was at a loss to control them, although there was some attempt at this (1 FC). Four months postoperatively his record suggested that there had been a diminution in the active process and that a more stable point had been reached. Schizophrenia was still very much in evidence, but some defenses had been established (3 FC responses, increased RT, F% increased). The record also showed some depressive tendencies—for example, in seeing unpleasant percepts (monstrosities) and verbalizing difficulty in seeing the percepts.

TAT: On preoperative testing all stories were told slowly and hesitantly. They were brief, and the patient required urging to give endings to two of them. There was a marked depressive tone; yet four of the five stories wound up with "eventually it ends happily," a conclusion quite out of keeping with what went before. No dominant themes were noted throughout, although in two stories people were seen as "brooding." Four months postoperatively the stories remained much the same in content and structure. There was slightly less description used, but otherwise the protocols were identical.

Psychomotor. The preoperative performance of this patient fell in the middle schizophrenic range, with a poor pattern of organization. Four months postoperatively no important changes appeared, but there was a small and consistent drift in the negative direction. In over-all view, this patient showed a small but consistent increase in the degree of psychosis present.

Systematic Behavior Rating. Little psychotic interference in test performance was seen preoperatively. Four months postoperatively there was a tendency toward alteration in the negative direction. In over-all view, there was no gross change in rated behavior. Both gains and losses were shown (5+, 9–). The average change from pre- to postoperative item value was –3.4. The largest changes (1 step) were decreases in both self-confidence and self-criticism.

Summary. Prior to stimulation this patient gave an average performance on intelligence tests. His memory-learning scores were below average. Personality measures showed a schizophrenic process and primitive emotional responses but fairly good reality contact. His psycho-

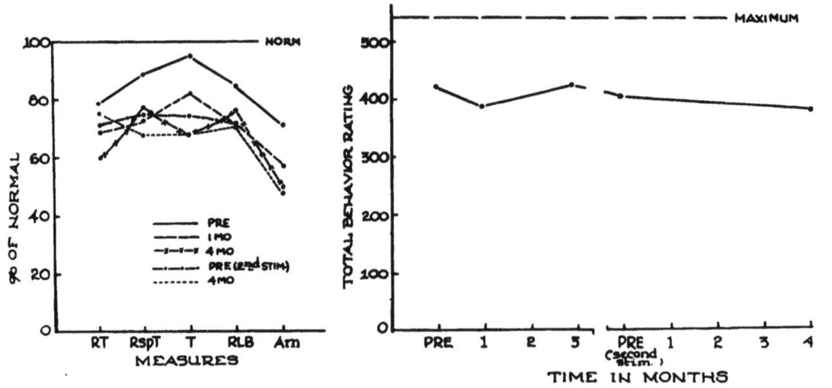

FIGURE XVI–3. Psychomotor performance (left) and total Systematic Behavior Rating (right) for Patient 8(15) at each test and for the same patient 15(8) on second stimulation

motor performance placed him in the middle schizophrenic range with poor organization. Behavior ratings indicated a slight degree of psychotic intrusion. Four months postoperatively he showed some general improvement in Wechsler-Bellevue scores and a decided loss in Porteus Maze score. There was general improvement in memory-learning performance. Personality measures showed schizophrenia still much in evidence, but the process appeared to be more stable. Some depressive tendencies were noted. The patient's psychomotor performance showed a small but consistent increase in the degree of psychosis. Behavior ratings revealed no gross alterations but suggested a tendency to greater psychotic intrusion in performance. The over-all picture is one of slightly increased psychosis. A graphic illustration of the changes in psychomotor and systematic behavior scores is given in Figure 3.

PATIENT 17

Aphasia. No disturbances were noted on preoperative testing. One month postoperatively the patient showed confusion on the identification of geometric forms but no other disturbance. Four months postoperatively no disturbances were noted.

Intelligence. Wechsler-Bellevue: This patient scored very low on all subtests preoperatively, and no change was noted either at one month or four months postoperatively.

Porteus Mazes: Scores were very low preoperatively and remained unchanged at one month and four months postoperatively.

Personality. Rorschach: The preoperative record presented the picture of a disturbed, confused person. The patient gave extremely vague responses, and was unable to specify their location. This reflected a loss of reality contact (which was also indicated by her low F+% of 59). Although she was very much aware of emotional stimuli (AR .72, blocking on color cards), she showed no capacity to deal with her own emotional states (no color responses). Her personality was severely constricted (extremely high F%), and she showed no inner resources (no M). Thought processes were disturbed (DW and Hdx) and quite stereotyped (high A%). Her reactivity was retarded (average T 1 R 19″), and she showed some anxiety (T unc: 27″; T col: 11″). One month postoperatively there were some changes in the record, although the majority of the elements remained the same. The patient's responses were still vague, with location impossible for some of them. Her contact with reality was somewhat strengthened (F+% 75). She was still unable to handle her own emotions (no color response) but was very much aware of them and more disturbed by them (complete rejection of Card X). Her personality was still highly constricted with no signs of inner resources (no M). The most striking change was the decrease in retardation (T 1 R 6″) and the dropping out of signs of anxiety. Four months postoperatively the patient's personality appeared little changed. There was less vagueness in her percepts, but the personality profile was not appreciably altered. There also seemed to be somewhat less confusion in thought processes, but there was an increase in stereotypy (extremely high A%). The increase in reality grasp was maintained but not increased. Reactivity was still much faster than it had been preoperatively but showed little change since the one-month testing interval.

TAT: Preoperatively little speech or performance was elicited on this test. After much urging, brief descriptions were given, such as "She's looking at him, he's looking someplace." One month postoperatively little change was noted in the protocol. On four months' postoperative testing more words were elicited, although urging was still required. Although the patient gave more descriptions than on previous tests, she could not be induced to produce any stories.

Psychomotor. The patient's preoperative performance fell in the low schizophrenic range. One month postoperatively her scores showed no important change, but there was some improvement in *Tapping.* The postoperative record was on practically the same level at four months as at one month. In general, the tests indicated a very disturbed patient who showed improvement in the worst aspects of her psychosis.

Systematic Behavior Rating. Preoperatively the patient showed definite psychotic interference in test performance. One month after operation there was no change in scores, but by four months there was a marked lessening in the degree of psychotic interference in test performance. In over-all view, there was a clear alteration in a positive direction (12+, 1−). The average change in item value from pre- to postoperative was +8.5. The largest changes (1 step) were increases in relevant verbalization, grasp of instructions, and attention to tasks and a lessening of psychotic intrusion during the testing period.

Summary. Preoperatively the patient earned very low scores on intelligence and memory-learning tasks. Personality tests showed a schizophrenic picture, disturbance in thought processes, and extremely poor reality contact. Psychomotor performance was in the lower schizophrenic range. Behavior ratings showed marked psychotic intrusion. One month postoperatively no changes were noted in intelligence or in memory-learning. On personality measures the patient showed improved reality contact. Psychomotor performance showed no important change. Behavior ratings remained the same. Four months postoperatively no changes were noted in intelligence or memory-learning. Personality protocols and psychomotor performance were much the same as at one month after operation. Behavior ratings showed clear alteration in a positive direction, indicating lessened psychotic intrusion in test performance. The over-all picture is one of psychosis in a patient of limited intelligence who showed a slight improvement following operation.

PATIENT 20*

Aphasia. No disturbances were noted at any test period.

*This patient had not yet reached the four months' test period when this report was prepared.

Intelligence. Wechsler-Bellevue: The patient performed at an average level preoperatively, with no change at the one-month test period.

Porteus Mazes: A low level of performance was given preoperatively, with a slight gain in score one month postoperatively.

Memory-Learning. The patient performed at a superior level on all tests preoperatively and showed no change one month postoperatively.

Personality. Rorschach: The patient presented a schizophrenic picture, but was in good contact with reality (F+% 86) and showed no bizarreness in thought processes (A% 35, P 5). She appeared to be an intelligent woman (R 37, varied content, good W, 3 M) with sufficient inner resources. She tended to be impulsive in her emotional responses (3 CF) but also showed a capacity for controlled, more mature type of responses (2 FC). There was some constriction in the personality (slightly high F%) and much anxiety (3 FY), some of which was connected with religious preoccupation (content of God). One month postoperatively the most striking change was an increase in autistic thinking and a tendency to live within the self (M/C:7/2). Contact with reality remained intact, as did the thought processes, which showed more conformity than ever (P 10). When the patient reacted emotionally, it was in an impulsive manner, and the more controlled response had dropped out. She still showed anxiety (5 FY, 1 FV) and some religious preoccupation.

TAT: At preoperative testing the stories produced had brief but well-developed plots. Four of the five concerned death and the sorrow of people still living. There was, however, a hopeful note in the consolation to be derived from religion. In one story the Virgin Mary actually appeared to a bereaved girl. Throughout, the religious theme was dominant. One month postoperatively the stories obtained were similar. The religious preoccupation had diminished, being seen in only one story. The stories were more concerned with interpersonal relationships, and two of them concerned rejected love. In each case the ending was happy. The patient identified herself with one girl, saying, "She is emotionally upset and so am I."

Psychomotor. The patient's preoperative performance was in the middle of the schizophrenic range. One month postoperatively there was a small but consistent loss on all scores. The limited information available to date indicates a slight but consistent increase in the degree of psychosis.

Systematic Behavior Rating. Preoperative scores indicated a moderate psychotic intrusion. The scores showed a slight increase in the degree of psychotic intrusion one month postoperatively.

Summary. Preoperatively this patient showed average performance on Wechsler-Bellevue scores but performed poorly on the Porteus Mazes. Her performance on memory-learning tasks was superior. Personality measures showed a schizophrenic picture, with good reality contact but with much anxiety and religious preoccupation. Her psychomotor performance placed her in the middle of the schizophrenic range, and behavior ratings showed moderate psychotic intrusion. One month postoperatively there was a slight gain in Porteus Maze scores but no change in Wechsler-Bellevue scores or in memory-learning tasks. The personality protocols showed a marked increase in autistic thinking, although reality contact remained intact. The patient's anxiety and religious preoccupation were unchanged. Psychomotor performance reflected some consistent increase in psychosis, and behavior ratings also indicated a slight increase of psychotic intrusion. This patient is still in the immediate postoperative period and any over-all comment on her status at this time would be premature.

SUMMARY

It appears from these records that of the nine patients studied:

Two were much improved—Patients 2 and 12.

Two were slightly improved—Patients 13 and 17.

Four were unchanged—Patients 6, 7, 14, and 20.

One became slightly worse—Patient 8(15).

We have approached the analysis of these records in still another way, in which we have tried to tie together the word pictures given in the records above. We wanted, if possible, to place together in some way the results of all the different tests given to see what agreement was achieved in following the postoperative course. The major obstacle to so doing was the fact that the projective tests of personality are analyzed by patterns of response and regularly defy quantification. To make the comparison we had in mind, however, required an over-all interpretive result rather than quantification of every score contained in the tests.

To this end we made a scale on which to score the total performance of each individual. The minimal obtainable performance was scored at one end and normal performance at the other, with anchor points in between. Table 4 shows the Rorschach scale with its extremes and anchor points.*

We used this scale with the records of patients not included in the present project, correcting and changing until the steps seemed to fit, and then scored each Rorschach test protocol of this series by means of it. Table 5 shows a similar scale for the TAT, evolved in the same fashion, again with minimal obtainable performance at one end and normal performance at the other.

The records of this series of patients were evaluated by means of this scale. We then ranged the psychomotor total score on a line of the same length, with minimal obtainable performance at one end and normal at the other, and did the same with the behavior ratings. Since these were already quantified scores, no scaling was necessary. The scores obtained by the above scaling methods were noted graphically, as shown in Figure 4. This notation permits inspection of changes in status from one test interval to another. We were aware that the zero points and units of scale for the different tests are only approximately equated, but the scheme appeared to be workable. Figure 4 shows the patterns so derived for the various patients concerned.

To take one further step, in order to get a single inclusive score, we averaged the separate but roughly comparable scores. These averages, shown in Table 6, indicate again that different patients follow different courses postoperatively. The greatest gains are seen in Patients 2 and 12; some gains can be seen in Patients 17 and 13; there is no great change in Patients 6, 7, 14, and 20; and Patient 8(15) becomes worse.

This agrees in every particular with the conclusions drawn from the word pictures and gives us greater confidence in our interpretation of the changes noted.

The intellective tests did not appear in the totalizer for comparison with the other tests because we found that scores on these tests did not have the same range of possible variation as the others, being subject

*In selecting the Rorschach referents for the normal anchor point, we used data from the Spiegel sample[15] as a base.

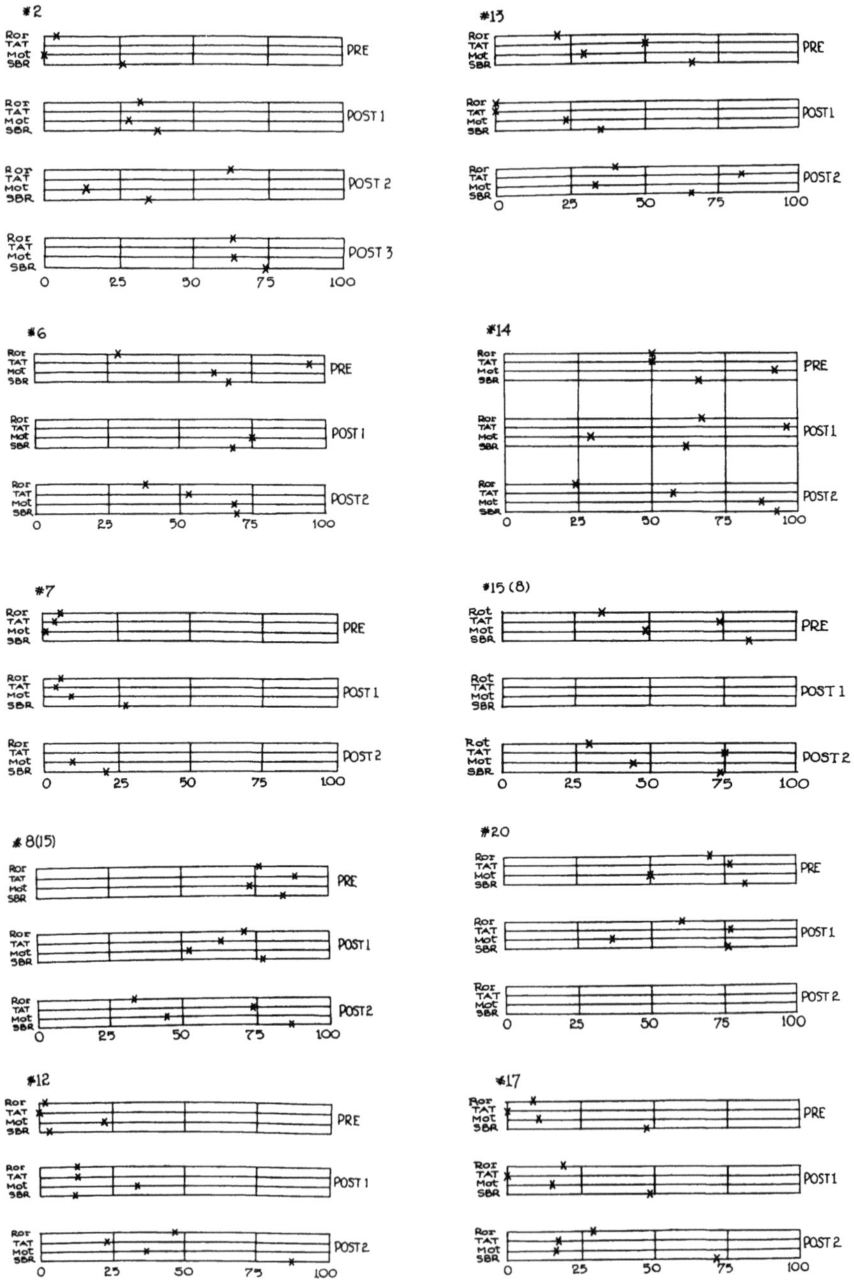

FIGURE XVI-4. Pre- and postoperative "totalizer" scores for each patient included in this series

TABLE XVI–4. Rating scale on the degree of psychosis as judged by Rorschach test performance

0	10	20	30	40
Completely disorganized, mute, extremely disturbed, loss of reality contact, thought processes bizarre	Somewhat disorganized, poor reality contact, some disruption of thought processes, affectively very flat or labile	Some integration of personality, but distortions in one area or another (e.g. thought processes, marked anxiety, lessened reality contact)	Well integrated, adequate reality contact, may be emotionally somewhat flat, show neurotic overlay	Normal
Severe schizophrenia	*Strong schizophrenia*	*Moderate schizophrenia*	*Mild schizophrenia*	*No schizophrenia*
May show: some rejection very low F + % low P pure C responses no C responses color-naming perseveration low productivity	May show: low F + % pure C responses high A % more than 3 s responses abstract responses no M	May show: high or low lambda FY and/or FV marked low A % M/C high on C	May show: adequate F + % high lambda color shock low C	Shows: 2–5 M M/C ambiequal CF larger than FC few C A % 33–59 P 5–9 lambda 57–83 F + % 69–89

TABLE XVI–5. Rating scale for Thematic Apperception Test performance

0	10	20	30	40
Protocol brief, merely description, urging required minimal performance	Some attempt to tell stories, attitudes of characters	Stories told, but in a rambling, indecisive way; not cohesive	Adequate stories with brief development of plots	Well-developed stories with cohesive plots

TABLE XVI–6. The average totalizer scale values for each patient at each testing interval

Patient	*Preop*	*Post 1*	*Post 2*	*Post 3*
2	9	32	36	67
6	63	72	57	
7	8	11	10	
8 (15)	80	66	60	
12	7	17	48	
13	42	15	55	
14	65	63	65	
15 (8)	60	—	56	
17	17	21	33	
20	70	64	—	

to only minor changes in the reflection of alterations in psychiatric status. There were some changes which indicated better functional use of the intelligence when the general psychiatric status of the patient was improved. No such changes were noted for the unchanged patients or for the patient who became worse.

Our general conclusions, then, are that in some instances the stimulation procedure improved the status of patients as measured by psychological tests, in some instances has been ineffective, and in one instance resulted in impairment. Although still subject to modification and improvement, the battery of psychological tests appears to have been effective and sensitive to changes in the status of the patients under study.

REFERENCES

1. The Columbia-Greystone Associates. *Selective Partial Ablation of the Frontal Cortex; A Correlative Study of its Effects on Human Psychotic Subjects,* edited by F. A. Mettler. Hoeber, New York, 1949.
2. The Columbia-Greystone Associates (second group). *Psychosurgical Problems,* edited by F. A. Mettler. Blakiston, New York, 1952.
3. The Columbia-Greystone Associates (second group). *Psychosurgical Problems,* vol. 2. *J. Nerv. & Ment. Dis.* (in preparation).
4. Eisenson, J. *Examining for Aphasia.* Psychological Corp., New York, 1946.
5. Wechsler, D. *Measurement of Adult Intelligence.* Williams & Wilkins, Baltimore, 1944.
6. Porteus, S. D. *The Porteus Maze Test and Intelligence.* Pacific Books, Palo Alto, 1950.

7. Wechsler, D. *A Standardized Memory Scale for Clinical Use.* Psychological Corp., New York, 1946.
8. Benton, A. L. *A Visual Retention Test for Clinical Use.* Psychological Corp., New York, 1946.
9. Beck, S. J. *Rorschach's Test,* vols. 1 and 2. Grune, New York, 1949.
10. Murray, H. and others. *Thematic Apperception Test Manual.* Harvard Univ. Press, Cambridge, 1943.
11. King, H. E. Psychomotor aspects of the orbitofrontal cortex. *Federation Proc.,* 9:70 (1950).
12. King, H. E. Psychomotor performance and psychiatric status. *Bull. Tulane M. Fac.,* 11:34–37 (1951).
13. King, H. E. *Psychomotor Aspects of Mental Disease* (in press).
14. Malamud, W., and S. Sands. A revision of the psychiatric rating scale. *Am. J. Psychiat.,* 104:231–237 (1947).
15. Beck, S. J., A. I. Rabin, W. G. Thiesen, H. Molish, and W. N. Thetford. The normal personality as projected in the Rorschach test. *J. Psychol.,* 30:241–298 (1950).

TABLE XVII–1. Summary of therapeutic results with schizophrenic patients. The operation was repeated on Patients 5 and 8.

Patient	Months (as of June 1952) Post-stim.	Out of hosp.	Working	Improvement rating (see text)	Complications c = coma s = seizure f = fever
1*	26	0	0	0	0
2	20	16	9	3+	S–C
3*	17	0	0	0	F–C
4	16	14	0	2+	0
5(24)	16(2)	12(0)	0(0)	2+(1+)	0(0)
6	15	11	2	2+	0
7	14	12	0	2+	S
8(15)	13(6)	6(1)	0(½)	2+(2+)	0(S–F)
9	13	0	0	0	0
10	12	0	0	0	F
11	9	5	2	2+	S–C
12	8	4½	4½	3+	S
13	8	5	0	3+	S
14†	7	1½	½	3+	F
16	6	0	0	2+	0
17	6	1½	0	3+	F
18	5	0	0	2+	0
19†	5	0	0	?	F–C
20	5	0	0	1+	F
22*	3	0	0	1+	0

*Considered technical failure.
†Died.

KEY TO RATINGS

4 + = normal adjustment; no defect
3 + = out of hospital; working; minimal defect
2 + = significant improvement; psychosis still evident
1 + = questionable improvement
0 = no improvement

CHAPTER 17

PSYCHIATRIC OBSERVATIONS

RUSSELL R. MONROE
ROBERT G. HEATH

As specific therapy is the aim of most research, we should like to be in a position to demonstrate conclusively that the behavioral changes observed in our group of twenty schizophrenic patients were due to septal stimulation rather than to adventitious factors. (Consideration of the control patients is excluded from this chapter.) Although we do indeed believe that our data suggest a causal relationship, we realize that they must be cautiously interpreted for several reasons. The most obvious is that twenty patients constitute only a small sample. Moreover, as explained in Chapter 8, each patient was selected on the basis of a poor prognosis, and the group as a whole therefore cannot be considered a true cross-section of the diagnostic category schizophrenia. Many variables were introduced by changes in the method of electrode implantation as the technique was gradually improved during the course of the experiment. As we were exploring an entirely new area it was thought inadvisable to set up rigid controls in this preliminary research program. In a sense, each patient must be evaluated separately rather than as one-twentieth of a group. Nevertheless, we feel that some generalizations, if not definite conclusions, can be drawn from our observations.

GENERAL THERAPEUTIC RESULTS

Table 1 shows a summary of the therapeutic results as of June 1, 1952.* In the left-hand column the patients are numbered according to the sequence of operation. Two patients, 5(24) and 8(15), had second operations; the results of the second operation are given in parentheses, following those of the first. The improvement ratings in column five (from 0 to 4+) are crude representations of the patients' over-all psychiatric status. Grade 4+ indicates a normal adjustment without any residual defects. As will be explained later, none of our patients

*Addendum F extends the follow-up period 12 months.

seemed to fit this category. Grade 3 + means that the patient was out of the hospital and working or effectively assisting with the household chores. Although showing some defects in adaptation, he would not be institutionalized for psychotic behavior. Grade 2 + indicates significant improvement in behavior; some patients so rated had left the hospital, the others had at least been shifted from the acutely disturbed ward to the open ward. Improvement in these cases was unquestionable, but evidence of overt psychosis remained. Grade 1 + indicates questionable improvement. In the two cases thus rated in Table 1, there seemed to be little change in the degree of psychosis, although the patients had become tractable. Also listed in the summary of therapeutic results are certain complications—namely, coma, convulsions, and fever, all of which are or have been used in the treatment of schizophrenics with variable results. The possibility that these complications were responsible for the patients' improvement will be discussed later.

In the group of twenty patients one died five weeks after operation. Of the remaining nineteen, eleven left the hospital, two subsequently returning to receive a second stimulation. One of these left the hospital following the second procedure. Thus, out of the nineteen patients, ten left the hospital. Nine at present are being followed in the out-patient department, one having died 1 1/2 months following his discharge. Table 1 reveals that eight of the nineteen received their last stimulation over 12 months ago. Seven received their last stimulation more than 5 months ago, and the remaining four have received their last stimulation within the past 5 months.* Discharged patients have been out of the hospital for periods of 1 to 16 months. By clinical standards, five are considered to have shown marked improvement, eight others significant improvement, two questionable improvement, four no improvement at all, and one could not be evaluated. All the patients, regardless of their present status, were felt to have shown some improvement during the first 6 weeks following stimulation. However, such improvement was difficult to evaluate, as there was always the possibility that it reflected a nonspecific response to either the operative or the rehabilitative procedure or to a combination of both. Figures 1–4 illustrate this improvement as measured clinically by the Malamud-Sands rating scale.

*As of June, 1952. See Addendum F, which extends the follow-up period 12 months.

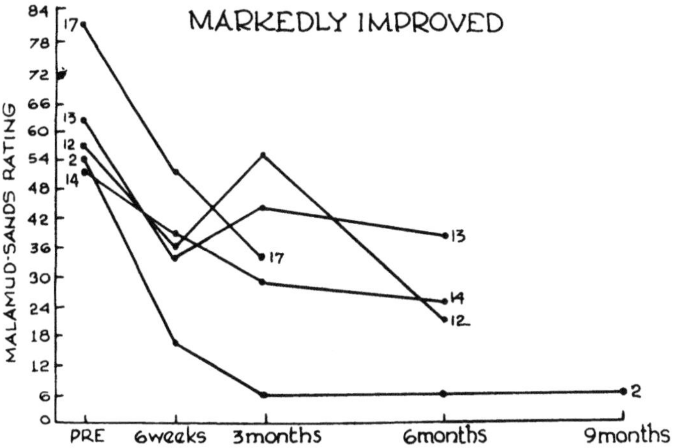

FIGURE XVII–1. Degree of improvement shown by Patients 2, 12, 13, 14 and 17 during 9 months following stimulation

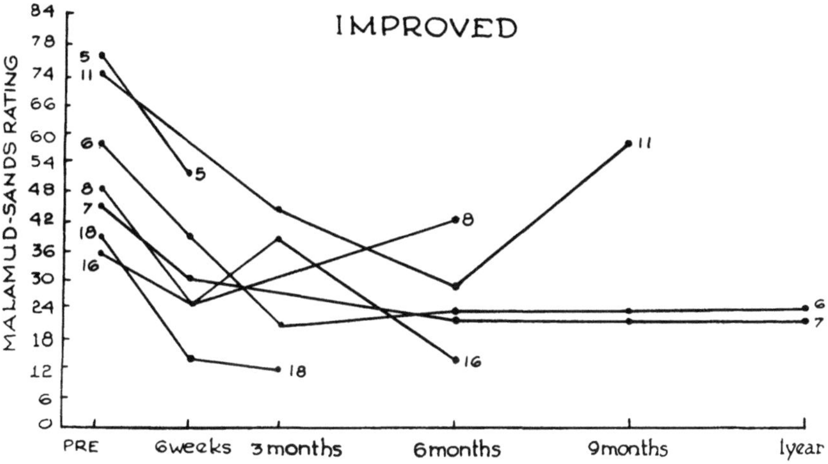

FIGURE XVII–2. Degree of improvement shown by Patients 5, 6, 7, 8, 11, 16, and 18 during the year following stimulation. Patient 4 was not rated because she was not seen regularly at the clinic

IMMEDIATE REACTION TO STIMULATION

The physiological reactions of the patients to stimulation have already been reported. Psychologically, most of the patients who were considered technical successes showed definite and immediate changes in behavior, as well as dramatic changes in emotional responsiveness. At times they became less tense and fearful, and at other times angry or frightened. Frequently one noticed a pleasurable reaction to stimulation. The patients became more alert—opening their eyes, gazing about the room, and for the first time indicating recognition of their therapist and awareness of distracting noises. There were also increases in motor activity and spontaneous production. Although previously almost inaudible or expressionless, speech became louder and enunciation clearer and inflection more appropriate. Sometimes these responses would be sustained following stimulation and other times they would subside quickly.

During the stimulations several of the patients reported subjective sensations. Patient 6 described a sensation of "being warm" and later said that he thought he heard the voice of God telling him not to masturbate. Patient 18 complained that he was going to "faint." This was also the complaint of Patient 20, who subsequently described other feelings, such as, "I feel more normal," or, "I have a glowing feeling. I feel good." Patient 17 reported, "I feel queer," and expressed considerable anxiety. Patient 14 was obviously frightened, expecting that he was to receive electroshock therapy. Three of the patients showed no objective signs (Patients 1, 3, and 9), and two could not be evaluated (Patients 2 and 19). Five of the patients who had been mute or underproductive before talked for the first time or showed more elaboration during the stimulation (Patients 6, 7, 11, 12, and 16). Thirteen showed a definite increase in alertness (Patients 4, 5(24), 6, 7, 10, 11, 12, 13, 14, 16, 17, 18, and 20), three an increase in tension (Patients 8(15), 14 and 22), while two others reported a decrease (Patients 7 and 20). One was obviously less productive during the stimulation (Patient 8(15)). As the final stimulation was applied within 24 to 54 hours after surgery, it could be argued that the alerting response noted during stimulation might be related to postanesthetic cortical depression rather than to any immediate change in the basic psychotic process. We do not feel this is the case for several reasons. Stimulation was postponed as long as possible, usually being done after most EEG evidence of barbiturate effect had disappeared and the patient had clinically returned to his approximate preoperative behavior. In the chronic experiments on monkeys (see Chapter 13) it was noted that the animals became much more alert and responsive during septal stimulation, although they had

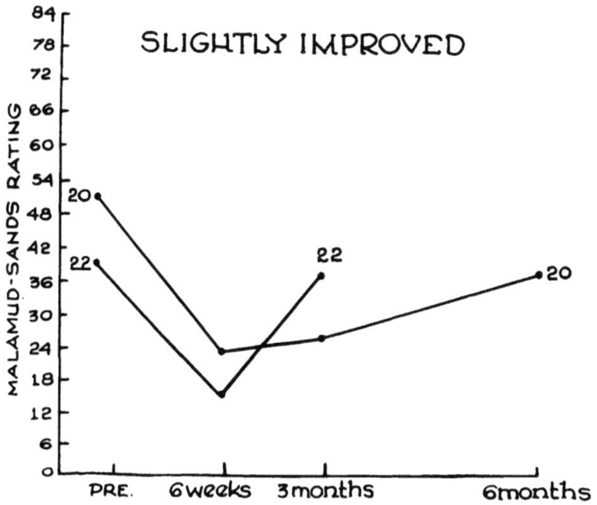

FIGURE XVII–3. Degree of improvement shown by Patients 20 and 22 during 6 months following stimulation. Patient 19 was not rated because of early death

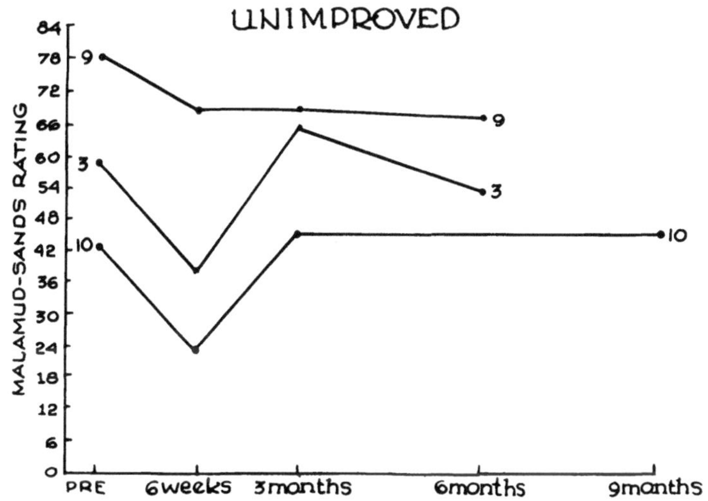

FIGURE XVII–4. Degree of improvement shown by Patients 3, 9, and 10 during 9 months following stimulation. Patient 1 was not rated

had no recent anesthesia or drugs. However, this point is now being investigated, as the new technique (see Addenda C and D) allows one to stimulate the patient several days or weeks after the operative procedure.

BEHAVIOR DURING THE FIRST TWENTY-FOUR HOURS

During the 24 hours following stimulation, improvement was generally maintained. Although delusions remained, the patients often seemed less preoccupied with them and occasionally expressed doubt as to their validity. Seven patients became definitely more alert (Patients 4, 6, 11, 12, 16, 18, and 19). Four showed dramatic changes in affect (Patients 7, 8(15), 14, and 16), one having tears in his eyes and a mournful expression (Patient 8(15)). Patient 14 expressed delight with the doctor's gift of ice cream. As he finished the last spoonful, he smiled broadly, saying, "Good to the last drop." Patient 16 greeted visitors with a friendly smile, whereas she had previously been hostile and uncooperative. Patient 8(15) showed a marked increase in the self-consciousness which had been present before operation. Two showed definite changes in their symptomatology, one dropping many of his bizarre mannerisms (Patient 6), while the other, who had previously demanded antiseptics whenever anybody touched him, discontinued this demand (Patient 14). Three of the patients showed little or no immediate change in behavior (Patients 1, 3, and 9), while two others could not be evaluated because they were in coma (Patients 2 and 19).

SUBSEQUENT CLINICAL COURSE

On the second or third day after operation the above-mentioned changes were overshadowed by the general dulling of affect, lethargy, confusion, and disorientation that are the natural consequences in any craniotomy. With a disappearance of the craniotomy effect, a steady improvement, lasting from three to six weeks, was noted in all patients. This was true even of those patients who subsequently relapsed to their preoperative status (see Figures 1–4). However, the course was a fluctuating one, varying from day to day. In those patients who showed the greatest improvement, the outstanding changes were: ability to relate to other people, increased responsiveness to pleasure, gradual appearance of a sense of humor, and more overt expression of anxiety and ambivalence. Less negativism was displayed and less autistic preoccupation; everyday problems were approached more realistically and more interest was shown in ward activities. Underproductive patients became talkative. Intellectually, most patients seemed to be better motivated in performing simple test problems. Speed was improved, but many still showed serious impairment compared with their prepsychotic status. Although hallucinations sometimes dramatically disappeared, delusions were maintained for several months. One could see the gradual development of doubt, with growing insight. By the fifth or sixth week after operation, patients who continued to improve were permitted to visit their homes. Those who were discharged left the hospital from 2 to 5 1/2 months postoperatively. Marked affective responses followed visits and discharges, the patients showing either intense pleasure or anxiety and depression.

Psychotherapeutic and rehabilitative programs were maintained at a superficial level. The immediate goal was that of increasing the patient's sociability and encouraging empathy with the family and hospital personnel. It was found that interpretation of unconscious motivation was usually of little help, even if it was attempted in an intensive manner as in the case of Patient 16. Sedatives and stimulants were given when appropriate. In retrospect we feel that some of the patients were pushed too hard, as several had to be readmitted to the hospital shortly after discharge, although they subsequently improved and have remained out of the hospital (Patients 8(15) and 12).

DETAILED EVALUATION OF THE POSTSTIMULATION COURSE

BEHAVIORAL CHANGES

Fourteen patients showed significant changes in their behavior during postoperative hospitalization (Patients 2, 4, 5(24), 6, 7, 8(15), 10, 11, 12, 13, 14, 16, 17, and 18). Patient 14, who had been so preoccupied with germs prior to operation that the ward personnel were required to bathe their hands in alcohol before they touched him, dropped this demand immediately, although he still refused to use the communal toilets or associate with other patients. With the change in his phobia, there was also a change in his behavior, as he was no longer negativistic or periodically assaultive. Patient 16 performed a number of obsessive rituals, such as stepping over lines when she walked down the hall. She felt this to be necessary, as she said, "Because my thoughts will kill somebody if I don't do this." Four months after operation, these obsessional traits were dropped periodically, although they intermittently but less frequently recur up to the present time. Before operation Patient 2 was preoccupied with her inner phantasy life to the point of almost complete inaccessibility. After operation she ate voraciously, gaining from 5 to 10 pounds a week. She socialized on the ward and began participating in occupational therapy. Patient 13 had a stereotyped mannerism wherein he would cross himself on the forehead and the mouth and then over the heart. After operation he gradually modified the procedure, making it look less and less abnormal, until it might appear to the casual observer that he merely had a tic. Patient 11, who prior to operation would sprawl on the floor, crawl about on his hands and knees, and hide his face behind his hands while he laughed in a bizarre manner, also gradually modified his behavior. After operation he still seemed somewhat embarrassed by the direct gaze of the therapist, but no longer hid his face behind his hands or giggled in a silly manner. Oftentimes he read magazines or even played cards with the other patients. Patient 8(15) had been very hostile, negativistic, and periodically assaultive before operation; afterward this aggressiveness diminished until he was generally friendly and cooperative on the wards. He still retained referential and persecutory ideas directed toward people in his environment and accompanied by intense rage, but he did not act on these ideas as before.

Five of the patients who had been relatively uncommunicative before operation became much more spontaneous afterward (Patients 2, 6, 11, 12, and 16). Patient 2, who had been almost mute, became talkative and later almost hypomanic. Patient 12 had shown no spontaneity before operation. If replying to questions at all, he answered with an almost inaudible "yes" or "no." Although he never elaborated on delusional or hallucinatory material after operation, he did show considerable spontaneity, particularly in talking of his feelings. He complained bitterly when his family returned him to the hospital, expressing the idea that he had been deserted.

Eleven patients showed significant differences in socialization (Patients 2, 3, 5(24), 6, 10, 11, 12, 13, 14, 17, and 18). In general, these patients had been idle, seclusive, and withdrawn before operation; afterward they participated actively in some or all of the ward activities. For instance, as Patient 6 improved, he showed an interest in relearning typing and shorthand. Although he was not capable of functioning well in this capacity, he was eager about trying and worked hard to relearn his old skill. Patient 10 had been on the back wards of a mental hospital for 18 years. Following stimulation he began playing checkers with his doctors and the other patients. Although his improvement lasted only 3 months, the change in the immediate postoperative period was significant. Patient 18, who had been confined to bed almost continuously for many months before operation, afterward became particularly interested in occupational therapy, building two porch chairs for his family. He constructed them rather quickly, but when it came to finishing them he showed a number of obsessive traits, sanding *ad infinitum.*

EMOTIONAL CHANGES

Even more dramatic than the behavioral changes were the changes in emotional responsiveness. Twelve patients showed significant improvement in their ability to relate to other people (Patients 2, 5(24), 6, 8(15), 10, 11, 12, 13, 14, 16, 17, and 18). Although Patients 5(24) and 10 relapsed to their prepsychotic state, the other ten maintained to a greater or lesser extent this improvement. Patient 6 had been afraid of homosexual attacks prior to operation, constantly backing up while conversing. He now developed a rather sticky dependency upon and identification with anybody who would show an interest in him. Patient 14 enthusiastically looked forward to visits from the ward personnel, whereas he had previously barricaded himself in his room, refusing to talk with them. He developed close attachments to both the nurses and the attendants.

One of the outstanding aspects of this change in emotional responsivity was the appearance of pleasurable feelings. Patient 2, who had shown symptoms similar to anorexia nervosa prior to stimulation, now expressed real delight at meals. Patient 5(24), who had shown disorganized sexual behavior with some sexual solicitousness, as well as fear, continued to show a sensual attachment to her male therapist but in a more realistic and subdued way. Patient 7, who was discharged from the hospital although showing only minimal changes in his behavior, expressed delight whenever praised by the therapist concerning his dress or his behavior.

After operation four patients manifested ambivalence, which had not previously been apparent (Patients 2, 6, 11, and 17). For instance, Patient 2, when shown any unusual attention, such as being taken to the movies by the ward attendants, would say, "I don't deserve all this. Sometimes it makes me feel bad. On the other hand, it makes me feel good, too."

Seven patients showed increased anxiety following operation, although this usually was transitory (Patients 6, 8(15), 11, 12, 16, 17, and 20). Before operation Patient 16 had periodic rages but had not expressed much anxiety. After operation she ran away from the hospital on two occasions, fearing that she was going to be killed. Patient 17 had two panic reactions, during which she hallucinated that one of the doctors was going to cut her arm off. When released on a pass, Patient 20 would refuse to come back to the hospital, fearing that the doctors were going to attack her sexually. In some patients anxiety was accompanied by depressive feelings. Patient 11, who had manifested self-derogatory ideas without appropriate emotion before operation, afterward showed intense feelings of unworthiness and depression when his family lost interest in him. Patient 12, whose affect was apparently flat before operation, showed a real depression postoperatively when his family found it necessary to return him to the hospital. At that time he expressed feelings of desertion.

Another important aspect of this emotional responsiveness was the development of humor. Nine patients demonstrated this dramatically (Patients 2, 5(24), 8(15), 10, 12, 13, 14, 18, and 20). Patient 13, who had been a completely "flat" catatonic before operation, afterward subjected his father to so much teasing that it became a rehabilitative problem, as his father reacts with outbursts of rage. It is undoubtedly true that this humor has an aggressive undertone, but it seems to be the best possible outlet for the patient's hostility. Patient 14 was particularly jovial after the operation, teasing the doctors and nurses constantly. Patient 18 showed a rather spontaneous, subtle wit, although his emotional responses did not seem to be as hearty as they might have been. Nevertheless, they were probably in keeping with his rather shy and reserved prepsychotic personality.

CHANGES IN IDEATION

Hallucinations and delusions were the last psychotic symptoms to disappear in those patients who continued to improve. In fact, the patients who improved most were those who had the least overt psychotic ideation. Seven patients have maintained most of their delusional symptoms up to the present time (Patients 3, 5(24), 7, 8(15), 10, 11, and 14), but three of them have shown dramatic improvement otherwise (Patients 8(15), 11, and 14). The best example of this is Patient 14, who had the germ phobia. Although postoperatively he was able to ride busses and streetcars, use public toilets, and mix in large crowds for the first time in 7 years, he steadfastly refused to mingle with the closed-ward patients, fearing contamination. He would not let his father bring his mother to the hospital, fearing that she too would be contaminated. These isolated phobias did not interfere with his departure from the hospital and subsequent employment, at which he worked satisfactorily until his sudden death a month and a half later. However, even a week before his death he refused to come back to the clinic because of his fear of contamination. Patient 11, who had left the hospital and was working as a dishwasher, still reported hallucinatory experiences which suggested self-mutilation or suicide.

Four patients reported a cessation of hallucinations and delusions (Patients 2, 6, 8(15), and 17) and did not seem to be responding to such, but there is the possibility that some were now capable of hiding these signs of abnormality. Patient 2 gave up all her ideas of oral impregnation, as well as the delusion of having been impregnated by Christ. Patient 6 dropped his hypochondriacal preoccupations and homosexual delusions, as did Patient 8(15), although the latter returned to them. As improvement progressed following stimulation, most of these patients showed gradual insight, often first expressing doubt as to the validity of their ideas. With constant reinforcement from the environment, they managed subsequently to drop them. Oftentimes patients would say, "I guess I am really crazy." More and more they would accept the real world about them, spending less time with autistic preoccupations. Nevertheless, it is our general impression at present that patients who respond particularly well to the stimulation procedure are the ones who have not developed highly systematized hallucinations or delusions but whose main abnormalities seem to consist of flattened affect or disturbed motor behavior.

As many psychiatrists feel that hallucinations and delusions are reparative symptoms resulting from a basic affective disturbance, it may well be that when a patient has had an opportunity for reality-testing over considerable period of time his hallucinations or delusions will disappear. Such a course is suggested already in the relatively short follow-up reports.

CHANGES IN INTELLECTUAL FUNCTIONING

Precise evaluations of intellectual functioning were made by the psychologists. Clinically, it seems that six patients had definite intellectual impairment severe enough to be suggestive of organic brain damage (Patients 6, 13, 14, and 17). In some of these patients it is possible that damage existed prior to operation. Patient 6, who had a topectomy, sometimes becomes confused. For instance, when walking down the rather complicated hallways in the psychiatric department, he will often make the wrong turn, although he has been there many times previously. However, in cursory clinical testing he performs at a highly abstract level, his memory seems intact, and he is fully oriented. Patient 13 shows a rather bizarre memory loss, which seems to vacillate in its severity. When seen in the clinic, he will not recall the names of the hospital personnel, nor will he recall the date of his last visit. However, when he meets the same people on the street, he will spontaneously call out their names. He is disoriented as to time, but not as to place and situation. He often goes to church during the week, thinking it is Sunday. He takes long walks, many times adventuring into strange parts of town. Although he always finds his way home, he sometimes forgets that he has recently been on a walk. As he was mute and uncooperative before operation, it is hard to tell whether his memory was faulty at that time. (Electrodes were placed unusually deep and caudal in this patient.) Patient 14, who had studied physics in college, was given several mathematical problems to solve when applying for a job following his discharge from the hospital. Although he could have solved these easily before he became psychotic, it was impossible for him to do so on the job test even with the aid of textbooks. Nine patients showed definite increase in motivation when presented with simple intellectual problems (Patients 2, 6, 8(15), 11, 12, 13, 14, 16, and 17). This same group seemed to perform the tests more rapidly and accurately than before stimulation.

THERAPEUTIC AND REHABILITATIVE PROCEDURES

Following operation we used a total-push therapeutic technique with the immediate goal of maintaining and extending the patient's increased affective responsiveness and realistic awareness. However, it must be pointed out that this therapeutic regimen is not limited to the present series of twenty patients but is a general one applied to all patients in the 70 beds which Charity Hospital puts at the disposal of the Tulane service. From four to eight residents are assigned to these 70 beds, and the hospital, compared with state hospitals in general, is well staffed with nurses and attendants. There is an active occupational therapy department for all patients, as well as social service facilities which are particularly useful in arranging for home care. Families are allowed to visit twice a week, and tractable patients are allowed frequent passes out of the hospital. Of the patients in this group, all but four (Patients 9, 10, 13, and 20) had been subjected to such a program without avail prior to their stimulation. In our research project it was not feasible to set up controls to evaluate the possible therapeutic effects that the enthusiasm of the participants might have on the patients. This would have involved carrying out all the steps of the combined operation and stimulation procedure except that of the actual electrical stimulation. It would have been necessary to hide this fact from all investigators except, of course, the electronics engineer who was actually giving the stimulation. We felt that we were unjustified in subjecting any patient to this regimen. It was believed that a long-term follow-up would expose any adventitious cures due to the optimistic enthusiasm of involved personnel. Seven of the patients in this group had been studied in a previous research project, in which electroshock therapy was compared with electronarcosis (Patients 2, 4, 5(24), 7, 11, 12, and 22). At that time they were subjected to numerous tests and much additional and sometimes enthusiastic attention but none showed any significant improvement in this experimental atmosphere.

We felt further justified in using a total-push technique because of our belief that a procedure such as subcortical stimulation would probably do no more than make the patient receptive to subsequent psychotherapeutic and rehabilitative measures. After all, for many years most of the patients involved had been living a bizarre, disordered life and consequently would need much guidance and education before it could be expected that they would make anything like a normal adjustment.

Within the first 24 hours after operation the therapist usually made an attempt to gain rapport by offering the patient something from which he could derive immediate pleasure. For instance, the therapist would find out the patient's favorite food or reading matter and on the first postoperative contact would present this to the patient. It was generally gratifying to observe the emotional response to this maneuver. Patients usually expressed real pleasure and deep appreciation. The therapist subsequently maintained an attitude of permissiveness wherever possible. Nevertheless, he also maintained a certain firmness, directly pointing out, over and over again, the inappropriateness of the patient's behavior and how it might be changed—for instance, saying, "Now you don't need to hide behind your hands any more, do you? You have nothing to be ashamed of." If the patient had an obsession or compulsion, the therapist would again actively participate—for instance, taking him on walks and encouraging him not to step over the tabooed lines. This approach had been used without success prior to the stimulation. To sum up, the approach was one of intensive attention, permissiveness, indulgence (particularly toward the patient's food preferences), timely correction of abnormal behavior, constant emphasis on reality, and over-all optimism toward the eventual outcome of the patient's illness.

Both the ward personnel and the patients' families were actively engaged in the rehabilitative procedure. Relatives were usually in constant attendance during the first few postoperative days and afterwards were encouraged to visit the patients frequently. As soon as it was feasible, patients were encouraged to leave the hospital in the company of their relatives. This usually resulted in mixed feelings. Pleasure was shown in anticipation of the outing, and obvious gratification and increase of self-esteem upon completing it successfully. However, the sudden change in routine would often elicit anxiety and occasionally depressive reactions. Such reactions did not postpone further outings; rather the therapist tried to persuade the patient to face the same situation again as soon as possible, hoping that repetitive activity would decrease his anxiety and begin to raise his self-esteem. Most of the time this worked. Yet on several occasions it apparently precipitated acute panic reactions, necessitating discontinuance of passes, and in two cases rehospitalization (Patients 8(15) and 12). In retrospect, it would seem that five patients were pushed beyond their limits, subsequently having exacerbations of their illness (Patients 8(15), 11, 12, 16, and 18). Seven patients responded successfully to this pressure, showing rapid improvement in their behavior and expressing considerable gratification that they were able to face problems that had not been attempted for some years (Patients 2, 4, 6, 7, 13, 14, and 17).

In several cases it was felt that maximum improvement was not obtained because the family failed in their rehabilitative efforts. This was particularly true of Patients 11 and 16. Patient 11 had only one close relative, a brother who could not provide adequate care. The latter's home was in a poor section of town, very overcrowded and offering no chance for supervision which would encourage gradual resumption of work and socialization. Patient 16, although of middle-class environment, could not go home because the members of her immediate family were too disturbed themselves to offer adequate care. As the project progressed, it became increasingly obvious that one of the criteria for selecting the patients should be the ability of the family to give extensive and prolonged rehabilitative supervision. The only other alternative would be to provide nursing homes for patients who cannot return to their families and who lack resources for private care.

Intensive interpretative psychotherapy was tried on two patients who were intelligent and particularly productive (Patients 14 and 16). Both had a large number of pseudoneurotic symptoms, including marked obsessions and hypochondriacal fears. One of us (R. R. M.) arranged to see them two or three times a week for hourly sessions. Patient 16, who performed certain rituals in order to avoid "killing" people with her thoughts, was seen on a number of occasions, when attempts were made to trace the origin of her obsessional ideas. She gained some insight, realizing that these might be connected with her own fears of retaliation or punishment, but she soon lost interest in keeping her appointments. She gradually refused to cooperate, claiming, "My physical condition won't allow me to walk that far." Patient 14 was superficially more ingratiating and cooperative, continuing to come to sessions, but he could not be induced to describe his subjective experiences. At each session he would repeatedly demand explanations of his numerous hypochondriacal fears, particularly those related to the operative procedure and the onset of his psychosis.

It should be emphasized that most of the patients in our series of twenty schizophrenics were incapable of subjective reporting. Even with intensive psychotherapy it was impossible to induce them to express their innermost thoughts and emotions. Interpretations of unconscious motivation were therefore necessarily based on symptoms appearing before and after stimulation. These interpretations are too sparse, we believe, to warrant discussion at this time. However, operative and stimulation techniques have now been developed to the point where they can be justifiably applied to pseudoneurotic schizophrenics who are more productive. Plans are underway for stimulation of several patients who have received intensive psychoanalytic therapy without benefit, and it is hoped that valuable introspective data can be obtained from them in regard to basic changes consequent to the stimulation procedure.

After the electrodes were removed, medications were used if they seemed indicated, but we avoided electroshock therapy, which we felt would complicate analysis of the results of stimulation.* Patient 12, who responded temporarily to sodium amytal prior to operation, was given sodium amytal postoperatively when he had a recurrence of marked anxiety with tachycardia and tremulousness. As before he became less disturbed and less tremulous, but there was a difference in his reaction to the drug in that the effect did not wear off in a few days. After his discharge from the hospital, it was gradually discontinued without any return of his anxiety. Patient 8(15) complained postoperatively of excessive tension and was placed on chronic sedation, which he had

*Patient 8(15) subsequently received EST.

required for many years prior to stimulation. Since he still complained of lack of energy, a feeling of hopelessness, and over-all depression, he was tried on dexamyl. When this failed to act as a euphorant, only increasing his tension, it was discontinued and he was placed back on sedation. Patient 18, after showing a rather marked improvement initially, again became quiet, seclusive, and withdrawn. He showed little interest in eating, appeared tense and anxious, and complained that everybody was "pushing" him. He was then placed on ambulatory insulin, to which he responded. At the present time he receives 45 units of insulin per day.* Patient 20, who showed periodic panic reactions, was tried on chronic sedation. However, on this regimen she became idle, seclusive, and bedridden; consequently, it was discontinued. Patient 17 also complained of fatigue and appeared underactive and retarded. She was placed on dexamyl during the latter part of her hospitalization. She showed increased interest in ward activities as well as less depression.

EVALUATION OF PATIENTS SHOWING MARKED IMPROVEMENT

Patients 2, 12, 13, 14, and 17 were considered to be much improved. As Patient 14 died 1 1/2 months after operation, psychiatric evaluation of his case is impossible. Considering the other four patients, we find that all were relatively young, ranging in age from 17 to 35. Three were diagnosed as catatonic and one hebephrenic. All had been sick for considerable periods of time—that is, from 2 to 7 years. All had shown relatively marked personality deviations prior to the onset of their psychoses. Patient 17 appeared quite schizoid and was possibly a mental defective. Patient 2 was extremely schizoid, in fact, might well have been diagnosed a simple schizophrenic many years before the onset of her catatonic symptoms 3 1/2 years ago (see Chapter 8, Table 1). All were emotionally flat, retarded, almost mute, idle, and seclusive. At times they were negativistic and uncooperative, although they did cooperate with the psychologist in performing their numerous and rather arduous psychological tests (Figure 5). None verbalized much in the way of delusional or hallucinatory material. It is interesting to note that such patients are considered to have a poor prognosis for psychosurgical

*See Addendum F for follow-up.

techniques and in fact have a poor prognosis generally if they have not responded to EST or insulin. Perhaps they will prove to be the type of patient who is most suitable for stimulation. As yet it is certainly too early to make any definitive statements on this subject. Four other patients presented a similar picture with a predominance of emotional flattening and motor retardation and little delusional or hallucinatory material. Two of these—Patients 4 and 5(24)—also left the hospital, but both have shown less improvement and Patient 5(24) has relapsed. Of the other two, Patient 22 was a definite technical failure and Patient 3 had minimal stimulation.

In view of our theoretical assumption that impairment of the facilitatory circuit was involved in schizophrenia, it seemed logical to infer that stimulation of the septal region might initiate clinical improvement. Do the clinical and neurophysiological data on these much improved patients substantiate this inference? In Patient 2, we have no definite proof in regard to placement of the electrode (since implantation was done manually under direct vision), but the neurologist, the neurophysiologist, and the surgeon concur that the electrode was placed in the rostral part of the septal region. In Patient 12, who showed the next most dramatic clinical improvement, the electrodes were placed in the lateral aspect of the ventricular wall, one definitely in the caudate near the internal capsule, and another deeper in the ventral aspect of the caudate nucleus. Stimulation of the latter initially produced the alertness that we associated with the facilitatory region. However, stimulation of the former, that in the caudate proper (hypothetical inhibitory circuit), produced diminished awareness resembling sleep. Patient 13 had one electrode placed deep in the caudal part of the septal region, another in the hypothalamus, and a third in the thalamus proper. On stimulation he not only became more alert, but showed marked anxiety and had numerous autonomic responses. Patient 14's electrodes were placed in the caudal part of the septal region; this patient showed marked fear as well as alerting and autonomic responses. Patient 17 had electrodes placed in the caudal part of the septal region, hypothalamus, and thalamus. Stimulation of the septal and hypothalamic electrodes produced marked autonomic responses, as well as an alerting reaction accompanied by fear. Thalamic stimulation resulted in cardiac dysrhythmia. The above data, which are taken up in detail in Chapter 13, do not conclusively demonstrate that stimulation of the septal region was responsible for the clinical improvement in these patients. It does seem certain, however, that they all had autonomic and immediate psychological responses. With one exception, these responses were in terms of increased responsivity, particularly fear and alertness. The one exception was the caudate stimulation of Patient 12, at which time the patient became sleepy. However, he did show an alerting response on stimulation of the other caudate electrode, which was near the internal capsule.

RESIDUAL SIGNS IN THE MUCH-IMPROVED PATIENTS

It would seem pertinent to review here the residual signs of impairment in those patients who have shown the most improvement. Patient 2, who was operated on 20 months ago, has been out of the hospital 16 months, and has been going to school for the past 9 months. She is one of the most dramatically improved patients in our series. Prior to operation, she had symptoms of anorexia nervosa, weighed only 58 pounds, had delusions of oral impregnation and hallucinations in which she felt that Christ was telling her that he had impregnated her. At the present time the patient weighs 116 pounds, obviously enjoys her food, is reasonably interested in her personal appearance, and particularly desirous of extending her social acquaintances, although she still shows rather marked anxiety in any new situation. She performs satisfactorily in school, having trouble only with arithmetic. She is self-conscious because she is considerably older than the other pupils in her classroom. She expresses a desire to go out with boys but has little opportunity to meet them, as she lives in a rather isolated community which lacks recreational opportunities. However, it is questionable whether she would make dates if she had the opportunity, as she says, "I'm afraid that the boys would think that I'm dumb. I don't know how to act with them, or how to talk with them." As the patient's home is far removed from any psychiatric or social service facilities, she has no chance for constructive rehabilitative guidance. She has a rather tenuous self-confidence, as best illustrated by a situation in her doctor's office, wherein the patient was intentionally given several problems that she could not be expected to solve. When she failed, the doctor mildly reprimanded her, saying, "Oh, you can do those problems." With this she became flushed, agitated, paced up and down in the doctor's office, and asked if it wasn't time for her to go. However, with minimal reassurance she immediately quieted down and resumed the interview. Her emotional responses, which had been notably shallow, have changed dramatically since operation. She appears somewhat hypomanic and euphoric, but her rather silly manner does not seem inappropriate when one considers that she is still adolescent.

Patient 12 has shown the next most outstanding improvement, 8 months having passed since he was operated on and 4 1/2 months since he was discharged from the hospital. He lives with his mother and father, brother, and sister-in-law on a farm in rural Louisiana. He works energetically at the farm chores, to which he makes a really significant contribution. For instance, he has learned how to drive a tractor, so that he is now able to plant and cultivate 20 acres of cotton. Before operation he was untidy, seclusive, and tremulous and periodically manifested outbursts of rage and destructiveness. At the present time, he becomes irritable whenever frustrated but does not show overt rage. Irritability is followed by a guilty fear, which leads to profuse apologies. Tachycardia and tremulousness have disappeared. The hallucinations which he experienced on one or two occasions prior to operation have not recurred. Nevertheless, in a social setting the patient shows a rather limited range of emotional responses, although there is no real inappropriateness. He is eager to socialize and broaden his recreational activities but as yet has been inhibited from doing so by his feelings of inadequacy, which limit his social activities to the family and close friends.

Patient 14, who was operated on 7 months ago, and was out of the hospital 1 1/2 months before his precipitous death from the rupture of a temporal lobe abscess into the ventricles, was the patient who had the marked germ phobia prior to operation—isolating himself in his room, constantly washing himself with alcohol or lysol but at the same time smearing feces and urine with abandon. Until shortly before his death he had been living with his family and working in a local defense plant. When he first started this job, he was criticized for slowness, as he obsessively checked and rechecked each part he was inspecting. However, within several days he was performing at high speed, although this was, of course, below his potentiality when one considers that he was a science major in college. He would ride busses and streetcars, use public toilets, and mingle with crowds, although for 7 years prior to that he had refused to do any of these things. Nevertheless, whenever seen by the therapist, he would go over the operative procedure again and again and demand an explanation of his illness, apparently trying to satisfy hypochondriacal anxiety. Circumscribed phobias remained in that he would not allow his mother to visit the hospital. Finally, still fearing contamination, several weeks after his discharge, he refused to see the doctors unless they came to his home or met him in some public place.

Patient 13, who still shows residual psychosis, has nevertheless markedly improved. He was operated on 8 months ago and has now been out of the hospital for 4 1/2 months. For many years prior to operation he had behaved in a typically psychotic way, being manneristic, mute, inaccessible, completely idle, and seclusive. At the present time he is living at home with his parents and siblings. He is not employed but does take an interest in the yard and crude carpentry work. He helps his mother with the housework, although he remains slow and inept at performing these tasks. He occasionally renews his interest in music and goes by himself to church and to movies, but so far he has not socialized at all with contemporaries. This is the patient who shows the memory impairment mentioned above. His mannerisms are much less obvious than before, although they still remain, now appearing as tics. Emotionally, he is quite flat, although more responsive than before.

Patient 17, a 26-year-old woman, had been negativistic, seclusive, retarded, and occasionally destructive for 2 years prior to operation. All her life she had functioned at a mentally defective level. Postoperatively she remained slow and retarded, slept excessively, and for some time required dexedrine to combat this lethargy. At the present time she is out of the hospital, visiting relatives in a nearby state. The family reports that she is as talkative as she has ever been, alert and interested in her surroundings, eager to participate in their social activities, and spontaneously offers to aid with the household chores. Before operation the patient and her mother quarreled constantly but now the two seem to be mutually dependent.

From this review of the five patients who have shown the most improvement following stimulation it is obvious that statements regarding the efficacy of the procedure have to be reserved. Even 20 months is a short follow-up, not to mention 7 and 8 months.* Patient 14 can hardly be considered a therapeutic success, as he died of a complication resulting from the procedure. It is also apparent that Patients 2 and 12, who no longer show psychotic symptoms, still have personality deficits—both showing excessive sensitiveness and a precarious self-esteem and Patient 12 also showing little improvement in emotional responsiveness. In Patients 13 and 14 psychotic symptomatology is still manifest despite the improvement in their behavior. With all these reservations, we nevertheless feel that a dramatic response to the procedure is evident when one compares the patients' present adjustment with their preoperative status.

EVALUATION OF NONSPECIFIC FACTORS

The 20 schizophrenic patients in our series were evaluated with regard to the following categories: cooperation on psychological tests, length of psychosis, length of present hospitalization, prepsychotic personality, Malamud-Sands rating, prognostic rating, emotional responsiveness, tractability, family history of disordered behavior, primary diagnosis, catatonic symptomatology, various types of complications, and postoperative EEG's (see Figures 5–17). This was done to see whether any intervening nonspecific factors might explain the therapeutic results.

It is a generally accepted psychiatric procedure to use discharge from the hospital as the most objective, although admittedly crude, measure of improvement. Likewise, length of previous hospitalization is used as the most objective criterion for the seriousness of the illness. We mentioned in Chapter 8 that the latter criterion is hard to apply in Louisiana, where mental hospital beds are limited and hence patients often remain at home even though they are seriously psychotic. It is also true that many families in this state will take patients out of the hospital despite the fact that they have shown little improvement following specific psychiatric treatment. Only in the case of Patient 4 did we feel that the family pressure led to early discharge from the hospital against medical

*See Addendum F, which extends the follow-up period 12 months.

advice. The patient's subsequent adjustment on the outside, although marginal, suggests that the family's insistence on discharge was justifiable, as the prediction of the psychiatric staff that she would require early rehospitalization has not proved true. On the other hand, Patient 16 would probably be out of the hospital now if the family were more cooperative. Despite these exceptions we shall use discharge from the hospital as the criterion for improvement in evaluating the factors mentioned in the preceding paragraph but in interpreting the data we shall keep in mind these two possible exceptions. Figure 6 indicates that no definite correlation can be made between clinical improvement and length of psychosis. Three of the five patients who were ill less than 3 years are now out of the hospital, as are two of the three who were ill between 5 and 10 years. However, none of the five patients whose psychosis had been overt longer than 10 years is now out of the hospital. Figure 7 indicates no relationship between discharge and length of hospitalization immediately preceding stimulation. Only one of the patients hospitalized for less than 3 months is now out of the hospital, but the same is true of those hospitalized for more than 18 months. As a short preoperative hospitalization is probably the best measure of the family's ability to tolerate psychotic behavior in one of their members, this figure illustrates that the family's acceptance of psychosis was not a significant factor in the ultimate discharge of our patients. In Figure 8 no definite correlation is apparent between discharge and prepsychotic personality. However, almost all our patients had severe adjustment problems prior to the overt manifestations of their psychoses. Patients 22 and 9 had allegedly normal prepsychotic personalities, but the history was not entirely reliable in either case, and it is more than likely that there was some disturbance of adaptation present long before the psychosis developed. Although the Malamud-Sands rating is a rather crude method of grading psychotic manifestations, Figure 9 indicates no correlation between scores on the rating scale and subsequent improvement. If anything, the reverse is true, as the three patients with scores of less than 40 are still hospitalized.

Although we have no really reliable indicators of prognosis for any type of therapy, we attempted a prognostic rating in the following manner: Four factors were evaluated—family history, prepsychotic personality, length of illness, and present psychotic behavior. Each one of these categories was rated from zero to 4. The ultimate rating on each patient was a summation. Thus, a maximum rating for any patient would be 16. The graduations from 1 to 4 were as follows:

I. Family history:
1. History of neurosis in the immediate family;
2. One member of the immediate family psychotic;
3. More than one member of the immediate family psychotic;
4. Identical twin psychotic.

II. Prepsychotic personality:
1. Transient or remitting neurotic symptomatology;
2. Outstanding character deviations or persistent neurotic symptomatology;
3. Previous psychotic breaks;
4. Continuously psychotic since an early age.

III. Length of illness:
1. Less than one year;
2. One to two years;
3. Two to five years;
4. Over five years.

IV. Present psychotic behavior:
1. Neurotic behavior with occasional depersonalizations;
2. Psychotic behavior with painful affect overt;
3. Affective responses inappropriate and silly;
4. Affective responses absent.

Figure 10 indicates no correlation between discharge and the prognostic rating as evaluated above.

On the basis of opinions of two or more observers, patients were next rated in a series according to the intensity and appropriateness of their emotional responses. The most appropriate as rated by us was Patient 19, and the least appropriate, Patient 9. In Figure 11, which gives the status of all the patients, there is no indication of a relationship between rated affect and subsequent discharge from the hospital.

In selecting the different variables which might weight the evidence in regard to discharge we felt that patients who were tractable before the experimental procedure might have been forced out of the hospital because of the optimistic enthusiasm of the research staff. Conceivably, these patients could then have remained out of the hospital without showing significant improvement. Figure 12 indicates no correlation between the patients who were discharged and those who were tractable prior to stimulation. From this it does not seem likely that those subsequently discharged were the patients who might have been discharged in a normal course of events if subjected merely to enthusiastic attention and optimism regarding the progress of their illness.

As seven of the ten patients who were discharged from the hospital had no family history of neurosis or psychosis, this evaluation would appear to have some prognostic significance (Figure 13). In the group of seven where one or more of the immediate family were psychotic, only two responded.

When the patients are divided according to diagnosis, it would appear that the catatonic schizophrenics responded somewhat better (Figure 14). All but two of the six catatonics (Patients 5 and 22) are out of the hospital, while only three of the seven hebephrenics and three of the seven paranoids were discharged. It also should be noted that of the two other catatonics Patient 5 left the hospital for a while but returned and Patient 22 was a technical failure. Breaking down the patient group into those who showed some catatonic symptoms and those who showed no catatonic symptoms (Figure 15), such a correlation becomes less clear. We find that four of nine who had no catatonic symptomatology responded, while the other six came from the eleven who showed some catatonic symptomatology. When the patients are classified by operative complications, some inferences are possible (Figure 16). Six of the eight patients who had convulsion or coma responded, while three of the seven who had fever responded, and two of the eight who had no complications responded. This, of course, immediately suggests that the therapeutic response might have been due to the convulsion or coma. However, all eight of these patients had had either electroshock or insulin coma therapy previously. Four had had EST, three EST and insulin, and another insulin (Chapter 8, Table 1). In view of the length of time these patients had been ill, it was highly unlikely that coma or convulsive therapy would have benefited them. In fact, five of the eight had had convulsive therapy immediately prior to stimulation (Patients 2, 3, 7,

EVALUATION OF PATIENTS BY NONSPECIFIC FACTORS (FIGURES 5–17)

FIGURE XVII–5 (right). Schizophrenics in patient group classified according to attitude toward psychological testing (cooperative or uncooperative). Discharged patients are indicated by circles

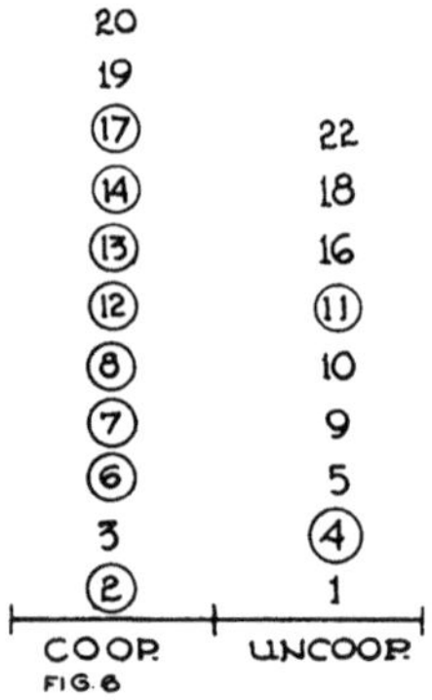

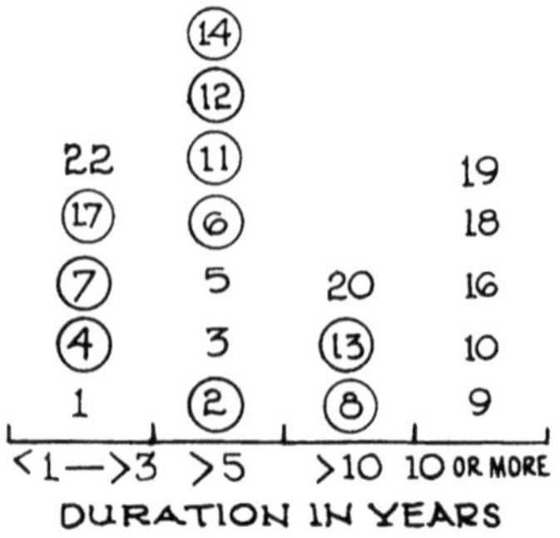

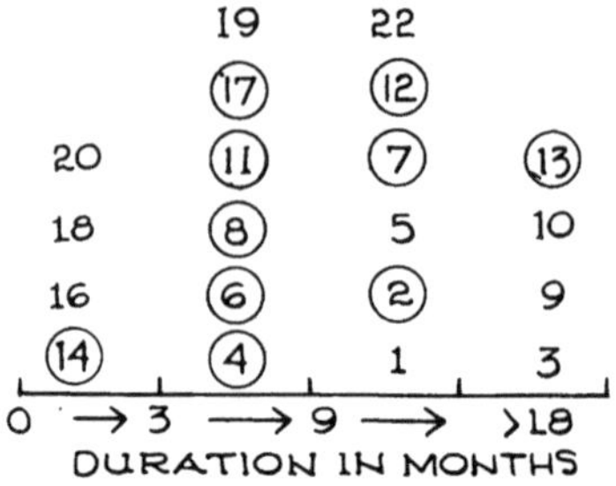

FIGURE XVII–6 (left). Schizophrenics in patient group classified according to duration of psychosis

FIGURE XVII–7 (right). Schizophrenics in patient group classified according to duration of most recent hospitalization

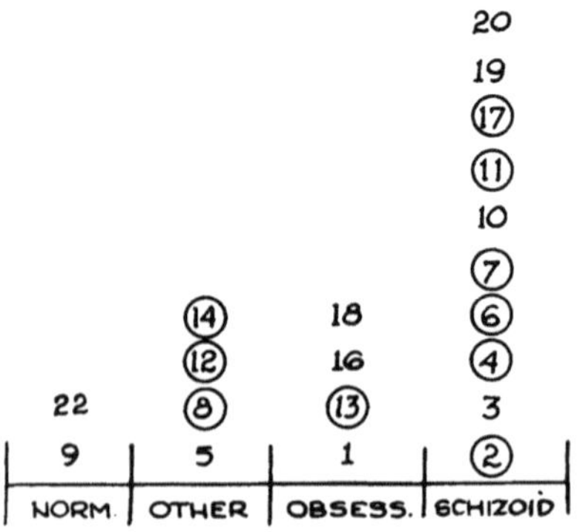

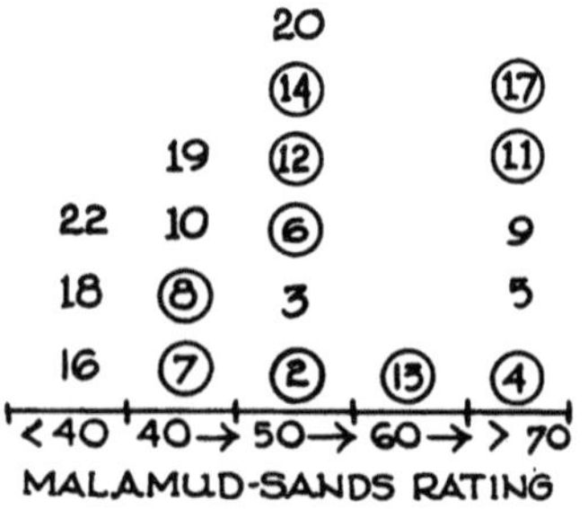

FIGURE XVII–8 (left). Schizophrenics in patient group classified according to prepsychotic personality

FIGURE XVII–9 (right). Schizophrenics in patient group rated on Malamud-Sands scale

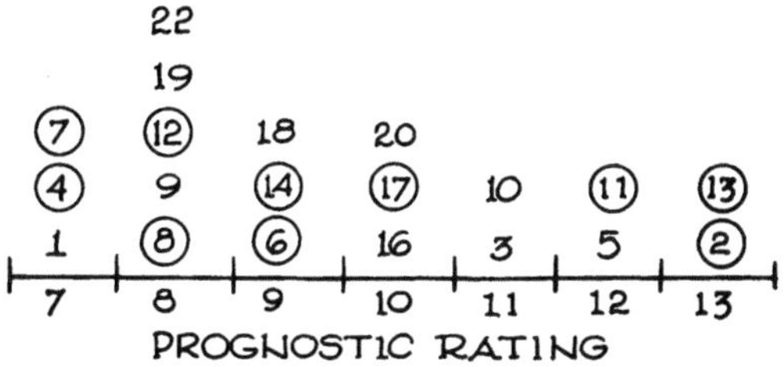

FIGURE XVII–10. Schizophrenics in patient group classified according to preoperative prognostic rating

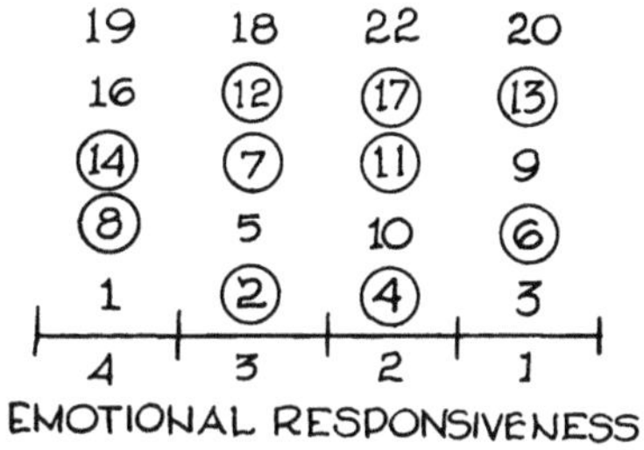

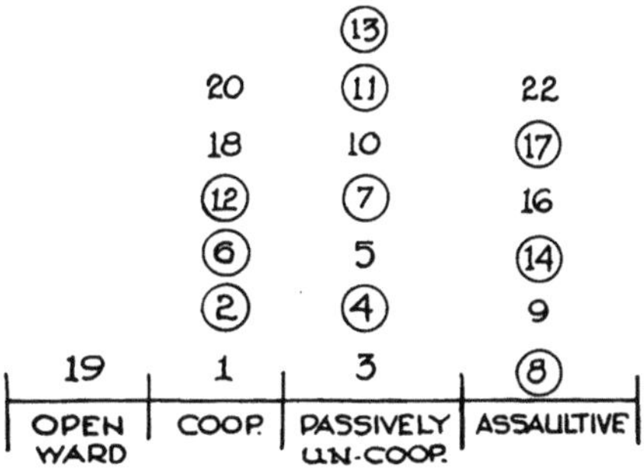

FIGURE XVII–11 (left). Schizophrenics in patient group classified according to emotional responsiveness. On the scale 4 = greatest, 1 = least

FIGURE XVII–12 (right). Schizophrenics in patient group classified according to tractability. The patients assigned to the open ward were considered the most tractable

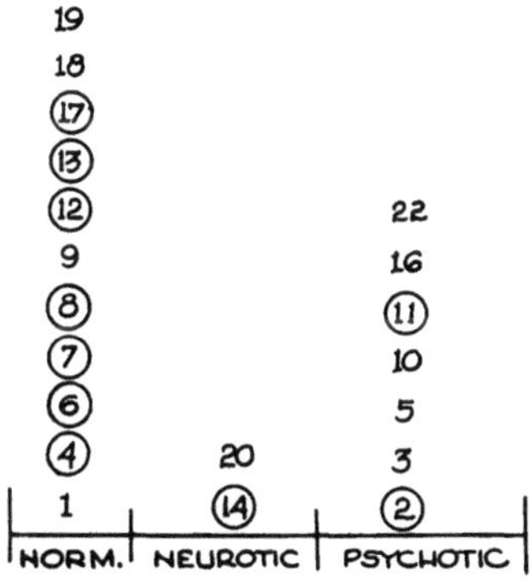

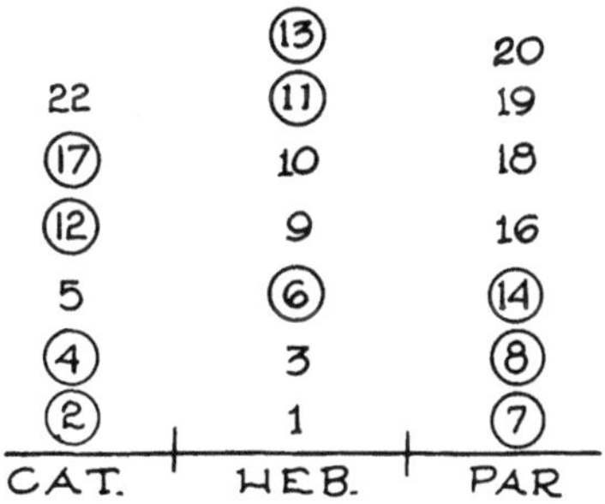

FIGURE XVII–13 (left). Schizophrenics in patient group classified according to family history

FIGURE XVII–14 (right). Schizophrenics in patient group classified according to primary diagnosis

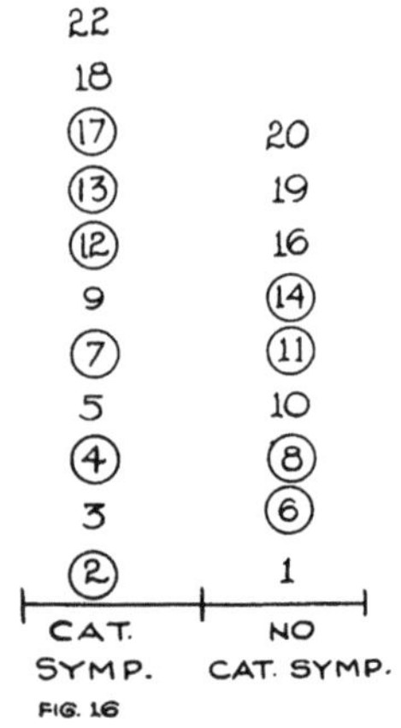

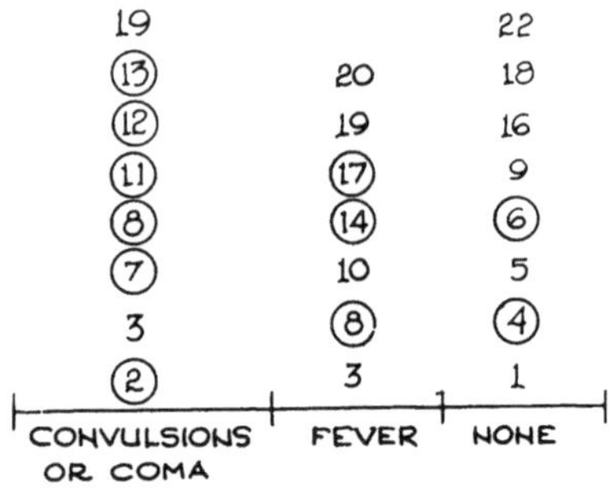

FIGURE XVII–16. Schizophrenics in patient group classified according to postoperative complications

FIGURE XVII–15 (above). Schizophrenics in patient group classified according to the presence or absence of catatonic symptoms

FIGURE XVII–17 (right). Schizophrenics in patient group classified according to postoperative EEG findings

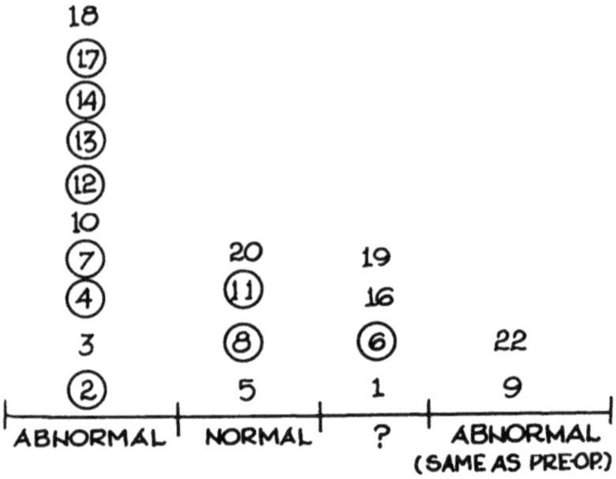

11, and 12). It must also be recognized that merely explaining the stimulation procedure in terms of focal electroshock therapy throws little light on the subject, as very little is known about the physiological mechanisms of EST or the reasons for clinical improvement following such treatment.

Perhaps there is one other suggestive correlation. If one divides the group into those who showed abnormal EEG's for a significant period postoperatively, those whose EEG's remained normal, those who for one reason or another had no postoperative EEG's, and those whose EEG's remained the same, but were abnormal, one sees that seven out of the ten who had abnormal EEG's are out of the hospital, while two out of the four who had normal EEG's are out (Figure 17). The other, Patient

6, had cortical damage, as he had a topectomy. This raises a legitimate question as to whether the therapeutic responses of some patients were due to activation of neurons by electrical stimuli or to brain damage consequent to electrode placement. Data from neurophysiology will have to be marshaled to clarify this point.

CORRELATION OF CLINICAL AND LABORATORY DATA

It is often most difficult to determine with any degree of exactness the reasons that patients with psychiatric disorders improve under treatment. In this series the patients have improved to varying degrees. There was one common denominator, namely, that all had failed to show lasting improvement with the conventional forms of therapy offered at this and other medical centers. Otherwise there were many variables, both in terms of the patients' illnesses and in the techniques of the therapeutic procedure. For this reason, as stated above, an exact statistical evaluation of the therapeutic effects of subcortical stimulation is impossible at the present stage of the investigations. However, at this point, in an attempt to correlate the clinical and the laboratory findings, we have summarized in outline form the clinical and laboratory data on the markedly improved, improved, and unimproved or only slightly improved patients, respectively (see Tables 2, 3, and 4). The factors selected for reference in the tables are the sites of electrodes which were stimulated, the intensity of the stimulation, the physiological responses, the stress response determined by eosinophilic or lymphocytic counts, and the immediate psychological response. Also included are changes in the scalp electroencephalograms following stimulation, as well as clinical neurological complications. Some of the pertinent laboratory correlations have been previously discussed.

The therapeutic hypothesis to be tested in this series of patients was whether stimulation to the facilitatory circuit would alter the patient's psychosis and lead to clinical improvement.

As we progressed through the first ten procedures we gradually made some tentative suppositions as to what might be immediate indicators of ultimate therapeutic success. We felt that the best immediate evaluation of the adequacy of stimulation might be the psychological response

TABLE XVII–2. Markedly improved patients*

Patient	*Site of electrode stimulated*	*Intensity of stimulation*	*Physiological response*	*Stress response*
2	Rostral part of septal region	Minimal (unique parameter)	Convulsion	Yes
12	(a) Caudate near internal capsule (b) Basal part of caudate near capsule and near facilitatory area	Moderate	Marked autonomic twitching spasms	Yes
13	(a) Septo-hypothalamic region (b) Hypothalamus (c) Thalamus	Maximum	Marked autonomic petit mal	Minimal
14	Septo-hypothalamic region	Moderate	Marked autonomic	Yes
17	(a) Caudal part of septal region (b) Ventral part of hypothalamus (c) Thalamus	Maximal	Marked autonomic and cardiac arrhythmia	Yes

*For details see clinical case reports in Section IV.

TABLE 2 (continued)

Psychological response	*Post-stim. EEG (scalp)*	*Neurological complications*	*Comments*
Coma	Random spike and slow wave	Prolonged coma	Best clinical result. Only patient with septal stimulation on operating table. Prolonged coma followed
(a) Transitory stupor or sleep (b) Alert; high intensity, stupor	Transitory random spikes	None	Next best clinical response. Both facilitatory and suppressor circuits stimulated as well as capsular region with capsular "fit"
Alert; fear	Right frontal slow wave	Transitory rt. Babinski & organic mental syndrome GM seizures 6 mos. after operation	Poorest result in this group. Present clinical course vacillates daily from psychosis to marked improvement
Alert; fear	Right frontal slow wave	Died 6 mos. after operation of temporal lobe abscess	Dramatic immediate improvement. Circumscribed phobia and intellectual inefficiency at death
Alert; fear	Right frontal slow wave	Meningitis; transient paresis of left leg	Satisfactory clinical result, although patient doesn't socialize

TABLE XVII–3. Improved patients*

Patient	*Site of electrode stimulated*	*Intensity of stimulation*	*Physiological response*	*Stress response*
4	High in septal region	Minimal	None	No data
5	Septal region	Minimal	None	No data
24	Septal region	Moderate	Autonomic; B P elevation	Minimal
6	Septal region (not verified by x-ray)	Minimal	Diffuse autonomic	No data
7	High in septal region	Minimal	None	No data
8	Septal region (not verified by x-ray)	Minimal	None	No data
15	Septal region (not verified by x-ray)	Moderate	GM seizure	Yes
11	(a) Septal region (area damaged during operation) (b) High in caudate or in corpus callosum	Moderate	Slight B P elevation	Yes (sodium retent.)
16	(a) Caudal part of septal region (b) Septo-hypothalamic region	Maximal	B P elevation	Yes
18	(a) Septal region (b) Septo-hypothalamic region	Maximal	Autonomic response	Yes

*For details see clinical case reports in Section IV.

TABLE 3 (continued)

Psychological response	*Post-stim. EEG (scalp)*	*Neurological complications*	*Comments*
Alert; talked	Slow wave for 2 mos. after operation		Patient out of hospital, improved but still overtly psychotic
Alert	No change		Good immediate response after 1st operation. Transitory response after 2nd operation. 9
Alert	Not done		mos. follow-up. No change
Alert	Not done	Post-topectomy	Out of hospital; unemployed but much improved and active
Alert	Bifrontal slow wave	None	Out of hospital, but idle and seclusive
Dull; confused	No change	None	Out of hospital with good clinical improvement. Both times partial relapse with depression
Explosive rage	No change	None	and referential behavior. No assaultiveness
Alert; coherent	No change	Transitory left hemiparesis; convulsion immediately after operation	Out of hospital, unemployed but active. Still hallucinating
Alert	Not done	Transitory left central facial paresis	Dramatic immediate improvement. Still definitely improved, but remains hospitalized because family is unwilling to assume responsibility for care
Alert; "faint"	Generalized slow waves	None	Slow but progressive improvement; out of hospital during the extended follow-up period

TABLE XVII–4. Unimproved or slightly improved patients*

Patient	Site of electrode stimulated	Intensity of stimulation	Physiological response	Stress response
1	Anterior thalamus	Minimal	None	No data
3	Septal region	Probably no stimulation as insulation failed	None	No data
9	Dorsal part of septal region	Minimal	Slight B P elevation	No data
10	(a) Caudal part of septal region (b) Corpus callosum	Moderate	Marked B P elevation	No data
19†				
20	(a) Septal region (b) Septo-hypothalamus	Moderate	Autonomic response—marked B P elevation	Probably slight response
22	(a) Subcortical white matter (b) Thalamus to septum (over 2 cm. between electrode)	Minimal	Minimal autonomic	None

*For details see clinical case reports in Section IV.
†Patient 19 omitted because of early death.

TABLE 4 (continued)

Psychological response	*Post-stim. EEG (scalp)*	*Neurological complications*	*Comments*
None	Not done	None	Only patient with stimulus to thalamus alone. No immediate or delayed effect
None	Rt. frontal slow wave. Rt. occipital. Sleep spindle	Meningitis with convulsions	Transitory improvement (?) after operation
Slight alert	No change (abnormal before operation)	None	Chronic, deteriorated patient with grossly abnormal scalp recording and moderate cortical atrophy
Alert coherent	Transitory random spikes	Meningitis	Immediate clinical improvement with gradual relapse 3 mos. after operation
Alert "felt pleasant"	No change	None	No change in delusional content. Socialized more freely
Excited	No change (abnormal before operation)	No change	Response to stimulation suggested spread to cortex. She probably received minimal subcortical stimulation, hence considered technical failure. Clinically became more tractable

of alerting and/or a physiological response, particularly elevation of blood pressure. At the same time we started measuring the stress response during stimulation, hoping that this might give us further indication of the therapeutic effectiveness of stimulation. Although we feel it is too early to rule out these initial suppositions, it is obvious from the above tables that no one factor or combination of factors seemed to be a reliable indicator of the patient's ultimate response to stimulation.

It is apparent from the tables that Patients 3 and 22, both technical failures, showed little or no change in the way of physiological, psychological, or stress response at the time of stimulation. The same is true of Patient 1, who was stimulated in the anterior thalamus. Therefore, it seems that stimulation in these cases was not effective either immediately or in terms of the ultimate clinical course; hence Patients 1, 3, and 22 are most useful in this series for indicating that in all probability such adventitious factors as craniotomy, frontal lobe damage, or the total push associated with the procedure were not effective in themselves as therapeutic measures.

The remaining patients showed some immediate responses to the stimulation, either physiologically or psychologically. In every case where the septal region or hypothalamus was adequately stimulated, there was also a stress response. None of these factors could be correlated with lasting clinical improvement. These patients did, however, show more than an immediate psychological response, manifesting to a greater or lesser extent some improvement during the first few months following stimulation, even though, as reported in the tables under Comment, many subsequently relapsed. This raises a logical question as to whether the type of procedure we are using is only capable of initiating improvement but not of sustaining improvement over a long period of time.

In view of the reported clinical improvements in schizophrenic patients following destructive types of brain surgery, evaluation of these patients in terms of brain damage is important but extremely difficult. All except Patient 22 had open operations, which meant there was unilateral frontal lobe damage, as direct exposure and visualization of the septal, caudate, and hypothalamic regions were necessary. This is reflected in the right frontal slow wave foci noted postoperatively in a number of patients. It is also apparent that a number of the patients had random spikes, which in some cases were transitory and in other cases have persisted. All five of the markedly improved patients showed EEG changes after stimulation, and four of the five also had some transient or persistent neurological symptoms. The sustained improvement in these cases might thus have been dependent upon the brain damage resulting from surgery. However, as will be pointed out in Chapter 18, there was no consistent pattern in the type or severity of the complications, in the time of their appearance, or in their duration. Moreover, three patients (Patients 4, 7, and 16) in the improved group and two (Patients 3 and 10) in the unimproved group also had evidence of brain damage without the sustained improvement of the first group. The present technique of electrode placement by the stereotaxic method, which reduces the brain damage to a minimum, will give us the answer to this particular question.*

It is pertinent here to mention that Patients 2 and 12 have shown the best and most sustained clinical improvement. In both of these cases there was something unique. In Patient 2 the site of stimulation was more rostral than usual, and also the parameters of current were unique (see Addendum D). In Patient 12 the site of stimulation was close to or in the capsule; on one occasion stimulation produced the usual alerting response accompanied by general twitching or spasm; on another occasion, transitory stupor or sleep. Patient 2 also had coma. One wonders whether improvement depends upon stimulation of the inhibitory as well as the facilitatory circuit.

A final factor which needs evaluation is the optimal type and intensity of current. We see from the tables no correlation between the intensity of the current and the clinical results, the improved group having had minimal to maximal intensities. At one time we felt that the early cases had received inadequate intensity of stimulation; hence we repeated the operation on Patients 5 and 8. The tables reveal that the second stimulation was of greater intensity and the physiological response, as well as the immediate psychological response, more marked. However, in both cases the clinical improvement was, if anything, less after the second operation than after the first.

We feel that our present inability to make a better correlation between

*See Addenda C and D.

the patients' clinical improvement and the various aspects of the procedure points up the need for improved techniques. This information must be considered against the background finding that patients with satisfactory electrode implantations invariably had a spiking abnormality in the septal region. At the present writing we are not certain whether septal spiking is characteristic of the schizophrenic process. If this question can be answered in the affirmative, recording over a long period of time may give us the necessary information for improving our therapeutic procedure. Since the June 1952 meetings we have established better and more exact techniques of implanting electrodes, as well as better techniques of stimulation and a more thorough method of testing the effects of stimulation in different regions of the brain. Progress in these respects is discussed in the addenda.

SUMMARY

1. Psychiatric evaluations have been made on twenty-two subcortical stimulation procedures performed on twenty patients. Eleven patients have been discharged from the hospital; two relapsed after discharge, but one improved after a second stimulation. Two patients died—one 5 weeks after operation and one 6 weeks after his discharge from the hospital. Nine patients are now followed on an outpatient basis.
2. Evaluation of the experimental group (see Chapter 8) reveals that the most optimistic prediction would have been that four patients of this group could be discharged without some intervening specific therapeutic procedure.
3. The most significant observation was the change in behavior immediately following stimulation.
4. No adventitious factors were found which played a discernible role in the therapeutic results.
5. The follow-up period, ranging from 36 to 15 months (see Addendum F), is too short for final evaluation of the therapeutic potentialities of this procedure.
6. Data from disciplines other than clinical psychiatry will be necessary to substantiate the basic theory.

CHAPTER 18

NEUROLOGICAL AND MEDICAL STATUS OF THE PATIENT GROUP

ARTHUR W. EPSTEIN
ROBERT G. HEATH
FREDERICK F. MILLSAPS, JR.

NEUROLOGICAL STATUS

Complete neurological examinations were performed on each member of the patient group preoperatively, postoperatively, and at intervals in the postoperative period. Of the twenty patients in the schizophrenic group (see Chapter 8), none showed abnormalities on the preoperative neurological examination. Ten of the patients in this group showed no clinical evidence of neurological complications either in the immediate postoperative period or thereafter, although Patient 8(15) had a generalized convulsion during stimulation.

The remaining ten patients showed some neurological complication. Two of these ten died (Patients 14 and 19). In the first, Patient 14, death occurred in the sixth postoperative month as a result of a left frontal-temporal brain abscess. This patient had had an earlier episode of acute meningitis, which subsided by the end of the second postoperative week. Patient 19, who had severe hypertensive cardiovascular disease, developed transient neurological signs in the fourth postoperative week and died in the fifth postoperative week. At autopsy, an abscess was found in the right frontal lobe, involving the septal region and extending to the base.

In all but two of the remaining eight patients the complications were limited to the immediate postoperative period. Of the six patients with such complications, three had meningeal reactions associated with wound infections (Patients 3, 10, and 17) and three had generalized seizures at some time in the immediate postoperative period (Patients 2, 3, and 11). In the case of Patient 3 the convulsions were associated with meningitis; Patient 11 had a transient left hemiparesis. Other transient signs included a monoparesis of the left lower extremity in Patient 17, who had a concurrent meningitis, and a left central facial weakness in Patient 16.

The complications in the two (Patients 7 and 13) whose neurological disorders appeared after the immediate postoperative period were grand mal seizures. Patient 13 had seizures six and eight months postoperatively, and Patient 7 had seizures eleven months postoperatively. Neurological examinations performed several days after the seizures revealed no abnormality in either. The electroencephalogram of Patient 13 showed a right frontal delta focus; that of Patient 7, scattered bifrontal slow activity and amplitude asymmetry in the occipital leads. Patient 13 demonstrated slight organic mental changes and a right Babinski sign in the immediate postoperative period. Both these patients have been discharged from the hospital, improved psychiatrically.

No definite conclusion can be reached concerning the relationship between psychiatric improvement and the occurrence of convulsions or other neurological complications. In the markedly improved group, consisting of Patients 2, 12, 13, 14, and 17, Patient 12 was the only one with no neurological complications. However, in the four cases in which complications did occur there was no consistent pattern in the type or severity of the complication, in the time of its appearance, or in its duration. Moreover, not all patients with convulsions or other complications showed significant psychiatric improvement, while others with no complications showed some improvement.

All three of the nonschizophrenic patients (Patients 21, 23, and 25) showed some abnormalities on the preoperative neurological examination—the first two, in the peripheral nervous system, and the third, Patient 25, in the brain. Patient 23 went into status epilepticus during stimulation. The others showed no neurological complications. All died. The autopsy of Patient 25, who had metastatic carcinoma of the breast, revealed a single, well-demarcated, metastatic nodule occupying almost the entire hypothalamus.

MEDICAL STATUS

Of the twenty patients in the schizophrenic group, only three (Patients 10, 18, and 19) showed some clinical evidence of medical disease before operation.

Patient 10 was reported to have had a labile hypertension for 15 years as well as diabetes mellitus, which was first discovered 4 months before admission and required from 20 to 40 units of protamine zinc insulin for regulation. However, preoperative studies did not confirm either of these diagnoses, although the glucose tolerance test indicated diabetes. Stimulation produced no definite change in the blood pressure or in the diabetic status. There was some alteration of the glucose tolerance curve in the direction of increased tolerance.

Patient 18 showed an abnormality on his chest roentgenograms, the first of which was performed slightly more than 27 months before operation. At that time, several tiny nodular densities associated with minimal fibrosis were noted in the right first and second interspaces. From their appearance and distribution, it was assumed that they represented an arrested tuberculous lesion. The next film was taken 22 days before operation. This again demonstrated the previously noted lesion and, in addition, a small area of soft density in the right second interspace, which had the appearance of a reactivation of the original lesion. The Mantoux test was positive, but because the new pulmonary lesion was discovered only a short time before operation, there was not adequate time to examine the sputum or gastric washings thoroughly for tubercle bacilli. Chest films taken 14 and 28 days after stimulation revealed essentially the same findings. The patient was followed with serial roentgenograms, and, on the film taken 56 days after stimulation, the chest area showed only the original fibro-nodular cluster. This has remained constant through the last examination, which was done late in the seventh postoperative month. It is felt that if the roentgenographic findings represented an active tuberculous process, the regression was unusually fast.

Patient 19 had marked hypertension, discovered about 10 months before admission, with hypertensive retinopathy (including some elevation of the disks), myocardial disease, and albuminuria. After operation, there were some episodes of cardiac decompensation and evidence of electrolyte depletion. There were no definite changes in the blood pressure. This patient died in the fifth postoperative week. Autopsy revealed an abscess to the right of the midline in the septal region, cardiac enlargement, atelectasis, and mild chronic bilateral pyelonephritis, indicating that the hypertension was secondary to renal disease.

Of the remaining seventeen patients in the schizophrenic group, only Patient 8(15) showed some medical complication during the postoperative course. This patient had an episode of epididymitis that began on the eleventh postoperative day and subsided in several weeks.

Of the three patients in the nonschizophrenic group, Patients 23 and 25 had metastatic carcinoma; Patient 21, far-advanced pulmonary tuberculosis. Patient 23, who had a primary carcinoma of the cervix, died on the third postoperative day after expelling a large amount of blood orally. Physical examination at that time suggested a pulmonary embolus. An autopsy was not obtained. Patient 25, who had carcinoma of the breast, died on the eighteenth postoperative day shortly after developing intestinal obstruction. Autopsy showed extensive metastases to the long bones and skull, as well as cerebral metastasis. Operation had produced no changes in these metastases. Patient 21 died in the fifth postoperative week after becoming increasingly cachetic. An autopsy was not performed. Stimulation apparently produced no definite changes in the tuberculosis. However, since the patient removed his electrodes on the second postoperative day, it is difficult to judge the effect of the procedure on the disease.

Section IV

CASE REPORTS

CHAPTER 19

INDIVIDUAL SUMMARIES OF CLINICAL AND LABORATORY DATA

ROBERT G. HEATH
RUSSELL R. MONROE
AND OTHERS

Patient 1

AGE AT OPERATION: 38
SEX: Female
MARITAL STATUS: Married
OCCUPATION: Housewife
RELIGION: Catholic (active)
INFORMANTS: Sister and husband
DIAGNOSIS: Schizophrenic reaction, hebephrenic type
OPERATION: April 18, 1950

Presenting Picture. On admission to the hospital in April, 1950, the patient had auditory hallucinations and paranoid delusions involving her family. She denied being ill, manifested an inappropriate affect for her ideation, giggling in a typically silly, hebephrenic way. Her appearance was described as resembling a "painted doll," as she was meticulously groomed but heavily made up.

Present Illness. The present illness began in August, 1948, when the patient became obsessed with the idea that a friend and the friend's children were going to be burned. She also developed a delusion that speakers and radios controlled by her mother-in-law were influencing her unfavorably. She was hospitalized and given electroshock therapy. This resulted in a partial remission and she was discharged from the hospital in February, 1949. Her first admission to Charity Hospital occurred in August, 1949. During that time she showed slight improvement after 25 insulin-coma treatments, being discharged in November, 1949 only to be readmitted in April, 1950, with the same symptoms.

Previous Personality Disorders. The patient became depressed following the death of her mother in 1933, and again upon the death of her brother in 1939 and her sister in 1946. However, she must have shown schizophrenic manifestations, as she received both electroshock and insulin therapy during her last hospitalization in 1946.

Family History. The patient was the youngest of four siblings born at 1-year intervals to a lower middle-class family. Her mother and father, as well as her brother and sister, died of hypertension. At the death of each, the patient became quite upset. The mother was described as a person whose behavior varied between strictness and angelical sweetness. The patient's sister commented, "Anna always reacted inwardly." It was claimed that the patient idolized her parents as well as her sisters.

Personal History. The patient was born in New Orleans in February, 1912. Little is known concerning her birth and early development. At the age of 5 she suffered a vaginal laceration which was to play a significant part in her subsequent psychotic delusions. Apparently it left her with a concept of mutilated genitals and inability to perform the usual feminine role, particularly that of child-bearing. She completed the first year of high school in the local parochial system; during this period she suffered much guilt over her masturbatory activity, which was enhanced by the strict discipline of the nuns. At home she had had ample opportunity to witness parental intercourse. This played a significant part in the patient's concept of sex as an act of violence. After being courted for 5 years, she married at the age of 21. She was quite concerned about pregnancies, feeling that she had to prove to her mother-in-law that she was a woman. Her first two conceptions resulted in miscarriages, which decreased her already precariously low self-esteem and augmented her sexual fears. She had her first child at the age of 26 and her second at 27.

Personality. Withdrawn, unambitious, irritable, and suspicious.

Physical and Laboratory Status. Physical findings were essentially negative. Blood pressure varied between 120/50 and 100/50. One EKG was suggestive of mild cardiac disease but the second was negative. X-rays of her skull and chest were normal. CBC, serology, and urinalysis were normal. Glucose tolerance and Thorn tests were within normal limits. EEG was read as "probably normal."

Hospital Course. The patient was in the hospital only 15 days prior to operation. During that period there was no significant change in her behavior.

Operation—Stimulation. April 18, 1950.

(a) Surgical technique—Open technique was used, with removal of electrode prior to closure of surgical wound.

(b) Electrode placement—A concentric bipolar electrode was placed in the anterior thalamus.

(c) Recordings—No physiological data were obtained.

(d) Stimulation technique—Stimulation at 8 volts was administered while the patient was on the operating table.

(e) Immediate physiological effects—No physiological response was observed.

(f) Immediate behavioral response—No psychological response to the stimulation was observed.

(g) Immediate chemical changes—No chemical data were obtained.

(h) Complications—None.

Follow-up Notes. One month after surgery the patient's physical condition was good. Her hebephrenic mannerisms and dereistic thinking had not disappeared, but her attitude toward them seemed to be one of indifference. She was given permission to return home on trial visits, but on such occasions she quickly reverted to her psychotic behavior. Four months after surgery, she was committed to the state hospital. No psychological data were obtained.

On June 1, 1953, 37 months after operation, the patient's condition was essentially unchanged.

PATIENT 2

AGE AT OPERATION: 17

SEX: Female

MARITAL STATUS: Unmarried

OCCUPATION: None

RELIGION: Catholic (active)

INFORMANT: Mother

DIAGNOSIS: Schizophrenic reaction, catatonic type

OPERATION: October 18, 1950

Presenting Picture. On admission to the hospital in October, 1949, the patient was quiet, withdrawn, and uninterested in her surroundings. She complained of persistent anorexia and was emaciated in appearance.

She behaved in a silly manner, expressed fears of oral impregnation, and was subject to vague auditory hallucinations of an accusatory nature. However, she was in contact with her surroundings, oriented in all spheres, and probably of normal intelligence. Mentally she was functioning far below her capacity.

Present Illness. Overt psychotic manifestations began 2 1/2 years prior to admission, during which period the patient sometimes refused to eat for periods as long as a week. She discontinued school and showed no interest in social activities, but occasionally she would read comic books and more rarely aid her mother in the housework. She was seen on an outpatient basis for 6 months, during which time she continued to complain of nausea and periodic vomiting and expressed a lot of hostility toward her mother for forcing her to eat. Clinic visits started in April, 1949; hospitalization became necessary by October of the same year as a result of malnutrition.

Previous Personality Disorders. The patient had always been considered "different," but she showed no overt psychotic manifestations prior to her present illness.

Family History. The patient's mother, aged 59, is a rigid, domineering woman who rules the home with an iron hand. The father is a farmer, aged 59, eking out a marginal existence. He is a mild man dominated by his wife and never showing any active interest in his children. The patient is the youngest of five children, all of whom have shown some psychiatric disability. The eldest is said to have been hospitalized for "sexual impotence," the actual cause being unknown. The second sibling, aged 25, is nervous, but, as a dentist, has nevertheless made the best adjustment of all the children. The third child has been hospitalized at a state mental institution and as an ambulatory patient is now receiving shock therapy. The fourth lives at home, being described as very nervous and dependent. The patient's father had two cousins who died in state hospitals.

Personal History. The patient's birth was normal, but her early development was definitely retarded. She was bottle-fed until 8 months; although toilet-trained before 1 year, she did not talk until 4. Quiet, withdrawn, and submissive, she was "the least attractive" child in the family. She sucked her thumb until the age of 10, performed poorly at school, and discontinued her education in the ninth grade at the age of 16. Menarche occurred at the age of 14 unaccompanied by any hygienic or sexual education. She has only the vaguest concepts of sexual intercourse and pregnancy.

Personality. The patient has always been quiet, withdrawn, seclusive, preoccupied with her religion, slow to develop, and considered eccentric in her behavior. Prior to operation she was described as "emotionally flat."

Physical and Laboratory Status. Physical examination revealed a small, emaciated female weighing 58 pounds. She had an acne-form rash over her face, back, and chest. Otherwise, physical and neurological findings were within normal range. CBC, serology, urinalysis, glucose tolerance test, BUN, EEG, chest and skull films were all normal. EKG was suggestive of myocardial disease with a low T2 and an inverted T3. Blood pressure varied from 110/70 to 80/60.

Hospital Course. The patient was started on electroshock therapy in February, 1950, receiving a total of 15 treatments. There was no significant change in her behavior, and so she was started on electronarcosis therapy in April, 1950, receiving a total of 15 treatments. Again there was no significant change. She continued to express ideas of oral impregnation and occasionally referred to auditory hallucinations of an accusatory nature. She constantly expressed feelings of unworthiness. There was marked retardation of psycho-motor activity.

Operation—Stimulation. October 18, 1950.

(a) Surgical technique—Open technique and local anesthesia were used. This was the only operation performed without general anesthesia.

(b) Electrode placement—A concentric bipolar electrode was placed in the septal region 11 mm. rostral to the foramen of Monro.

(c) Recordings—No physiological records were made during the procedure. Preoperative EEG showed random spikes presumably due to EST. Sharp spike focus noted postoperatively in scalp lead persisted through 12 months' follow-up. Slow wave activity likewise continued during the same period.

(d) Stimulation technique—Five septal stimulations of 30 seconds each up to 4 ma., at 6 volts, were given while the patient was on the operating table. Procedure terminated because of convulsion following stimulation.

(e) Immediate physiological effects—Multiple generalized seizures.

(f) Immediate behavioral response—No psychological changes were observed.

(g) Immediate chemical changes—Thorn test findings indicate very satisfactory pituitary-adrenocortical response.

(h) Complications—Convulsion followed stimulation, requiring termination of the procedure.

Follow-up Notes. During the next 24 hours the patient had several more convulsions; she was comatose for 2 days after operation. Except for transient bilateral Babinskis, there were no positive physical findings on neurological examination. Twelve days after operation the patient showed more spontaneous motor activity than she had exhibited in some time. She was eating well and gaining weight. Two weeks after operation she was considerably more spontaneous in her productions, showing an appropriate and labile affect. She was talkative and associated with other patients but frequently expressed ideas of unworthiness, saying: "I don't think I should get well, I don't deserve it." Ambivalent feelings were noted in complaints such as: "Sometimes I don't know how I should feel, happy or sad." Gradually during the next month she extended her activities and expressed fewer and fewer self-depreciatory ideas. She gave no evidence of auditory hallucination. Two months after operation she was enthusiastically going out of the hospital to eat lunch or to attend movies. Two and a half months after operation she went home for her first visit. The family was amazed, enthusiastic about her changed behavior, reporting that she was friendly, outgoing, spontaneous, and cheerful—in fact more so than she had ever been in her life. The patient was discharged from the hospital approximately 4 months after operation. EEG's taken 2 and 4 weeks after operation had revealed generalized delta activity, with occasional spikes in both occipital leads. Neurological examination upon discharge was negative, except for some slight left-right confusion. She continued to show a few spikes in occipital leads as well as generalized slow waves. During the subsequent period at home, the patient began many activities she had not even contemplated before, such as participating in social gatherings, visiting relatives, and learning to drive a car. Her appetite continued to be good; she steadily gained weight until she weighed 116 pounds 6 months after operation. It was noted on clinic visits that she was overtalkative, overactive, and excessively demonstrative. A year and a half after operation, the patient maintained her improvement. She returned to school, where she performed well scholastically. She expressed some feelings of inferiority because she was with younger children, but nevertheless had a number of girl friends, although socialization outside the school was limited because of her family's isolation and lack of transportation. She wanted to go out with boys but hesitated to do so. "They'll think I am dumb. I don't know how to act and don't know how to talk," she explained. Her precarious self-esteem came out when the therapist placed her in a situation of stress, where she was given problems she could not perform, and then mildly reprimanded her for failure. She became agitated, paced up and down the room, asked if she couldn't leave. Upon reassurance she sat down again and presently cooperated with the interviewer. Psychological data revealed marked postoperative improvement, although the record still showed a schizophrenic pattern.

On June 1, 1953, 31 months after her operation, she is still making an excellent social adjustment. She continues to go to school, now has an occasional date, and recently tolerated the sudden death of an older and much-admired sister with no more than the usual grief reaction.

PATIENT 3

AGE AT OPERATION: 20
SEX: Female
MARITAL STATUS: Single
OCCUPATION: Bookkeeper
RELIGION: Catholic (inactive)
INFORMANTS: Mother and sister
DIAGNOSIS: Schizophrenic reaction, hebephrenic type
OPERATION: January 18, 1951

Presenting Picture. On admission to the hospital in December, 1949, the patient was untidy, mute, and uncooperative. Her only verbal responses were statements such as: "Get out of here. Keep moving." While expressing this hostility, she often smiled in a bland, inappropriate manner. At times she became violent and destructive. Under amytal it was revealed that she was preoccupied with sexual delusions, involving Lucifer and a fictitious character named Murphy, who was subjecting her to sexual temptation.

Present Illness. In September, 1947, the patient experienced difficulty in keeping up with her work, finding that she made many mistakes which necessitated working late hours to complete the required tasks. At the same time her friends noticed she was gradually becoming withdrawn and would sit for long periods staring out into space while smiling inappropriately. When they addressed her, she would not respond. Nevertheless, she kept working in a menial capacity until early in 1948, at which time she was discharged for inefficiency. Following this, she would sit for many hours staring off into space, occasionally cried for hours, but refused to confide in anyone concerning her thoughts. She received 12 electroshock treatments on an outpatient basis. From July, 1948, to February, 1949, she received psychotherapy without avail, continuing to remain seclusive and withdrawn into her world of fantasy, which largely revolved around sexual and religious preoccupations.

Previous Personality Disorders. No previous psychotic episodes were reported.

Family History. The patient is the eldest of three children, having a sister 1 year younger and a brother 2 years younger. Her father is a middle-class businessman described as quiet, reserved and having little interest outside his home. He is dominated by his wife, who is described as an extroverted, independent person responsible for the upbringing and discipline of the children. The patient's sister is the leader of the siblings and closest to the patient. Her brother is at present a theological student. Both siblings are considered to have normal personalities and appear to be making an adequate social adjustment.

Personal History. The patient was born after 7 1/2 months' gestation, during which time her mother had developed nephritis. She was kept in an incubator for 6 months following birth. During infancy and early childhood she was cared for by a nurse whose chief concern was food intake and bowel regularity. The patient developed slowly, always behind her sister; she had to be coaxed to eat and received frequent purgatives for "constipation." She was considered a sickly child, dependent upon her siblings and submissive in her play relationships with other children. She was a poor student, having to work long hours to complete her work. She participated in few social activities and had no outside interests. Following graduation from high school, she and her sister got jobs together in a local bank. The patient performed satisfactorily as long as she had simple tasks in the same department with her sister. However, shortly after being transferred to a different department and being assigned to tasks requiring more skill and responsibility, her present symptoms developed.

Personality. The patient was a passive, submissive, withdrawn child, very dependent upon her family, particularly her younger sister, and uninterested in outside activities. She was very conscientious, working hard to attain a modest degree of adjustment in her social milieu. She has never shown any heterosexual interest.

Physical and Laboratory Status. Physical examination revealed an obese girl with a fat distribution involving principally the face and trunk. She had small feet and small hands with tapering fingers. There was a slight tendency toward hirsutism and questionable striae on the abdomen. However, the skin was of normal thickness and consistency. Blood pressure ranged from 110/80 to 180/110. The glucose tolerance test showed a tendency toward slight delay in return to normal levels. Both the oral and the Exton-Rose glucose test showed 160 mg/100 ml. at the end of 2 hours. The glucose tolerance showed 209 mg/100 ml. at 1 hour. All fasting blood sugar determinations, however, were within normal range. No sugar was found in the urine. BMR's were minus 1 and minus 6. X-rays of the skull revealed a calcification in the sella diaphragm but were otherwise negative. CBC, urinalysis, BUN, chlorides, and serology were all within normal range. Urinary 17-ketosteroids were 18 mg/24 hours. EEG and EKG were normal. Although the diagnosis of Cushing's syndrome was entertained, a definite diagnosis could not be made on the basis of laboratory studies.

Hospital Course. Following hospitalization in February, 1949, the patient received electroshock and insulin therapy without benefit. She was generally seclusive, withdrawn, unclean and untidy. She would lie in bed most of the time, moving her legs in a rhythmic fashion; she was mute and inaccessible except for occasional expressions of hostility which were often accompanied by inappropriate silliness. At times she was violent and uncooperative. Under amytal her productions were disconnected and illogical. The only consistent delusions that could be elicited were the ideas that she was taking a bath and being sexually stimulated by Lucifer and an imaginary man named Murphy. At one time she developed the idea that she was pregnant. She was discharged in February, 1949, but readmitted again in August, having made no significant improvement on her trial visit at home. During her last hospitalization she received a total of 8 EST's at irregular intervals.

Operation—Stimulation. January 18, 1951.

(a) Surgical technique—Open technique was used.

(b) Electrode placement—A bipolar electrode, with poles 2 mm. apart, was placed in the midline septal region. Small gauge copper wires insulated with enamel were used.

(c) Recordings—The few records obtained were considered questionable because of the technical failure noted below. They did show runs of paroxysmal, high voltage spiking. This may be of importance in the light of data gathered from later patients. The preoperative EEG was normal. Postoperatively a slow wave focus was revealed in the right frontal and a sleep spindle focus in the right occipital region. The records were followed for 4 months after operation.

(d) Stimulation technique—No effects were noted from stimulation. It was considered a technical failure because of a breakdown in insulation.

(e) Immediate physiological effects—No physiological response was observed.

(f) Immediate behavioral response—No psychological response to the stimulation was observed.

(g) Immediate chemical changes—No chemical data were obtained.

(h) Complications—Ventriculitis developed as a result of implantation. This was successfully treated with antibiotics.

Follow-up Notes. Following the operation, the patient showed some perseveration and seemed a little less negativistic. The next day her temperature reached 104°F. and physical examination revealed meningeal signs; there seemed to be a weakness in the sixth cranial nerve on the right. She appeared confused and frequently got out of bed and wandered around despite her general malaise and high fever. When

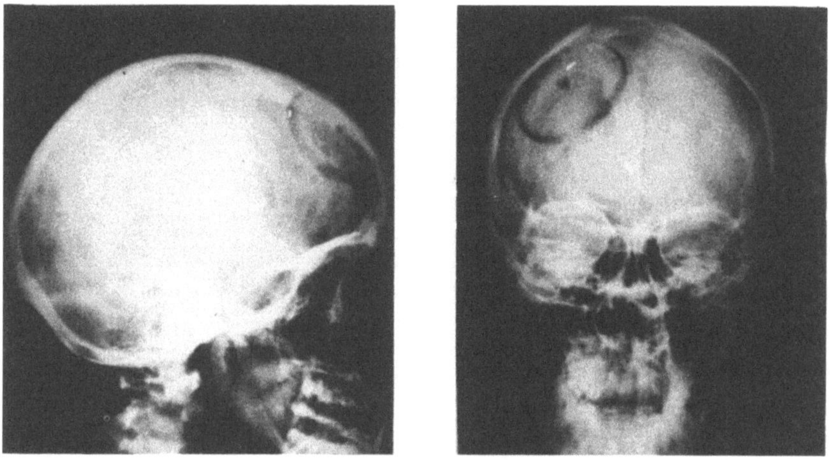

FIGURE XIX–1. Patient 3

purulent fluid was obtained from the subgaleal space, a diagnosis of ventriculitis was made; antibiotics were given, and within a week temperature was normal. During her acute febrile illness the patient's affective responses became more varied and appropriate; anxiety, tremor, and periodic crying were also noted. For a few weeks after operation she was able to hold a rational conversation with her doctor, if he initiated and maintained it. She expressed a desire to bake a pie and described in detail what she considered the proper method. She visited her family on frequent passes, expressed a desire to do so in the future, and appropriately responded with pleasurable emotion when describing these excursions. Two months after operation, the patient became periodically violent toward the ward personnel and reverted slowly to her preoperative status—lying in bed, hostile, negativistic, and mute. When she was productive, her speech was generally irrelevant and disconnected. Her appetite became voracious, and she gained 19 pounds in a period of several weeks. During the first month after operation, she had had two convulsive seizures, which were subsequently controlled by phenobarbital. As already noted, EEG revealed a right frontal S3 focus and a right occipital sleep spindle. In May, 1951, an attempt was made to repeat the surgical procedure and stimulation, but, upon opening the flap, it was discovered that the patient had a chronic osteomyelitis, and so the operation was postponed. No psychological data could be obtained.

As of June 1, 1953, 30 months after operation, the patient is quiet and seclusive, but more cooperative and active than before. Her appetite is controlled. Otherwise, there has been little change in her behavior. She is still hospitalized.

Patient 4

AGE AT OPERATION: 26
SEX: Female
MARITAL STATUS: Single
OCCUPATION: None
RELIGION: Baptist (active)
INFORMANT: Mother
DIAGNOSIS: Schizophrenic reaction, catatonic type
OPERATION: February 8, 1951

Presenting Picture. On admission to the hospital in June, 1950, the patient was mute and immobile, showing waxy flexibility as well as posturing. She made no spontaneous movements, although she would carry out simple motor acts, such as brushing her hair or teeth, if these were initiated by somebody else. Occasionally she would smile inappropriately or giggle. She withdrew slowly from painful stimuli.

Present Illness. In June, 1949, the patient fainted several times during her menstrual period. At the same time it was noted that she was tense, irritable, confused, and preoccupied. She was depressed and tearful, expressing guilty fears constantly and begging forgiveness for early childhood sexual transgressions. She was admitted to a private sanitarium in August, 1949, where she received electroshock therapy; in October, 1949, she returned home slightly improved. Shortly thereafter she developed a cancerophobia and again became preoccupied with imagined sexual transgressions. Hospitalization was precipitated when she made a feeble suicidal gesture with a rifle.

Previous Personality Disorders. There is no history of previous psychotic episodes.

Family History. The patient is the only child of a lower middle-class family that has always lived in small towns or rural communities. She expressed resentment toward her father, who as a traveling salesman is frequently away from home. Apparently there is a close relationship between father and daughter, although it was the mother who played the predominant role in her upbringing. The mother appears to be of low average intelligence but sincere in her affection for her only child.

Personal History. The patient's birth and early development were normal. The mother was strict in discipline, initiating toilet training at 2 months. The daughter has always been quiet, well behaved, and somewhat seclusive. She performed adequately at school, although she was particularly slow. She has always had numerous somatic complaints and frequent fainting spells; after graduation from high school she discontinued employment several times because of "delicate health." There were no overt manifestations of childhood sexuality, and during adolescence she showed little inclination to socialize with boys. Several years before the onset of her illness she was accosted sexually by a contemporary but managed to break away, avoiding physical harm.

Personality. The patient has always been quiet, obedient, retiring, a "good child."

Physical and Laboratory Status. Aside from the catatonic symptomatology, physical and neurological examinations were within normal limits. Blood pressure was 110/78. CBC, blood chemistry (including BUN and blood glucose), serology, urinalysis, chest and skull x-rays, EKG, and EEG were all within normal limits.

Hospital Course. On the wards there were no significant changes in the patient's behavior except under sodium amytal, when she would communicate in a limited way. She explained her inability to talk as a paralysis, complained about lack of attention from hospital personnel, and discussed some of her disappointment in not becoming a nurse or falling in love and marrying. She talked about how unpredictable and dangerous men were. In August, 1950, she was started on electronarcosis, receiving 15 treatments over the next 5 weeks. At first she showed a slight improvement, in that she took more interest in her personal hygiene and became somewhat more communicative. She remained emotionally flat, however, and at times inappropriately silly, at the same time continuing to hallucinate and to express ideas of persecution. Shortly after cessation of treatment she became mute and catatonic. Electroshock therapy was then administered, starting in October, 1950. Again she received 15 treatments during the following 5 weeks and responded as before, improving at first and then relapsing when treatment stopped. Her condition remained unchanged until the time of operation.

Operation—Stimulation. February 8, 1951.

(a) Surgical technique—Open technique was used.

(b) Electrode placement—A bipolar electrode was placed high in the septal region, about 6 mm. rostral to the foramen of Monro.

(c) Recordings—Physiological records made after operation but before stimulation were inadequate. Preoperative EEG's were normal. During the 2-month period after operation a slow wave (S3) focus was recorded over the right frontal region.

(d) Stimulation technique—There were six septal stimulations lasting 1 to 2 minutes at estimated peak currents of 2 to 5 ma. and 4 to 16 peak volts.

(e) Immediate physiological effects—No physiological response was noted.

(f) Immediate behavioral response—The patient appeared more alert and began to speak, answering questions for the first time, although she still did not elaborate on her statements.

(g) Immediate chemical changes—No chemical data were obtained.

(h) Complications—None.

Follow-up Notes. Immediately following operation the patient talked for the first time in several weeks, answering simple questions with a "yes" or "no" in a barely audible whisper and even talking spontaneously about her hostility toward her therapist. She seemed more alert and aware of her surroundings but showed no initiative or interest in participating in ward activities or occupational therapy. If urged she would passively accept invitations to go to the solarium for soft drinks with the doctors but during this time remained quiet, withdrawn, and unresponsive. She told her mother that she was afraid the doctors would seduce her on these walks. She expressed considerable resentment over continued hospitalization and begged her mother to take her home. Two and a half months after operation, in April, 1951, she was discharged to the care of her family. For the first 3 months at home she made a marginal adjustment, helping with the housework, responding to questioning and seeming to take an interest in things, although she remained shy, seclusive, and

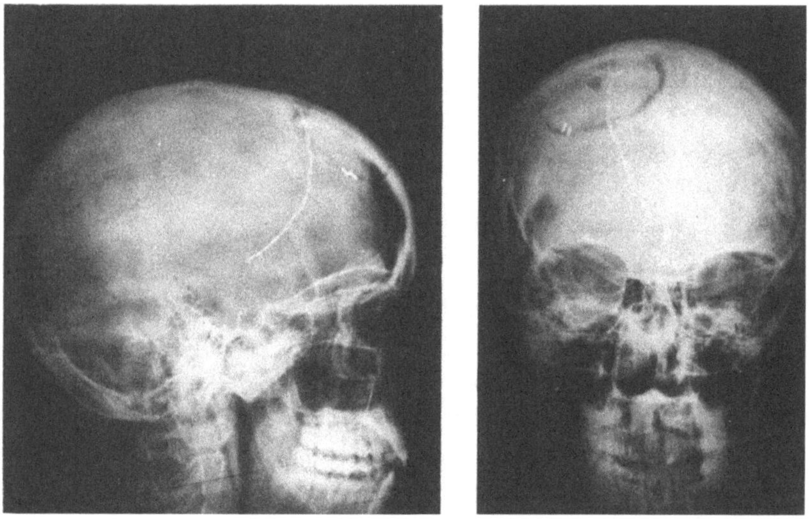

FIGURE XIX-2. Patient 4

lacking in spontaneity. Six months after operation she suddenly showed bizarre mannerisms and unusual postures. This was followed by 3 days of vomiting. At this time she was confined to bed, and subsequently she had to be fed, dressed, and bathed until 10 months after the operation, when she was again able to take care of her personal needs. During the latter part of 1951 she ate well and, in fact, gained 20 pounds. In December, 1951, she was still seclusive and idle, took little interest in her surroundings, and, except for periodic bursts of inappropriate laughter, remained almost totally mute. She seemed to be responding to hallucinations. Although oriented in all spheres, she was uncooperative for further testings of intellect and sensorium. A letter from her mother in April, 1952, 14 months after operation, revealed that the patient had again improved somewhat, as she now helped with the housework, seldom laughed to herself, seemed to take an interest in her personal appearance, and occasionally went by herself to visit her grandmother. She had continued to gain weight, was alert to conversations going on about her, and occasionally showed some spontaneity.

Slow improvement continues to be observed on June 1, 1953, 29 months after operation.

Patient 5 (24)

AGE AT FIRST OPERATION: 23
SEX: Female
MARITAL STATUS: Separated
OCCUPATION: None
RELIGION: Protestant (inactive)
INFORMANT: Mother
DIAGNOSIS: Schizophrenic reaction, catatonic type
OPERATIONS: February 23, 1951, and April 10, 1952

Presenting Picture. On admission to the hospital in May, 1950, the patient vacillated between withdrawn, seclusive, negativistic and friendly, outgoing, seductive behavior. She often laughed in a silly manner. She would be inaccessible for several days, then become animated and overproductive, revealing in minutest detail her sexual conflicts. She talked frequently of her guilt concerning masturbation, expressing the idea that she was an unwanted child inferior to her brother.

Present Illness. The patient's psychotic behavior began 4 years before her present admission, although she had shown behavioral disorders prior to that time. Psychosis was manifested by outbursts of temper and irritability toward her parents and by gradual seclusiveness and withdrawal. Periodically she became agitated and confused, wandering about the town at odd hours without her family's knowledge. She would sit by herself chain-smoking and often stayed up all night or went to bed with her clothes on. She was involved in frequent affairs with men. Recently she had been taken to a private physician who gave her electroshock therapy on an outpatient basis without definite improvement. Fourteen months prior to admission the patient was married but was totally unable to take care of her home, making life so difficult for her husband that he rejoined the Navy 3 months later. Shortly after this she attempted suicide and was admitted to the state hospital. There she was described as excited, sexually solicitous, and periodically assaultive, requiring restraint. After 21 electroshock treatments she showed some improvement but was discharged when it was discovered that she was pregnant. In November, 1949, she had her child. While she was on the maternity ward she again became acutely disturbed. Nevertheless, she returned home and remained there with no real change in behavior until she was admitted to the Charity Hospital, New Orleans, in 1950.

Family History. The patient, her brother, and two sisters, born to an economically lower-class family, have all shown marked emotional instability. The father is a heavy drinker, who often behaves irrationally. At times he rejects his children; at other times he intervenes when his wife attempts to discipline them. The patient's mother is described as a good housekeeper who puts up with her husband's abuse, developing acute abdominal complaints whenever his demands are excessive. The patient's sisters have made poor adjustments; her brother was unable to complete the sixth grade in school. He consequently gets much attention from his mother, who feels particularly protective toward him.

Personal History. The patient was born in New Orleans in 1928. Her developmental years seem to have been normal, although she was often teased because of her appearance. During early life she took an active part in school activities, played with the other children and was self-assertive to the point of being considered belligerent. At school she did very well, showing some talent at drawing. She first felt attracted to a boy at the age of 15. Shortly thereafter she began to worry about catching tuberculosis from men, crossing the street to avoid any possible contamination from passing too close to them. At this time she became preoccupied with sex, avidly reading literature on the subject, but being particularly interested in homosexuality. After menarche, which did not occur until 17 1/2, she vacillated between frequent dates and fearful withdrawal from all contacts with men.

Personality. The patient was described as a difficult child, belligerent, self-assertive, and given to frequent tantrums. She made no close emotional attachment to either her family or colleagues.

Physical and Laboratory Status. Physical and neurological examinations were within normal limits. CBC, BUN, blood sugar, glucose tolerance, serology, and urinalysis were all within normal limits. Chest plate and skull films were all negative and EEG revealed normal alpha rhythm (10 c/sec.). Blood pressure has always been within normal range.

Hospital Course. The patient was started on electronarcosis treatment in July, 1950, receiving 3 treatments per week for a total course of 15. During the treatment there was little change in behavior, except that she seemed slightly more responsive to her environment and more concerned about her personal appearance. She was started on a course of electroshock therapy in October, 1950, again receiving 3 treatments a week for a course of 15. During this period there was still no significant change in her behavior. On one occasion, following a visit from her husband, the patient walked around in a dazed fashion and showed posturing as well as waxy flexibility. Just prior to her operation her mental status was much the same as upon admission. Affect remained shallow and inappropriate with frequent outbursts of silly laughter. Alternately she was withdrawn and friendly, hostile and erotic. Her stream of productions was disconnected, at times incoherent. Her delusions continued to center around sexual matters.

First Operation—Stimulation. February 23, 1951.

(a) Surgical technique—Open technique was used.

(b) Electrode placement—A bipolar electrode was placed in the septal region.

(c) Recordings—Scalp recordings were normal before stimulation and continued normal throughout the follow-up period. Spikes were noted in the deep recordings. Emotional stimulation appeared to produce alterations in the deep recordings. The follow-up recordings are incomplete.

(d) Stimulation technique—There were two septal stimulations of 1 minute each, at 2 ma. and 6 volts.

(e) Immediate physiological effects—No appreciable physiological response was noted.

(f) Immediate behavioral response—There was a good behavioral response to stimulation, the patient becoming more alert and responsive.

(g) Immediate chemical changes—No chemical data were obtained.

(h) Complications—None.

Follow-up Notes. Three days postoperatively the patient was well oriented and seemed in good contact with her environment and less erotic. She still showed occasional bursts of inappropriate laughter. Two weeks later she was making numerous inquiries about other patients she had known, and her family remarked that she had "lost her glassy stare." Three weeks after operation she was much friendlier and more outgoing and talkative. She complained about her mother's strict super-

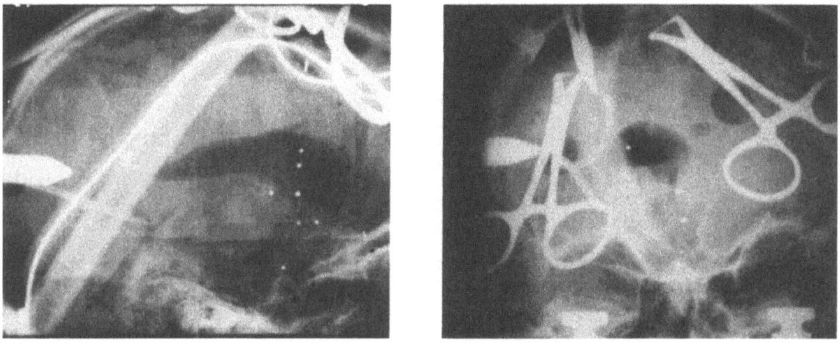

FIGURE XIX-3. Patient 5(24)

vision. Gradually she became more spontaneous and showed less hostility. At times, speaking rapidly, she revealed remnants of her previous bizarre ideation, such as, "Sometimes I think I am a Negro and they are trying to make me work for them." A month after operation she was even more spontaneous, related well to the ward personnel, was friendly to all doctors, and often went for walks with them in the halls. Sometimes she still attempted to be seductive, but in a reserved, more realistic manner. She was discharged from the hospital in May, 1951, approximately 11 weeks after operation. At that time she was neat, interested in applying make-up, and generally related in a friendly, appropriate manner to those around her. She was much less preoccupied with inner conflicts and more responsive to immediate needs. She was making realistic plans to separate legally from her husband. Some bizarre ideation appeared to remain, but she was reluctant to talk about it. She often said, "I was in a dream world before—sometimes I wish I could get back in it, but not really." During her first month at home she continued to progress although she still remained frightened and confused regarding her sexual role. She could be friendly and outgoing with her family but was unable to maintain this gain outside the home. For the next several months her condition was essentially unchanged. She did no work, not even aiding with the housework. She showed no desire to socialize, spent most of her time listening to the radio or reading movie magazines, and was apparently preoccupied with her fantasy life. When seen in the clinic, she attempted to avoid the doctors, showed little emotional response, and when questioned about her fantasies, gave scattered and evasive answers. She denied having hallucinations or paranoid trends. No psychological data could be obtained.

Psychotic Exacerbation. In March, 1952, the patient became acutely disturbed, threatened various members of her family, and began breaking up the furniture. This behavior required immediate rehospitalization. At that time the patient was completely negativistic, uncooperative, periodically excited, and assaultive. She recognized her former doctors but refused to talk with them. She was disheveled and untidy in her appearance and showed none of the spontaneous erotic behavior that had been apparent on her first admission. She displayed far less emotional response than previously. As before, physical and laboratory examinations were within normal limits except for the scar and the skull defect which had resulted from her previous operation.

Second Operation—Stimulation. April 10, 1952.

(a) Surgical technique—Stereotaxic technique was used.

(b) Electrode placements—Seven unipolar electrodes were placed in subcortical structures of the left cerebral hemisphere; three in the septum, two in the hypothalamus, and two in the caudate nucleus.

(c) Recordings—A recording taken the day following the operation revealed spikes in the septal leads. The patient forcibly removed her own electrodes, making further recordings impossible.

(d) Stimulation technique—The patient received three septal stimulations. The first two were to leads 12 and 13 for 10 minutes at 18 and 32 ma. The third stimulation was to leads 11 and 13 for 13 minutes 40 seconds at 34 ma.

(e) Immediate physiological effects—One stimulation to the septal electrodes (leads 12 and 13) produced a change in blood pressure from 110/76 to 144/110, with marked tachycardia, flushing, and sweating; another stimulation (leads 11 and 13) produced a blood pressure response of 150/100, with marked tachycardia and alternating movements of both hands, upon manual reversal of polarity of the stimulus.

(f) Immediate behavioral response—There was an obvious increase in alertness.

(g) Immediate chemical changes—The chemical data are not clearcut. There is a possibility that there was a down dip on the return of the lymphocyte count toward the preoperative level. This possibility is significant because it came at the time that lymphopenia usually appears, namely, between 1 1/2 and 2 hours following stimulation. In this instance the lymphocytes appeared to have been returning to normal level. The count was 800 before the first stimulation but rose to a level of 1,850; 1 1/2 hours after stimulation it was down to 1,176, then apparently began to climb again. Within 4 hours after stimulation it reached a peak of 2,374. No significant change in plasma electrolytes took place.

(h) Complications—None.

Follow-up Notes. For the first 2 days after operation the patient remained quiet and negativistic, at times combative, requiring restraint. Her temperature rose to 103.5°F. but subsided immediately. There were no abnormalities on physical and neurological examination. Eleven days after operation she showed her first change in behavior, becoming more cooperative with the nurses and freely verbalizing her hostility toward her female therapist. Two weeks after operation she responded for the first time to the therapist's invitation to go for a walk and to get a "coke." At that time she smiled appropriately and initiated conversations. Her productions were coherent and logical. She began expressing erotic interest in the male doctors and continued to be hostile toward her own therapist, a female physician. Three weeks after operation, although she preferred to be alone most of the time, she occasionally mixed with the other patients and expressed some interest in occupational therapy. Six weeks after operation her behavior was still improving. Her emotional responses were shallow but more appropriate. She was less preoccupied with her fantasy life, although she expressed mild referential ideas. She continued to be erotically interested in the male doctors, asking them for kisses on several occasions. At the same time she was hostile toward and resentful of the female physicians. She had a transitory depression from which she recovered. No psychological data could be obtained.

The patient's postoperative course appears to be similar to that following her first stimulation. However, no further improvement has been noted, and she remains hospitalized on June 1, 1953, 13 months after her second stimulation.

Patient 6

AGE AT OPERATION: 28

SEX: Male

MARITAL STATUS: Single
OCCUPATION: Unemployed
RELIGION: Catholic (active)
INFORMANTS: Patient and previous hospital record
DIAGNOSIS: Schizophrenic reaction, hebephrenic type
OPERATION: March 15, 1951

Presenting Picture. On admission to the hospital in January, 1951, the patient was shy, effeminate, fearful, childlike, dependent, illogical, and manneristic. He talked in a rambling, circumstantial manner about his sexual and religious problems.

Present Illness. Although this patient has always been considered peculiar, it was only late in 1946 that he became openly psychotic. At that time he was panicked because of the lack of privacy caused by the limited sanitary facilities in his home. After one such experience he became acutely agitated, hit and threw water on his mother, and then beat up his brother when the latter interceded. At approximately the same time his first and only homosexual experience took place. Shortly afterward he entered a state hospital, where he received electroshock therapy. Seven months later, although unimproved, he was discharged at the request of his family. Shortly after his release he got up during a mass and publicly denounced the priesthood for taking money from the poor. He was talking in an irrational, confused manner and consequently was returned to the state hospital for further EST. Again at the family's request he was discharged, only slightly improved. He remained fearful, seclusive, and preoccupied with ideas of homosexuality. In 1949 he was admitted to the Charity Hospital.

Previous Personality Disorders. Before the onset of his present illness in 1946 the patient had no overt psychotic episodes.

Family History. The patient is the second of three children born in Louisiana to a French family of low economic status. Apparently there was little affection between the parents and children, for the patient was sent away to parochial schools at an early age. He has expressed a good deal of resentment toward both parents, but particularly toward his mother, who in his description is a very rigid, authoritative figure. His older brother and younger sister are both married and apparently adjusting well.

Personal History. Little is known about the patient's birth and early development. He was sent at the age of 5 to a Catholic home for children and at 12 to a seminary, where he stayed until he was 18. He was always submissive and obedient, avoiding trouble by "avoiding the priests." He always had difficulty with his scholastic work and did not form any strong emotional attachments. Resentful of extreme discipline, he nevertheless did not revolt against it. While he was at the seminary he apparently had a number of homosexual preoccupations but engaged in no activity. Following his graduation he went to a monastery, left there to work for several months at a CCC camp, and then tried to attend a small college, where he remained for only 5 weeks because the pace was too fast. He worked at a number of menial jobs, finally ending up as a stenographer for the Port of Embarkation. At this last job he had to work with a number of women; this finally became too much for him, with the result that he returned home "because of his nervousness." It was at this time that his present illness started.

Personality. Extreme ingratiation covered underlying intense resentment. Guilty fears and training made him preoccupied with religious and philosophical concepts while interfering with any close or lasting emotional ties.

Physical and Laboratory Status. Physical examination revealed a well-developed, well-nourished young man with no significant abnormalities. On one previous examination under rectal manipulation he had become quite excited and disturbed. Laboratory findings, including CBC, BUN, glucose tolerance, serology, urinalysis, and chest and skull films, were all negative. Two EEG's were normal, and two showed random spiking.

Hospital Course. When he was admitted to this hospital in 1949, the patient was extremely fearful of all personnel, backing away from them and holding them at arm's length as if expecting a sexual attack. He complained that people could smell his genitals and expressed the fear that something terrible would happen to him if he exposed himself in any way. After receiving a total of 18 insulin-coma treatments without improvement, he had a topectomy in November, 1949. The only change noted postoperatively was that he became even more talkative and more preoccupied with religion and sex. His fears and seclusive behavior continued. While he was in the hospital he wrote numerous letters to the doctors, frequently addressing them as gods, and in a very vague, disconnected, symbolic manner discussed all kinds of philosophical and religious problems. Prior to the operation of March, 1951, the patient's behavior changed little. He was shy, friendly, polite, fearful, and ingratiating by turns. He showed a number of bizarre mannerisms, such as pulling at his shirt, grimacing, and backing up in short, fast steps. He continued to be overtalkative, frequently conversing with the other patients about his most intimate problems. His productions were illogical, circumstantial, and at times incoherent and bizarre. In addition to religious and philosophical problems they included some obsessive reminiscences about his mother's and sister's lack of propriety. Generally he was euphoric but at times became irritable and angry.

Operation—Stimulation. March 15, 1951.

(a) Surgical technique—Open technique was used.

(b) Electrode placements—Three bipolar electrodes were implanted; but their positions were not adequately checked by x-ray. One electrode (lead 1) was reported to be in the caudate nucleus, another (lead 2) in the septal region, and the third (lead 3) in the anterior thalamus.

(c) Recordings—The data are inadequate because of the apparatus used at that time. Four preoperative EEG's were made; two showed random spiking and two were normal. No scalp leads were recorded postoperatively.

(d) Stimulation technique—There were two septal stimulations of 2 minutes each. Estimated peak currents ranged from 1 to 3 ma. The current between the electrodes was not measured at that time; in the light of later information it appears likely that the current fell to 1/5 of the estimated peak value in the course of 30 seconds. There was no reversal of polarity.

(e) Immediate physiological effects—Minimal physiological effects of a diffuse sympathetic type were noted.

(f) Immediate behavioral response—The patient complained of remembering voices he had previously heard reprimanding him for perverted sexual activity. He said he had felt a "shocklike or warm feeling" during the stimulation. He seemed euphoric and became more responsive and alert.

(g) Immediate chemical changes—No chemical data were obtained.

(h) Complications—None.

Follow-up Notes. The day after the operation the patient described the previous night's experience as if he had had an hallucination: "The voice of the Lord was talking to me." He also described the sensation as a feeling of warmth and pleasantness at one time and as a "shock" at another time. A week after the stimulation he seemed a little quieter and able to tackle his difficulties in more realistic fashion, but he continued to ask bizarre questions about religion and sex. Six weeks later there was little definite change. He was quiet on the ward, neat and tidy, more coherent in his productions, and appropriate in his emotional responses to the doctors and nurses. He was much more discreet in his behavior, not discussing his problems with the other patients—in fact showing reluctance to talk about them even with his own therapist. Placed on an open ward, he expressed concern over the future, particularly the preoccupying problem of continuing in the Catholic religion or shifting to another. He related warmly to anybody who showed some interest in him, immediately forming a strong identification and dependency. With the ultimate hope of getting a job as a secretary, he began typing and studying shorthand. Two months after operation he tried typing for the hospital on a voluntary basis but found it difficult to keep his margins straight and to spell correctly. At this time he showed his first self-assertive behavior when he told a Protestant minister who was trying to convert him to stay away.

The problems that preoccupied him were concerned with the immediate future, such as finding a job and supporting himself. He got a job on his own initiative, working as a waiter. For several weeks he lived in the hospital until he acquired enough money to make arrangements for a furnished room. In July, 1951, 3 1/2 months after operation, he was discharged from the hospital to live in a small furnished room and work for $26.00 a week plus tips at a local coffee shop. For 2 months he functioned surprisingly well on this job. He was subjected to many stresses, as his fellow employees, who were for the most part psychopaths, took advantage of him by borrowing money from him and involving him in perverted sexual activities. He performed fellatio several times, assuming the female role without expressing excessive guilt, but then showed realistic, self-assertive behavior by refusing to participate in this activity in the future. He was particularly untidy and unclean at that time but on the insistence of the therapist, on whom he was very dependent, began to take an interest in his personal appearance.

In October, 1951, largely to extricate himself from his psychopathic colleagues, he returned to his home in rural Louisiana. Since then he has not worked, complains of rather severe headaches, writes frequent letters to the doctors in the hospital, and continues monthly visits to a local mental hygiene clinic. He remains emotionally unstable and still preoccupied with religion and sex but not in a delusional way. Numerous hypochondriacal complaints prevent him, he feels, from working on a steady job, although he is putting to use some of the handicraft skills he learned in occupational therapy at the hospital. He is rather unrealistically resentful over "exploitation" by his family, who utilize his invalidism to get extra welfare aid. At times he seems to show some recent memory defects and confusion; however, intelligence-testing reveals that he can function on a relatively high level in abstract thinking and perform rather complicated mathematical problems. At present his general demeanor is that of childlike ingratiation and dependency. Psychological testing showed little change in his schizophrenic pattern.

On June 1, 1953, no change in the patient's mental status was noted. He is not working regularly, although he does aid with the farm chores. The follow-up period now covers 25 months.

Patient 7

AGE AT OPERATION: 35
SEX: Male
MARITAL STATUS: Single
OCCUPATION: Teacher
RELIGION: Baptist (inactive)
INFORMANT: Mother
DIAGNOSIS: Schizophrenic reaction, paranoid type
OPERATION: April 25, 1951

Presenting Picture. On admission to the hospital in May, 1950, the patient was seclusive, hostile, and generally uncommunicative. He seemed to be hallucinating and occasionally expressed delusions of bodily injury, particularly to the effect that he was being poisoned. At times he was completely illogical in his productions, and occasionally he also showed bizarre mannerisms and posturing.

Present Illness. In November, 1949, the patient had a severe asthmatic attack, which was followed by fear of impending death. He began hallucinating, warned his mother not to go outside because somebody would harm her, and expressed the opinion that he was going to be shot. He also said that he was under the influence of some radio or atomic waves. His condition remained essentially unchanged until he was hospitalized in May, 1950.

Previous Personality Disorders. No previous psychotic episodes were reported.

Family History. The patient is the only child of an economically lower-class Negro family. The father spent little time with his family and moved away from home in 1942. The patient became agitated and resentful at that time. His mother, a high school graduate of above-average intelligence, has always worked as a domestic. She seems sincerely concerned over her son's illness.

Personal History. There was nothing remarkable about the patient's birth and early development. He developed asthma at the age of 5 and has had frequent attacks since then. He was a small, unathletic, seclusive child predominantly interested in books, and his lifelong desire was to be a teacher. He did well in school, graduating from college and subsequently taking postgraduate work in sociology. Following this, he was a substitute teacher for several years and then a union secretary for a year and a half. During the latter period he did typing to make extra money but was dissatisfied with this work, as he preferred to teach. When he failed to get a permanent teaching appointment, his asthma was exacerbated and he became seclusive, lost interest in girls, and finally developed hallucinations and delusions.

Personality. The patient has always been a quiet, shy, retiring individual, intellectually inclined. Although superficially friendly and occasionally sociable, he was never lighthearted or jovial.

Physical and Laboratory Status. Physical examination revealed a small, undernourished, Negro male weighing only 95 pounds. His blood pressure was 120/70. Otherwise physical and neurological findings were within normal limits. Laboratory studies, including CBC, blood chemistry, glucose tolerance, serology, urinalysis, chest and skull films, EKG, and EEG, were all normal.

Hospital Course. On the wards the patient was preoccupied, hostile, and negativistic. He refused to be questioned, would not respond to any psychotherapeutic procedures, and often wandered off to stare out of the window. He was evasive about his previous delusions and at times he denied hallucinations, but repeated questioning did elicit a vague description of paranoid trends. He also expressed some resentment about his hospitalization. He remained in good contact with his surroundings, his memory did not seem to be impaired, and superficial testing suggested high intelligence. In July, 1950, he was started on electroshock therapy, receiving 3 treatments a week for a total course of 15. Afterward he continued to be uncooperative; he ate poorly and spoke freely of his delusion that the food was poisoned. He also complained of hearing voices that threatened to harm him. He received little benefit from EST and consequently, in October, 1950, was started on electronarcosis, again receiving 3 treatments a week for a total course of 15. He became more illogical and incoherent in his productions and showed some grandiosity, saying, "I am the master of all the world." His seclusiveness and preoccupation remained. Although encouraged to go home on passes, he refused to do so, expressing despair about his ultimate recovery.

Operation—Stimulation. April 25, 1951.

(a) Surgical technique—Open technique was used.

(b) Electrode placements—Three bipolar electrodes were implanted: one (lead 1) in the caudate, another (lead 2) apparently somewhat high in the septal region, and a third (lead 3) in the anterior thalamus.

(c) Recordings—There were infrequent spikes from lead 2, but no spiking abnormalities were recorded from the other two leads. No change appeared in the records immediately following stimulation. However, frequent, sharp, high voltage spikes were noted, about 6 hours after stimulation, in lead 2. The preoperative EEG was normal. The first postoperative scalp EEG, made 1 month after surgery, showed a slow wave focus in the right frontal region, but 2 months after surgery the record was normal. An EEG taken after the generalized seizure occurring about a year postoperatively showed a bifrontal slow focus and amplitude asymmetry in the occipital regions.

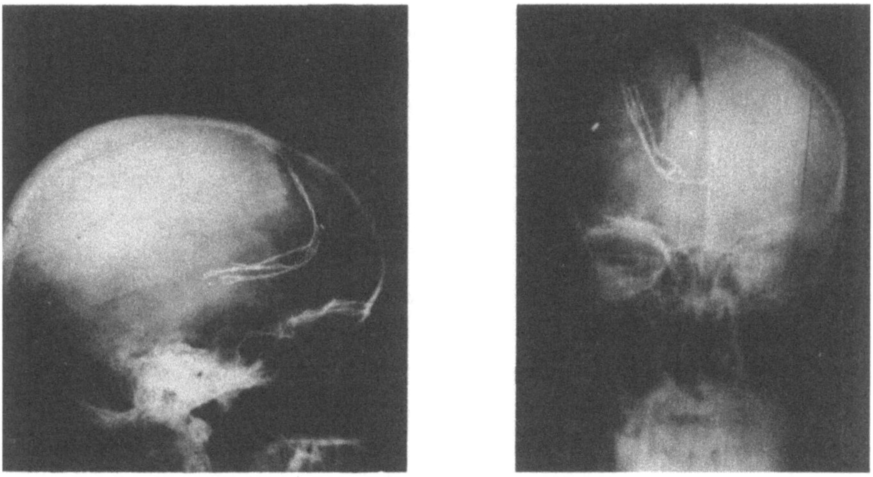

FIGURE XIX-4. Patient 7

(d) Stimulation technique—There were two septal stimulations, the first for 2 minutes, the second for 1 minute. The peak current of the first was estimated at 3 ma.; in a short period this dropped to 1 ma. The second started at 6 ma. and dropped to 1 1/2 ma.

(e) Immediate physiological effects—Stimulation to the septal electrode (lead 2) produced no apparent physiological response.

(f) Immediate behavioral response—The patient showed an increase in alertness, marked by much more animation and spontaneous elaboration.

(g) Immediate chemical changes—No chemical data were obtained.

(h) Complications—About a year after operation the patient had a grand mal seizure.

Follow-up Notes. One week following operation, the patient seemed definitely more alert and responsive. He got out of bed and for the first time accompanied the doctors to the solarium. He would talk about everyday events, even though he still remained evasive concerning his illness. Although he never socialized freely, he did walk about the wards and occasionally participated in ward activities. He denied having hallucinations; in fact, he professed inability to recall previous hallucinations and delusions. Three weeks after operation, he consented to go home on a pass to visit his mother, something he had refused to do prior to operation. He remained somewhat hostile and depressed, claiming that the operation had not helped him and expressing his old ideas that he would never get well or be allowed out of the hospital. Despite encouragement to leave the hospital on passes, he remained seclusive, despondent, and uninterested in his surroundings. He was, however, more responsive emotionally than before, showed fewer mannerisms, and apparently no longer had hallucinations or at least was now capable of covering them up. Nine weeks following stimulation he was discharged from the hospital and since then has been coming regularly to the outpatient clinic, always accompanied by his mother. He is perfectly cooperative but appears emotionally shallow and uninterested. Psychological tests revealed very slight improvement.

On June 1, 1953, 24 months after operation, the patient shows little spontaneity or initiative, producing only in response to direct and repeated questioning, although occasionally he does respond to praise and interest by the therapist. At home he remains idle and seclusive, spending most of his time listening to the radio, reading newspapers, or daydreaming. He still denies having hallucinations but is so evasive that one questions his denial.

PATIENT 8 (15)

AGE AT FIRST OPERATION: 41
SEX: Male
MARITAL STATUS: Married
OCCUPATION: Baker
RELIGION: Catholic (inactive)
INFORMANTS: Patient, patient's wife, mother
DIAGNOSIS: Schizophrenic reaction, paranoid type
OPERATIONS: May 2, 1951, and December 6, 1951

Presenting Picture. The patient was transferred to this hospital in October, 1950, from a private sanitarium where he had been since 1949. At that time he was depressed and agitated, displaying periodic aggressive and uncooperative behavior. He projected most of his difficulties onto his wife and expressed homosexual preoccupations.

Present Illness. Although the patient had had several breaks previously, his continuous illness dates from 1945, when he was hospitalized because of psychotic behavior. At that time he was particularly preoccupied with quarrels with his wife. He was discharged after receiving EST but in 1947 and periodically thereafter received further EST on an outpatient basis. During this hospitalization he revealed numerous obsessive-compulsive traits, constantly washing his hands, imagining that he saw semen in the bathtub water, and expressing fears of contamination by sperm which would make him a "queer." He expressed numerous ideas of reference and talked in a derogatory way about the "Jews" and the "Dagos." His symptoms were exacerbated by the death of his mother in 1948 and the death of his father in 1949. In the latter part of 1949 he was admitted to a private sanitarium, where he received both insulin shocks and EST without marked benefit. Since his transfer to the Charity Hospital he has continuously remained depressed, agitated, and preoccupied with homosexuality, ideas of reference, and feelings of persecution.

Previous Personality Disorders. The patient first showed psychotic symptoms in 1931 at the age of 20. While dating his first girl he became preoccupied with his inability to perform sexually and developed obsessional ideas and suicidal fantasies. He tried to relieve his anxiety by reading all of the available psychoanalytic and sexual literature. He feared that he was "an unconscious homosexual." He was briefly hospitalized without treatment and subsequently made a marginal social adjustment until 1938. At that time he sought psychiatric help for a psychotic symptomatology, which had been precipitated by a divorce from his first wife and one homosexual experience. After receiving metrazol treatment, he improved enough to be discharged from the hospital in 1939. Subsequently he manifested abnormal behavior by his insistence on numerous operations, his continuous preoccupation with masculinity, and frequent requests for hormonal treatments. Nevertheless, he made a marginal economic adjustment, running his own bakery. He remarried in 1941, and performed well enough sexually to have two children by this wife. Since 1945 he has either been hospitalized or receiving outpatient psychiatric care.

Family History. The patient is the second of four children, having an older sister and two younger brothers. The family members are hard-working, lower-class artisans. They are stern, devout Catholics and very prohibitive in sexual matters. Parental discipline was extreme, leaving the patient with many early memories of severe physical punishment.

He has several memories of severe beatings by his father; his mother, too, although at times protective, was generally strict and often physically abusive. He was often told by his father that he was circumcised by jerking off the foreskin. The patient felt that the other children were treated better than he was. There has always been and still is constant bickering among the siblings.

Personal History. As far as is known, the patient's birth and early development were normal. However, he soon became preoccupied with his bodily integrity and sexual drive. His outstanding early memories are of harsh discipline with occasional violent retaliations on his own part. During childhood and adolescence he was strong physically and participated actively in sports. In playing football or boxing he combated fears by charging blindly in a rage, often in a very inept, self-destructive manner. He was always shy with the opposite sex and never really dated girls until the onset of his first psychosis as described above.

Personality. Even before his first psychotic episode, the patient was generally suspicious and often became depressed and tearful. In his rare moments of euphoria he became aggressive and hostile. As a rule, he tended to be seclusive and withdrawn.

Physical and Laboratory Status. Physical examination revealed no abnormalities except for labile blood pressure, which was usually in the normal range but at times varied from 140 to 160 systolic and from 90 to 110 diastolic. Laboratory findings, including CBC, BUN, serology, urinalysis, and EKG, were all within normal limits.

Hospital Course. The patient received psychotherapy during the first 7 months of his hospitalization. His paranoid ideation, referential feelings, and preoccupation with homosexuality all continued. On numerous occasions he expressed feelings of hopelessness, shame, and unworthiness but he persistently denied any hallucinatory experiences. He was obsessively reminiscent concerning his past. Throughout his hospitalization, the patient was completely oriented and in good contact with his surroundings, showed excellent recent-remote memory, and performed well in all intelligence-testing. When operation was finally decided upon, he became particularly tense and irritable and expressed numerous hypochondriacal complaints.

First Operation—Stimulation. May 2, 1951.

(a) Surgical technique—Open technique was used.

(b) Electrode placements—Three bipolar electrodes were implanted, but the locations were not adequately checked by x-ray. According to the surgeon's report one electrode was in the caudate nucleus (lead 1), another (lead 2) was in the septal region, and a third (lead 3) in the rostral part of the thalamus.

(c) Recordings—Moderate spiking showed in the septal lead. The recordings were not significantly affected by the stimulation; the spikes occurred as frequently at the termination of the procedure as before stimulation.

(d) Stimulation technique—The patient was stimulated once through the septal lead for 2 minutes at an estimated peak current of 5 ma., which dropped to 1 ma. by the end of the stimulation. This is the first patient in whom actual current measurement was made between the two poles of the stimulating electrode.

(e) Immediate physiological effects—Stimulation to the septal electrode (lead 2) produced no apparent physiological response.

(f) Immediate behavioral response—There was little in the way of psychological change. If anything, the patient was retarded and became dull and somewhat confused.

(g) Immediate chemical changes—No change in serum electrolytes was shown.

(h) Complications—None.

Follow-up Notes. During this stimulation and directly afterward the patient was subjected to direct and intense questioning regarding his many delusions. He reacted with extreme hostility, threatening to kill doctors once he was well. One week after surgery his hostility had subsided considerably, much to the relief of the patient, not to mention the doctors. There was decreasing need for sedation and less hypochondriacal preoccupation. Although many of his delusions persisted to a lesser degree, the patient was obviously more friendly, outgoing, cooperative, and under considerably less tension. However, he appeared somewhat depressed, asking, "If the tension is relieved, why don't these ideas go away?" He was discharged from the hospital in June, 1951, 7 weeks after operation. At home he gradually became more depressed and suspicious. He was seclusive, would not look for a job, showed marked ideas of reference, and developed feelings of persecution which started with his wife and then involved a neighbor and finally even his children. He voluntarily requested readmission to the hospital in December, 1951.

Readmission. The patient's mental status was similar to that noted at the time of his first hospitalization, except that he was now neater and more cooperative, perhaps because he was more depressed. He remained suspicious, evasive, and predominantly referential. Insight into his illness was apparent this time, as he realized his tendency to misinterpret and project. He expressed fears that he would be committed to a state institution because of his failure in the previous treatment. Sensorium remained intact, and again he performed rapidly and correctly on abstract reasoning.

Second Operation—Stimulation. December 6, 1951.

(a) Surgical technique—Open technique was used, with reopening of the previous incision.

(b) Electrode placements—An attempt was made to place electrodes in the same areas—i.e., septal region, caudate nucleus, and rostral part of the thalamus, but the placements were not checked by x-ray.

(c) Recordings—The prestimulation record showed frequent spikes of high amplitude, which were most prevalent when the patient was drowsy or in light sleep and which were limited to lead 2, not appearing in other deep leads. Records on one of the milder stimulations showed what appeared to be a subcortical seizure pattern at the site of the stimulation, which did not spread to the cortex and which was not accompanied by loss of consciousness. When cortical seizure patterns were recorded several minutes later, they were accompanied by a grand mal seizure. Following one stimulation, the spikes from lead 2 were considerably reduced in amplitude and frequency of occurrence and were reversed in polarity. Consequently, stimulation was applied again to this lead. At the end of the second stimulation spikes were still present but were considerably reduced in size and appeared with much less frequency. Pre- and post-operative scalp EEG's for both operations were normal.

(d) Stimulation technique—There were four stimulations of 3 to 10 minutes through the septal lead. The currents ranged from 4 to 10 ma. Current was monitored at this time, and there was no polarization.

(e) Immediate physiological effects—Stimulation to the septal electrode produced a slight rise in blood pressure from 140/80 to 160/86. There was a slight increase in heart rate, and the patient gradually became cyanotic and then apneic. Tonic movements of the right arm and leg were noted, and the patient appeared to be disoriented. Several minutes after stimulation he had a generalized convulsion.

(f) Immediate behavioral response—A few minutes after the generalized convulsion the patient reacted in an explosive manner, demonstrating some confusion and disorientation. During the stimulation he had reported that he felt tension disappearing. He smiled and seemed more emotionally responsive to the interviewers.

(g) Immediate chemical changes—There were no changes in serum electrolytes. The eosinophils, as is always the case, diminished as a result of the operation. There was a 73 per cent drop in lymphocytes with the stimulation. Maximum drop occurred 1 hour and 15 minutes after the last stimulation and 4 hours after the first stimulation. The lymphocytes climbed to their prestimulation level 1 1/2 hours after the maximum drop.

(h) Complications—Stimulation was followed by a generalized convulsion.

Follow-up Notes. The patient recovered his memory the day following the operation except as it related to events of the day of operation. Four days postoperatively he was quiet and friendly, although still expressing paranoid ideas. He became preoccupied with the smallness of his penis and the largeness of his breasts. By the sixth day he definitely decided that he was a "queer" and that everybody knew it. However, he continued to improve in his affective responses and seemed to relate better to the therapist. On the sixteenth day he developed epididymitis, which surprisingly did not seem to disturb him. He continued to be suspicious of the ward personnel, often rejecting medicine, as he felt they were trying to "trick" him. Gradually he became more friendly, particularly with the doctors, and 5 weeks after operation went home on a pass. He returned in a rage because of difficulties with relatives, still expressing his ideas of persecution. However, he was pleased because for the first time in many years he had enjoyed intercourse without premature ejaculation. Six weeks after operation, since he continued to show considerable improvement, he was discharged to live at home and report to the clinic. At home he was in good spirits, slept well with slight sedation, bragged about his appetite, had little feeling of inner tension, and made active plans for reopening his bakery. He did notice that one beer made him unsteady and confused. When he was seen in the clinic 2 1/2 months after operation he appeared somewhat euphoric. He brought with him pies which he had baked for the various doctors. Eleven weeks after his operation he tried to open up his bakery but ran into numerous practical difficulties. Each frustration led to more tension until finally he had several outbursts of rage directed against his family. At the same time his wife had to be hospitalized, leaving him at home to take care not only of the bakery but also of his children. Under this excessive burden the patient became tense, fearful, angry, confused, and depressed. He lost his billfold, set the grease in the bakery on fire, flooded the house with the washing machine, began drinking heavily, and finally set the house on fire when he accidentally fell asleep while smoking. When the firemen arrived, he became so disturbed that he had to be taken to the police station. The hospital was called and the patient was readmitted in March, 1952. On the wards he was hostile, uncooperative and destructive, requiring seclusion and restraint. At times he would become depressed and fearful over his failure to make a go of the bakery, expressing concern over his wife's illness and operation. His rage and destructiveness gradually changed to hypomanic euphoric behavior, with periodic outbursts of irritability and uncooperativeness. As this behavior gradually subsided, he was given several passes, during which adjustment at home was satisfactory. After 2 months of this rehospitalization he was discharged. At home he was placed on sedation, still complained of persistent tension, seemed moderately depressed and retarded, and preferred to be idle and seclusive. Accompanying his feelings of depression was a return of many of his delusional ideas. Two weeks after release from the hospital he was shifted from sedation to dexamyl to see whether the depression and inactivity would lessen. As this did not help, he was placed on outpatient EST. His depression lifted, but anxiety and referential ideas continued. EST was discontinued in March, 1953.

It is of interest that psychological tests revealed an increase in psychotic signs after stimulation on both occasions despite some clinical improvement.

On June 1, 1953, 18 months after the second operation, he still is out of the hospital, but anxiety and depression keep him from working. However, delusions are minimal and insight remains.

Patient 9

AGE AT OPERATION: 39
SEX: Male
MARITAL STATUS: Single
OCCUPATION: None
RELIGION: Jewish (active)
INFORMANTS: Mother, brother, hospital records, social service
DIAGNOSIS: Schizophrenic reaction, hebephrenic type
OPERATION: May 24, 1951

Presenting Picture. When this patient was transferred from the state hospital in May, 1951, he presented a classical picture of a chronic, deteriorated schizophrenic. He was mute, inattentive, uninterested in his surroundings, and retarded in motor activity; he was usually cooperative but at times negativistic and resistive. Periodically he would burst forth with loud laughter and grimace in a bizarre way.

Present Illness. The patient's illness had begun insidiously 20 years before, at which time he gradually became suspicious and seclusive, expressing ideas of persecution. He was periodically belligerent and assaultive. He lost all interest in his personal appearance, refused to eat, and finally became so inaccessible that hospitalization was necessary. Although he was taken out of the hospital several times by his family, he never showed any real remission but continued to be suspicious, withdrawn, untidy, delusional and hallucinated. He often impulsively struck out at the family or other patients. At the beginning of his long hospitalization he was given a diagnosis of "dementia praecox, catatonic type." During this time he had numerous courses of electroshock treatments, with only slight and temporary improvement. The last EST was terminated 2 months before his admission to this hospital.

Previous Personality Disorders. There were no previous psychotic episodes.

Family History. Both the parents are Russian Jewish immigrants of lower middle-class status who have maintained this economic level by constant work and driving ambition. The father, now 70 and suffering from Parkinsonism, worked during virtually all his waking hours and consequently participated little in the upbringing of the children. The mother was the disciplinarian in the family, always demanding good deportment and satisfactory educational performance of her children, insisting that they either be or marry professional men. The patient has two older and four younger siblings, all of whom are satisfactorily adjusted and moderately successful, although one sibling seems extremely anxious and self-conscious. The mother, in her contact with the hospital, manifested numerous paranoid traits.

Personal History. The patient was born in New Orleans in 1912. Birth and early development were uneventful, except for the fact that his mother became depressed when he was 3 months old and required hospitalization for 6 months. Although the patient was not particularly attached to any member of his family, he had a large circle of friends, was considered a good mixer, participated in team sports, and during adolescence even coached athletic teams in his spare time. He completed all but 3 months of high school, at which time he insisted on leaving to go to work, despite his mother's plea that he continue schooling and become a dentist. He worked as a bill collector for about a year prior to the onset of his illness at the age of 18. During childhood he participated in some mutual masturbation with one of his brothers. He was considered "highly sexual" by his family, who would not elucidate further.

Personality. Prior to the onset of his present illness, the patient is said to have been an alert, mildly self-assertive person with considerable interest in social activities.

Physical and Laboratory Status. Physical examination revealed a well-developed and well-nourished male in no acute physical distress, the only positive finding being keloid formations on both temporal regions, apparently the result of long-term electroshock therapy. Neurological findings were within normal limits. Laboratory tests, including CBC, blood chemistry, serology, and urinalysis, were all normal, as were EKG and chest and skull films. EEG revealed generalized S2 and S3 activity of the paroxysmal type, possibly the result of continuous EST. Pneumoencephalogram suggested minimal cortical atrophy and hydrocephalus ex vacuo, probably consistent with the history of repeated electroshock treatments. Daily blood pressure varied from 130/98 to 110/80.

Hospital Course. During the 16-day period prior to operation, the patient's behavior remained the same as on admission.

Operation—Stimulation. May 24, 1951.

(a) Surgical technique—Open technique was used.

(b) Electrode placements—Three bipolar electrodes were implanted. Postoperative x-rays showed that the electrode intended for the caudate nucleus (lead 1) was probably in the lateral ventricle. Lead 2 was 8 mm. rostral to the foramen of Monro in the midline and 1 cm. dorsal to the foramen in the septal region. Lead 3 appeared to be in the corpus callosum.

(c) Recordings—A grossly abnormal EEG, a semistuporous record, was found preoperatively; in view of the history this was attributed to prolonged EST. Deep recordings showed moderate spiking from lead 2 exclusively. These occasionally appeared in bursts with high voltage. Spikes continued through the stimulation and persisted until the end of the period of deep recording. The scalp EEG's remained semistuporous throughout the patient's hospitalization.

(d) Stimulation technique—There were two septal stimulations of 2 minutes each, at a current of 5 ma. in one and a current of 8 ma. in the other. Constant measurements of currents were made, so that the intensity of stimulation could be controlled throughout the duration of the stimulus.

(e) Immediate physiological effects—Stimulation to the septal electrode produced a blood pressure rise from 120/86 to 150/106 without any other apparent physiological effect.

(f) Immediate behavioral response—The patient appeared to brighten up and spoke a few words during the stimulation.

(g) Immediate chemical changes—No chemical data were obtained.

(h) Complications—None.

Follow-up Notes. Immediately after the operation it was thought that the patient seemed more alert and responsive to his environment, although he generally remained mute and inaccessible. On the second and third nights he became acutely disturbed, again showing his impulsive destructive behavior. On the fourth day he spoke his first sentence and subsequently increased his verbal productions until, 12 days after operation, he could be contacted at will, although persistent prodding was required. His silly smiling and bizarre mannerisms lessened significantly. Ten days after surgery he went out on a pass with his family. During this visit he seemed to appreciate passively what was going on about him but did not enter into the family activity. On the ward, for the first time, he would smoke cigarettes and show interest in games and occupational therapy, but only as an observer. During the third postoperative week he maintained his gains but showed no further improvement. This was the point of maximum improvement; gradually, over the next few weeks, he returned to his preoperative status. Finally he was transferred back to the state hospital, unimproved, 6 months after operation. Psychological data could not be obtained.

Follow-up on June 1, 1953, 24 months after operation, reveals no change in the patient's status.

PATIENT 10

AGE AT OPERATION: 56
SEX: Male
MARITAL STATUS: Single
OCCUPATION: Stenographer-bookkeeper
RELIGION: Catholic (inactive)
INFORMANT: Brother
DIAGNOSIS: Schizophrenic reaction, hebephrenic type
OPERATION: June 7, 1951

Presenting Picture. The patient was admitted to the psychiatric wards of Charity Hospital in May, 1951, as a transfer from a nearby veterans' hospital. On admission he was generally idle and seclusive. For long periods he sat by the window staring out into space. When approached, he was often friendly though somewhat silly; at other times he was hostile and negativistic. His productions were generally cryptic and illogical and sometimes totally incoherent, but at other times childishly concrete or symbolic. Somatic delusions dominated his thoughts.

Present Illness. The patient has been continuously hospitalized for 17 years. His first psychotic symptoms were delusions that his food was poisoned and that people were accusing him of various sexual perversions. He became confused, untidy, and disorganized in his behavior. At that time he was actively hallucinating. Hospital records reveal that throughout the years his behavior would vary from untidy, mute, inaccessible negativism (during which he had to be tube-fed to avoid emaciation) to neat, tidy, hostile, aggressiveness with elaborate paranoid delusions.

Previous Personality Disorders. There is no history of psychotic episodes before the onset of the present illness.

Family History. The patient was the eleventh of thirteen children born to a strict Catholic family of low income. The father made a marginal living as a salesman and merchant. According to the informant there was little love or affection shown to any particular sibling, as the mother was "too busy caring for all the children." An older brother is at present hospitalized with a diagnosis of schizophrenia.

Personal History. The patient was born in New Orleans in 1895. No specific information is available regarding his birth and early development, although they were presumably normal. At school he completed the eighth grade but took no part in group activities and showed no interest in girls. He apparently formed no strong attachments to members of his family. At the age of 20 he left home to work as a clerk-stenographer for the Government, a job he resumed after an honorable discharge from the Army during World War I. He was engaged to be married at one time but broke the engagement for unknown reasons and has displayed no interest in the opposite sex since.

Personality. Always considered shy and withdrawn, the patient, unlike his siblings, was not interested in sports, outdoor activities, or social events. Although he has had virtually no heterosexual contacts, there is no history of homosexuality.

Physical and Laboratory Status. The patient is a well-developed, moderately obese male with a history of hypertension for the past 10 years and diabetes requiring 40 units of protamine zinc insulin per day for the past 6 months. On physical examination it was found that his blood pressure varied from 100/70 to 130/90, although during the previous hospitalization his blood pressure, quite low during mute, inaccessible periods, had been generally significantly elevated during more lucid paranoid periods, varying from 160/105 to 150/100. On transfer to the Charity Hospital, his hypertension disappeared and his diabetes markedly improved. During the previous hospitalization the glucose tolerance test revealed a blood sugar rise to 500 mg/100 ml. and his fasting blood sugars had been as high as 274 mg/100 ml. with 4+ sugar spilled in the urine. Even under insulin his blood sugars averaged around 200 mg/100 ml. and he continued to spill sugar. In this hospital his fasting blood sugars were all within the normal range. On the Exton-Rose test his fasting blood sugar was 145 mg/100 ml. At 30 minutes, 1 hour, and 2 hours the determinations were respectively 240, 345, and 324 mg/100 ml. Neurological findings were normal, and CBC, serology, urinalysis, and EKG were all normal. Chest films showed slight cardiac enlargement; skull films revealed pineal calcifications; and EEG showed low voltage fast waves.

Hospital Course. On the ward the patient was generally idle, seclusive, and unkempt. He spent most of his daylight hours staring out of the window. When approached by hospital personnel he generally smiled in a silly way, replying to the question, "How are you?" by saying, "I'm alive." He often resisted ward routine and at times became openly belligerent and assaultive. His mood was rapidly variable, including periods of depression, anger, resentment, suspicion and silly friendliness. Usually cryptic and illogical, his productions were at times completely incoherent and at times understandable in a childishly concrete or symbolic way. Although generally terse and unproductive, when aroused he would have a rapid flow of disconnected associations. Mental content centered around somatic delusions, of which he said, "The people downstairs are affecting my brains" or "I don't hear through my ears, no air around here." There was no significant change in his behavior during the two weeks prior to operation, but throughout this period it was considerably more psychotic than it had been at the other hospital. There the patient had been in much better contact with his surroundings, and he had seemed more friendly, outgoing, productive, and cooperative. He would go into minute details concerning his early life, showing an astounding memory concerning names, addresses, and small episodes that had occurred during early childhood. It was at this time, also, that he had had persistent hypertension and diabetes.

Operation—Stimulation. June 7, 1951.

(a) Surgical technique—Open technique was used.

(b) Electrode placements—Three bipolar electrodes were implanted. X-ray study showed lead 1 in the caudate nucleus and lead 2 about 3 mm.

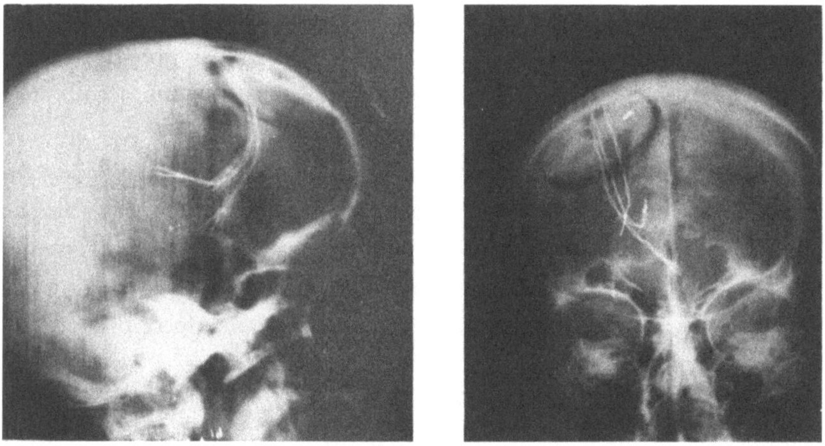

FIGURE XIX-5. Patient 10

rostral to the foramen of Monro in the septal region. Lead 3 was angulated toward the thalamus but appeared to be too high to be in the thalamus and too far caudal to be in the anterior thalamic region; it was therefore assumed to be in the corpus callosum.

(c) Recordings—Prestimulation deep recordings showed a few spikes in the septal lead 2. They were particularly prominent in records made while the patient was asleep (i.e., had not recovered from anesthesia). In poststimulation recordings the spikes appeared to be reduced; it was difficult to obtain samples over a long period, since the patient was not likely to remain asleep while a record was being made. Preoperative EEG's were normal. After stimulation random spikes appeared in the scalp recordings and lasted for 2 1/2 months; the patterns then returned to normal.

(d) Stimulation technique—There were four stimulations to the septal electrode (lead 2), lasting from 2 to 11 1/2 minutes at peak currents of 10 ma. In addition there was one stimulation to lead 3 (the lead intended for the anterior thalamic region but actually placed in the corpus callosum), lasting 2 minutes at a current of 4 ma. Current was measured and maintained throughout the period of stimulation.

(e) Immediate physiological effects—Stimulation to the septal electrode (lead 2) produced a rise in blood pressure from 116/82 to 186/124 without any other apparent physiological effects. Stimulation to lead 3 produced no apparent physiological effect.

(f) Immediate behavioral response—There was no response from stimulation to lead 3, but a marked change in psychological status occurred during the septal stimulation—the patient becoming more alert, less disorganized in his thought processes, and much more coherent.

(g) Immediate chemical changes—The eosinophil count dropped from 140 to 20 per cu. mm. following operation, and there was a further drop (from 20 to 5 per cu. mm.) following stimulation. The lymphocyte count did not change significantly.

(h) Complications—Following implantation an infection developed which responded to removal of the bone button.

Follow-up Notes. On the second day after operation, the patient continued to be more alert, recognized his doctor readily, and showed mild hypertension, with a blood pressure of 140/94. Urine was negative for sugar. He was less resistive to ward routine and laboratory procedures but complained about pain in his head. Tears were noted in his eyes, suggesting a somewhat more intense and appropriate emotional response. Subsequently, he again became more withdrawn and delusional, maintaining that he had not been operated upon but had merely received a "haircut." At first he did not take an interest in the ward activity, but within 1 month after surgery he was on the open ward, showing more interest in what was going on around him and appearing friendlier. He was certainly more cooperative. However, the transfer to the open ward stirred up numerous fears and uncertainties; the patient looked like a scared rabbit in his new environment. He gradually became friendlier, would wave to various doctors when they walked by, and eventually showed some initiative in walking down the hall to the solarium. He enjoyed visits with his family, although, as before operation, he denied that they were really his family, saying, "Not relatives, just associations." Frequently he now forgot not to address them as brother, sister, and so on. At this time the Exton-Rose test revealed a fasting blood sugar of 80 mg/100 ml. At 30 minutes, 1 hour, and 2 hours the determinations were respectively 143, 167, and 200 mg/100 ml. A similar result was obtained on examination 2 months later. During the month of August the patient vacillated between warm, friendly, cooperative behavior, participating in games with ward personnel and playing checkers with his therapist, and seclusive, negativistic, hostile moods, during which he would lock himself in his room. These swings occurred at 2- or 3-day intervals. Gradually, during the fourth month after operation, his regressive episodes became more frequent and of longer duration, until it became necessary to transfer him to the closed ward for more intensive supervision. By the fifth month he had regressed to the point where his behavior was almost identical with that noted preoperatively.

During this period the patient's fasting blood sugar fluctuated between a minimum 59 and 91 mg/100 ml. His blood pressure also showed minor fluctuation. During the second month he had a low-grade fever and complained of frontal headaches. Neurological examinations revealed no complications, and he responded to antibiotics. He was transferred back to the veterans' hospital 6 months after operation, with no improvement in his psychosis. At that time EEG was normal. Psychological tests were not obtained.

Follow-up on June 1, 1953, 24 months after operation, reveals no change in the patient's status.

PATIENT 11

AGE AT OPERATION: 19
SEX: Male
MARITAL STATUS: Single
OCCUPATION: None
RELIGION: Protestant (active)
INFORMANTS: Brothers
DIAGNOSIS: Schizophrenic reaction, hebephrenic type
OPERATION: September 20, 1951

Presenting Picture. The patient was brought to Charity Hospital in June, 1951, in a comatose condition after having ingested an unknown quantity of barbiturates.

Present Illness. The onset of the patient's illness was insidious. He had always been considered peculiar by his relatives and associates and since adolescence had been completely dependent, financially and socially, on his family. Three years prior to the present hospitalization he was actively hallucinating. In March, 1950, he was admitted to the psychiatric service of this hospital following a suicide attempt similar to the one which he made in 1951. After a course of 15 electroshock treatments and 15 electronarcosis treatments, which resulted in only slight remission, he was discharged in December, 1950, to the care of his brother. During the subsequent 6 months he became progressively more seclusive and made repeated bizarre attempts at self-mutilation. At times he showed marked inappropriateness of affect, especially silly giggling.

Previous Personality Disorders. Six and 7 years prior to his present admission, the patient had been admitted to the medical wards of this hospital because of dehydration and vomiting. No definite diagnosis was made at either time, nor was there any personality evaluation.

Family History. The patient was the third from the youngest of fourteen siblings born to a lower-class Negro family who subsisted as farm laborers in Mississippi. When the patient was 6 years old the mother died of pneumonia. Subsequently he lived with various step-siblings. Social and economic standards in the family have always been marginal.

Personal History. The patient was born in February, 1932. There is no information concerning his birth and early development. None of the informants recall any serious illness or notable developmental retardation. He was considered of average intelligence, having completed the sixth grade in 5 years. However, he has never held a steady job and after 3 months of military service in 1948 was discharged for ineptness. At one time he was arrested for vagrancy and committed to a juvenile reform institution for 8 months.

Personality. The patient is described as being submissive, withdrawn, inept, and totally dependent upon others for planning or foresight. Any initiative he did show was overly ambitious and unrealistic. His failures have always resulted in withdrawal and seclusiveness.

Physical and Laboratory Status. Except for poor muscular development and sparse hair over the body, the findings of the physical examination were within normal limits. Blood pressure was 102/66. Chest and skull x-rays, EKG, EEG, and glucose tolerance curves were all within normal limits. CBC, blood chemistry, and serology were normal.

Hospital Course. The patient continuously attempted bizarre self-mutilation, remained silly, grimaced frequently, uttered peculiar guttural laughing noises, made desultory attempts at aiding with the ward chores, was quite uninterested in his physical appearance, and often sprawled

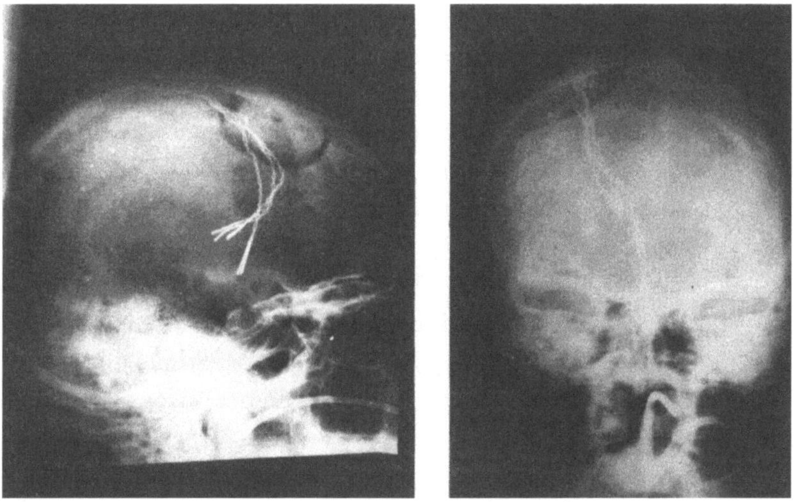

FIGURE XIX-6. Patient 11

out on the floor or crawled about on his hands and knees to secluded corners. He complained of insomnia, had a poor appetite, and often refused to eat for several days. By turns he was either resistive to or overdependent on the ward personnel. He spoke about inferiority feelings and he seemed preoccupied with sexuality. It was apparent that he had hallucinations although he would not discuss them. He did openly express paranoid trends and somatic delusions.

Operation—Stimulation. September 20, 1951.

(a) Surgical technique—Open technique was used.

(b) Electrode placements—Three bipolar electrodes were implanted. On the follow-up x-rays, lead 2 was at the base of the anterior horn of the ventricle about 3 mm. lateral to the midline in the septal region. The other two leads, 1 and 3, were slightly to the right of the midline. It was difficult to determine their exact positions, but both appeared to be high in the caudate nucleus or corpus callosum.

(c) Recordings—Preoperative recordings were inconclusive, but the EEG appeared to be normal. Deep recordings made approximately 8 to 10 hours following the stimulation revealed many slow spikes from the area adjacent to lead 2. On the sixth postoperative day the scalp showed a right frontal delta focus which was present but less marked, with a spread to the right temporal region, on the twelfth postoperative day. One month after operation the scalp EEG was normal.

(d) Stimulation technique—There were two stimulations to the septal region, one for 2 minutes and one for 15 minutes at currents of 8 and 14 ma., respectively. There was one stimulation to a lead in the corpus callosum or the caudate nucleus; it was given for 1 minute at a current of 8 ma.

(e) Immediate physiological effects—Stimulation to lead 2 (in the septal region) produced a mild blood pressure rise from 124/80 to 148/100. There were no other physiological effects. Stimulation to lead 3 (in the caudate nucleus or the corpus callosum) was without any apparent physiological effects.

(f) Immediate behavioral response—The patient became alert and more coherent.

(g) Immediate chemical changes—This was the first patient in whom urinary excretion of electrolytes was followed. Preoperatively the ratio of potassium to sodium was 0.67. On the fourth day postoperatively the ratio was 1.18. We considered this change important in the light of the seizures at that time, since it indicated sodium retention or potassium excretion. There was diuresis of 4.55 liters on the first postoperative day.

(h) Complications—The patient had convulsions with hemiparesis 4 days after operation.

Follow-up Notes. For the first 3 days after operation the patient continued to be more alert and less preoccupied with somatic complaints despite the craniotomy. However, on the fourth postoperative day he had a generalized seizure followed by eleven more seizures occuring in the next 12 hours. This was followed by a 24-hour period wherein the patient was comatose and showed a right flaccid paralysis with a positive Babinski. On the seventh postoperative day the patient became responsive and asked for nourishment. He had no subsequent convulsions. The right-sided paralysis gradually disappeared until, 3 weeks after operation, neurological findings were within normal limits. By the twelfth post-operative day he was showing some initiative and appeared more social and spontaneous. He waved and smiled appropriately to everybody who passed, his appetite improved, and he became more demanding and self-assertive. He showed some interest in occupational therapy. He continued, however, to have self-deprecatory and self-mutilative ideas and occasionally a recrudescence of inappropriate laughter and grimacing. Four weeks after operation the patient expressed some depression, complaining that his family showed no interest in him. At the same time he asked one of the nurses for nail polish, painted his fingers red, assumed girlish poses, and proudly displayed his feminine mannerisms before the other patients. He continued, though to a lessening degree, to have hallucinations. He said that "voices" told him to commit suicide and made several bizarre exhibitionistic attempts to follow out these commands. Five weeks after operation he went on his first pass. He seemed elated upon his return, but, periodically thereafter he lapsed either into moods of depression or into homosexual acting-out, his affective responses were still shallow, and residuals of inappropriate silliness were apparent. Nevertheless, his emotional responses showed much improvement postoperatively. His depressions abated in both frequency and extent, and he now made a conscious effort to participate in activities whenever he felt a "blue spell" coming on. He continued with mild self-deprecatory ideas and expressed some referential trends. His EEG was normal at the time of his discharge, 17 weeks after operation, to the care of his brother, who, as the only available relative, had to be coerced into taking the patient. The home environment was highly unfavorable; the patient lived in the most primitive circumstances, sharing a bed with several small children. His brother tended to be exploitive and was often physically abusive. Nevertheless, the patient secured employment washing dishes, at which he worked satisfactorily for 6 weeks. He gradually became more depressed and complained of his old referential paranoid ideas, somatic delusions,. self-mutilative preoccupations, and auditory hallucinations.

These gradually subsided and on June 1, 1953, 20 months after operation, he was living with other relatives, aiding with the housework but showing little interest in seeking employment. He occasionally hears voices but says, "They don't bother me as before."

PATIENT 12

AGE AT OPERATION: 23

SEX: Male

MARITAL STATUS: Single
OCCUPATION: Student
RELIGION: Catholic (active)
INFORMANTS: Mother and father
DIAGNOSIS: Schizophrenic reaction, catatonic type
OPERATION: October 11, 1951

Presenting Picture. On admission to the Charity Hospital in November, 1950, the patient was withdrawn and seclusive. He smoked incessantly, neglected his personal appearance, and remained uncommunicative except for meeting his immediate needs. He showed bizarre mannerisms, such as facial grimacing, tugging at his chin, and staring at his fingers, which were held in an unnatural extended position. Occasionally he would become hostile and negativistic.

Present Illness. Four years before admission the patient discontinued his college work without explanation. He sought and obtained employment but quit work several months later, dissatisfied with his occupation. He returned to school but was unable to function intellectually and therefore took a job as a railroad hand. Although he was withdrawn, seclusive, and irritable, he functioned satisfactorily on the job until he became involved in a weekend escapade with some of his fellow employees. During this weekend he became intoxicated and contracted a gonorrheal urethritis which required medical attention. At that time he became agitated, confused, and then uncontrollably destructive, finally requiring hospitalization and electroshock therapy. He was discharged slightly improved but at home he seemed depressed, continued to be seclusive, and occasionally threatened suicide. He was rehospitalized for another course of EST and discharged in August, 1950, slightly improved. At home he remained idle, seclusive, depressed, and grossly tremulous. He seemed confused and disoriented. When he was seen in one of the local mental hygiene clinics, hospitalization was suggested for a diagnostic work-up, as it appeared that he might have neurological complications.

Previous Personality Disorders. Although the severity of the patient's illness has fluctuated since the fall of 1946, he has been persistently psychotic during this time. Prior to that date he had had no psychotic episodes.

Family History. The patient is the fourth of six siblings born to a large French Catholic family living in rural Louisiana. The other children are all females who have made satisfactory social adjustments. Most of them are married and all have college educations. The father is described as a meek, affectionate man who makes a marginal living operating a small shop. The mother is an obese, cooperative, friendly woman, affectionate toward her children and rather indulgently protective.

Personal History. The patient was born in 1927 after a full-term, uncomplicated pregnancy. His early development seemed normal in every respect, except that he had enuresis until the age of 6. Although described by the family as a colorless child, he was not considered abnormal in his social or scholastic adjustment. From the parents' description it would seem that the patient preferred to be a follower in play with his contemporaries and was excessively dependent upon the family. He graduated from high school and attended college without showing any particular interest in education—merely following the family tradition in a passive way. At 14 he accidentally shot himself, but there is no evidence that this was an attempt at self-mutilation. He was popular in the community and had close friendships with several boys. He showed the usual interest in girls during adolescence and had his first coital experience at that time.

Personality. The patient is described as a passive, conforming, overly dependent individual. He was an average student but showed little initiative or ambition.

Physical and Laboratory Status. Routine physical examination showed no abnormalities. Neurological examination revealed mild cogwheel rigidity in the upper and lower extremities, slightly greater on the left. There was also suggestive dysdiadochokinesis and weakness, again on the left. Pneumoencephalograms, x-rays of the skull, EEG, EKG, urine, CBC, serology, and BUN were all normal. Subsequent neurological examinations revealed no definite or persistent abnormality. The patient showed an eosinophil response to cortisone but not to epinephrine or ACTH.

Hospital Course. On the ward the patient remained seclusive, withdrawn, hostile, and negativistic. He responded well to 15 electronarcosis treatments in March, 1951, but 6 days following cessation of treatment returned to his previous status. In May, 1951, a craniotomy was performed for the stimulation procedure. Cortical incision and electrode placement were not carried out because an anomalous vein was encountered on the cortex. Arteriograms demonstrated anomalous superficial cerebral veins but no arterial abnormalities. Maintenance electroshock therapy was started in July, 1951, and discontinued in September, 1951. Immediately following cessation of shock therapy the patient was slightly less withdrawn and more cooperative. However, this improvement rapidly disappeared. At the time of his second operation he was uncommunicative, untidy, continued with his bizarre mannerisms, smoked incessantly, and showed little emotional response except for anxiety manifested predominantly by tremulousness and tachycardia. His face was immobilized, suggesting perplexity and confusion, and he spoke in a flat, soft monotone. Rarely he would show outbursts of anger and assaultiveness. Under sodium amytal he became more communicative, complained about "losing my sense," and admitted to one or two episodes of vague auditory hallucinations. He was tried on intermuscular injections of sodium amytal and responded to this regimen by becoming more friendly, cooperative, and communicative. However, this improvement gradually subsided despite persistent medication. He appeared to be grossly oriented and seemed to have no recent or remote memory defects but was uncooperative for further intelligence testing.

Operation—Stimulation. October 11, 1951.

(a) Surgical technique—Open technique was used.

(b) Electrode placements—Three bipolar electrodes were implanted. They were, however, misdirected into subcortical structures of the left cerebral hemisphere. All were placed in the lateral wall of the left ventricle instead of the medial wall of the right ventricle. Air studies after operation aided in locating the actual placements. The uppermost electrode (lead 3) was farthest lateral and clearly in the capsule. The other two electrodes were close to the capsule. Lead 2 was probably in the caudate nucleus close to the capsule. Lead 1 was likewise close to the capsule but was deeper than lead 2, probably touching the gray matter of the ventral aspect of the ventricle (possibly the ventral caudate). All were caudal to the foramen of Monro. The farthest forward (lead 2) was still a few millimeters behind the foramen.

(c) Recordings—Six preoperative EEG's were all normal. Deep re-

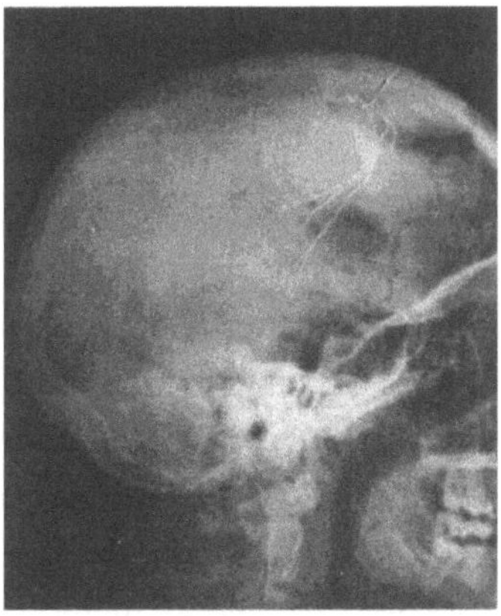

FIGURE XIX–7. Patient 12

cordings prior to stimulation showed no spikes and nothing of particular interest except spindles corresponding to a clinical state of drowsiness or sleep. Slow waves and sleep humps likewise appeared from time to time. There were four postoperative scalp EEG's. The first two, covering a period of 2 1/2 months, showed abnormalities characterized by random spikes; the last two were normal.

(d) Stimulation technique—Many stimulations were carried out, because two of the leads gave tonic movements suggestive of capsular stimulation. Subsequent stimulations were made at low frequency as a check on the capsular placement. Lead 2 (the deep electrode), when stimulated at 100 c/second on the first two occasions, produced a diminished state of awareness resembling sleep. Lead 1 which appeared to be in the ventral aspect of the caudate, produced the most pronounced awakening effect and was therefore stimulated more than the others, with an intensity of 4 to 12 ma., lasting from 2 to 4 minutes. During this stimulation the patient appeared to be somewhat more alert.

(e) Immediate physiological effects—Stimulation to the deep electrode (lead 1) produced autonomic effects including flushing, sweating, dilatation of the pupils, and increased respiration. The most pronounced effect, however, was a tonic movement of the right arm and leg, a turning of the body to the right, and a rolling of the eyes outward and upward to the right. This was followed by a period of stupor. Stimulation to lead 3 (in the caudate near the capsule) produced similar but less pronounced effects. Stimulation to lead 2 produced dilatation of the pupils and at first a generalized increase in motor activity, which gradually blended into a decreased state of awareness indistinguishable from sleep.

(f) Immediate behavioral response—There was increased alertness during the stimulation of the ventral aspect of the caudate (lead 1).

(g) Immediate chemical changes—Preoperatively the patient did not respond to the Thorn test made either with epinephrine or ACTH; he responded only to cortisone. He did react to the stress of surgery with a loss of eosinophils. The Thorn test was continued for 7 months following stimulation, with only one response on November 14. This patient remains a classic non-responder. Urinary electrolyte excretion studies showed that for the period including operation and the immediate stimulation, the potassium-sodium ratio was 0.85, which is considered within normal range. Another urinary excretion study done 5 days following stimulation showed a ratio of 2.8, indicating considerable retention of sodium. There were no changes in plasma electrolytes.

(h) Complications—None.

Follow-up Notes. The most immediate and pronounced postoperative changes in the patient were marked emotional responses. At first he showed marked hostility, expressed by striking out or spitting at the ward personnel, but 2 weeks following operation this gradually disappeared and the patient became quite amiable and pleasant. For the first time he showed some spontaneity, mixed freely with the other patients, called the nurses by name, and took an interest in his personal appearance. Three weeks after operation his anxiety and resentment returned. From time to time he became negativistic and gradually lost interest in the ward activity, although retaining his increased spontaneity and emotional warmth. One month after operation he left the hospital on his first pass and responded to this experience with obvious delight. Upon his return, however, he seemed somewhat depressed and negativistic. Five weeks after operation he went home on a visit for the first time. There he seemed keenly aware of his surroundings, commented about changes in the house, and asked about old friends, although showing considerable anxiety and blocking. Nevertheless, the family was impressed with his improvement and asked for his release from the hospital 1 1/2 months after operation. When he was seen 2 weeks later in the clinic he showed extreme anxiety, marked tachycardia, tremulousness, and irritability and complained that he was doing too much and felt pressed at home. His anxiety mounted until, 1 month after his discharge, he became assaultive and destructive and made an abortive attempt to mutilate himself with a knife, thus precipitating rehospitalization. A really intense depression became evident for the first time. He expressed the feeling that his family had betrayed him by returning him to the hospital and for some time he was negativistic and uncooperative. He was again placed on sodium amytal (3 grains intramuscularly three times a day) and responded readily to this treatment, becoming pleasant and cooperative, less fearful, and less tremulous. Soon he expressed a desire to return home. Five weeks after readmission and 13 weeks after operation he went on a 3-day visit, during which he adjusted satisfactorily. He was discharged for the second time 1 week later. At that time the family stated that he seemed better than he had been for years. He showed spontaneous interest in the farm, displayed initiative in aiding with the chores, took care of his personal needs, and entered actively into social conversations. For the first 2 weeks at home he was maintained on oral sodium amytal. He has used the amytal medication once since. Seven months postoperatively, 2 1/2 months after his second discharge, he continued to make excellent adjustment at home. He planted twenty acres of cotton, milked the cows, ran the tractor, and had only rare outbursts of anger when frustrated in his work performance. He reacted to these outbursts with guilt and repentance. He rarely socialized outside of the family and expressed ideas which suggest that he would take it as a personal failure if adverse weather conditions led to a crop failure. His EEG showed random spikes 2 1/2 months postoperatively but by 3 months was normal. He still showed no eosinophil stress reaction, except for one occasion when he was taking sodium amytal. Psychological testing revealed marked improvement in his records, although there was still evidence of psychotic material.

As of June 1, 1953, 19 months after operation, he continued to maintain his dramatic improvement.

Patient 13

AGE AT OPERATION: 35
SEX: Male
MARITAL STATUS: Single

OCCUPATION: Musician
RELIGION: Catholic (active)
INFORMANTS: Mother, sister, brother, previous hospital record
DIAGNOSIS: Schizophrenic reaction, hebephrenic type
OPERATION: October 23, 1951

Presenting Picture. The patient was transferred to Charity Hospital from another hospital in October, 1951. At that time he was withdrawn, uncommunicative, manneristic, passively cooperative, and emotionally flat.

Present Illness. In 1944, while the patient was serving in the armed forces overseas, he became preoccupied with death and religion. He was withdrawn, confused, and uninterested in his personal needs. Being incapable of active duty, he was hospitalized and evacuated to the States, where he recovered enough to receive an honorable discharge. Upon returning home, however, he was idle, seclusive, and preoccupied with the idea of becoming a priest. He finally entered a Catholic school to accomplish this goal, but he failed to keep up with his studies and was generally untidy and unkempt in personal appearance. Hospitalization became necessary in the fall of 1947 when he refused to eat. At that time he was diagnosed as showing a schizophrenic reaction, paranoid type. He received subcoma insulin and electroshock therapy, following which, though unimproved, he left the hospital against medical advice. Several months later, in June, 1948, he became assaultive and uncontrollable, was rehospitalized, and received insulin-coma therapy and maintenance shock treatments. In the hospital he varied between assaultive, paranoid behavior and mute, negativistic, semicatatonic behavior; in both phases he presented a feeding problem. He frequently indulged in posturing and bizarre ritualistic mannerisms and at times exhibited a rapt, ecstatic preoccupation. After 61 insulin comas the patient gave up his bizarre mannerisms and no longer went into catatonic trances. Although he had no insight into his illness, he was placed on a full schedule of rehabilitative activity. Within several months, however, he had reverted to his former behavior. Periodic assaultiveness required assignment to the disturbed ward. At the time of transfer he was receiving custodial care only.

Previous Personality Disorders. There had been no previous psychotic episodes.

Family History. The patient is the youngest of five children born to an immigrant Catholic family in which discipline was strict and parental authority unquestioned. There was a great deal of religious tension in the house—the father leaving the Church and returning to it several times. The father was able to provide an adequate income for the family from his own business in which he was aided by his wife, the children being left in the care of a maid. The father is irritable and easily provoked to violent outbursts of rage. The mother is a strict, controlling woman, always correcting her children but doing so in a "sweet and gentle way." She seems sincerely interested in her family and openly affectionate. All the siblings are making a satisfactory social adjustment.

Personal History. The patient was born at full-term with no complications. Early physical development was normal. His mother states that he was toilet-trained at the age of 2 months. He had few friends but was an average student, graduating from high school at the age of 16. He became an accomplished musician but had few other outside interests. Although he played off and on in dance bands, he never held a steady job prior to his entrance into the army in 1940 at the age of 24. He enlisted voluntarily and finally obtained the rating of sergeant. He never showed sustained heterosexual interest.

Personality. The patient has always been a quiet, somewhat seclusive, obedient person, generally friendly and agreeable but not outgoing. He was excessively preoccupied with cleanliness. Prior to his psychosis he did not express any unusual interest in religion.

Physical and Laboratory Status. Results of the physical and neurological examination were within normal limits. Laboratory tests, including urinalysis, CBC, blood glucose, serology, chest x-rays, EEG, and EKG were all normal. He did not react to the Thorn test.

Hospital Course. On the wards the patient remained untidy, unkempt, and uninterested in his surroundings. He was passively cooperative but easily distracted. He used many bizarre, stereotyped gestures which suggested that he was constantly crossing himself. He fingered his genitalia, giggled in a silly manner when vaguely reporting his hallucinations, and was scattered and illogical in his productions. He performed simple problems without difficulty but could not deal with more complicated ones because of his short attention span. Abstract problems were usually solved in a bizarre, personalized manner involving his religious preoccupation. He was only partially oriented and showed some memory impairment.

Operation—Stimulation. October 23, 1951.

(a) Surgical technique—Open technique was used.

(b) Electrode placements—Three electrodes were implanted. Leads 1 and 2 were both placed about 2 mm. lateral to the midline. Lead 1 was close to the base of the brain, directly below the foramen of Monro (in the hypothalamus). Lead 2 was 2 mm. rostral to the foramen of Monro, about 3 mm. from the base of the brain (in the septo-hypothalamic region). Lead 3 appeared to be slightly forward of the middle of the thalamus, 8 mm. to the left of the midline.

(c) Recordings—Two preoperative EEG's were normal. The first postoperative scalp recording, made approximately 1 month after operation, showed on both sleep and waking a delta focus in the right frontal and to a lesser degree in the right temporal region. Six months after operation there was a right delta focus indicative of symptomatic epilepsy. Just prior to this EEG the patient had one generalized convulsive seizure. On deep recordings, lead 2 showed high amplitude spikes very frequently. Very sharp high amplitude spikes were also obtained from lead 1. Lead 3, which was more lateral than the spiking leads 1 and 2, showed none of the characteristic spikes. Stimulations to lead 2 (septo-hypothalamic) showed a petit mal pattern through the deep recordings. No scalp electrodes were in place at the time. After this pattern had been evident for a matter of a minute or two, there were some clinical manifestations of a petit mal seizure characterized by a diminished awareness and twitching of the thumb. Following stimulation to lead 3 there was marked increase in the spikes in lead 2. Following many of the stimulations there was a temporary reduction in the occurrence of spikes. The next day they were found to be still present, coming through quite strongly though perhaps slightly reduced.

(d) Stimulation technique—A total of thirteen discrete stimulations were administered, ranging in intensity from 2 to 12 ma. and in duration from 30 seconds to 17 minutes.

(e) Immediate physiological effects—Stimulation to the hypothalamic electrode (lead 1) produced an initial rise in blood pressure from 148/92

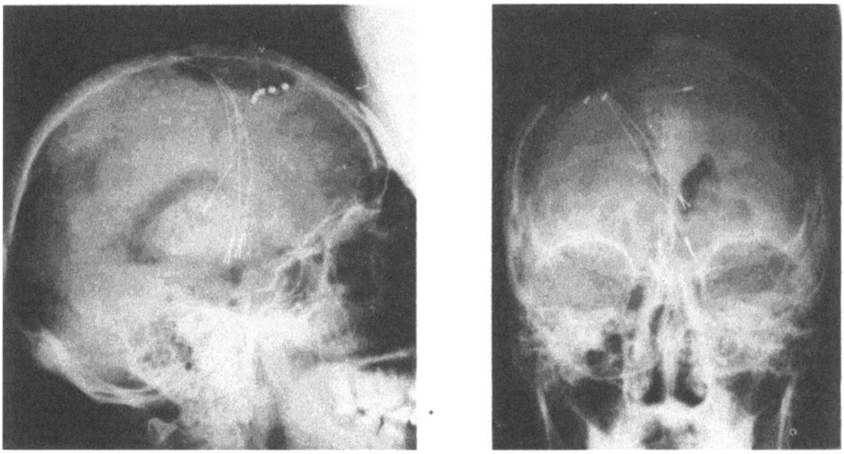

FIGURE XIX–8. Patient 13

to 175/115 along with a diffuse sympathetic discharge, a clonic movement of the right arm and leg, and left internal strabismus followed by convergence as the current was increased. The patient complained of nervousness, urinary urgency, and chills. Stimulation to the septo-hypothalamic electrode (lead 2), produced no immediate blood pressure response, but as current was increased, pressure rose from 140/70 to 190/108. Tachycardia of 180, flushing, sweating, and dilatation of the pupils were noted; and as stimulation was continued, there developed a clonic 3-per-second movement of the right thumb with what appeared to be a petit mal variant seizure. Stimulation to the left midthalamic electrode (lead 3) produced apnea and an associated decrease in awareness.

(f) Immediate behavioral response—Two minutes after the petit mal EEG pattern appeared, some clinical manifestations of a petit mal seizure occurred, characterized by a diminished awareness and twitching of the thumb. On septal stimulation the patient become more alert and productive.

(g) Immediate chemical changes—Preoperatively there was no response to the Thorn test. Only three lymphocyte counts were taken on the day of stimulation. The level after operation but before stimulation was 2,590 per cu. mm. The second count, at the time of stimulation, was 2,788 per cu. mm. The third count, taken 6 hours after the last stimulation, was 1,510 per cu. mm. In the light of data on other patients this drop may be considered significant. Six days following stimulation the count was 925 per cu. mm. Urinary excretion studies showed that the potassium-sodium ratio was 0.56 on the day of operation (i.e., the 24-hour period beginning at the outset of the operation). One day after stimulation it was 0.53, and 2 days after stimulation it was 0.78. There were no changes in plasma electrolytes.

(h) Complications—The patient had convulsions 6 and 8 months postoperatively. Transient right-sided neurological signs were noted for 4 to 5 days after operation.

Follow-up Notes. During the first 3 days postoperatively the patient was febrile and somnolent, having to be fed by vein. During this period he had one generalized convulsion. By the end of the week, however, he was out of bed feeding himself, though openly masturbating and occasionally defecating on the floor. At that time he was mute, often seen kneeling and praying. Two weeks after operation he went to occupational therapy, played cards with the other patients, and talked spontaneously for the first time. Three weeks after operation there was a definite increase in his emotional responsivity. He appeared more cheerful, did not seem as preoccupied with his religious ideas, and engaged in such ward activities as ping-pong and dancing. One month after operation he left the hospital on his first pass. Throughout this period he displayed rather extreme mental confusion and disorientation, which had probably been present before operation but less apparent because of his limited productivity. He continued to improve during the second month, was less gluttonous, and would occasionally help with the ward chores. However, he often reverted to his previous stereotyped religious mannerisms and remained relatively sparse in his production, answering the doctor's questions in as few words as possible. On January 22, 1952, 3 months after operation, he was discharged. He continued with his religious preoccupation but seemed in better contact with his surroundings and more responsive to his family. He socialized freely, talked spontaneously with the therapist, and even demonstrated some humor in teasing his father. During the fourth and fifth months after operation he began to take more interest in the home, caring for the yard and doing minor crude carpentry work. Although his disorientation and severe memory impairment continued, he would surprise his family by finding his way around town even in strange sections. He went to the movies by himself and gradually dropped his stereotyped mannerisms or modified them so that they appeared more like tics. He was neat and clean, though somewhat restless, and showed some return of his prepsychotic intelligence—that is, his speech reflected his relatively high scholastic achievements. He was able to perform simple arithmetical problems rapidly and accurately and responded to the similarities test and proverb-interpretation test at a highly abstract level. He still carried a catechism with him and attended church regularly but no longer openly expressed religious delusions. In describing his personality changes, his mother said, "It certainly is a miracle, although I do hope his memory comes back." Postoperative EEG's have shown persistent right frontal delta (S-3) focus. On two occasions, 6 and 8 months after operation, he had a seizure. For this he was placed on phenobarbital 8 months after operation. Psychological tests revealed slight improvement.

In November, 1952, the patient's old symptoms returned to such an extent that hospitalization was required. However, on custodial care, occupational therapy, and minimal psychotherapy he regained his previous improvement, being discharged April, 1953. On June 1, 1953, 19 months after operation, his adjustment at home was the same as that described.

PATIENT 14

AGE AT OPERATION: 22

SEX: Male

MARITAL STATUS: Single

OCCUPATION: Student

RELIGION: Catholic (active)

INFORMANTS: Mother, father, and the patient. Information also obtained from previous hospital records.

DIAGNOSIS: Schizophrenic reaction, paranoid type

OPERATION: November 20, 1951

Presenting Picture. The patient was admitted to Charity Hospital in September, 1951. He was shabbily dressed, wore his hair in long ringlets, and had a stringy moustache and a goatee that gave him a messiah-like appearance. Despite the sedation given him by a private physician because he refused hospitalization, he was in a panic—barricading himself in his room and refusing to cooperate with the ward personnel.

Present Illness. The patient became acutely psychotic in June 1951, when he refused to eat or leave his bed. He demanded that his food be sterilized or boiled in Lysol, bathed both his feet in Lysol, and sprayed Lysol on his genitals. He would not allow his dirty clothes to be touched, fearing that the germs might be disturbed and thus might contaminate the air. To meet the coercive demands of his germ phobia, his parents had moved from the city to an isolated country home.

Previous Personality Disorders. In 1948, while a senior student in college, majoring in physics, the patient suddenly found that he had difficulty in performing work that had previously been easy for him. At this time he became frightened of dirt and spent many hours under the shower scrubbing himself. He was hospitalized and received a series of electroshock treatments which were followed by marked improvement lasting 10 to 12 months. He again relapsed and received further EST followed by insulin-coma therapy. Again he improved, but this time relapsed shortly after his discharge in June, 1950.

Family History. The patient is an only child, born to an upper middle-class Catholic family. The father made a substantial living, despite a limited education. He is somewhat effeminate in mannerisms. The mother appears especially meek, constantly complaining that she feels left out. She is afraid to drink water away from home, and whenever she uses a public toilet will sterilize the seat with a bottle of iodine carried in her purse. The father was stern, yet affectionate; both parents were indulgent and overprotective of their son, who responded by excessive dependency on their approval and praise.

Personal History. The patient was born by a breech delivery in February, 1929, after a normal pregnancy. He had a "wry" neck for the first month of his life. He was breast-fed on a schedule, based on the then-popular "let them cry" technique. As a child he was relegated to the basement to play so that he would not disrupt his mother's meticulous housekeeping. He performed well in parochial school, socialized readily, and was interested in sports and dances. In college he seemed to make a normal, if somewhat inhibited, adjustment. He did exceptionally well scholastically, had many friends among the men, with whom he drank regularly. He had occasional dates but never did any "heavy necking." His present illness began in his senior year when he suddenly discovered that he was becoming "dumb" and failing in his courses; he then developed systematized obsessional delusions.

Personality. Prior to the onset of his psychosis, the patient appeared to be an obedient, dependent individual, overly attached to his parents but nevertheless making a satisfactory social adjustment and being accepted by his colleagues. He has always shown a preoccupation with death and abhorred the killing or harming of defenseless animals.

Physical and Laboratory Status. Physical and neurological findings were within normal limits. Blood pressure was 120/80. Blood glucose varied from 89 to 111 mg/100 ml. EKG, EEG, urinalysis, CBC, and serology were all within normal limits. On the Thorn test the patient did not react.

Hospital Course. On the ward the patient remained completely isolated, barricading himself in his room to prevent other patients from contaminating him with "nerve germs." Whenever approached by patients, he would shout at the top of his voice, "Keep that queer away from me!" He refused to use the common toilet facilities—remaining unbathed and unshaven in his room, which was strewn with dirty clothes and feces. However, he cooperated with the physicians, because he felt that he was in the hospital for laboratory tests which would prove his sanity to his parents. When it became obvious that he was going to be operated on, he became assaultive and destructive. Toward the hospital personnel he maintained a haughty, condescending air, but became demonstratively affectionate whenever his father visited him. Although he appeared to be of superior intelligence, he could not perform even the simplest abstractions without becoming involved in his concrete personal delusions.

Operation—Stimulation. November 20, 1951.

(a) Surgical technique—Open technique was used.

(b) Electrode placements—Three electrodes were implanted. Lead 1 was 1 cm. to the right of the midline at about the depth of the foramen of Monro and probably in the caudate nucleus. Lead 2 was about 15 mm.

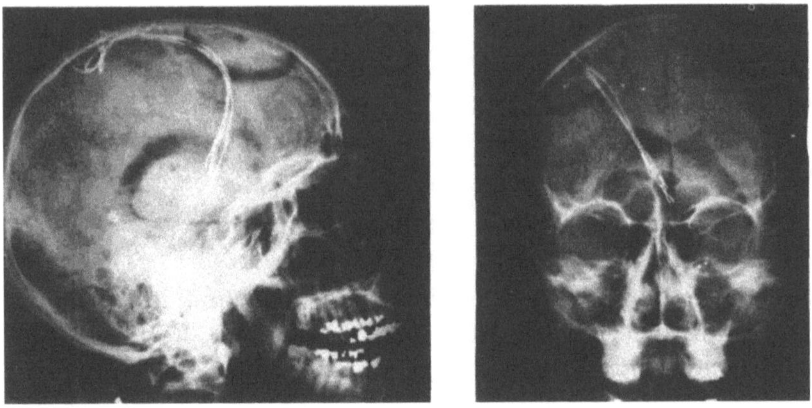

FIGURE XIX–9. Patient 14

ventral to the foramen of Monro and 2 mm. lateral to the midline (in the septo-hypothalamic region). Lead 3 was also close to the midline, about 1 cm. dorsal to lead 1.

(c) Recordings—Two preoperative EEG's were normal. One post-operative scalp recording 4 1/2 months after stimulation showed a slow wave focus and sleep spindle depression. Focus was in the right frontal region. Prestimulation deep recordings showed occasional slow spike and wave patterns in lead 2 when the patient was drowsy or asleep; these were not present when he was awake and alert. Spikes were limited to this lead. There was some suggested correlation between emotional stimuli when the patient was being interviewed and activity on the deep leads. Immediately following one stimulation there was spike and flat-top activity, some slow waves, and high voltage activity limited to the region adjacent to lead 2. During the course of these recordings the patient developed a chill, and interesting records of cortical and sub-cortical activity were subsequently obtained. It is not clear whether the chill, marked by chattering of the teeth and shaking of the body, was related to the previous stimulation, since it did not follow immediately. The subcortical activity began in lead 2 and spread to other subcortical leads. The correspondence between subcortical and scalp activity was striking, the activity showing first in subcortical leads and spreading to the scalp leads. At the conclusion of the period of deep recording no further spiking was seen in the deep leads but this fact is of doubtful importance, since the patient did not become drowsy or go to sleep during this period.

(d) Stimulation technique—There were four septo-hypothalamic stimulations. The duration was 2 to 10 minutes, with currents of 2 to 8 ma.

(e) Immediate physiological effects—Stimulation to the septo-hypothalamic electrode (lead 2), at 2 ma. produced an initial rise in blood pressure from 120/86 to 210/160. This response was a maximal one; as the stimulation was continued the pressure dropped to 160/90. There was tachycardia of 174; flushing, sweating, tremor, dilatation of the pupils, and increased rate of respiration were noted.

(f) Immediate behavioral response—The patient verbalized great anxiety and appeared frightened for some minutes following stimulation. However, he seemed more alert and in better contact with his environment.

(g) Immediate chemical changes—Preoperatively this patient did not respond to the Thorn test, the eosinophils going up after the administration of epinephrine. Following the surgical procedure he responded very promptly and dramatically, the eosinophils dropping 60 per cent and 80 per cent in response to the epinephrine. Following stimulation there was an immediate and very dramatic drop in lymphocytes, which reached a maximum decrease of 80 per cent by 3 3/4 hours after the first stimulation (1 hour after the last stimulation). By the time, on the second day, that the patient was given another stimulation the lymphocytes had climbed to approximately their preoperative level. With that stimulation there was a second drop of 70 per cent. Results of the plasma electrolyte studies are rather indefinite.

(h) Complications—The superficial wound infection which developed postoperatively responded to removal of the bone button, but the patient died suddenly 6 months later with a brain abscess.

Follow-up Notes. The day following operation there were obvious changes in the patient's behavior. He continued to be alert and responsive. He was not so preoccupied with his fear of contamination. When he was offered an ice-cream sundae by the physician, he responded with obvious pleasure, remarking after he had finished, "Good to the last drop." Although he was easily distracted, his general attitude represented a continuation of his previous phobia about contamination. He continued to urinate and defecate in his room. On the sixth postoperative day he developed a fever of 102°F. He was started on antibiotics, and by the eighth day his temperature was normal. On the twelfth day his wound became infected and meningeal signs appeared. On the fourteenth day he was taken to surgery, where the wound was reopened and the bone flap removed. Despite this, his psychiatric condition steadily improved, so that on the twenty-seventh day after operation he was moved to the open ward. He still refused to associate with the other patients but was not afraid of contamination by the doctors or ward personnel. He formed a number of warm attachments with the personnel and liked to joke with them. He expressed some sexual interest in the nurses and was known to have secretly masturbated. Thirty-five days postoperatively he spent Christmas at home. For the first time in many years he rode on buses and streetcars without fear of contamination; however, this increased self-confidence resulted from an omnipotent concept of his father, who would protect him from such a catastrophe. The therapist encouraged identification with his father with partial success. Two months after operation the patient still had no insight into his illness, maintaining steadily that his difficulty was due to "a brain germ." He was approached directly on the subject and informed that there were no germs known to involve the brain in such a manner and that he was a psychotic patient like the rest of the people on the ward. He responded at first with anxiety but subsequently began to mix freely with open ward patients whom he thought were like himself. Four months postoperatively he was spending 6 days out of 7 at home, where he socialized freely with the family and their friends, occasionally had contemporaries in to visit, worked around the house, and began to make plans for subsequent release from the hospital. He was discharged 5 1/2 months after operation and 2 weeks later secured a position as an inspector in a local defense plant. For several days on the job his output was exceedingly low because of the obsessive carefulness. Within a week, however, he was performing satisfactorily and was praised as an exceptional worker by his immediate superior. One week later, approximately 6 months after operation, he discontinued work because of a severe headache. On the following day, when a fever of 102°F. developed, he was immediately admitted to the Charity Hospital (May, 1952). His headaches and fever continued, and he showed mild meningeal signs. During that evening he lapsed into coma. Aspiration of the ventricles through the old operative defect revealed pus. The patient expired shortly after this procedure. Post-mortem examination revealed an abscess in the temporal lobe. Four and a half months postoperatively his EEG had shown right frontal mixed delta, theta focus, and general sleep spindle depression.

Psychological tests had revealed no significant changes despite the definite social recovery.

PATIENT 15. See Patient 8.

PATIENT 16

AGE AT OPERATION: 47
SEX: Female
MARITAL STATUS: Single
OCCUPATION: None
RELIGION: Episcopalian (inactive)
INFORMANT: Mother
DIAGNOSIS: Schizophrenic reaction, paranoid type
OPERATION: December 11, 1951

Presenting Picture. On admission to Charity Hospital in October, 1951, the patient was moderately agitated and uncooperative. She expressed numerous somatic delusions and had fixed referential ideas.

Present Illness. The patient has probably been continuously ill, with periodic exacerbation, for at least 32 years. During this time she has had ten hospitalizations, the first occurring in 1927. During adolescence, prior to the first hospitalization, she developed symptoms suggestive of anorexia nervosa, complaining of loss of appetite, nausea, vomiting, weight loss, and cessation of menstruation, as well as experiencing delusions of oral impregnation after a kiss by one of her boy friends. Subsequently she had numerous obsessive-compulsive traits but until 1935 was hospitalized only for a 6-month period in 1927. In 1935 she spent 3 months in a hospital with a diagnosis of schizophrenic reaction, simple type. She reported only two vague hallucinatory experiences at that time. From 1935 until 1940 she was under the care of a private physician who saw her daily in psychotherapeutic sessions. During this period she was periodically assaultive and uncooperative, both toward her family and toward her therapist. She was again hospitalized in 1940, diagnosed as showing a schizophrenic reaction, hebephrenic type, and was discharged 1 year later without treatment, unimproved. She was rehospitalized in 1946 with the same diagnosis. At that time she was given electroshock therapy, but this was discontinued after 3 treatments because of her marked anxiety. She was shifted to insulin, but after 3 comas escaped from the hospital. At home she was seclusive, hypochondriacal, periodically uncooperative, and habitually silly and giggling. Anxiety and depression were reported, as well as two suicidal attempts. In 1948 she was first admitted to the Charity Hospital with somatic delusions centered around her gastrointestinal tract. She was subsequently committed to a state institution, then readmitted to the Charity Hospital psychiatric service in 1949 with a diagnosis of paranoid schizophrenia. At that time hypochondriacal preoccupations, hostility, uncooperative behavior, referential ideas, and paranoid trends were all noted. Several months later, after slight improvement on psychotherapy, she was discharged from the hospital under the care of her mother. At home she gradually became uncontrollable and was readmitted to this service in July, 1950, at which time her referential delusions were quite fixed. She explained her obsessive behavior on the basis of preventing her thoughts from "killing other people." On the wards she varied between obsequious ingratiation and agitated rage. There was no evidence of intellectual deterioration. She showed some slight insight into her illness, saying, "Something is wrong with my mind. I feel it dimming out." She was again tried on a home visit in August, 1951, but soon became unmanageable and was rehospitalized for her present and tenth hospitalization in October, 1951.

Previous Personality Disorders. The patient has probably been psychotic from the age of 15. Prior to that there were no overt psychotic manifestations, but she did have numerous hypochondriacal preoccupations and phobias.

Family History. The patient is the elder of two children of a middle-class family of moderate means. The father was a railroad man and subsequently a merchant. He is described by the patient as a "crude Irishman." The mother, now 72, seems psychotic and senile; she is irascible and difficult to deal with. At times she accepts the patient's delusions as reality. The patient's brother, three years her junior, works for a contractor, has never been married, and appears rigid, hostile, and extremely insecure. He refuses to visit the hospital because, he says, "The smell makes me feel sick."

Personal History. The patient was born in July, 1904, in New Orleans. Little is known about her birth and early development. Her earliest memories of her parents are that they were excessively strict, showed a preferential attitude toward her brother, were always fighting, and generally created an unpleasant home atmosphere. She admits that she had difficulty getting along with people and did not mix freely with the other children. She can recall having vague disquieting anxieties at the age of 5, stimulated by vividly colored pictures of Hell and the Devil in one of her children's books. At 10 her abdominal complaints began. Of these the patient says, "I soon compensated by being gluttonous." From that time the patient was a chronic invalid, using her gastrointestinal complaints to explain her lack of social participation. On graduation from high school she remained home for several years, "doing nothing but reading and thinking." Subsequently she had several menial jobs but held none of them for more than 3 or 4 months. She has never married, nor has she ever shown strong interest in the opposite sex. Most of her life has been spent either in hospitals or in a dependent state with her family.

Personality. The patient's personality apparently has been deviate since early childhood. She herself has always recognized that she was peculiar and different but denies having been insane. She remembers vague feelings of anxiety and unrest at a very early age and has had continuous somatic complaints since the age of 10.

Physical and Laboratory Status. Results of physical and neurological examinations were within normal limits, as were CBC, urinalysis, blood glucose, EKG, EEG, and x-rays of the skull and chest. Blood pressure varied from 80/60 to 112/80. There was no response to the Thorn test.

Hospital Course. In the hospital the patient continued with her somatic delusions and ideas of reference. There was no evidence of hallucinations. She showed no insight into her illness, denying that there was anything wrong with her except "ptosis of my stomach." She was alternatingly ingratiating and docile, then angry and destructive. She showed no obvious intellectual deficits.

Operation—Stimulation. December 11, 1951.

(a) Surgical technique—Open technique was used.

(b) Electrode placements—Three electrodes were implanted. Lead 1 was 3 mm. rostral to the foramen of Monro and about 6 mm. lateral to the midline in the base of the right anterior horn of the right lateral ventricle (septal region). Lead 2 was within 2 mm. of the midline in the caudal aspect of the septal region (septo-hypothalamic region). Lead 3 was in the anterior thalamus very close to the midline.

(c) Recordings—There were three normal EEG's before operation. The patient was too uncooperative for postoperative scalp recordings. Deep recordings made between operation and stimulation showed very strong spiking from leads 1 and 2. The spikes in lead 1 appeared more frequently and were of greater amplitude; in fact they were among the largest of any seen in the entire patient series, approaching 300 microvolts. After stimulation spiking was markedly reduced and large amounts of slow wave activity appeared in the subcortical leads. Near the end of the record, several hours after stimulation, spikes occurred rarely and were far less sharp than early in the record.

(d) Stimulation technique—There were five stimulations to the septal region (lead 1), lasting 1 to 5 minutes, at currents of 2 to 16 ma. There were also four stimulations of the septo-hypothalamic region (lead 2), lasting 2 to 10 minutes, at currents of 4 to 16 ma.

(e) Immediate physiological effects—Stimulation to the septal electrode (lead 1), produced a slight rise in blood pressure from 120/87 to 130/98. Stimulation to the septo-hypothalamic electrode (lead 2), produced a rise in blood pressure from 118/80 to 178/110. The patient became agitated.

(f) Immediate behavioral response—Increased alertness and responsivity were noted.

(g) Immediate chemical changes—Before operation the patient did not respond to the Thorn test. When the septal region was first stimulated (lead 1), the lymphocyte count was still low as a result of the operation. The lymphocytes then began to increase, and 1 hour later the count reached a peak of 1,702 per cu. mm. About this time the septo-hypo-

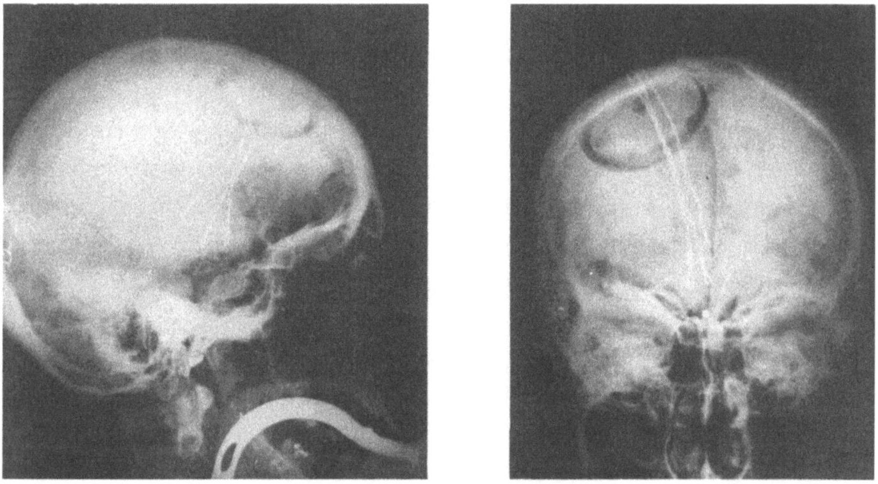

FIGURE XIX-10. Patient 16

thalamic region (lead 2) was stimulated. Two hours after stimulation to lead 1 and 1 hour after stimulation to lead 2, the count dropped to the minimum of 800 per cu. mm. No plasma electrolyte studies were made.

(h) Complications—None.

Follow-up Notes. The day after operation the patient's affective responses seemed definitely more appropriate. She expressed some pleasure and anticipation in seeing her doctor. One of her first remarks following the stimulation was, "Now I don't have to be perfect." Five days later there was definitely less hostility and the patient continued to respond to her doctor with a rather warm smile, saying, "The backseat driver in my brain has now been removed." In 2 weeks she was removed to an open ward, began getting out of bed, and seemed less preoccupied with her delusions. Three and a half weeks after operation she left the hospital on her first pass. The comment by the surgeon at that time was, "The most remarkable improvement I have ever seen in any patient suffering from any disease." One month after operation she was noted to be secretly masturbating. She continued to have a good sense of humor and seemed to appreciate her mother's visits for the first time. Five weeks after operation she developed several acute panic reactions, fearing that the doctors were going to kill her. She ran away from the hospital on two occasions, having to be returned by friends or relatives. After this she showed no interest in leaving the hospital, continued to complain of stomach upsets, and spent most of her time in her room in bed with the door shut. She would not read, complained that her eyes were bothering her, demanded a refraction, but refused this when it was offered. She subsequently refused all diagnostic or therapeutic procedures which would aid in her rehabilitation. An attempt was made to persuade her to go across the street for psychotherapeutic sessions, but after several trials she refused to continue on the ground that it upset her stomach. Nevertheless, the patient's attitude is pleasant, and she has developed considerable insight, saying, "I certainly am crazy." For the first time she has expressed some hope of getting well and seems quite pleased when her obsessions leave her for a few hours, then becomes depressed when they return. Much of her obsessional behavior has gradually disappeared, although she still prefers to remain isolated in her room.

In essence, her improvement seems to have been that she is emotionally more responsive, pleasant, and cooperative, although still isolated and withdrawn. She has somatic complaints which she utilizes for secondary gain. However, she is not so preoccupied with them as before, nor does she interpret them in a delusional way. Her obsessive rituals have gradually been dropped. Her main difficulty at this time is that neither her mother nor her brother is willing to or capable of taking her home and aiding in her rehabilitative process.

No further changes were noted in the patient's condition on June 1, 1953, 18 months after operation.

PATIENT 17

AGE AT OPERATION: 26
SEX: Female
MARITAL STATUS: Single
OCCUPATION: None
RELIGION: Greek Orthodox (active)
INFORMANTS: Father and mother
DIAGNOSIS: Schizophrenic reaction, catatonic type
OPERATION: December 10, 1951

Presenting Picture. At the time of admission to Charity Hospital in

June, 1951, this patient was mute and negativistic. She remained seclusive and showed psycho-motor retardation with occasional outbursts of destructive behavior.

Present Illness. The family have always regarded the patient as different from other children but noticed a definite change in her behavior 2 years prior to her admission. At that time she refused to leave her room, was unable to perform even the most elementary tasks, such as combing her hair or brushing her teeth, and periodically became excited and destructive. After 15 electroshock treatments on an outpatient basis, she improved slightly but relapsed within 2 weeks after cessation of treatment.

Previous Personality Disorders. There were no previous psychotic episodes.

Family History. The patient is the younger of two daughters born to parents who were naturalized Americans of European extraction. The family have rigidly abided by the restrictions of their religion and nationality. All relatives have been successful in the restaurant business except the patient's father, who has repeatedly failed and is now employed as a waiter. The mother is described as a nervous, demanding person whose unreasonable extravagances were considered an important factor in her husband's failures. The patient and her elder sister were reared by their maternal grandmother. The sister was more aggressive in her social relationships and considerably more successful scholastically.

Personal History. The patient was born in October, 1925, in New Orleans, following a full-term gestation and normal delivery. Developmental retardation was obvious, as she did not walk until 23 months nor talk coherently until 4 years of age. She was quiet, withdrawn, and sensitive about being different from other children, constantly praying to God that she might change and be like her contemporaries. She was slow in school, spending 2 to 3 years in each class. Informants state that although she seemed able to learn lessons adequately the night before, by the following morning she had forgotten most of what she had learned. She was constantly agitated over this inability to perform, finally discontinuing school at the age of 15 in the fifth grade. Menarche occurred at 14, but menstrual periods have been irregularly spaced at 2-, 3-, or 4-month intervals. The patient has always been fond of and dependent upon her older sister, whose marriage and moving to another state are felt to have been precipitating factors in the patient's present illness. The parents attribute the patient's psychotic behavior to her open masturbation, which has persisted since early adolescence.

Personality. The patient has always been retarded in her development, sensitive, shy, seclusive, withdrawn, and unable to compete intellectually with her colleagues. Before her illness she was excessively submissive.

Physical and Laboratory Status. Results of physical and neurological examinations were within normal limits. Laboratory studies, including EEG, chest x-rays, urinalysis, CBC, fasting blood sugars, BUN, and serology, revealed no abnormalities. Preoperative EEG showed random spikes and hypersynchrony, interpreted as indicative of remote brain injury. There was no response to the Thorn test.

Hospital Course. On the ward the patient barricaded herself in her room, required 4 to 5 hours to complete her meals, would not respond to questioning, and was at times uncooperative about routine ward care. She usually submitted when attacked by other patients but occasionally became assaultive without provocation. Four months after hospitalization she would make simple demands and occasionally participated in occupational therapy or social games with the other patients although incapable of following even the simplest instructions. She enjoyed leaving the hospital on passes as long as she did not return home, which always precipitated acute anxiety and destructive behavior. She remained slovenly, retarded, and emotionally flat except for an occasional inappropriate smile. She was completely oriented, showed no memory defects, and was able to do simple calculations correctly but slowly. She expressed somatic delusions such as "Food goes into my empty head to fill me up" and mild ideas of reference—"Everybody makes fun of me and talks about me."

Operation—Stimulation. December 10, 1951.

(a) Surgical technique—Open technique was used.

(b) Electrode placements—Three electrodes were implanted. Lead 1 was in the ventral part of the hypothalamic region 5 mm. to the right of the midline. Lead 2 was farther down in the caudal part of the septal region. Lead 3 was in the medial group of thalamic nuclei.

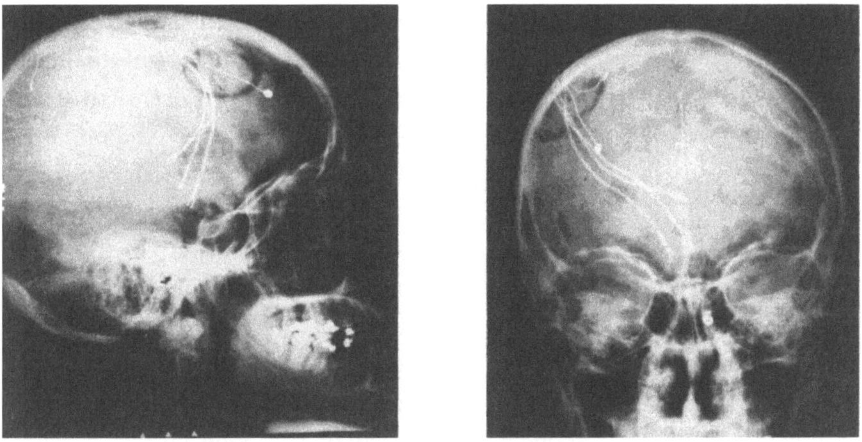

FIGURE XIX-11. Patient 17

(c) Recordings—There were two abnormal preoperative EEG's with random spikes and hypersynchrony in the occipital region. Deep recordings prior to stimulation showed moderate spiking from leads 1 and 2, somewhat greater in lead 1. There may have been some changes on the record during interview prior to stimulation. A postoperative scalp EEG showed right frontal delta focus. For some time following the last stimulation there was a reduction in spikes, whether the patient was asleep or awake.

(d) Stimulation technique—There were three stimulations in the caudal part of the septal region (lead 2), lasting 2 to 6 minutes, at currents of 4 to 12 ma. Five stimuli were administered to the ventral part of the hypothalamic region (lead 1), lasting 2 to 5 minutes, at currents of 2 to 14 ma. One thalamic stimulation, to lead 3, was given for 1 minute 35 seconds at a current of 6 ma.

(e) Immediate physiological effects—Stimulation to the septal electrode (lead 2) produced a rise in blood pressure from 110/70 to 180/100. The sustained effect was erratic, there was tachycardia of 162, a startle reaction appeared, both eyes opened, and the patient expressed fear. Stimulation to the hypothalamic electrode (lead 1) produced a marked rise in blood pressure from 140/80 to 200/120. Again the maintenance of this pressure was erratic, and there were a marked tachycardia and a startle reaction, the eyes opened, and a right external strabismus occurred. Following stimulation there was a marked cardiac arrhythmia. The patient again complained of fear. Stimulation to the thalamic electrode (lead 3) produced no apparent physiological effect whatsoever.

(f) Immediate behavioral response—The patient appeared more alert and now verbalized coherently; however, she did complain of feeling anxious.

(g) Immediate chemical changes—There was no response to the Thorn test before operation. The maximum lymphopenic decrease was 32 per cent at 2 hours and 18 minutes after the first stimulation and about 20 minutes after the last stimulation.

(h) Complications—A superficial wound infection which developed following operation responded to removal of the bone button. During the third week postoperatively she developed a meningitis which responded to antibiotics.

Follow-up Notes. During the first week after operation the patient remained negativistic but no longer mute. She verbalized her complaints and openly refused to cooperate. Three days postoperatively she displayed some posturing and waxy flexibility. By the second week she was more spontaneous and productive but still autistic and obsessively reminiscent. Her eating habits became gluttonous. The meningitis that developed in the third week after operation was accompanied by more seclusive and withdrawn behavior. She vomited, showed abdominal distension, nuchal rigidity, and sustained ankle clonus on elicitation of the left patellar reflex. Culture of the cerebral spinal fluid revealed Aerobacter strain. She was placed on antibiotics, and 1 week later the results of neurological and general physical examinations were negative and her temperature was normal. Following this there was steady improvement. The patient was enthusiastic about participating in the ward activity, showed more affective responsiveness to her environment, and became enthusiastic when offered the chance to leave the hospital on passes. But while at home she isolated herself, and upon return to the hospital she appeared retarded, withdrawn, and seclusive. She had several acute panics in which she reported visual hallucinations of being attacked by one of the doctors in an effort to cut off her arm. She also complained because the furniture in the home was moved. Nevertheless, her course was one of continued improvement. The outstanding abnormality noted was the extreme psycho-motor retardation. Because of this, 2 months after operation she was placed on 5 mg. of dexedrine twice a day. She responded immediately to the drug with an increase in physical activity and alertness. At the same time she showed her first real initiative in that she dressed herself and attempted to leave the hospital, stating, "I just decided I'd take a pass on my own." Despite her mother, who was a hostile, overprotective, nagging individual, the patient's adjustment on her passes gradually improved. At home she helped occasionally with the household chores and entered into conversations, although she showed little interest in socializing outside the home. She no longer expressed hallucinations or delusions. She repeatedly asked her therapist if she might not be discharged from the hospital. Four and a half months after operation she was discharged, much improved. Psychological tests indicated slight improvement.

On June 1, 1953, 18 months after operation, the patient was still making the marginal adjustment which one would expect on the basis of her prepsychotic personality.

PATIENT 18

AGE AT OPERATION: 39
SEX: Male
MARITAL STATUS: Single
OCCUPATION: Technician
RELIGION: Presbyterian (active)
INFORMANTS: Father and brother
DIAGNOSIS: Schizophrenic reaction, paranoid type
OPERATION: January 8, 1952

Presenting Picture. On admission to the Charity Hospital in December, 1951, the patient appeared depressed and retarded. He was resistive to hospitalization, stating that he had entered for a rest cure only. Concerning his ideation, he was uncommunicative, except to ruminate about his hypochondriacal preoccupations. Despite his negativism, he was superficially polite, cooperative, and at times ingratiating, although his emotional responses were shallow and unsustained.

Present Illness. In 1939, 12 years prior to hospitalization in December, 1951, the patient returned home from an expedition abroad where he had been in a situation of considerable real danger. Upon his return he was actively hallucinating, and expressing numerous ideas of reference and persecution involving his employer. For the next 2 years he was treated on an outpatient basis with electroshock therapy. Despite this treatment his symptoms progressed, and he finally required hospitalization and further EST, which proved unavailing. As his case had now become a feeding and management problem, he was committed to a state hospital in 1942, where he remained until his discharge, slightly improved, in 1945. Subsequently he made a marginal adjustment on the family farm, although he was unable to do even the simplest chores, remaining idle, seclusive, and at times uncooperative and destructive. In 1949 he was again hospitalized for a period of 12 months and again received EST therapy. He returned home slightly improved and was able to perform menial household chores, but again became hallucinatory and assaultive, apparently acting on referential and persecutory ideas involving the Catholic Church and his previous employer.

Previous Personality Disorders. Prior to the onset of his illness in 1939, the patient had had no overt psychotic episodes.

Family History. The father, who has developed a close, companionable relationship with the patient, is a professional man of moderate means. He has remained devoted and seriously concerned with his son's welfare during his illness. The mother, active in community organizations, has had little time for the patient, either during his present illness or in his early childhood. There are two much younger siblings who have always looked up to and admired him. The parents are strongly religious, opposed to drinking and smoking, but not excessively autocratic.

Personal History. The patient was born in Salt Lake City in 1913, after a full-term gestation and normal delivery. His development, social adjustment, and scholastic achievements were all superior. The only psychiatrically important trait reported during his childhood was his "excessive neatness." During high school he dated girls, joined a fraternity and a debating team, had many friends, and was considered quite a jokester. He showed initiative and other qualities of leadership. He attended college for 1 year but because of financial reverses during the depression left college to study as an apprentice to his father. Father and son worked together in a spirit of close comradeship.

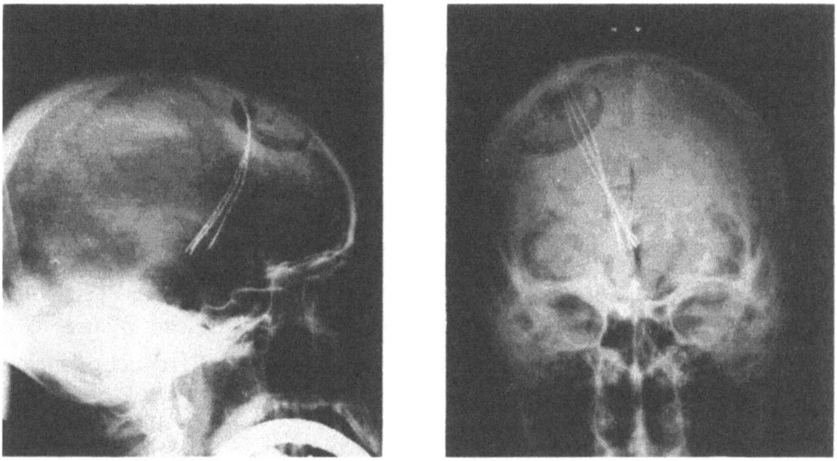

FIGURE XIX–12. Patient 18

Personality. The outstanding personality traits reported by the father were the patient's rather obsessively conscientious behavior and his lack of any serious heterosexual interests.

Hospital Course. During his month's stay in the hospital prior to operation there was almost no change in his behavior. He spent most of his time in bed, ate poorly, but did take care of his personal needs. He remained superficially passive and ingratiating, but stubbornly resisted any suggestion that he needed further treatment.

Physical and Laboratory Status. Physical examination revealed a thin, pale, rather sickly looking male whose chest x-rays showed findings compatible with tuberculosis in the right lung. This was similar to the lesion noticed during his previous hospitalization 2 1/2 years before. Mantoux skin test was positive in 48 hours (1 to 10,000). It was impossible to do smears and sputum cultures because the patient had no cough. Gastric washings were negative. Preoperative blood pressures varied from 140/90 to 120/80, and neurological findings were within normal limits. EEG, EKG, urinalysis, CBC, blood glucose, and BUN were also within normal range. The patient responded to the Thorn test.

Operation—Stimulation. January 8, 1952.

(a) Surgical technique—Open technique was used.

(b) Electrode placements—Three electrodes were implanted. Lead 1 was close to the midline directly ventral to the foramen of Monro near the base of the brain (septo-hypothalamic region). Lead 2 was in the midline, dorsal and a few millimeters caudal to lead 1. It may have lain in the rostral aspect of the third ventricle. Lead 3 was the most rostral. It was 8 mm. in front of the foramen of Monro and 3 mm. lateral to the midline in the septal region.

(c) Recordings—There were three preoperative EEG's. One was normal; two were mildly abnormal. Four months after operation scalp recordings showed generalized slow wave activity. In the deep recordings before stimulation there was moderate spiking from lead 3 and to a lesser extent from lead 1. Spikes were present, but less frequent, during the psychiatric interview. It was felt, although these findings have not been completely analyzed, that there were changes in the deep recordings which could be correlated with emotional reactions precipitated by the interviews. The deep recordings made after stimulation showed rather pronounced seizure patterns, but this did not reach the cortex. On one of the stimulations to lead 1 there was spread to other subcortical leads, which subsided before any scalp activity was noted. After the last stimulation occasional high voltage, slow waves appeared over a period of 1 hour and 15 minutes. It is questionable whether any spikes were seen during this period of continuous recording.

(d) Stimulation technique—A total of seventeen stimulations were given. There were six stimulations between the two poles of the septo-hypothalamic electrode (lead 1), lasting 2 minutes to 10 minutes at currents of 2 to 4 ma. There were eleven stimulations to the septal electrode (lead 3), lasting 2 to 32 minutes, at currents of 4 to 22 ma.

(e) Immediate physiological effects—Stimulation to lead 3 produced a mild rise in blood pressure from 116/76 to 142/96. This response was maintained. Tachycardia was noted, the patient became pale and sweaty, and both pupils were seen to dilate. Stimulation to the septo-hypothalamic region (lead 1), produced a marked blood pressure response of 180/120. At the same time tachycardia of 192 was noted; the patient flushed, sweated, and complained of faintness. His pupils dilated first on the right side and then bilaterally.

(f) Immediate behavioral response—Despite the fact that he felt faint after stimulation of the septo-hypothalamic lead, the patient seemed more alert and responsive.

(g) Immediate chemical changes—Preoperatively the patient had shown a good response to the Thorn test; postoperatively on two occasions he failed to respond. The maximum lymphopenic response following stimulation was a 38 per cent drop 6 1/2 hours after the first stimulation and 35 minutes after the last stimulation. On the urinary electrolyte excretion studies there were three preoperative determinations. The ratios were 0.39, 0.44, and 0.67. Over a 24-hour period beginning at the conclusion of operation and running through the stimulations and into the next day the ratio was 1.08. There were no significant changes in plasma electrolyte.

(h) Complications—None.

Follow-up Notes. Immediately following the stimulation the patient's emotional responses seemed more appropriate, both in quantity and quality. He was warm and friendly, mixing more actively with the other patients, participating in the ward activities, and taking an interest in occupational therapy, in which he constructed several porch chairs for his family. He developed some insight by the second week, admitting that he must be mentally ill and that his physical complaints were largely the result of this condition. On intelligence testing his responses were much more rapid than before. Although more friendly, he still showed a residual shyness in that he had difficulty in looking the examiner in the eye, walked with a slow, shuffling gait, and consistently rejected the idea of moving to an open ward where he would have more freedom. Two weeks after the operation he left the hospital on a pass with his father, expressing for the first time a desire to see his brother and sister. One month after operation his condition continued to improve, the most outstanding residual abnormality being his constant concern over a feeling of pressure, which he attributed to the ward personnel and his obsessive preoccupation with time. Whenever he would go on a pass he constantly watched the clock so that he would not overstay his allotted period. He developed more and more anxiety until, 2 months after operation, it was felt advisable to put him on sodium amytal. He showed some immediate improvement on 3 grains three times a day, but a month later he relapsed and became depressed, resentful over the pressures of the ward routine, and uninterested in his former activities and therapeutic sessions. He spent most of his time in bed, ate poorly, and continued to lose weight. At that time he was taken off amytal and placed on ambulatory insulin to see whether his anxieties could not be allayed and his appetite stimulated. He began to improve, being discharged from the hospital October, 1952. Before operation an infiltrative lesion was noted in the right first and second interspace. The patient had no sputum and two gastric washings were negative. However, x-ray findings were compatible with active TB. One month after operation there appeared to be minimal fibro-calcific changes representing improvement over the preoperative films. Follow-up films to March 17, 1953, indicate no further change in the lesion.

Although still somewhat hypochondriacal, seclusive, and withdrawn, the patient aids his family with the farm chores and occasionally socializes with the neighbors. Mild referential ideas which recurred when first discharged have disappeared as of June 1, 1953, 17 months after operation.

PATIENT 19

AGE AT OPERATION: 32

SEX: Male

MARITAL STATUS: Single

OCCUPATION: None

RELIGION: Catholic (inactive)

INFORMANTS: Parents, sister, former hospital records

DIAGNOSIS: Schizophrenic reaction, paranoid type (with malignant hypertension)

OPERATION: January 22, 1952

Presenting Picture. The patient was admitted to the surgical service of Charity Hospital in September, 1951, because of malignant hypertension. He was considered a possible candidate for a thoraco-lumbar sympathectomy. When tests revealed persistent hypertension with levels ranging from 250/150 to 190/120, the prognosis for sympathectomy was considered poor. As the medical history revealed that the patient had been hospitalized several times for overt psychotic behavior, the psychiatric service was consulted. On interview the patient appeared tense, fearful, and suspicious, revealed mild referential ideas, and showed considerable disorganization in his thinking, particularly on abstraction. As it was felt that a sympathectomy would be of no avail, in fact might precipitate an open psychosis, he was transferred to the psychiatric ward for observation in October, 1951. On the ward the patient showed no overt psychotic manifestations except under amytal.

Present Illness. At some time between 1942 and 1944 the patient was hospitalized for a short time on a psychiatric ward. Information concerning this hospitalization is unavailable; the patient was reluctant to talk about the details. He did mention in a delusional way that while in the Army he was under the influence of a psychiatric hypnotist. Informants first noticed abnormal behavior after his discharge from the service in 1945. He refused to accept employment, became progressively more seclusive until he would not leave his parents' home, refused meals, did not sleep for days, and expressed numerous ideas of persecution. He had the fixed somatic delusion that he was a victim of pediculosis, acting on this delusion in such a way that he burned his skin with caustic agents, destroyed his clothes, and set fire to his mattress. He became homicidal and, after firing a rifle at his brother, was admitted to a state hospital. Two weeks later he escaped, returned home, where the family tolerated him until September, 1948, when he was admitted to a local veterans' hospital. At that time his symptoms consisted of auditory hallucinations of a persecutory nature and a now well-developed delusional system with ideas of reference and persecution. The diagnosis of schizophrenia, paranoid type, was made and he received a course of insulin-coma therapy with good results. He was allowed to leave the hospital in April, 1949, on a trial visit but returned voluntarily in September, 1949, because of a recurrence of hallucinatory experiences and insomnia. During this hospitalization he developed a sensitivity to insulin, so that further coma therapy could not be given. However, his condition seemed to improve and he was allowed to leave again on a trial visit in February, 1950, and discharged 9 months later. Many of his former symptoms reappeared. He remained at home, complained of numerous somatic ailments, refused to seek employment or to socialize, and was irritable and seclusive in his behavior. Although he would not express them spontaneously, when interrogated he revealed some somatic delusions, such as having bubbles in his blood, having lice, and coughing up "the bones" of his larynx. He also had vague persecutory and referential ideas concerning his former associates in the Army. He denied, however, a recurrence of his previous hallucinatory experiences.

Previous Personality Disorders. Prior to the onset of the patient's present illness no psychotic episodes occurred.

Family History. The patient is the ninth of thirteen children born to a French family making a marginal subsistence on a small farm in Louisiana. The parents are both living but suffering from chronic medical illnesses. They are apparently affectionate, proud of their family, devout Catholics, and respected in the community. All of the siblings except one brother obtained a high school education, although most of them now work at rather menial occupations. There is a family history of asthma, diabetes, hypertension, glaucoma, and tuberculosis, but no mental illness.

Personal History. The patient had a normal birth following a full-term gestation. Infancy and early development were considered normal and free from serious illness. The patient entered school at the age of 6; he studied conscientiously but made only average grades. In high school he participated in athletics, particularly boxing. It was noted by his family that while taking part in sports he observed excessively strict hygienic routines. Following graduation, at the age of 17 1/2, the patient helped his father on the farm until his eighteenth birthday, at which time he enlisted in the Army. He was out of the country from January, 1942, until March, 1944. He received an honorable discharge from the Army in April, 1945.

Personality. The patient is described by his family as having been obedient, helpful around the house, devoutly Catholic, particularly sensitive to any dissension within the family, and frightened by minor physical injuries. He avoided smoking and alcoholic beverages. He enjoyed community parties in high school but dated only casually and never became deeply attached to any girl.

Physical and Laboratory Data. Physical examination revealed Grade II retinopathy with marked spasms of the arterioles, moderate AV nicking and arteriosclerosis with one small flame hemorrhage in the left eyeground, and some edema residue in both eyegrounds. There was a low-pitched diastolic murmur best heard near the edge of the sternum in the fourth left intercostal space, with some increase in the mitral second sound. A soft mitral systolic murmur was transmitted to the pulmonary valve area. Blood pressure was 242/150. Otherwise, physical and neurological findings were negative. Urinalysis showed a specific gravity of 1,010. Albumin was either negative or 1 plus, and fine granular casts were occasionally seen on microscopic examination. PSP excretion was 80 per cent at the first hour. Fishberg concentration showed the highest specific gravity of 1,010 in 2 hours. Urea clearance was 168 per cent. BUN was 16.4. Total serum sodium was 135 meq/L. (on salt-free diet). Cardiac-thoracic ratio was 14.9/30.5. There was slight x-ray evidence of cardiac enlargement and pulmonary congestion. Intravenous pyelograms showed normally functioning kidneys. EKG showed definite evidence of myocardial disease compatible with left ventricular hypertrophy and anterior-lateral myocardial ischemia.

Sodium amytal, benzodioxen, splanchnic block, cold pressor, and etamon chloride test did not lower diastolic pressure significantly. Preoperatively circulation time was 25 seconds (decholin); venous pressure, 130 ml. of water.

Hospital Course. The patient was on the surgical ward for 3 weeks and on the psychiatric ward for 2 1/2 months while he was worked up from the medical and psychiatric standpoints. He did not seem to resent this long delay in specific procedure and was not afraid of surgery despite his hypochondriasis, as he was more concerned about his persistent hypertension. On the wards he was untidy and unkempt for several weeks, even refusing to take baths, but later became cooperative and pleasant. He seemed content to live in the protected hospital atmosphere. Overt psychotic behavior was not manifest, although under sodium amytal he again expressed delusions that an Army officer had him under posthypnotic suggestion and control and was taking away some phenomenal intellectual capacity that he had once possessed. When given abstract problems to solve he reacted in a very bizarre, circumstantial way, formulating the problems and answers in a concrete, personalized manner. He reacted with extreme hostility to his female therapist, expressing so much resentment that in order to keep the patient in the hospital it was necessary to transfer him to a male therapist. As the day of operation approached, his hypochondriacal complaints increased. To a large degree these complaints were justified, since his physical condition also deteriorated. His outstanding complaint was nocturnal dyspnea. Chest films at that time showed minimal pulmonary congestion. There was no ankle edema and it was thought that many of his breathing difficulties were of an asthmatic nature, as his physical examination showed numerous expiratory rhonchi. He made a poor response to the Thorn test.

Operation—Stimulation. January 22, 1952.

(a) Surgical technique—Open technique was used.

(b) Electrode placements—Lead 1 was deep in the rostral part of the hypothalamus, almost at the base of the brain. Lead 2 was dorsal to lead 1, 14 mm. lateral to the midline, possibly in the rostral part of the thalamus. Lead 3 was in the midline near the rostral part of the hypothalamus.

(c) Recordings—This patient had three normal preoperative EEG's. There were no postoperative scalp recordings. Very little was obtained from attempts at deep recording during stimulation except slow wave activity from all leads. Occasional spikes were noted, especially during sleep, but the spiking was minimal and questionable. There was nothing remarkable about poststimulation recordings on the deep leads.

(d) Stimulation technique—There were three stimulations to lead 2 (in the thalamus), which was laterally placed. The current was between 1 and 15 ma. There were two stimulations to lead 1 (deep in the hypothalamus) with currents between 2 and 14 ma. There were three stimulations to lead 3 (higher in the rostral part of the hypothalamus near the septum) with currents between 2 and 40 ma. Duration of stimulations varied between 2 and 33 minutes.

(e) Immediate physiological effects—Stimulation to one rostral hypothalamic electrode (lead 1) produced a marked slowing and deepening in respiration. Stimulation of the other rostral hypothalamic electrode (lead 3) had no apparent physiological effect other than a marked internal strabismus. Stimulation of the rostral thalamic electrode (lead 2) had no apparent effect.

(f) Immediate behavioral response—This patient was relatively alert prior to stimulation. It is questionable whether there was any response to stimulation, although he may have become slightly more alert.

(g) Immediate chemical changes—Preoperatively the patient made a poor response to the Thorn test but a good response to ACTH. No Thorn tests were taken after operation. The maximum lymphopenia represented a 54 per cent drop, which occurred 1 hour and 44 minutes

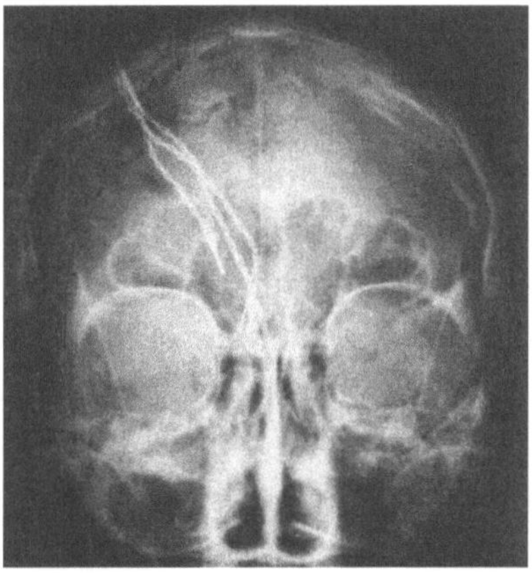

FIGURE XIX-13. Patient 19

after the last stimulation. Plasma sodium and potassium values showed some change over the period of time the patient was followed. Two preoperative sodium-potassium tests were done here. On the first reading the sodium was 145 meq/L. and the potassium 3 meq/L. On the second reading the sodium was 135 meq/L. and the potassium 2.8 meq/L. Fourteen days after stimulation the sodium was 118.5 meq/L. and the potassium was 2.6 meq/L. Chloride was 68 meq/L. The patient had been on a low sodium diet up to this time. It was decided then to switch him to a normal salt intake, with a high carbohydrate, high protein diet, as he was quite cachectic. He was given intravenous fluids, including sodium by clysis and potassium by mouth. This dietary regimen was continued until death. On February 18, when 14 days had passed after the previous low reading and the start of the new dietary regimen, the sodium was 124 meq/L. and the potassium 4.8 meq/L. This was the last analysis. No further plasma electrolyte studies were made.

(h) Complications—The patient experienced acute cardiac failure immediately after operation and was given digitalis rapidly. He was exhibiting a pulsus alternans at the time of stimulation. Blood pressure was 250/150; pulse rate was 168; respiration was 32. There was a stormy postoperative course terminated by death; autopsy revealed a right ventricular abscess.

Follow-up Notes. Because of the minimal psychiatric symptoms and the patient's rather extreme physical illness, psychiatric evaluation was overshadowed postoperatively by medical considerations. He did seem to respond well initially, talking in a coherent, pleasant manner despite high temperature the day following operation. He claimed that he felt better despite numerous physical disabilities and organic symptomatology. Shortly thereafter he became confused, disoriented, and restless. One month after operation he complained of visual and olfactory hallucinations of an organic type. He was completely disoriented and delirious at this time. During the delirious episodes he was sexually uninhibited and at the same time expressed intense hostility toward women in general.

The patient's medical condition proved a dilemma to the treating physicians. He began producing copious amounts of urine, with specific gravity of 1,002 and albumin of 4 plus, occasional red blood cells and 5 to 10 white blood cells—cellular and granular casts all being seen on microscopic examination. Urinary chloride excretion was 10 meq/L. in 24 hours. He was obviously putting out excessive amounts of salt. The plasma sodium 2 weeks after operation was 118.5 meq/L. and plasma potassium 2.16 meq/L. He was taken off the salt-free diet and given intravenous fluids, after which he developed a rather marked peripheral edema.

At the same time he had several syncopal attacks and developed a labored respiration, some basal rales, and many expiratory squeaks and a grossly irregular peripheral pulse of 96 per second. Medical consultants decided the patient had extra supraventrical systoles, but did not feel that it was the result of overdigitalization. Three weeks after operation the patient began vomiting, and consequently was given intravenous sodium and potassium. At first he showed improvement but 3 days later developed cardiac failure. Nevertheless, he was given desoxycorticosterone, following which he became particularly dyspneic. Desoxycorticosterone was discontinued, and 2 days later he was shifted to cortisone, 50 mg. per day. His condition steadily became worse, with physical and laboratory findings suggesting both cardiac and renal failure. Five weeks postoperatively he expired. Terminally the patient showed dilatation of the right pupil, weakness of the right latero-oblique occular muscle, and a deviation of the tongue to the right. Autopsy findings showed the two following significant pathological changes: evidence of an old chronic pyelonephritis and, on sectioning of the brain, evidence of chronic brain abscess extending from the fronto-cortical surface to the third ventricle in the region of the anterior commissure.

PATIENT 20

AGE AT OPERATION: 37
SEX: Female
MARITAL STATUS: Single
OCCUPATION: Teacher
RELIGION: Catholic (active)
INFORMANT: Mother
DIAGNOSIS: Schizophrenic reaction, paranoid type
OPERATION: January 31, 1952

Presenting Picture. On admission in January, 1952, the patient was quiet, seclusive, withdrawn, and preoccupied with her delusions that she was bisexual, could impregnate herself, had already been artificially inseminated, and had given birth to several children, as well as to dogs and cats. She showed no spontaneity, although she would smile amiably when addressed, and was perfectly cooperative toward the ward routine. Unless urged to get up, she would spend most of her time in bed.

Present Illness. Eight years previously, when the patient was 27, she had become moody and developed ideas of reference and feelings of persecution directed toward the nuns of the convent where she had been residing for 3 years. At that time (1944) she was hospitalized, given a course of 12 electroshock treatments, and discharged to the care of her family, slightly improved. Over the next 6 years she became gradually more and more disturbed, and finally uncontrollable. Throughout this period she had been under the supervision and constant care of her mother. Again she was committed to an institution, this time in February, 1951. She then had paranoid delusions and was actively hallucinating. However, 2 months later, at the insistence of her family, she was again discharged even though she was unimproved. She was manageable at home, but her delusions expanded until she felt that all her family were dead and that those around her were merely wearing masks. The family, finally accepting the necessity of further hospitalization and treatment, sought admission for her in January, 1952.

Previous Personality Disorders. During the patient's junior year in college she suddenly found herself unable to concentrate. Although the work had been easy for her before, she could now pass her courses only by making a supreme effort. She recalls no other symptoms. The family apparently were not aware of her difficulty.

Family History. The patient was the youngest of four daughters in a closely knit, lower middle-class Catholic family manifesting marked mutual interdependence and restrictive discipline. The children were allowed little initiative, were restricted socially, and were given absolutely no sexual education. The mother commented, "We never brought up the subject of sex. I kept them right under my eye all the time."

Personal History. The patient was born in February, 1915. Both gestation and delivery were uneventful; the baby was described as "the finest of all." However, the mother added that the patient had been an extremely quiet child, always obedient and ingratiating. As she grew older, it was noticed by the family that she had a "languid and gloomy nature." At 15 months she showed a peculiar preference for an old umbrella, which she would actively seek out and enjoy sitting under for long periods. At 2 years she had an attack of colitis and at 4 of influenza, but there were no serious complications to these illnesses. She was always religious, quiet, seclusive, and superior intellectually, showing a preference for reading or playing with animals rather than mixing with other children. She did well scholastically, graduating from college at the age of 21. Subsequently she taught school but had few friends, did not mix heterosexually, and at the age of 24 decided to join a convent. It was 3 years later, while she was in this convent, that her present illness began.

Personality. As described by the family, the patient was a quiet, seclusive, underactive individual, predisposed to moody spells and generally languid. She would attempt numerous tasks but tire of them quickly. She was intensely pious, and seemed uninterested in the opposite sex, never showing the usual feminine interest in marrying and having a family.

Physical and Laboratory Status. Examination revealed an extremely obese female with a blood pressure of 134/90 but no other positive physical or neurological finding. EEG revealed T-wave abnormality suggestive of myocardial disease. Serum cholesterol was 315 mg/100 ml. Three BMR's were −15 and −17 and −12 per cent, respectively. X-rays were negative, except for many minimal osteoarthritic changes in the lumbar spine.

Hospital Course. During the month prior to operation, the patient maintained the delusions reported on admission. She denied, and showed

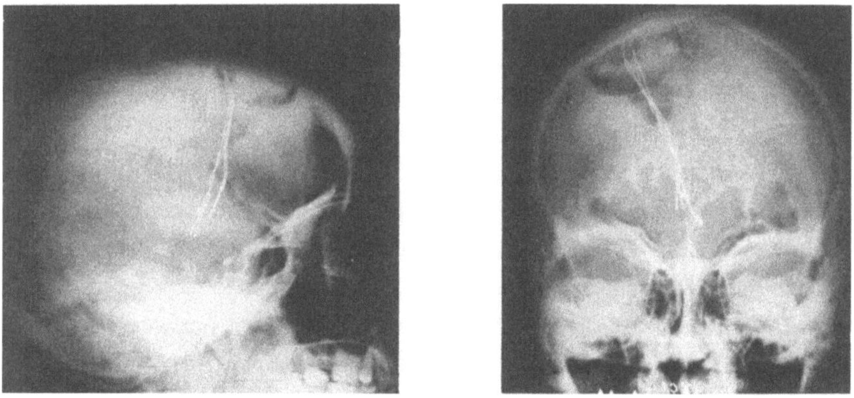

FIGURE XIX–14. Patient 20

no evidence of, hallucinations but remained shallow and silly emotionally. On the wards she was neat and tidy in her appearance, though seclusive and idle. She was oriented in all spheres and seemed of superior intellect. Her abstract thinking seemed unimpaired, although her answers were usually circumstantial.

Operation—Stimulation. January 31, 1952.

(a) Surgical technique—Open technique was used.

(b) Electrode placements—Two bipolar electrodes were implanted: one (lead 1) was placed 11 mm. directly ventral to the foramen of Monro at the midline in the septo-hypothalamic region, the other (lead 2) was placed 6 mm. rostral to the foramen of Monro and 2 mm. lateral to the midline in the septal region.

(c) Recordings—There was one normal EEG before operation and one normal scalp recording after operation. Deep recordings before stimulation showed a large amount of slow activity which tended to obscure frequent spiking. Most of this was in lead 1. Spiking, though present to a marked degree, was somewhat unusual in that it was ragged, of high voltage, and inconstant in form. This patient showed correlations between emotional reactions and recordings through the deep leads. On several occasions the subcortical patterns almost resembled fit activity during a period when the patient said she was panicky over fears of death. Deep subcortical recordings were followed continuously for 35 minutes after the last stimulation. There appeared to be less spiking than before stimulation.

(d) Stimulation technique—Four stimulations were given. Three were to the septal electrode (lead 2), lasting 3 to 10 minutes at currents of 2 to 10 ma. One stimulation was to the septo-hypothalamic electrode (lead 1), lasting 8 seconds at a current of 4 ma.

(e) Immediate physiological effects—Stimulation to the septal electrode (lead 2), produced an initial rise in blood pressure from 130/80 to 200/120. There was a generalized sympathetic discharge; the patient said she felt warm and faint. Stimulation to the septo-hypothalamic electrode (lead 1) produced a marked blood pressure rise. The stimulation was kept on for 4 seconds, during which time there was a diffuse sympathetic discharge and the patient said she felt "pins and needles" all over. Blood pressure continued to be elevated for some time following stimulation.

(f) Immediate behavioral response—The patient brightened somewhat during both stimulations and said that she was "warm and faint" but that it was a "pleasant feeling."

(g) Immediate chemical changes—Maximum lymphopenic response was a 16 per cent drop, which may be more significant than would at first appear. As a rapid rise had occurred 3 1/2 hours after the last stimulation, indicating that the trend had been distinctly upward, the drop probably indicates a marked dip in the curve. No additional chemistry data were obtained.

(h) Complications—Four weeks after operation the patient ran a low-grade fever and showed slight bulging at the operative site. On antibiotics the temperature returned to normal.

Follow-up Notes. Immediately following stimulation the patient's ideational content was the same as before. At times, however, she suggested that there might be some doubt concerning its validity, saying, "Well, I know those may be preconceived ideas, but I feel that they are correct." At other times she would talk rationally about her mother, and only when directly questioned would again express her delusional idea that the latter was an impostor wearing a mask. There was an obvious increase in the warmth and friendliness of her attitude toward the ward personnel and physicians. During the next 3 weeks this affective change disappeared somewhat, but she still seemed more responsive than before. At the same time, she openly expressed anxiety centering about the idea that she would be artificially inseminated in her sleep. Three weeks postoperatively she left the hospital on her first pass and showed some reluctance to return, saying, "They will impregnate me." For the first time since the night of stimulation, she talked of impending death. The family felt that during her visit she showed more emotional contact with her surroundings and socialized more freely with her relatives and reported that she had expressed open irritability concerning the protective attitude of her mother. As her anxiety increased 6 weeks after the operation, she was put on sodium amytal, 3 grains t.i.d. However, she became so somnolent that this was discontinued. As her delusional fears of artificial insemination increased, it was necessary to place her on a closed ward to keep her in the hospital.

As of June 1, 1953, 16 months after operation, the patient's delusional content is much the same as on admission. She still responds emotionally in a more spontaneous manner, mixes more freely with the other patients, and expresses her delusions more reluctantly, but the improvement has been minimal.

PATIENT 21

AGE AT OPERATION: 58
SEX: Male
MARITAL STATUS: Married
OCCUPATION: None
RELIGION: Catholic(?)
INFORMANT: Mother
DIAGNOSIS: Involutional melancholia; far-advanced pulmonary tuberculosis
OPERATION: March 6, 1952

Presenting Picture. At the time of transfer to the neuropsychiatric service in February, 1952, the patient was agitated, depressed, morose and preoccupied. He consistently requested the doctors to end his life because he did not want to burden anyone. He paced restlessly up and down in his isolation room, frequently asking for water. He was disheveled and preoccupied with numerous gastrointestinal symptoms. He interpreted hospitalization as punishment.

Present Illness. Psychiatric consultation was first requested in December, 1951, because of varied bodily complaints which included back pain, hip pain, abdominal pain, shortness of breath, intolerance to heat and cold, weakness, etc. At that time it was noted that the patient was depressed. No specific therapy was recommended. His depression deepened; he began to lose weight, prayed frequently, appeared nervous, and expressed numerous suicidal ideas.

Previous Personality Disorders. There is no history of previous personality disorders which required treatment by a psychiatrist.

Family History. When the patient was 3 months old his father died of pneumonia. By his mother's second marriage he has one stepsister. The patient's wife is described as a nervous person who is critical and hostile toward the hospital personnel. They have five children, four sons and one daughter, all of whom are living. The eldest son has been treated for active tuberculosis, which is now arrested. The youngest son has stomach ulcers. The other members of the family have no significant medical history and appear to be making a satisfactory adjustment.

Personal History. The patient was born in New Orleans in September, 1893. Little is known about his early childhood. He had virtually no formal education, starting to work regularly at the age of 19 in the pressroom of a local paper. He stayed on the same job for 33 years, advancing to the position of press foreman. In World War I he was a private in the Army. He had numerous friends and enjoyed the pastimes of fishing and of building furniture in his home workshop, where he spent a great deal of time.

The patient was first hospitalized for tuberculosis in October, 1949. His illness, discovered after that of his son, was then diagnosed as active, far-advanced pulmonary tuberculosis, on the basis of chest x-rays which revealed a large cavity 7 cm. in diameter located in the apex of the right lung. There were other scattered areas of soft infiltration in the right upper lung and right hilar region. Sputum examinations were repeatedly positive for acid fast. The patient was placed on a course of complete bed rest and 1 gm. of streptomycin daily for 90 days. His fever subsided, his respiratory symptoms decreased, and he gained 19 pounds. However, his sputum remained positive for acid fast, and there was no change in the cavity or infiltrative process. He refused pneumonectomy and was given a second course of streptomycin, but the chest cavitation increased in size. In June, 1950, the patient had daily hemoptysis, which continued until pneumoperitoneum was induced in July, 1950. However, the hemoptysis returned and continued despite further courses of streptomycin therapy. The patient finally consented to lobectomy, which was carried out in May, 1951. Reactivation of the disease followed, with a spread to the left lung. In July the patient was given a course of tibione therapy, and in October pneumoperitoneum was induced for the second time. There was some remission in his illness, sputum being only intermittently positive for acid fast. At this time however, his physical and mental status began to deteriorate, with increasing depression, suicidal trends, agitation, and subsequent reactivation of his tuberculosis.

Personality. The patient was always considered a compulsive, hard-working, overconscientious person, dependent upon his family.

Physical and Laboratory Status. Aside from the findings related to his tuberculosis, as mentioned above, the patient had a blood pressure of 150/110 and a pulse of 64. Respiration was 18. Hematocrit was 40 per cent, WBC 9,000, and urinalysis normal. Serology was negative, blood glucose 87 mg/100 ml., and BUN 13.4. Spinal tap revealed protein of 12 mg/100 ml., glucose 95 mg/100 ml., chlorides 710 mg/ 100 ml., and a 0011000000 colloidal gold curve. A 30-minute, 10-lead EEG revealed the principal waking frequencies of 5, 6 and 7 per second, sinusoidal in form and normal in range and amplitude. No sleep record was obtained. The patient was not allowed to hyperventilate because of his pulmonary condition. The diagnostic impression was given as generalized moderately slow activity suggestive of epilepsy or related disorders.

Hospital Course. Prior to operation the patient was extremely agitated and continued with numerous somatic complaints centered about the upper respiratory system. He was self-deprecatory and asked that he be killed. He was disheveled, agitated, uncooperative, and belligerent.

Operation—Stimulation. March 6, 1952.

(a) Surgical technique—Stereotaxic technique was used.

(b) Electrode placements—Four unipolar electrodes were placed in the septal region; the most caudal was at the level of the foramen of Monro. All were within a few millimeters of the midline.

(c) Recordings—One preoperative EEG showed generalized slow activity. One scalp recording 2 weeks after operation showed a frontal slow focus in addition to the generalized slow wave activity. On the deep recordings there was no spiking from any of the leads. They were featureless except for some interesting changes with sleep. There was no significant change in the deep recordings after stimulation. The scalp recordings looked very much better the day after stimulation, showing less slow wave activity. This response reversed very rapidly, however, when on the second postoperative day the patient pulled out his own electrodes.

(d) Stimulation technique—There were eight stimulations. Seven were between the two rostral leads. One was between the two caudal leads. Duration of stimulation was from 1 1/2 to 12 minutes on the different stimuli, with currents of 2 to 40 ma.

(e) Immediate physiological effects—Stimulation to the rostro-septal electrode produced a rise in blood pressure from 118/68 to 170/110, accompanied by an increase in pulse rate, dilatation of the pupils, and a generalized tremor. Stimulation to the septal electrode produced no blood pressure response, but the patient flushed and there was an increase in pulse rate.

(f) Immediate behavioral response—At the higher intensity of stimulation the patient ceased to show any signs of depressive ideation, became bright and jovial, and told many jokes.

(g) Immediate chemical changes—There was a drop in eosinophils as a result of surgery, but it was not so great as that seen after the open operation. Maximum lymphopenic decrease was 56 per cent. This decrease appeared twice, separated by 2 1/2 hours, in association with different stimulations. There were no changes in plasma electrolytes.

(h) Complications—Death followed about 6 weeks postoperatively, without autopsy. However, cerebral trauma incident to the patient's pulling out the electrodes was felt to be a contributing factor.

Follow-up Notes. There were no significant changes in the deep recordings after stimulation. It was thought that the recordings looked much better on the day following stimulation, as there was less slow wave activity. This condition reversed very rapidly, however, when on the second postoperative day the patient pulled out his own electrodes. Subsequently, evidence of clinical improvement disappeared, and many of the old depressive symptoms of psychosis returned to persist until the patient's death, approximately 6 weeks following surgery.

It was felt that the patient's tubercular symptoms improved for a few days following operation inasmuch as the clot disappeared and one sputum examination during this period was negative. X-rays suggested possible slight improvement, as reported on March 19, 1952: "In comparison with film of 3/5/52, there is suggestive slight decrease in the size of several of the smaller nodular densities in the left central lung field."

PATIENT 22

AGE AT OPERATION: 21
SEX: Female
MARITAL STATUS: Married
OCCUPATION: Housewife
RELIGION: Baptist (inactive)
INFORMANTS: Aunt and uncle
DIAGNOSIS: Schizophrenic reaction, catatonic type
OPERATION: March 25, 1952

Presenting Picture. On admission in September, 1950, the patient was mute and negativistic. She showed evidence of marked weight loss and would occasionally laugh in an inappropriate, silly manner.

Present Illness. The patient's illness began in August, 1949, shortly after the birth of her fifth child. At that time she felt depressed, feared impending death, neglected her household duties, and complained of her husband's behavior. After a temporary remission, the patient again relapsed, refused to eat, spent most of her time lying in bed, laughed in a peculiar manner, seemed preoccupied, and totally neglected the care of her children. She was nursed by an aunt for approximately 9 months while awaiting admission to the hospital.

Family History. The patient was the eldest of six children born to an impoverished Negro rural family. Her mother developed paranoid schizophrenia following the birth of her last child and has been hospitalized for the past 17 years. The patient was raised by her maternal grandmother.

Personal History. Neither of the informants has any information concerning the patient's birth and early development. She obtained an eighth grade education, discontinuing school to marry a man who was 8 years her senior. Her first four pregnancies were uncomplicated. Little is known about her relations with her husband except that he frequently left home and has shown little interest in the patient since she has been hospitalized.

Personality. The patient's prepsychotic personality is described as bright, friendly, quiet, conscientious, perhaps a little shy.

Previous Personality Disorders. There were no previous psychotic episodes.

Physical and Laboratory Status. Results of physical and neurological examinations were within normal limits. Laboratory findings, including CBC, blood sugars, serology, urinalysis, EKG, AP and lateral x-rays of the skull were all within normal limits. Chest film revealed prominence in the basal markings of the right lung, suggesting chronic bronchial disease, apparently inactive.

Hospital Course. Even under the influence of sodium amytal the patient remained uncooperative and negativistic, refusing to reveal any of her delusions, hallucinations, or paranoid conceptions, although at times she appeared to be acting on such ideas. Electronarcosis was started in November, 1950, but had to be discontinued after 6 treatments when a lung abscess developed in the right middle lobe. In January, 1951, electronarcosis was started again, but was discontinued a second time when pneumonitis developed. In August, 1951, after oral surgery, the patient was started on electroshock therapy, receiving 20 treatments over the next 7 weeks. On this regimen she showed transitory improvement and became more cooperative on the wards. However, shortly after cessation of treatment she reverted to her silly, uncommunicative, seclusive behavior. Continuously throughout this time she incorrectly identified people on the wards, often referring to them as if they were relatives. She occasionally admitted auditory hallucinations and persistently demanded to be sent home. From time to time she became assaultive, requiring restraint. Because of this, in November, 1951, the patient was put on maintenance shock therapy, receiving 1 treatment per week until the time of operation. On this regimen her behavior was at least tractable. Preoperative EEG revealed a basic waking frequency of 11 per second as before, but the record was filled with 5 and 6 per second waves typical of postelectroshock records.

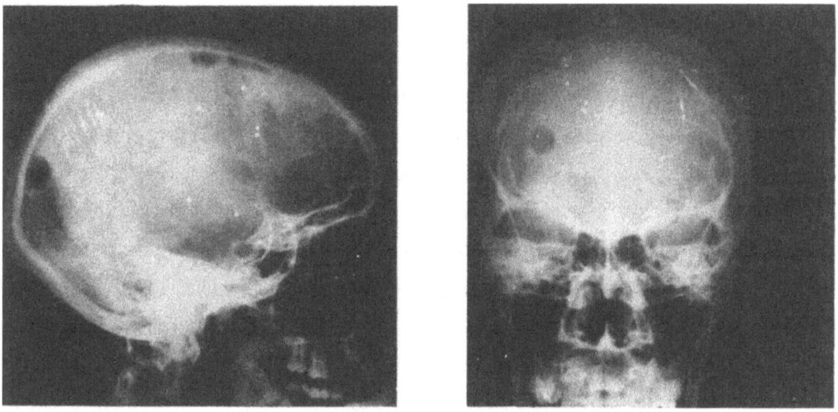

FIGURE XIX–15. Patient 22

Operation—Stimulation. March 25, 1952.

(a) Surgical technique—Stereotaxic technique was used.

(b) Electrode placements—Eight unipolar electrodes were implanted in the septal region, caudate nucleus, and thalamus. They were checked with x-ray and found to be in excellent locations. During closure, however, five of the deep electrodes were pulled up to the level of the cortex or into the subcortical white matter. Only two remained in their original positions. One was in the septal region; the other in the thalamus, more than 3 cm. away.

(c) Recordings—The distance of over 3 cm. which separated the two electrodes made meaningful recordings from these leads impossible. Preoperative EEG was abnormal, with diffuse slow wave activity. The abnormality continued essentially the same in postoperative scalp recordings.

(d) Stimulation technique—Despite the technical difficulties encountered at the time of operation, twelve attempts at stimulation between the two electrodes were made. There was some blood pressure response to these stimulations.

(e) Immediate physiological effects—Stimulation of the displaced electrodes (cortical and subcortical) produced motor responses which were characteristic of areas 6 and/or area 8. These involved complex movement of the eyes, arms, legs, and of the left and, in some cases, the right side of the face. Associated with this movement was generalized autonomic discharge. Stimulation between the remaining deep electrodes (septum to thalamus) resulted in mild increase of blood pressure.

(f) Immediate behavioral response—On stimulation to the displaced electrodes the patient became excited, fearful, and uncooperative. Stimulation between the remaining deep electrodes produced some alerting.

(g) Immediate chemical changes—The stimulations produced no lymphopenic response. Urinary electrolyte studies were made. Before operation the potassium-sodium ratio was 0.43; during the 12-hour period between operation and stimulation it was 0.72. A 12-hour urine specimen taken during the deep stimulation, which was undertaken 1 and 2 days following the implantation of electrodes, showed a potassium-sodium ratio of about 3.6. There was a slight but continued rise in plasma sodium beginning the day following operation and coinciding with the first deep stimulation. The level was 135.9 meq/L. before the deep stimulation 1 day after operation. Beginning a few hours after stimulation and carrying through for 24 hours, the sodium level was measured at regular intervals and showed an increase from 135.9 to 140 meq/L.

(h) Complications—None.

Follow-up Notes. There was no change in the patient's behavior for 3 days after operation. She remained withdrawn, negativistic, periodically assaultive and uncontrollable. However, on the fourth day she began to improve, becoming more responsive to her surroundings and taking part in the ward activities for the first time. She seemed more alert and remembered names better, but she still mumbled vaguely about hallucinations and continuously talked in a very unrealistic manner about going home. Improvement continued for the next 3 weeks as she became continuously more responsive and friendly. EEG revealed mixed alpha-theta activity with inconstant delta activity in all leads. Three weeks after operation the patient began to regress. Again she became seclusive, retired to her room, and was generally uncooperative as far as the ward routines were concerned. She remained more responsive emotionally and continued to address people by their right names but, gradually becoming belligerent and assaultive, had to be placed again on electroshock therapy. No psychological data were obtained.

On June 1, 1953, 13 months after operation, the patient is still hospitalized. Although no longer assaultive, hence not requiring maintenance EST, she is completely withdrawn and inaccessible.

PATIENT 23

AGE AT OPERATION: 26

SEX: Female

MARITAL STATUS: Married

OCCUPATION: Housewife

RELIGION: Protestant (active)

INFORMANTS: Husband and brother

DIAGNOSIS: No psychiatric diagnosis. Medical diagnosis, metastatic carcinoma, probably epidermoid tumor of cervix.

OPERATION: March 27, 1952

Presenting Picture. The patient was first seen in consultation in February, 1952, for relief of intractable pain due to metastatic carcinoma. At that time she was suffering intensely, febrile, emaciated, and obviously in the terminal stage of her illness.

Present Illness. In August, 1951, the patient complained of low back pain, which extended down her thigh to her great toe. This was associated with numbness and tingling exacerbated by jarring or sneezing. These symptoms progressed until the patient was referred to the outpatient clinic of Charity Hospital in November, 1951, where she was seen in the orthopedic clinic and admitted to their service in December, 1951, with a presumptive diagnosis of herniated intervertebral disk.

Family History. The patient is the youngest of four children born to an impoverished rural Mississippi Negro family. Little data could be obtained concerning the emotional relationships within the family except that the patient and her brother say their parents were good to them. Their primary social activity was the church. There was no mental illness in the family.

Personal History. Little information is available because the patient was unable to talk for long periods. Her brother could tell very little, since he had left home during her infancy. There were no abnormalities in her birth or early development. She had 3 years of schooling and subsequently worked in a factory near her home. At the age of 15 she had an illegitimate child; at 23 she married her present husband. Shortly before the onset of her illness there was a rift in the marriage which neither the husband nor the patient would discuss. No children were born to this marriage.

Personality Disorders. No personality disorders were reported.

Physical and Laboratory Status. Physical examination revealed a temperature of 102°F., slight thyroid enlargement, tachycardia, lower quadrant tenderness, moderate scoliosis, moderate muscular atrophy of the left thigh and calf. A grapefruit-sized mass in the pelvis had pushed into the vagina, displacing the cervix to the right. The hematocrit was low, requiring several blood transfusions. In February, 1952, x-rays showed areas of decreased density in the lower ilium, the ischial remi, the acetabulum, and the proximal left femur, which were thought to represent changes due to extension of the carcinoma.

Hospital Course. Shortly after admission to the hospital a large pelvic mass was discovered. In January, 1952, a culpotomy was performed. Biopsy revealed a malignant tumor, probably epidermoid. It was discovered that there was extension to the left hip and upper shaft of the left femur. She had daily elevations of temperature and extreme pain. Pelvic surgery was ruled out because of the extensive metastasis. The patient was given a formal mental status test to rule out any possibility of psychosis. Despite her severe pain the patient managed to smile frequently and seemed to be alert and of average intelligence. At first she was suspicious of the interviewer, fearing manipulations, which had always been painful, but later became relaxed and friendly. At times she was uncooperative because she resented being questioned about her emotional problems and her past life when her suffering was so intense. Nevertheless, her emotional reactions seemed to be appropriate. Her thought content centered around her present illness and discomfort. She spoke rather reminiscently of her home life and husband, for whom she now expressed considerable love. She apparently had no realization of the seriousness of her illness and hoped to rejoin her husband and child and resume her household duties. Her chief areas of interest lay in gardening, flowers, caring for the house, and listening to the radio. She was oriented in all spheres, showed no memory defects, and performed conceptual problems compatible with her intelligence and third-grade education.

Operation—Stimulation. March 27, 1952.

(a) Surgical technique—Open method was used.

(b) Electrode placements—Three bipolar electrodes were implanted. One (lead 1) was placed at about the level of the foramen of Monro but 1 cm. lateral to it, probably in the caudate; another (lead 2) was

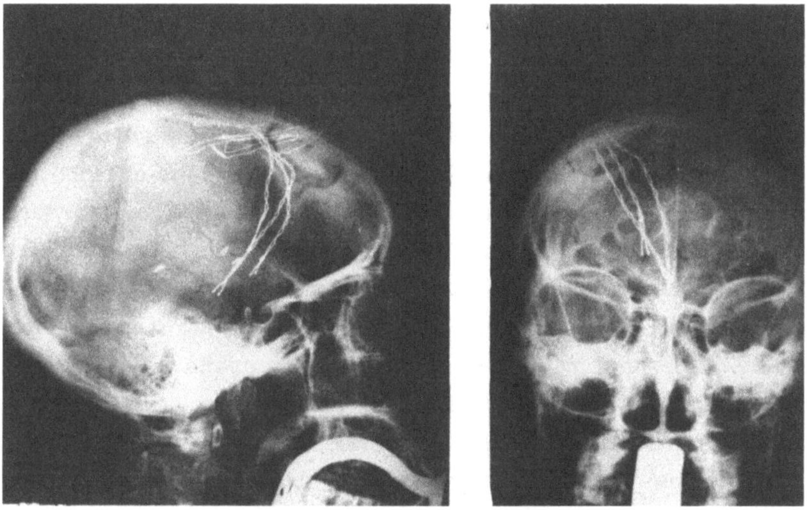

FIGURE XIX-16. Patient 23

placed in the septal region, 1 1/2 cm. rostral to the foramen of Monro, 1 cm. beneath the foramen, and 2 mm. lateral to the midline; the remaining one (lead 3) was placed in the midline about 2 cm. directly beneath the foramen in the septo-hypothalamic region.

(c) Recordings—No EEG's were taken prior to operation. Before stimulation recordings were taken from the scalp as well as from the deep electrodes. These showed a mild degree of slow wave abnormality. There was no spiking from scalp or subcortical electrodes. Prolonged stimulation to lead 2 at high intensity resulted in a seizure. The seizure began in the subcortical leads when the stimulation was terminated and did not appear in the scalp leads until about 1 minute later. When the cortex became involved a clinical seizure with tonic and clonic movements occurred. Subsequently large slow waves appeared in paroxysmal bursts at frequencies of 2 to 5 per second in the subcortical leads. These were not reflected in the scalp leads. At this time the scalp leads showed definite generalized slow wave activity. Electrical abnormalities, both cortical and subcortical, persisted for several hours.

(d) Stimulation technique—Four stimulations were made: three to the septal electrode (lead 2), lasting 4 1/2 to 10 minutes, at currents of 2 to 18 ma., and one to the septo-hypothalamic electrode (lead 3), lasting 7 minutes and 45 seconds, at a current of 2 ma.

(e) Immediate physiological effects—Stimulation to the septal electrode (lead 2), produced a rise in blood pressure from 134/76 to 160/105. Tachycardia and flushing were noted and preexisting tremor was seen to stop. The patient became euphoric. Stimulation to the septo-hypothalamic electrode (lead 3), produced an initial rise in blood pressure at 2 ma. from 140/80 to 180/135. There was marked tachycardia of 172. The patient went into a brief episode of auricular fibrillation; flushing, sweating, and dilation of the pupils were noted; and the eyes were seen to converge. A repeated stimulation to the septal electrode (lead 2) threw the patient into a generalized convulsion.

(f) Immediate behavioral response—During stimulation the patient became very relaxed, even slightly euphoric, and stated that she no longer felt the intense pain. Her facial expression relaxed, and it was apparent on objective observation that she was relieved of her pain.

(g) Immediate chemical changes—Maximum lymphopenic response was 76 per cent 1 1/2 hours after the last stimulation and 3 1/2 hours after the first stimulation. Eosinophil response to surgery was a drop to 8.3 per cu. mm., which is not so great as is sometimes noted. Plasma electrolytes were unchanged. Urinary electrolyte studies were of little value because the patient received infusions of normal saline.

(h) Complications—A generalized convulsion occurred during the stimulation procedure.

Follow-up Notes. On the morning following stimulation the patient was still semistuporous. Her eyes were open, however, and she responded to commands from the physician. Two days after the operation the patient still appeared to be comfortable. Her vital signs were normal. She carried on a conversation with her physician and replied to questions, saying that she had no pain at all. However, she died at 7:25 P.M., on the following day. Permission for an autopsy was not obtained.

PATIENT 24. See Patient 5.

PATIENT 25

AGE AT OPERATION: 39

SEX: Female

MARITAL STATUS: Married

OCCUPATION: Housewife

RELIGION: Catholic (inactive)

INFORMANT: Husband

DIAGNOSIS: No psychiatric diagnosis. Medical diagnosis, metastatic carcinoma (breast)

OPERATION: May 1, 1952

Presenting Picture. The patient was admitted in April, 1952, for intracranial surgery in an effort to relieve intractable pain caused by widespread metastatic breast carcinoma.

Present Illness. A left radical mastectomy was performed on the patient in 1947, followed by deep x-ray therapy. There were no particular symptoms until 4 years later, when she began complaining of severe pain in her hip and leg. At that time it was found that she had bony metastases. After that time her course was rapidly downhill. Between September and December, 1951, she showed temporary symptomatic improvement while she was receiving large doses of testosterone. However, in December of 1951, the beneficial effects of testosterone could not be maintained. Subsequently she was on steadily increasing doses of narcotics, until, just prior to hospitalization, she was receiving 1/32 of a grain of dilaudid every 4 hours. Because of her debilitated condition, she was hospitalized elsewhere for 2 months prior to her admission to Charity Hospital. Recently she had shown periodic confusion and disorientation.

Family History. The only informant is the patient's present (second) husband, who has almost no information concerning her past. So far as he knows there is no history of nervous or mental disorders. Both the patient's mother and grandmother died of carcinoma.

Personal History. Again little information is available because the informant has no knowledge of the patient's past life. Apparently birth and early development were normal. She graduated from high school, married at the age of 18, and had one daughter by her first marriage, which ended in divorce after a few years. Seventeen years ago the patient remarried. The couple had two children, a boy, now 16, and a girl 13. Although separation and divorce have often been considered, the patient and husband have remained together "for the children's sake." In 1949 the patient had a hysterectomy. The reasons for this are unknown, although the husband says, "She was very irritable and thought this would help her."

Personality. The patient is described as easily irritated and at times a heavy drinker. However, she was considered to be a good mother, although not a particularly attentive wife.

Personality Disorders. There is no evidence of previous mental disorder.

Physical and Laboratory Status. The patient was an emaciated white female appearing seriously and chronically ill. There were firm subcutaneous nodules from 1 to 3 cm. in diameter scattered over most of her body. Generally these nodules were not tender, but some were movable, while others were fixed to the underlying tissue. The left breast had been removed and the right breast was filled with hard, irregular masses. The abdomen felt full of the same nodular masses. Neurological examination revealed, besides the organic dementia reported below, bilateral optic atrophy. It was believed that the patient probably had intracerebral metastases. RBC was 4,000,000, hemoglobin 12.5 Gm. per cent, hematocrit 37.5 per cent, WBC 8,500, blood glucose 105 mg/100 ml., BUN 22.2, serum protein 7.55 Gm. per cent, creatinine 2.8 mg/100 ml., serology negative, urinalysis negative. Cerebral spinal fluid revealed a quantitative protein of 248 mg/100 ml. and glucose of 105 mg/100 ml. A 30-minute preoperative EEG showed the principal waking frequency was 7 and 7.5 per second; the sleep record showed a generalized spindle; there was no hyperventilation record. The diagnostic impression was generalized moderately slow activity. Findings were consistent with a clinical diagnosis of early moderate increase in intracranial pressure. AP's and laterals of the skull revealed extensive osteolytic metastases to the skull. Other x-rays revealed metastases to most of the skeleton. EKG was within normal limits.

Hospital Course. The patient lay in bed, moving rarely, complaining of severe headaches and nausea. She vomited after almost every meal, a reaction that could be controlled by the administration of sodium amytal prior to eating. She was incontinent of urine and feces. She was so weak that she had to be fed. Her mood seemed to be generally one of depression. She complained constantly of pain all over her body. Sensorium was clouded. At times she was disoriented and confused, not recognizing her husband or friends. However, on one occasion, she discussed impending surgery in an intelligent manner.

Operation—Stimulation. May 1, 1952.

(a) Surgical technique—Stereotaxic technique was used.

(b) Electrode placements—Five unipolar electrodes were implanted, all within a few millimeters of the midline. The most rostral one was deep in the septal region; three of the others were likewise in the septal region. The fifth electrode, the most caudal, was in the rostral hypothalamus. The electrode leads were numbered from 1 to 5, lead 1 being most rostral and lead 5 most caudal. See Chapter 10, Figure 4.

(c) Recordings—One EEG 3 days prior to operation showed generalized slow wave activity and suppression of sleep spindles. On the evening of operation there were many slow waves in the deep recordings made prior to stimulation, but nothing in the way of clear-cut spikes until after the stimulation. The postoperative recordings from the deep electrodes indicated continuing abnormality, characterized by occasional spiking through the septal region.

(d) Stimulation technique—Sixteen stimulations were given during the course of 8 days. There were five stimulations the first night. The first two were intraseptal stimulations, lasting from 1 1/2 to 8 minutes at currents of 2 to 22 ma. The next two stimulations were to electrodes slightly farther back but still within the septal region; one lasting 1 minute, the other 12 minutes 15 seconds, at currents ranging from 6 to 24 ma. The fifth stimulation involved one electrode in the caudal part of the septal region and one in the rostral part of the hypothalamus; it lasted 3 minutes 15 seconds at currents of 4 to 20 ma.

The next group of five stimulations occurred 4 days later. There were three stimulations to electrodes in the rostral part of the septal region, for periods of 12 seconds to 20 minutes at currents of 2 to 24 ma. A fourth stimulation was given through the other two leads within the septal region, lasting 10 minutes at currents of 8 to 20 ma. A fifth stimulation, between the caudal septum and the rostral hypothalamus, lasted 3 minutes 40 seconds at currents of 6 to 20 ma.

On the following day, the fifth day after operation, the third series of stimulations, three in number, was administered. The first was intraseptal and lasted for 22 minutes at currents of 8 to 22 ma. The second, applied to the far rostral part of the septum, lasted 6 minutes 20 seconds at currents of 2 to 18 ma. The third, administered broadly across the septum, lasted 4 minutes 45 seconds at currents of 4 to 26 ma.

Eight days after the first stimulation the last two stimulations were administered, both through the septum. Duration was 5 minutes on one occasion and 10 minutes on the other, at currents of 4 to 24 ma.

(e) Immediate physiological effects—Stimulation of septal leads 2 and 3 produced an initial rise in blood pressure from 135/80 to 140/90. Pressure rose to 190/100 as current was increased. There was marked tachycardia. Stimulation of septal leads 3 and 4 produced an initial blood pressure response of 160/100; as current was increased the pressure rose to 200/115, accompanied by marked tachycardia. Stimulation of the hypothalamic electrode (lead 5) produced an initial blood pressure response of 200/110; again there was marked tachycardia and, in this case, an internal strabismus. The patient said she felt tense. Subsequent stimulation of these anatomical regions gradually lost effectiveness. On the seventh postoperative day there was a reversal in effect; the patient showed a slowing of pulse rate and a drop in blood pressure on septal stimulation.

(f) Immediate behavioral response—The patient complained of fear and tightness in the chest.

(g) Immediate chemical changes—In the first stimulation series, lymphopenic response was not marked, the lowest drop being 24 per cent. The eosinophil response to surgery was less than usual, being in the neighborhood of 50 per cent.

There was no increase in blood sugar on any of the stimulations, indicating that the procedure evidently did not release epinephrine. There was no significant lymphopenia on any of the later stimulations. As some of the earlier electrolyte studies were complicated by the use of saline infusions, a deliberate attempt was made to dispense with them in the last series. Twenty-four hours after this series was completed the plasma potassium increased from 4.1 to 5.3 meq/L. and the plasma sodium from 130 to 149 meq/L. During this time the potassium-sodium ratio in the urine did not change. However, on the following day it increased from 0.69 to 2.43, while the plasma sodium and potassium remained essentially the same. On the third day the urinary potassium-sodium ratio was still high, ranging from 1.54 to 1.74; the plasma potassium varied between 4.2 and 4.7 meq/L., and the plasma sodium rose to 160 meq/L. On this day the patient was given by clysis 1,000 cc. of 5 per cent dextrose in normal saline and 1,500 cc. of 5 per cent dextrose in water. There was marked alteration in the quantity of urine excreted at various times in association with stimulations.

Follow-up Notes. Postoperative recordings from the deepest septal electrode indicated continuing abnormality characterized by occasional spiking. Throughout this period the patient showed signs of organic dementia. During the few days preceding her death, however, there seemed to be some psychological improvement. Although she remained weak and showed a poor memory, at no time did she have a recurrence of her pain and disorientation was somewhat lessened. Just before she died she began projectile vomiting of coffee-ground material. Death occurred 18 days after operation; according to the postmortem the primary cause was intestinal obstruction. Examination revealed metastases in virtually all the bones of the body. The skull was invaded, and there was extensive intracerebral metastases which had virtually wiped out the hypothalamic and upper mesencephalic area. There were also metastatic lesions in the pituitary.

Section V

DISCUSSIONS

Participants in the Discussions*

PSYCHIATRY

Daniel Blain, M.D., *Medical Director, American Psychiatric Association*
Douglas D. Bond, M.D., *Professor of Psychiatry*
Western Reserve University
Herbert S. Gaskill, M.D., *Professor of Psychiatry*
School of Medicine, Indiana University
George C. Ham, M.D., *Professor of Psychiatry*
School of Medicine, University of North Carolina
David M. Levy, M.D., *Attending Psychoanalyst*
Psychoanalytic Clinic for Training and Research, Columbia University
Sandor Rado, M.D., *Clinical Professor of Psychiatry, Columbia University*

INTERNAL MEDICINE

J. W. Johnson, Jr., M.D., *Medical Director*
Interstate Life and Accident Insurance Company

PSYCHOLOGY

John C. Eberhart, Ph.D., *Chief*
Research and Fellowship Grants, United States Public Health Service
Carney Landis, Ph.D., D.Sc., *Professor of Psychology*
New York State Psychiatric Institute and Hospital, Columbia University

PHYSIOLOGY

George H. Bishop, Ph.D., *Professor of Neurophysiology*
School of Medicine, Washington University (St. Louis)
John C. Lilly, M.D., *Associate Professor of Medical Physics and of Experimental Neurology, School of Medicine, University of Pennsylvania*

BIOCHEMISTRY

R. A. Cleghorn, M.D., *Associate Professor of Psychiatry*
Faculty of Medicine (Allan Memorial Institute), McGill University

ANATOMY

Fred A. Mettler, Ph.D., M.D., D.Sc., *Professor of Anatomy*
College of Physicians and Surgeons, Columbia University
William F. Windle, Ph.D., Sc.D., *Professor of Anatomy*
University of Pennsylvania

NEUROSURGERY

James B. Campbell, M.D., *Associate in Neurological Surgery*
College of Physicians and Surgeons, Columbia University

*Affiliations and titles are given as of June, 1952. Guests are listed alphabetically under their major disciplines, and the Discussions in Section V follow this order.

Discussion*

HERBERT S. GASKILL, M.D.
Professor of Psychiatry
School of Medicine
Indiana University

Dr. Heath and his associates have presented a new therapeutic approach to the treatment of schizophrenia. In doing so they have clearly outlined the theoretical concepts which led to the formulation of this new treatment. Psychiatrists always have been interested in this disease and have been accumulating data in regard to every aspect of this illness. Unfortunately, much of this has remained isolated with little attempt to piece together fragments into a meaningful whole. Such an attempt with considerable success has been done by Dr. Heath and his group. They have not depended on one approach but have integrated the known facts from both the psychic and the somatic aspects of this illness, and more important they have made many new observations. As was to be expected from such sound research methods, important new discoveries were forthcoming.

The amount of data which has been presented has been enormous and I shall limit my remarks to two aspects—first, to the electroencephalographic spike, which has been discovered in the schizophrenic patient, and, secondly, to the clinical results of the electrostimulation.

Some years ago Dr. Stanley Cobb suggested that much basic data might be discovered if electrodes could be placed in the midbrain and in other deeper structures of the brain. If further study substantiates the fact that this spike is found in all or nearly all schizophrenics and not in other illnesses, then an important fact concerning this disease will have been uncovered. From there it will be necessary to learn a great deal more as to what such a discharge phenomenon means.

*For obvious reasons no editorial changes have been made in the text of any of the Discussions included in Section V.

The clinical importance of these studies must not be minimized since they may help to differentiate the various types of schizophrenia and assist in making more accurate predictions as to the ultimate prognosis of the individual case. These studies may assist in differentiating between environment.

The clinical aspects of this therapeutic approach are impressive. After having heard a discussion of the clinical results, seen a number of patients in sound film, pre- and post-operatively, and subsequently interviewed a number of these patients themselves, and finally to have participated in an actual operative and stimulation procedure, leaves little doubt in our minds that something fundamental happens to the patient. The withdrawn, affectless individual whose thinking is so autistic and irrational when samples can be obtained, during the process of stimulation shows an immediate and perceptible change in his psychic and somatic responsiveness. This change is so dramatic and so real that one is reminded of the fairy story of "The Sleeping Beauty." The patient who has been so remote, living in a dream world with little evidence of awareness of his or her environment and with diminished responsiveness in feeling, which is mirrored in the lessened autonomic responsiveness, shows immediate changes in all of these spheres.

The changes enumerated above appear to persist in those patients who have been followed post-operatively insofar as the follow-up period permits of evaluation. This period is still too short to be extremely significant in any study of schizophrenia.

The number of patients treated is relatively small and the follow-up period too short to permit a definite statement in regard to the therapeutic effect of electrostimulation. From the statistics given it would appear that approximately 50 per cent of the patients were markedly improved. From a statistical point of view there is some question as to whether this is sufficient to credit the electrostimulation with any specificity in regard to the therapeutic change. Figures of from 30 to 50 per cent of cures have been given many times in the past in regard to various treatment methods in schizophrenia but many of these patients after a follow-up period of 5 years have shown an increasing tendency towards relapse.

In conclusion I should like to emphasize that I do not believe the significance of this study should be primarily determined on the clinical results. Any new approach to the study of schizophrenia with a breadth of vision and imagination which this research study has shown is of inestimable value and is making a basic contribution to the study of this disease. Few questions have been answered with any definiteness in the study thus far. Much new information has been obtained but this is primarily in the development of new leads which will need further exploration and evaluation, not only from this research group but from many other research groups, before any definite opinion can be formed about this contribution. This was an extremely stimulating conference and gives us hope of more definite answers in the near future.

Discussion

GEORGE C. HAM, M.D.
Professor of Psychiatry
School of Medicine
University of North Carolina
Chapel Hill

In opening my remarks, I pointed out that a good deal of what I would have to say would be presumptive, based on several factors. First of all, the quantity of material that was presented was such that it was almost impossible to do any type of objective integration of it during the actual conference itself. Secondly, that a good deal of what was expressed by the various presenters included a great deal of experience which was not formulated or could not be formulated as yet, yet which probably contained a great many truths which were pertinent.

I then pointed out that I would be speaking largely to the clinical situation in regard to the change in clinical state of the patients, but that I wished to make a few remarks about some of the more fundamental physiological, biochemical and psychological research. As you will recall, I broke the presentation down into three days and used a musical analogy. I suggested that the presentation of the theoretical framework, the psychodynamics, the neurophysiology and so on were excellent, stimulating, broad in scope and yet to the point and very plausible, based on a great deal of research by the Tulane group as well as the studies of others. I likened this part of the presentation to a Beethoven quartet. The second day, in which the description of the surgical technique was presented, its development and the description of the procedures, was likened to Wagner; and I made the facetious remark that possibly this was like the entrance of the gods into Valhalla. The third portion, namely the actual testing and recording and stimulating of the patient following operation, reminded me of Honegger or Stravinsky, and added the suggestion that it might be something like

Moussorgsky in his music "A Night on Bald Mountain." All of this carried with it some feeling about the changing sharpness and objectivity of the procedure and the increasing number of factors that were impinging into the situation as we progressed from the theoretical framework through the actual pre-operative, pre-stimulative physiologic and biochemical measurements and the surgical intervention to the intense activity, tension and interest that were present during the period following recording and stimulation.

There is unquestioned evidence of the marked metabolic changes in both the animal experiments and in man. These, I think, are of extreme importance and indicate a new and extremely valuable understanding of total functioning. This demonstration alone will have lasting and very important significance. The fact that the concept grew out of the collaboration of many different disciplines and approaches, was developed through animal experimentation and shown to occur in man, was in itself an example of a beautifully conducted piece of scientific reasoning and study. The surgical problem, although great, was handled with skill and is improving in its sharpness and exactness all the time. The relationship of clinical improvement to the subcortical spikes and their disappearance following stimulation of the septal area was, in my opinion, less sharp. I suggested that even though the concept of inhibition and facilitation had been clearly shown in relationship to the motor and metabolic changes, other factors may be involved in what clinical improvement occurs in addition to functional changes in the septal area and the metabolic sequelae. Among these are, of course, the fact that there is a tremendous motivational investment by the investigating group in this problem; there is an intense interest and attention to the patient during the post-operative stimulating phase; the whole procedure is one of extreme black magic and omnipotence with rather intense narcissistic reward to the individual for improvement. Experiences in many fields of psychosomatic study now indicate that factors other than the specific physiologic change or pharmacologic stimulus must be taken into consideration in measuring clinical improvement. The history of Bargen and Bargen's serum in which he was able to get a statistically significant improvement in ulcerative colitis, yet others failed to get the same result even with his own material, was one of the early indications of this. The increasing knowledge of the relationship of improvement, clinically, in hypertension as related to the physician's attitude, even though it be the unconscious attitude of the physician, rather than to the drug, is becoming data of widespread knowledge (Ferris et al.). Obviously, the experimental control of such a situation is extremely difficult inasmuch as any type of control that you consider even up to the one of putting in the electrode and not stimulating but giving everything else runs into the difficulty that actually the basic motivation and interest of the investigators is changed. I think, however, that before a great deal of meaning is attached to the clinical improvement in schizophrenia, a good deal of thought must be given to other factors in addition to the facilitation of this local septal area alone.

I also mentioned the fact that the clinical psychiatric formulations did not indicate inclusion of the specific nuclear conflicts of these individuals nor was there a psychodynamic formulation which presented the lifelong instinctual problems and the typical defenses for this individual. The descriptions were more phenomenological than genetic and dynamic, and it occurred to me that the different reactions, clinically, of the patients might be related to the specific differences in the basic nuclear personality dynamics as they respond to the procedure, to the particular therapist, and to the meaning of the rather gross intervention, stimulation and interest. I suggested that each patient, if possible, be studied to such a point that a clear-cut psychodynamic formulation as mentioned above could be formulated so that one would know what to expect of a given patient in his reaction to interpersonal relations as accurately as one would know what to expect of his cortico-steroid production.

I closed by stating that I have nothing but admiration for the excellence of this scientific study, for the persistence, for the devotion of the entire group to this goal, and considered it an outstanding example of integrated research of the type which will bring us the kind of knowledge we need to know about total adaptation both for further research and for clinical application. I considered it a privilege to have the opportunity to join the group and see this presentation. I hope that in the future I may have even more intimate and detailed knowledge of further progress.

Discussion

DAVID M. LEVY, M.D.
Attending Psychoanalyst
Psychoanalytic Clinic for Training and Research
Columbia University

I

The implantation of electrodes in certain areas of the brain and the stimulation of these areas was followed by a remarkable change in all but a few of twenty schizophrenic patients. These patients were selected on the basis of severity of illness.

The discussion and the presentation of data by the staff engaged in the new operative procedure and by their guests, was devoted largely to the technical and anatomic aspects of the problem. This seemed appropriate in a first large conference on the subject since the improvement of the surgery and the electrostimulation, and electroencephalographic recording are the first and still the foremost problem. Refinement and simplification of these procedures will enhance their value by reducing the damage of brain cells to a minimum, by determining the optimal sites and surgical technique for implantation of electrodes; possible reduction of their number; and optimal method, time and frequency of stimulation.

II

The finding of "spikes" in the E.E.G. recordings highlighted the discussion in regard to the neurophysiology. The "spikes" offered the tempting theory that schizophrenia resulted in or from dysfunction of the facilitatory and/or suppressor centres in the brain stem, and that elimination of the "spikes" was followed by restoration of function. What function? If the cells that are stimulated "tune up" the organism, what does this mean in relation to schizophrenia? Does it mean that schizophrenia is an energy disease and that a temporary lift in energy is the spark that carries the patient out of himself into social activity? If an energy theory were accepted a number of psychological theories would be necessary to bolster it. These would involve a theory as to the kind of personality that responds to the dysfunction in the schizophrenic way, and a theory to explain why some schizophrenics and not others progress satisfactorily after the initial "lifts."

The physiologic functions of the f. and s. centres particularly need further explanation in quest of an answer to the "lift." So far the explanations must remain in the form of "energizing," as it affects alertness, attention-span, muscle tone and ACTH effects. It is the basic social function, without which the individual is not related to other human beings, that remains elusive. The experimental work thus far has been limited to the effects on the behavior of the animal, without knowledge of the animal's previous social relationship. Experiments that can tell us the effects on the relationship of monkey A to monkey B, a relationship carefully studied beforehand, might help. It is not too difficult to produce experimentally a monkey who remains isolated from the others, though not schizophrenic. The "experimental neurosis," as produced by Lyddell, is closer, I think, to schizophrenia than to neurosis. In any case it is a combination of experimental psychology and neurophysiology that might lead us to an understanding of some function in the f. and s. centres more directly related to social drive, a drive that impels organisms to seek each other, a drive basic to the sexual and maternal. Aside from the problems dealt with in this study, the finding of a physiologic function that is essentially basic to social linkage would certainly be a fundamental discovery.

III

Theoretically if the change observed during the postoperative period of stimulation were a permanent one, the large majority of cases would, in a practical sense (self maintenance and social adjustment in the community) be cured.

Actually, about half the number of patients showed evidence of change throughout follow up periods, and half of these (one-fourth of the total) were cured, in the sense of cure employed.

Calling the results failures, partial improvement and favorable improvement, some of the failures were explained as technical failures; i.e. failures due to poor placement of electrodes or inadequacies in stimulation.

Favorable results may be related to the type of patient as classified in the hospital. Thus, the most favorable results were found in catatonics, next in the paranoid, least in the hebephrenics.

Simple tabulation of the case abstracts resulted in the finding that all cases characterized as "silly" or "dilapidated" or "actively hallucinating," which comprised in all one half of the series of twenty cases, contained most of the failures.

From this finding one might explain the results as a measure of potential capacity for social response, or, a measure of the intactness of the personality that remains in spite of the disease. From that point of view one would regard the hebephrenics' silly, deteriorated behavior as evidence of regression or/and an original (preschizophrenic) immaturity of the severest degree. The catatonic would be regarded as remaining behind the facade of negativism the most intact of the three. We are dealing with people who have protected themselves from their fellow beings or who, as a result of their failure in relationships with them, have broken or made impossible, contact with them. The hebephrenic, it would appear, is incapacitated from the start. A study of the prepsychotic social experiences of the schizophrenics as a prognostic factor would be worth doing. The catatonic's defense is an oppositional barrier; the paranoid's defense is an active attack. In terms of interpersonal relationship the hebephrenic can't; the catatonic won't; the paranoid will but only to dominate and destroy. When the latter is actively hallucinating it would mean that he is in a state in which the fears involved in the feelings of the danger of his fellow men are too intense, too acute, for favorable change. It may be found that operative procedures must wait for a more quiescent period. (Research problems: initial postoperative response as prognostic indicator. Are there any special features in the quality of the response that will aid in prognosis: for example, Heath's idea that it is a favorable sign when a patient can talk about his psychotic symptoms with a sense of humor?)

IV

When a patient has responded favorably to stimulation, why should he continue to respond favorably thereafter? Does it follow that one or two or several series of stimulations should have a "permanent" effect? In every case other forms of therapy were utilized before and after the electrosurgical therapy. It was evidently taken for granted that the electrostimulation alone would have no permanent value. The suggestion of a control group composed of patients receiving the surgical procedure (using the term to include electrostimulation) alone, i.e. with no further therapy than nursing and the previous custodial type of care, was regarded as quite unnecessary. The point of view as expressed by the clinical psychiatrist was apparently shared by the other members of the research team. The reasoning runs as follows: (1) How can you expect anyone who has been inside an institution for years to embark on a new venture requiring a marked upheaval of by now an old way of life, without help? (2) Even if the patient's contact with psychiatrist and social worker continued after release from the hospital, the expectations of the patient's family, assuming there is a family to receive him, might be (as it often was) excessive. They, the family, might expect the patient to assume responsibility immediately, as though he had suffered nothing more than a fractured bone which was now completely healed. (3) Under the requirements of the "controlled" experiment, a patient might leave the hospital to join a family containing psychotic members (as actually happened), or a family that had enjoyed for years the freedom of a burden whose return they were now strongly resisting (as also happened) or to have no family to go to, no prospective employment, no social contacts.

Accepting the obvious conclusion that psychiatric and social therapy are essential, the loss of a "controlled" group is not a serious one, since there are numerous studies that can serve in the same capacity: series of cases of schizophrenics treated by various forms of psychosurgery, shock therapy or insulin therapy, or by intensive psychotherapy alone.

The problem of duration of change produced by the electrostimulation is difficult to solve, however, by clinical study. When a failure is explainable by environmental difficulties following release from the hospital, the question of permanent or temporary stimulation effects becomes relatively unimportant. With a very large body of case material it will be feasible to correlate "permanency" of change with such factors as placement of electrodes, intensity, duration, frequency of stimulus, also surgical skill. Such correlations can then be measured against different post-hospital conditions, scale-rated from favorable to unfavorable.

V

From the preceding paragraph the inference is clear that a transitional period of care is an important phase of therapy. The operative procedures activate the organism in a manner that induces socialization. The patient's symptoms are in abeyance. He appears friendly, talks agreeably, and for the time being, has recovered his sanity. The closed door has been opened. The psychiatrist is aware of the need for frequent contact at this stage. Psychotherapy is chiefly in the form of emotional support. Psychoanalytic forms of intensive psychotherapy are not employed. The reasons presumably are fear of probing (which might possibly upset the applecart) and practical considerations. The latter involve economy of time and personnel. If simpler forms of psychotherapy work the method has wider application. The psychiatrist believes also that the type of patients seen, in terms of intelligence and schooling, were poor prospects for intensive psychotherapy.

Once the door has been opened and the patient aided in developing sufficient initiative to walk out, he needs a place to go to. This place has been determined in a sense by the social worker. She has had contact with members of the patient's family, has discussed prospective employment with them, etc.

The social worker, as well as the psychiatrist, have meanwhile tried to develop an attitude of acceptance and encouragement on the part of those who have a responsible relationship to the patient. Post operative support and the receiving environment are evidently important factors in therapy. Important also is a transitional stage where for whatever reason transportation from hospital to home cannot or should not be made without a period of partial protection. This would involve workshops, rooming houses and various facilities which could probably be built up through existing social agencies. The transitional phase, the phase in which the patient resides outside the hospital under special conditions, before he makes the complete break, is indicated, obviously, for numerous patients besides those considered in this group. It is especially indicated for patients who have undergone the special operative procedure because of the abrupt nature of the cure, in contrast with the usual slow recovery and easing into outside activities, when recovery occurs in patients who have received no more than "ordinary" state hospital care.

VI

The operative procedure is an advance over other forms of psychosurgery because it entails much less destruction of brain cells and because it is physiologically a rational rather than an empirical procedure. It is rational presumably because it is an attempt to stimulate areas previously found by experimental work with animals to be intimately connected with vegetative function. Greater exactitude of location, connection, and function of these areas is a current investigation. In contrast with lobotomy it stimulates rather than destroys, and ideally, should have none of the unfortunate aftermath of intellectual deterioration and loss of sustained goal behavior so commonly involved with the former procedure. Psychological research starts with the advantage of known weaknesses in the thoroughgoing testing methods used in the Columbia-Greystone project. The availability of a new test, developed at Tulane, gives promise of a reliable measure of intellectual deterioration following the new operation. It will aid in the work on improving the method of implanting electrodes with minimal cell damage. Without the benefit of special tests, clinical observation shows clearly now, that adverse intellectual and personality changes are generally less frequent and less severe than after lobotomy.

The disadvantage of the Tulane procedure (which will probably be its rubric) is the special skill, the training, and the length of time involved. That is also, however, a decided advantage. It will be difficult for any surgeon to enter the skull for the purpose of almost random slashing of the brain after the new method is well established.

VII

It is interesting that in the Tulane project the surgery is far in advance of the psychotherapy. The latter consists largely of emotional support and aid through social workers in regard to family acceptance and community contacts. If it works well that way, so much the better. However, Sullivan's results with schizophrenics at the Shepard Pratt Hospital through psychodynamic training of nurses and attendants produced a majority of cures over twenty years ago. He dealt, however, only with young schizophrenics whose breakdowns had been recent. Further the proportion of cures were greatly reduced after he left the hospital. For his project a careful selection of personnel was necessary. Under prevailing conditions in state hospitals the method now used at Tulane is less demanding, hence more feasible. It must be borne in mind always that the patients selected for therapy in the Tulane experiment were the least promising. Nevertheless, it would be valuable for therapy as well as research to select certain cases for more intensive study. At least some good introspective accounts of the change in feeling of the patient as a result of the operation would be available.

Discussion

J. W. JOHNSON, JR., M.D.
Medical Director
Interstate Life and Accident Insurance Company

Without in any way detracting from the technical and observational accomplishments of Dr. Heath and his group it seems to me that the most important thing in evidence during these three days has been method. In spite of a heritage of schism within his particular discipline to which, of course, he in no small part contributed, I have a hunch that a mind as curious and as interested as Freud's would have been not only delighted to see analytical and physiological techniques of investigation constituting a single research method but really rather relieved to find that devotion to such method could bind together a group for as long as even one academic year. That there has apparently been none of the dissociation which has rendered ineffective and uncomfortable much of the research in psychiatry is probably less a tribute to Dr. Heath and Tulane than to method. Actually, method was the one thing that made possible the gathering together for three days in New Orleans in June of as polyglot a group of physicians as sit around this table. I've sat here as an internist, interested in the methods of insurance medicine, concerned with what psychiatry may add to a framework from which I can work effectively and comfortably, the while listening to the discussion of a theory, description of techniques and report of observations. It has impressed me that a spectrum of participation broad enough to include Rado and Lilly, or Levy and Campbell and not spill over into either ultra-violet or infra-red is again a testimony to method.

A short while ago Dr. Rado referred to his participation in this panel as that of a sidewalk superintendent watching, I felt with affectionate interest, the construction of a building by a group whose competency to plan, he recognizes, but whose competency at execution he is required to criticize by the very nature of the undertaking and his own training. This it has seemed to me has been the general attitude of the panel participants. As I look back at the start of the panel three days ago I felt rather more like a sidewalk bum required by limitations of background to look through those various peep-holes, provided by management for the curious and which were not being used by others. I have a definite impression that on the first day I looked for a peep-hole, found most of them occupied and lay claim to one, apparently unoccupied, by muttering something about "actuarial methods," "biostatistical approach" and "contemporary clinico-projective techniques of underwriting." The panel discussion began as a matter of fact with a good deal of such peep-hole perception of the whole, but by discussion amongst those of us on the sidewalk, by movement, as it were, from perspective to perspective, it seems to me that after three days of participation, we on the sidewalk are beginning to acquire an overall appraisal of the construction framework. This again would constitute evidence supporting method and it is such evidence that must ultimately establish the value of the proffered theory.

As I understand the theory or framework to which these methods of study are being applied, it seems rather straightforward and orderly, and to be based on a body of objective data of reasonable size. Though the pressure of presenting data has perhaps obscured the presentation of theory which Dr. Heath offered us the first morning, I persist in an impression that the framework is neither so rigidly constructed as to blunt the instruments of objective exploration nor so ephemeral as to permit of no contact with such instrument.

Dr. Heath and his group seem to begin with something of a Heraclitean concept of movement and then enter the field of biology with the idea of relating movement to survival, of working one's way back, as it were, from response to stimulus, from muscle via mind, the Sherringtonian "controller of muscle," to that which prods the organism to assume a second equilibrium. The hedonic levels of pleasure and pain, I gather, reflect success or failure in achieving such equilibrium. Proceeding philogenetically they enter the area of actual application of method at the level of the cat where data point to a less intimate integration of cortex to forebrain and muscle. The group then moves on via the monkey, an experimental animal with a more intimate integration, to study schizophrenic man and man making other, more or less successful, efforts at survival.

Their efforts at study center around forebrain relationships and forebrain-cortical relationships, their methods of study comprising both inspective and, within the limitations of communication, introspective techniques. Again, it has seemed to me, the orientation has been philogenetic and the tools of psychology, neurophysiology, and biochemistry have been applied to broaden the opportunity for inspection and those of psychoanalysis to broaden the opportunity for communication and introspection.

The acquisition of distance receptors, of memory, judgement, projection, of thinking, realistic or autistic, of levels of feeling more highly integrated than the hedonic levels, of metabolic drives integrated variously with philogenetically higher central nervous system levels, might well require for survival varying delay in response, or what is probably more important, make possible a delay in response. If then Dr. Heath offers us his pleasant little doodle that $Eq\ (t) \rightarrow N \rightarrow A \rightarrow Eq_2\ (t')$ which he translates as Equilibrium at a given time, leads (if for no other reason than that the damned thing is alive and time's awastin'—i.e., metabolic) to Need (tension) to Activity (pleasure) and so to a Second Equilibrium at a successive time, it behooves Dr. Heath and the group who are associated with him either to stick to the philogenetic level of the paramecium or design methods sufficiently inclusive to apply that formula to higher philogenetic levels. They have apparently elected to stop short at a level just a little lower than the angels and to apply a method as inclusive as is available in 1952.

I can't, however, agree with Dr. Mettler's statement last night that this is just another cruise of *The Beagle,* vintage 1952. It seems to me that the method itself is a function of theory with the advantages and limitations that such an integration implies. What is to be found here at Tulane is neither Darwinian nor Freudian, inspective nor introspective, but an effective awareness of varying degrees of integration not simply an effort at integration. It is certainly not eclectic. The abhorrence by nature of a vacuum would seem to parallel the abhorrence by our hosts of dissociation. As a private practitioner of internal medicine, I am perhaps particularly aware of certain advantages of dissociation and can, therefore, express an appreciation of a group which is not seduced by those advantages.

An extraordinary amount of technical and observational material has been gathered. It has obviously been quite difficult to prepare and present. Its acquisition has required a vast amount of work by a very devoted group. The framework is up, to refer again to Dr. Rado's analogy, but there are a goodly number of unbolted girders and in the upper stories some of the girders are not only precariously balanced but a few seem supported by sheer force of personal magnetism. So far as I can see, in considering the data presented in this preliminary report to the panel, the technical and observational accomplishments of Dr. Heath and his colleagues consist of:

1. The placing, with increasing skill and accuracy, of exploring and stimulating electrodes within designated centers of the human forebrain.
2. The observation, by exploration, of anterior septal spiking in schizophrenics.
3. The application, with increasing knowledge, of electrical stimulation to human forebrain centers.
4. The observation, by stimulation, of so far ill defined integrations which have perhaps been well described as facilitatory circuits in the anterior midline or septal regions and as repressive circuits in the dorso-lateral or caudate regions.
5. The confirmation, from stimulation, of a relationship between the central mid-line or hypothalamic regions to changes in steroid and electrolyte mechanisms, so far ill defined as to direction and subsequent impact on the total organism.
6. The observation, from anterior-septal stimulation in schizophrenics sufficient to decrease the frequency of spiking, of an alteration in movement and hedonic capacities which tends towards compensation of such patients and a greater capacity for the utilization of what has been variously referred to here as "Tincture of Heath" or "Total Push."
7. The observation, from exploration and stimulation, of other integrations or circuits, not yet defined but which when related to theory

enables the various members of the panel group to maintain a fairly high titre of participation for these three days and provides the active group with enough drive to look forward to a great deal of work yet to be done.

At times during the past few days most of us here have questioned the wisdom of presenting this material at this time. All of us, hosts and guests, would like to see the areas of integrations more firmly established, the lines of investigation more sharply drawn, the opportunities for critical appraisal more clearly defined. However, Dr. Heath has not opened the door to a small room, certainly not to a room of his own. Rather a very large territory is being opened and I would hold it neither inappropriate, unwise, nor immodest for the openers to invite others skilled in surveying to explore it with them. It certainly looks like fertile country.

Discussion

CARNEY LANDIS, PH.D., D.SC.
Professor of Psychology
New York State Psychiatric Institute and Hospital
Columbia University

Three aspects of the reports which we have heard seem to me to deserve further comment. These are the development of the cooperative research method which is now called the *combined operation procedure,* the role of theory in combined operation projects and the results themselves. One of the earliest extensive non-military combined operation projects in the medical sciences was the first Columbia-Greystone Project. It was the good fortune of several of the investigators here at Tulane, as well as several of the guests including myself, to have been associated with that project. It was for all the Columbia-Greystone Associates a new sort of cooperative venture where methods of coordination and research were developed as the work progressed. All of us were enthusiastic with this general approach to a major problem in medical science—particularly in psychiatry—and congratulated ourselves on having had a part in this new development. The second Columbia-Greystone Project encountered numerous difficulties. The New York State Brain Research Project was a failure so far as it was supposed to be a cooperative research venture. This led to considerable disillusionment with what we had hoped might develop into a new highway for psychiatric research and a mental re-evaluation of the combined operation idea.

The very evident success which has attended this Tulane venture is indeed heartening and illustrates that combined operation research in psychiatry is possible and that the first Columbia-Greystone Project was not a serendipity phenomenon. I am still unable to define with any degree of accuracy those elements which lead to success in a combined operation project and which elements lead to disaster. I wish that it were possible to state more precisely the role which is played by interpersonal relations, by preconceived theory, by youth and enthusiasm, and by the nature of the problem itself.

The application of the method of logical deduction from theory or hypothesis to psychological experimentation has never impressed me. The least possible preconceived theory coupled with the greatest possible knowledge of previously established factual observations has always seemed the best way of moving into a research venture. The extensive and somewhat involved theoretical basis, which Dr. Heath supplied as the basis of this Tulane combined operation project, seemed to me largely unnecessary, at least so far as the psychological discipline was concerned. Indeed I am ready to believe that Dr. King was essentially untouched by the theorizing in planning and carrying out those parts of the work for which he was responsible. If I may speculate at this point, I would guess that Dr. King chose to utilize the particular experimental procedures employed from the experience which he had gained from his connection with three previous brain research projects. He selected procedures which he or others had found to be workable with uncooperative mental patients and which seemed to yield changed scores following brain surgery. In addition, as he said, he continued the use of parts of standard intelligence tests and projective techniques so that ready reference points might be available. In any event the theoretical construction of the psychiatric discipline neither led to the selection of functions to be measured or to the psychological evaluation of the findings.

The theory then seems to have been of value to the thinking of Dr. Heath. It may have been of utility in administration and in public relations. That the theory as such has added anything to the explanation of the changes which were brought about seems dubious to me, nor do I see where the theory has aided in the explanations offered by the investigators in the clinical disciplines.

Psychology is the latest experimental discipline to be added to medical research teams. It has proved its worth in the brain research projects. The excellent report which Dr. King gave shows that experimental psychology has just begun to make real contributions to a combined operation of this variety. It must be emphasized that what Dr. King has done is experimental psychological research in the true tradition of the discipline. It would have been all too easy to include that art now called "Clinical Psychology" in a project of this sort and have achieved nothing. Clinical psychology as practiced at present is primarily an art of aid and assistance in diagnosis and therapy. So far it has made few if any contributions to the elucidation of the basic problems of psychiatry. One should also recognize that Dr. King is an experimental psychologist of outstanding ability and that the ingenious methods which he has devised place him in the front rank of his psychological colleagues.

So far as the psychological research in this project is concerned, the Tulane group has a working team of proved ability. Dr. King can be counted on to carry on in the further development of the work without any suggestions on my part. My advice to his collaborators in the other disciplines is, "Don't try to foist your psychological theories on to him."

Dr. King has been very careful not to intrude psychological investigation during the acute phase of the "treatment." He has based his report on tests given well in advance of surgery and a month or so after surgery has been completed. I hope that as this project continues methods may be devised for the doing of psychological measurements during the acute phase of this procedure, namely after surgery but immediately before and after stimulation. Of course everyone else wants to work with the patient during this interval and there are no very promising ready and obvious methods of psychological measurement available which would immediately justify cutting down on the time now utilized by other disciplines whose methodology is better organized. I do believe that it would be of value to have psychological measurements pushed into this period even though such measurements may be fragmentary.

Dr. Levy has made two criticisms of Dr. King's work which I believe deserve comment. He has restated the conviction held by so many clinical observers that frontal lobe surgery must of necessity lead to intellectual damage or deficit. It has been regularly found by every psychologist who has had the opportunity of applying intelligence tests before and after psychosurgery that there is no permanent damage to intellect, learning, or memory so long as the more posterior portions of the frontal lobe were not involved by the surgery. It is true that the Porteus Maze Test usually shows a loss in M.A. score immediately following operation.

However, when the Porteus is administered six months to a year following operation a complete return to preoperative level of function has been uniformly found. The myth that the frontal lobe tissue mediates higher intellectual processes dies hard. Dr. Levy also objected to the use of an outside-of-the-hospital-normal-population as a standard for comparison for the psychotic patients on the motor performance tests. If I understood him, Dr. Levy would rather have had the comparison made with patients in hospitals suffering from one or another physical disability without mental involvement. It is doubtful that anything would have been gained by using a hospitalized control group, and I think that much would have been lost. Not every otherwise normal human being who is in a hospital for injury or physical disease is normal in the everyday sense of the word. Physical illness and hospitalization certainly detract from his "normality." Dr. King was trying to contrast the psychotic population with a truly normal population. If he had compared the psychotics with another hospitalized population, he would have introduced the unknown effect of physical illness plus hospitalization. These additional variables themselves would have had to be isolated and measured before he could have said how nearly his psychotics had returned to normal following treatment.

Dr. King has found that his performance scores for psychiatric patients (based largely on reaction time and tapping) are quite significantly below the standards set by his normal population. Indeed the differences are such that they may well serve as indicators or even measures of the degree of mental disorder. Furthermore they reflect the progress of recovery from mental pathology. These findings are thought provoking. The tests employed are exceedingly simple calling for a minimum of motor skill and of "mental" coordination. It is common to say that psychoses and neuroses are expressions of disorders of the higher mental processes. Perhaps they are but no sort of objective measuring device so far administered by experimental psychologists or by investigators from any other scientific discipline has given any regular and consistent indication of disorder of higher mental processes. Now Dr. King has demonstrated that the *simplest* sort of performances do reflect a decreased efficiency. Psychosis and neurosis slow down simple habitual movements by a very significant amount and as the disease process is ameliorated the efficiency again approaches normal standards. *This is new* and has potentialities of its own which are quite as important as are the dramatic results of the stimulation of the septal areas. Where it will lead no one can say, but there is no doubt in my mind that Dr. King has opened a field of immense potentialities.

If I may violate my own advice to the other disciplines to leave psychology alone, I would like to make some suggestions to both the investigators in neurophysiology and in biological chemistry. It is, of course, most interesting to know that spike potentials are obtained from the septal area in schizophrenic patients and that such spikes were not found in patients suffering from other ailments. But, we should know what such spikes indicate. The statement that they are an expression of the simultaneous discharge of many neural units is a description and not an explanation. The appearance of the large slow waves in sleep or in the catatonic state likewise deserves explanation which goes beyond description. Most probably the spikes and the slow waves are an expression of chemical or metabolic processes which are of importance in their own right, and which, if isolated would lead on to further investigation in the realm lying between chemistry and neurophysiology.

It seems to me that a more intimate analysis should be made of both the spikes and the slow waves so that their precise electrical properties might be known more accurately. If these properties were known it might be profitable to stimulate the brain with electric potentials which are as nearly as possible similar to the spikes or to the slow waves. Biologically speaking there is no particular virtue in using a square wave stimulator. Gastaut (*EEG. Clin. Neurophysiol.*, 1949, 1:205), and Walter, Dorey and Shipton (*Nature*, 1946, 158:540) have registered the EEG of persons who were potential epileptics and have used the EEG to control "photic driving" of the flicker variety finding that such modulated photic driving precipitated seizures. From this grows the suggestion that in place of using square wave stimulation one might well use spike potential or slow wave stimulation applied at various frequencies and intensities to those portions of the brain where they occur spontaneously. One might also apply such stimuli 180° out of phase from their normal mode of appearance. It is, of course, impossible to predict what might be the outcome of such "patterned" stimuli but the results might be interesting.

My own knowledge of biological chemistry is sketchy; hence the report of Dr. Price did not convey very much knowledge to me. One hopes that in the published reports Dr. Price will be able to show the meaning and the significance of determinations which he made. I am at a loss to know whether or not the changes which he has found are limited to each patient as an individual or whether any generality is to be attributed to them.

It seems to me that this is a "midstream" conference. The Tulane group has carried on from where the Columbia-Greystone group left off. They have made real progress although no one can really say just yet where the work is leading. It is difficult to envisage the totality and the significance of their findings at the present time. In a way this conference reminds me of a story concerning Professor Whitehead of the Philosophy Department at Harvard. Shortly after the professor had joined the Harvard faculty, he was a member of an examining committee for a Ph.D. candidate in psychology whose thesis was concerned with the technical problem involving the kinesthetic components of affective experience. At the end of the examination, after the candidate had been excused, the chairman of the Examination Committee turned to Professor Whitehead and asked him his opinion of the candidate's defense of his thesis. Professor Whitehead replied, "First rate, first rate, I never understood a word of it, but it certainly sounded like the proper sort of nonsense."

Discussion

GEORGE H. BISHOP, PH.D.
Professor of Neurophysiology
School of Medicine
Washington University (St. Louis)

There are two contrasting approaches to research; one an overall attack on a general problem, necessarily guided by a preconceived theory, which is then pursued into its ramifying details; and the other, a start at some specific point, from which one more or less follows his nose, as the program develops. The former rather more ambitious approach has its complications, and one of these is that any uncertainty in the plan of attack can compromise many of the conclusions.

There are a variety of ways to be sure of validating such a theoretical interpretation as lies back of this work. One is a search for rather specific overall correlations between a given procedural maneuver and a change in patient behavior. Another is the more direct step by step investigation by appropriate means of the mechanisms presumed to be involved in the condition under study, and those actually involved in the experimental procedures. The first method is that which has met with considerable success in the use of the EEG record, which still lacks any adequate fundamental interpretation however. But the work under consideration is also employing the other approach. It is this second approach which would seem to a neurophysiologist to merit further emphasis. The problem might thus be more securely tied down to its obvious neurological moorings.

For instance, what are the actual neurological connections of the subseptal region; e.g. of the nucleus acumbens and the medial septal nucleus? Is there in fact a connection between this region and cortex, or in the reverse direction; how specific is it, and does it in fact "reverberate"? This term has been widely used, and rather loosely. Whether any given circuit does in fact reverberate its activity is a matter to be demonstrated.

The question of the relation of this region to activity elsewhere is complicated by a second question. What is the type of stimulation employed here doing to the tissues affected, and what tissue is in fact involved? A rough estimate of the current density between electrodes is that at 5 ma. total current, one ma. per square mm. cross section would not be an unreasonable value. The current density per cross section of the whole brain applied in shock therapy (0.5 ampere total through a cross section of roughly 10,000 sq. mm.) comes out at 0.05 ma. per sq. mm., or smaller than the currents routinely employed here by a factor of twenty. When currents up to 30 ma. are applied this factor indicates that at the point of application, over 100 times shock therapy current is flowing. The results to be expected of such current strengths, especially when applied over many minutes instead of a few seconds as in shock therapy, would be rather drastic; some damage at the site of application would seem certain, and wide spread of current to surrounding regions might be as significant a factor as the more local effect.

The frequent occurrence of results such as usually are associated with hypothalamic activation suggest such spread of stimulating current. Lack of evidence of serious destruction at the site of application might indicate that pulses of only 1 msec. duration are less destructive, while still stimulating, than longer pulses; or it might indicate that any damage caused at the immediate locus of application was either not extensive enough, or not important enough, to materially affect behavior, and that any effect induced was assignable to the effects of current flow to the larger area included at some distance from the electrodes, a possibility of sufficient significance to the guiding hypothesis to merit consideration.

One would like to know therefore what effects currents of the values employed have both on the loci of application, and on loci at varying distances from this; in terms both of tissue damage, of permanent destruction, and of stimulating effectiveness.

Complicating this question is the circumstance that at any locus in the central nervous system lie structures of many different susceptibilities to stimulation by electric current; axons of various sizes and types, dendrites, cell bodies, etc., are present, and must respond at quite different thresholds. The range of such thresholds in optic cortex for instance is at least 20 to 1, and in terms of voltage threshold, the more sensitive are capable of responding to less than 0.1 volt, as compared to the many volts applied in the stimulating procedures employed here. In fact it seems possible that the existence of known differences of sensitivity of different elements in the central nervous system might be made use of as a means of their differential stimulation, in further analysis of what the stimulus is doing to the structures to which it is applied.

Aside from the neurological and neurophysiological considerations, is the question of adequate controls. It is perhaps a good deal to ask for blank experiments of so drastic a character on human subjects, but if the problem justifies itself in general, controls are as justifiable as the procedure intended to be effective. Especially in a procedure where by no means all experiments show the looked for results the obvious ideal would be one control operation for each full experimental procedure. Short of this, at least as many controls of some significant degree of pertinence—perhaps merely involving the handling of a number of comparable patients without operation in essentially the same way as those operated—would be required to give what must eventually amount to a statistically significant estimate of the many factors involved in the patients' response to the procedures in question.

Such comments are intended as suggestions for further procedures, rather than as objections to current interpretations, which latter under the circumstances would seem premature. The surprising feature of this work is not that present shortcomings can be found in it, but that it should be done at all.

Discussion

JOHN C. LILLY, M.D.
Associate Professor of Medical Physics and of Experimental Neurology
School of Medicine
University of Pennsylvania

A. INTRODUCTION

I find this project to be rather surprising: it is my first experience with a work in which people with such a diversity of trainings cooperate enthusiastically on such manifold activities of the central nervous system. Dr. Heath deserves a large amount of credit for organizing and inspiring such a large group effort. Tulane Medical School, especially in the person of Dean Lapham, is to be congratulated on its support of such a unique project.

I am glad to see any new effort being made to find a less damaging, less sacrificial means of dealing with mental disorder than are lobotomy, leucotomy, gyrectomy, thalamotomy, and other intentional destructions of nervous structures. On a first view, this project appears to be such an effort in principle—on a closer inspection it appears not to be in reality—I'll defer this point till later. Meanwhile, let me add that I feel that this project can become less damaging to brain tissue as it proceeds, and some of the possible routes are indicated below.

B. TECHNIQUE

The technical progress realized in the last two years on this project gives me pleasure. The improvements in operative technique and in the methods of psychological and physiological evaluation and observation are particularly noteworthy. The present stereotaxic technique and implantation of electrodes is a greatly appreciated advance over the older, vastly more traumatic "open-type" operation.

My suggestions for improvement in this region of the project are as follows:

(1) The parameters of stimulation should be changed; their effects should be tested on a more systematic basis. The problem here is to be above the threshold for stimulation and to minimize electrolytic injury to tissue. Since neither the threshold phenomena nor the injury effects have been worked out in animals, this is a difficult problem.

What are the criteria for threshold currents? If the regions of interest act, when stimulated, at all like motor cortex does, we can say that at least 5 parameters must be fixed before we can define the responses accurately.* The current strength, the pulse duration, the pulse repetition frequency, the train duration, and the train repetition frequency each exert their effect on the threshold. In a given parametric region, a given system may have a lower threshold than another system, but in another parametric region have an equal or lower threshold. Now that chronic implantations of electrodes are being done in these cases, it may be possible to take time to obtain different types of responses from the same electrode loci by merely changing these parameters. But first, I suggest doing another set of experiments on animals—experiments designed to quantitate the injury due to current flow through tissue.

(2) In some published experiments* and in some unpublished ones, we have found that rectangular, unidirectional waveforms injure brain tissue. The parameters of this injury process have not been fully explored. We suggest* that the injury is due to electrophoretic transport of proteins and other constituents of nerve cells, electro-osmosis, electrodialysis, electrolysis of electrodes, changes in pH and the concentration of other molecular and ionic species in the vicinity of the electrodes. To a first approximation we suggest that the extent of these processes is proportional to the total coulombs passed through the tissue in one direction during any given period of continuous stimulation. Thus we conclude that the preferred region of stimulation parameters is that which gives minimum coulombs at threshold; this region happens, in the case of cortex, to be short pulse durations, fairly low frequencies, train durations up to 20 seconds, and low-train repetition frequencies.

*Lilly, John C., Austin, George A., and Chambers, William W., *Journal of Neurophysiology*, vol. xv, no. 4 (July 1952).

Following this line of reasoning, a bidirectional waveform with a short pulse in each direction should reduce the transport coulombs nearly to zero and should be less injurious than a unidirectional one. We found this to be true in unpublished experiments on sensorimotor cortex. In addition, we found that the current thresholds (when the opposing pulses were a millisecond apart) were not significantly increased over those of the unidirectional waveform, in the analogous parametric region.

(3) It is suggested that more attention should be paid to the avoidance of noxious stimuli. The arterial puncture for blood pressure pickup at present looks very disturbing—some sacrifice in accuracy of measurement can be made for the comfort of the patient without serious loss of data; some form of flexible tubing in the artery, or a non-puncture method of measurement may help.

Other stimuli and situations in these experiments, which are not noxious to a non-psychotic person, can be noxious to a psychotic patient. The skin temperature leads, the EEG leads, the recumbent position, and the small observation room are outstanding in their strangeness; potentially, at least, these features can represent realization and re-inforcement of psychotic fantasies in a somewhat bizarre fashion.

The recumbent position plus the interrogator at the head of the litter (effectively, over the patient's head, where the leads come in) can lead to fantasies in the psychotic patient of castration, rape, impregnation, "control of the mind," etc. These stimulated fantasies may exert a rather profound effect on the psychological outcome; such stimuli lead to ambiguity in interpreting the results of electrical stimuli running concurrently.

C. DESIGN OF EXPERIMENTS

(1) Apparently there are at least 2 major working hypotheses at present in this group. The first (A) is that electrical "stimulation" of the "septal region" somehow temporarily breaks down the schizophrenic's barrier to communication with the interviewer and changes his emotional behavior and feeling to a less psychotic and more normal pattern. The second (B) is that electrical "spikes" recorded from the "septal region" correlate with the schizophrenic mental activity as opposed to normal mental activity.

From the evidence presented, I'm not convinced that either hypothesis is valid. I suggest the following experiments to test their validity:

Test of hypothesis (A): the whole procedure be carried through as it is done now, with one exception: the stimulating current is to be controlled by one person. He runs an experiment on the rest of the group, (1) by sometimes turning the current on when requested by the interviewer and (2) sometimes not turning it on; but in each case the interviewer and the rest of the group must believe it was turned on; and the converse, turning it on without the knowledge of the group to see if they can pick up the reactions of the patient said to be characteristic of the response to electrical stimuli. The evaluation of the effects on the patient are recorded immediately after each real and "control" stimulation. This test may necessitate running a patient all the way through with no current being passed at all (again, without group knowledge)—to see how much the rest of the variables (operation, interview, environment, etc.) contribute to the clinical result.

Test of hypothesis (B): by recording concurrently the speech in the experiment room on a tape recorder and in one channel of the EEG ink-writer and the electrical activity of the "septal region" on another EEG channel, it may be possible to show whether or not there is a correlation between "spikes" and emotionally and psychotically important verbal material. Even more convincing would be a sound motion picture of the patient, combined with a picture of the spikes on one EEG channel and speech on another. A frame by frame analysis of facial expressions, speech, and "spikes" by an observer who knows the patient very well would give the critical data for testing this hypothesis.

There is a third hypothesis which seems to me to be invalid on theoretical and logical grounds. This hypothesis (C) is that (1) the "spikes" can be abolished by electrical "stimuli" into the same electrodes from which they are picked up and hence (2) that the schizophrenic reactions will be concurrently abolished. By electrically *damaging* tracts and nuclei, maybe one can abolish the possibility of the electrodes picking up the "spikes," but they still may exist in adjacent regions. Until the existence of a correlation between the "spikes" and the schizophrenic reactions is demonstrated, I do not think this hypothesis can be tested adequately. Talk of breaking of feedback circulation of neuronal activity had better wait until an adequate demonstration is made of such circulation and of methods of breaking it up. The difficulty in using electrical damage to "abolish" any nervous activity is that around such a lesion one may set up a wide zone of spiking neuronal discharge and/or slow wave activity which is highly pathological. It may be that such zones carefully placed in the correct region and of the correct shape and size are what will give the desired therapeutic result—but this is yet to be demonstrated.

D. THERAPEUTIC RESULTS WITH THE FIRST 19 CASES

To date (first 19 schizophrenic patients), there have been, in my opinion, too many variables varying from one case to the next to explain either the therapeutic successes or the failures. The trauma (psychic and organic) of the open type of operation and its sequelae of convulsions, spiking EEGs, etc., is an enormous set of variables in itself: different areas in each patient firing differently complicate this picture. The variability of electrode placement and of the parameters of the electrical current from one case to another is too great to estimate the influence of the current itself. The changes from one interviewer to another, the changes in technique, mood and interest of each interviewer with one case and from case to case are an extremely complex set of variables which apparently have not been controlled with this set of patients.

I bring up these points because obviously this group wants to introduce improvements and because I wish to add to their list of things to be done which I feel are necessary. I thank the group for this opportunity to share their data, their hopes, their successes, and their failures; rarely does one meet with such esteemed frankness and honesty in such complex research. I wish them the best of luck and the hope that they reach their therapeutic goal in our lifetime.

Discussion

R. A. CLEGHORN, M.D.
Associate Professor of Psychiatry
Faculty of Medicine
(Allan Memorial Institute)
McGill University

It has been an encouraging and stimulating experience to hear the results of this combined attack on the psychological and physiological investigation of lesions in the forebrain of man and other animals. My present comments will be confined to the results reported on cats.

At first sight the parallelism between the effects of adrenalectomy and those of bilateral destructive lesions at the base of the septum is most striking. When one tabulates the likenesses and the differences to adrenal insufficiency the picture becomes more complicated. The likenesses consist in the survival time, 3 to 14 days in 4 cases, the hyponatremia and hyperkalemia, terminal hypoglycemia, weight loss and gastro-intestinal changes. The differences shown by the animals with septal injury are the early lethargic behaviour pattern, the early hyperglycemia and poikilothermia, the drop in the red cell count and the presence of intact hypertrophied adrenals. .

It is not unlikely that one is dealing with at least two successive groups of changes which one may term phases. Immediately following the operation the picture is one of disturbed central nervous system integration with the psychic picture being one of pathological lethargy and the physiological one of disturbed homeostasis involving control of body temperature and another function in which the autonomic participates, namely, control of the blood sugar level. The hyperglycemia is reminiscent of Bernard's piqure which was shown by Donhoffer and Macleod in 1932 to be mediated through the autonomic but requiring adequate adrenal cortical hormones for its exhibition.

It is possible that during the early poikilothermia and hyperglycemic phase there is concurrently an excessive discharge of ACTH. This would account for the hypertrophied adrenals at death. It is conceivable that this leads to a change in adrenal secretion so that sodium and nitrogen loss occurs and the final picture is fictitiously like that of adrenal insufficiency. On the other hand the apparent early excessive secretion of ACTH and adrenal hyperfunction may be succeeded by diminished ACTH secretion and real adrenal insufficiency. The evidence of Tokay who found in 1931 that stab wounds in the caudate area led to a salt loss by way of the kidney is evidence which may support the adrenal insufficiency theory. On the other hand one has not ruled out other hormonal (posterior lobe of the pituitary) or autonomic effects on the kidney which may lead to the appearance of renal salt loss. The pathological picture shown by the gut at death is very like that in adrenal insufficiency. Similar changes are found after extensive burns, wound shock and prolonged adrenalin infusion. What one would like to know is whether hypertrophy of lymphoid tissue is found in these septal-injured cats as in adrenal insufficiency.

Whatever the ultimate outcome of these studies, no matter what mechanisms may finally be shown to account for the observed changes the stimulus supplied by the present findings can have nothing but a beneficial and salutary influence. It is a privilege to have been present at this presentation.

Discussion

FRED A. METTLER, PH.D., M.D., D.SC.
Professor of Anatomy
College of Physicians and Surgeons
Columbia University

The presentation before us consists of a number of communications which have been united by the thread of theory. The reaction of the reader to this will vary, depending upon his personality and training. From the long-range point of view, it probably makes little difference whether one commences the investigation of a problem from the deductive or inductive points of view, provided, in the first case, that a theoretical approach is not allowed to straiten the objective accumulation and interpretation of data and, in the second case, that an effort is made to arrive at the general from the particular. Nevertheless, the dangers inherent in the deductive approach are greater than those in the inductive insofar as it is not always possible to return to objective facts if the initially adopted and conditioning theory proves to be wrong. Contrariwise, it is often feasible for the same or other individuals to complete, at some subsequent time, an incompletely developed, inductively oriented study. There is in the present communication, I think, some evidence that the theoretical preconceptions have tended to constitute a bed of Procrustes in which the reported data have at least been invited to recline if not made to conform. Thus, the data reported in individual communications do not all deal with the septum, with the septal nuclei nor even with the septal region. In interdisciplinary relationships, however, this rather fundamental fact is glossed over and it is implied that the basic material is relatively homogeneous. From my point of view, no sound basis has been advanced here for the assumption that schizophrenia is due to specific septal pathophysiology or that this condition is influenced by manipulations of this region. It therefore becomes necessary to examine individual communications for their own particular informative value and, as nearly as possible, independently from the theoretic background.

The fundamental difficulty in many of the separate communications (apparent from those aspects of Hodes and Peacock's observations which have already appeared in print) is the unclear nature of the proximal experimental factor referred to above. No data have been presented to document the location and extent of the lesions reported by Heath in cats under the heading of chemistry and behavior after ablational studies. (It is somewhat disturbing to find, in some instances where, as in Case 25, postmortem material is available, that the authors' morphological terminology does not entirely agree with accepted anatomic usage.) Similarly, how is it possible to know where the electrodes were placed in the patients in terms of the small, powerful, contiguous structures which lie in the general area attacked? Further, even if one knew where these placements were, how have the numerous physical difficulties inherent in the changing methods of stimulation and recording been surmounted and why would it not have been advisable to reject, from the raw data, those instances the interpretation of which is somewhat obscured by complicating factors? Satisfactory supporting data and explanations may be available to answer each of the above questions, but they have not emerged here, and unless the reader is presented with this information it is unfair to expect him to reach a conclusion which, if adequate objective data had been brought forward, he might very well have naturally accepted. Since it is clear that the motivation of the investigators is serious and laudable and since they have labored with industry, such a conclusion must be reached with regret. That Heath found disorders of motor and metabolic function in his cats is obvious, but what caused these is far from clear. Not only have satisfactory anatomic data establishing the loci of the lesions not been brought forward, but the factor of functional disturbance at a distance from the lesions and due to ventricular pathology or vascular interference has not apparently been controlled. There is further no clear one-to-one relationship between the reported metabolic disturbances and the lesions, whatever their nature. Such metabolic disturbances might have been the algebraic result of a train of events related to the lesions only in an indirect and circuitous manner.

Those parts of the chronic animal studies dealing with the increase or decrease in awareness, provide interesting confirmation of the existing literature and extend this to the degree that they indicate the commonly observed EEG phenomena accompanying sleep probably represent only one limited aspect of the data available on the temporal and locational aspects of the electrical correlates of somnolence and that the primary process may begin at deeper levels. Dr. Hendley's presentation also represents a contribution to existing knowledge. The long latencies found in this work indicate the direction in which it should be extended.

Although the schizophrenic component of the patient group contains one or two individuals, the malignancy of whose condition is not so obvious as is that of the remainder, the average prognostic expectation was certainly poor. It is unfortunate that more complete records of the early psychiatric history of these cases could not be obtained. Lacking these the preoperative period of psychiatric observation might perhaps have been profitably extended. Certainly the same energetic supportive techniques which were employed after operation should have been utilized prior to it.

The surgical procedures described fall into two groups, open and closed techniques. The former, which amounts to the insertion of one or more continuously connected electrodes into the walls of the anterior horn of the lateral ventricle and through a restricted unilateral lobotomy, is certainly not an operation of choice. According to the consensus of the authors, it is now only of theoretic and historical interest. However, this is the procedure employed on nearly all the patients for whom relatively complete data are available and its disadvantages must necessarily be reflected in those data.

The second procedure consists of implanting a continuously connected fine wire electrode by carrying it into the substance of the brain on a tube which is later withdrawn. The stereotaxic instrument employed is that manufactured by the Labtronics Corporation. Placement has been estimated according to roentgenographic methods. A completely satisfactory human stereotaxic instrument has still to be devised and so is an antemortem method of determining the placement of stereotaxically oriented electrodes. The authors entertain the hope that satisfactory coordinate mensuration may ultimately be developed from an atlas—a hope not shared by this commentator in view of the historical development of this subject.

It is probable that greater facility and flexibility can be achieved with other instruments previously described. It is certain that the electrode situation is susceptible of great improvement. It is by no means certain that a high degree of reliability of electrode placement will ever be achieved. This being the case, and lacking the possibility of anatomic verification of such placements, the best that can be done in the future will be to determine what the factor of error for particular placements is and to carry work forward on a statistical basis. Such a methodology has obvious disadvantages for psychiatric research but it would be unwise not to recognize the existence of a very palpable factor of error in the roentgenographic method (which is the best we are likely to have for a long while) of locating stereotaxically placed foci in the human.

According to Dr. Hodes, abnormal spiking may be found in certain schizophrenic patients in the region of the diencephalon. Such spiking is augmented during sleep and may possibly make its way to the cortex. Heath regards this as evidence of a fundamental manifestation of pathophysiology in what he calls "the septal area" and as a characteristic of schizophrenia. Hodes' data are clear and appear to show that such spiking is unrelated to any possible local pathology which might result from placement of the deep electrodes. Heath's interpretation of the data, however, appears premature. Heath further assumed that if his original set of hypotheses was correct, so-called septal stimulation should abolish such peculiar deep spikes, at least one gathers, in cases where the patients' clinical psychiatric pictures were considered to have been improved. Hodes reports that in some instances deep stimulation did tend to obliterate such abnormal spikes but only for a relatively brief period and only in some patients. Because the original data are presently unavailable to me it is not possible to see whether there was any correlation between such occasional temporary obliteration and reported clinical improvement. By referring to the pertinent printed material the reader should be able to determine this for himself.

Mr. Becker's description of the stimulation technique is a straightforward account of a progressively improving methodology. In general it is undesirable, of course, to record through electrodes through which high current densities have previously been run, but in the present instance it is not easy to see how this could have been avoided. A question of combined-operations procedure should be mentioned here. I have previously been somewhat concerned about the effect which "combined-operations" research might have upon individual research and have pointed out, after consideration of some of the effects of this that a "combined-operations" project may very well (a) provide material for subsequent individual research which material might otherwise not have become available and (b) contribute new significance to research problems eminently suitable for individual research and which might not otherwise be considered worth the expenditure of great labor and significant funds. I now perceive that combined-operations research may very well not only stimulate but indeed require individual research, especially at the local level, before the major project is launched. Such research might well be in the nature of restricted scouting activities into portions of the territory which the entire party is subsequently to explore.

Drs. Peacock and Price's data and, to some extent, that of Drs. Epstein and Millsaps introduce an interesting note into the general presentation. The phenomena reported by the two former agree rather well with what one would expect to result from hypothalamic discharge and/or lesion. One would be interested to know therefore at least which electrodes, said to be elsewhere, were really in the hypothalamus, whether current was spreading to it or whether some neurological mechanism was discharging in an hithertofore undetermined manner. The latter explanation appears to controvert the logical law of parsimony. To the present commentator the data presented by these four workers appears to compose the essential advance of the project. The observations are quite objective, have a high degree of internal consistency and, providing the anatomic discrepancies noted above are taken into consideration, appear to demonstrate that the large body of data already accumulated by experimental physiologists who have studied these portions of the forebrain is directly applicable to the human. Some information has, of course, been available for the human from previous neuropathological and neurosurgical studies and it is gratifying to see this extended.

Dr. King has brought forward a practical testing procedure for patients of the present type in situations like this one. His approach is full of common sense, provides an interesting application of the rating scale technique to the psychological testing situation and also to the results of the tests themselves. We have here a clear picture of what those eight patients which were susceptible to examination by his methodology were doing. He has very dexterously avoided a considerable number of pitfalls and entanglements in which he might easily have become involved. It is therefore not without some misgivings that we find some of his data reinterpreted by Dr. Monroe.

Dr. Monroe is obviously enraptured by the theoretical considerations advanced by Dr. Heath and appears convinced that the methodology employed has been responsible for a phenomenal degree of improvement in the cases under his observation. He has approached his subject with vigor and near-evangelical enthusiasm, his patients with a confident and buoyant spirit and their relatives with support in his left hand and the fell force of the law in his right. His patient group has made a good over-all record, but whether this record is a reflection of his own buoyant confidence and his vigorous manipulation of their environment or whether it is to some extent related to the experimental procedure seems to me quite unanswered. It is true that the patients in question were subjected to preoperative total push, but I should not be surprised if the EMF equivalent of this had different values, depending upon whether Dr. Monroe was or was not himself convinced that he had at his disposal a completely effective therapeutic weapon.

The reader may gain from the preceding comments the impression that I regard the work reported herewith as rather inconsequential. This is by no means the case. If work of this type were easy to do, it would have been done long ago. It is true that I consider the theoretical superstructure of the project a hindrance rather than a help, the general conclusions drawn from data overextended, the plan of execution inconstant and somewhat diffuse and some technical aspects susceptible of great improvement, but it is of the greatest importance that interdisciplinary work of this sort shall be carried forward not merely, though especially, in psychiatry, but in all fields of medicine. It should also be pointed out that great industry and a high sense of integrity have characterized the execution of the project. It is not difficult to present a bland tableau of accomplishment if integrity is to be compromised. If the accurate workings of any progressive enterprise are examined certain defects can always be found and there is always room for improvement.

There must have been some very difficult administrative moments for Dr. Lapham during the execution of this work and some hard decisions to be made by the agencies supporting it. To him and to them I offer my congratulations for equally sharing a courageous sense of scientific responsibility. The workers themselves I wish good fortune as they carry these difficult problems forward into clearer focus, and in Dr. Heath, a former student of mine, I do indeed take pride even though (let it not be forgotten), I do not agree with him.

Discussion

JAMES B. CAMPBELL, M.D.
Associate in Neurological Surgery
College of Physicians and Surgeons
Columbia University

This report is rendered after considerable reflection and repeated study of notes taken at the meeting. This auditor still has enthusiasm for the pioneering spirit of the group who carried out the experimental procedures and admiration for their daring to persist in the face of technical risks. It should not be the province of the surgeon to criticize the psychiatric aspects of the study, or data accumulated and interpreted by the electroencephalographer, chemist, or psychologist. This will, doubtless, be done by the auditors from the other disciplines. This project cannot help but to contribute to basic medical knowledge if it continues, and the data are consistently accumulated and objectively interpreted.

This auditor, however, feels that certain changes in procedure and methodology might further the project. It is fortunate that placement of electrodes under direct vision by means of an open operative attack through the frontal lobe and underlying structures, has been given up. The morbidity caused by the procedure, doubtless, clouded some of the results that might have been obtained, because of coincident damage to structures not under investigation. Certainly, the stereotaxic placement of electrodes is a step forward. Nevertheless, a word of caution in the interpretation of results obtained by this means of electrode placement seems to be in order. It is well-known by all who have worked with this methodology in animals and man, that the structure aimed for may not be the structure reached. Therefore, in the human, autopsy verification of position of the electrodes is of paramount importance. Since it is the aim of this project to benefit and cure patients, great delay in obtaining objective data goes without saying. Nevertheless, certain patients will die and come to autopsy, which will make it possible to correlate the psychologic data with the physiologic and anatomic data recorded in the completed protocol. Data available from living patients in the project, can only be used in the most guarded manner after sufficient autopsies have been performed.

Just as there was a great morbidity from infection, and in some cases, mortality, with the placement of electrodes at open operation, there, doubtless, will be a repetition of these factors if the leads are brought out through the skin at the time of operation. Therefore, it is suggested that when stereotaxic placement of the electrodes is made, that the electrodes then be collected in a small length of polyethylene tubing, and left buried beneath the scalp for at least three weeks. It should be possible to distinguish the leads by knotting wires, or by marking them by some other means. After there has been thorough wound healing, the polyethylene tubing could be located by palpation and under novocaine anaesthesia, and aseptic technic brought out to the surface. By this time, there should be a well-sealed tract around each lead, and a thin, firm capsule around each electrode. This should make the whole procedure safer from the point of view of sepsis. In addition, during this delay for wound-healing and encapsulation, valuable observations might be forthcoming concerning results obtained from the mere presence of an electrode in a vital subcortical structure, and it is just possible that this portion of the procedure alone, might be fairly significant. Then stimulation could be instituted. The patient would have been rested and the chance for morbidity or even mortality should be greatly minimized, and the results of stimulation freed from the confusion of surgery and anaesthesia. If the connections with these leads were handled in an aseptic manner, it should be possible to even replace them beneath the scalp and to wait for another month or so, if such seemed to be desirable as the project progresses. Of course, remote control stimulation, which has been possible in animals for some years, would be the most desirable of all technics, and, doubtless, will be done before too long with the rapid advances that are being made in the field of electronics.

This auditor has had some experience with the placement of electrodes and electronic apparatus within the body of animals. It seems appropriate to mention that silver solder is a highly irritating substance that breaks down within the body, and it is suggested that the electrodes be made out of a noble metal or one of the stainless steel alloys that is known not to react within the body. It is possible the chemical reaction alone, caused by contact of a silver solder electrode with body fluid, may be of some significance. Certainly, the characteristics of the stimulating current must be such that the matter of hydrolysis in the region of the electrode must be minimized. If not, results obtained from stimulation will again be clouded by extraneous factors. It has been the experience of our laboratory, that insulating materials present a very great problem. Nylon, in our experience, has been a most unsatisfactory insulator, because of the fact that most nylons are hygroscopic and quite irritating when in contact with living tissue because of solvents that "bleed out." It is, therefore, suggested, that the members of the project give serious consideration to using a more inert substance as their insulator, such as polyethylene, kel-f, or teflon. All of these substances, of course, must be absolutely free of plasticizers, in order to obviate chemical irritation all along the tract. These suggestions are not offered in criticism, but merely to help, since they have found their origin in experience accumulated in our laboratory.

Section VI

ADDENDA

ADDENDUM A

CASE HISTORY OF THE PATIENT OPERATED UPON IN JUNE, 1952

ROBERT G. HEATH
RUSSELL R. MONROE
AND OTHERS

PATIENT 26

AGE AT OPERATION: 27
SEX: Male
MARITAL STATUS: Single
OCCUPATION: None
RELIGION: Catholic (inactive)
INFORMANT: Mother
DIAGNOSIS: Schizophrenic reaction, hebephrenic type
OPERATION: June 13, 1952

Presenting Picture. The patient was readmitted to Charity Hospital in May, 1952. At that time he was apathetic, seclusive, and hallucinating.

Present Illness. The onset of the patient's illness had been insidious. It was reported that he had been "nervous" since early adolescence and had been rejected for military service 10 years before for psychiatric disability. During this period he was idle and seclusive, having almost no social relationships. He had never worked steadily and was often depressed for several months at a time. He expressed mild suicidal ideas, saying he had "nothing to live for." Overtly bizarre symptoms started in September, 1950, when the last of his three younger brothers entered the military service. Since that time he had remained in his upstairs room. He consulted numerous physicians for somatic complaints which included dizziness, low blood pressure, weakness, insomnia, "weak stomach," nausea, vomiting, and aches and pains in his extremities. He was slovenly in his personal habits and became obsessively preoccupied with reading a set of encyclopedias from A to Z. Whenever left alone in the house he became fearful, locking all the doors and windows. In August, 1951, the family said that he became "crazy," by which they meant that he talked in an unintelligible, incoherent manner, usually cursing the priest, the Church, and his family. At the same time he manifested threatening behavior toward those in the house.

Previous Personality Disorders. There were no previous overtly psychotic episodes.

Family History. The patient is the second oldest of five sons born to parents of low economic status, whose marital adjustment has always been poor. The father drinks heavily, while the mother, who was orphaned at the age of 11, has established deep dependent relationships with her sons. Only the eldest son has married and seems able to maintain a home and family of his own. Two of the younger brothers have required psychiatric care, one being hospitalized for a period of 6 months while in the Coast Guard.

Personal History. No significant abnormality is reported in the patient's birth and early development. Throughout childhood he was a "good boy," causing less trouble than any of his siblings. The family felt that his physical health suffered when at the age of 4 he had pertussis and a tonsillectomy. He attended school and made satisfactory marks until he stopped at the age of 13 in the seventh grade. Although he occasionally joined in group activity with other children, he seemed to play a passive role and preferred to be by himself and stay close to home. During adolescence he drifted from one job to another, never working for more than 3 or 4 weeks on one job. He offered no excuse for quitting jobs except to say that he was "fed up with them." He showed no interest in the opposite sex until the age of 20, when he began dating a widow considerably older than himself. The family objected to this relationship. At the time that he became seclusive and withdrawn, he broke off with this woman and subsequently had no heterosexual contacts, although he showed interest in girls by watching them from the window of his home.

Personality. The patient was described as quiet, withdrawn, and lacking in ambition. He was sensitive, nervous, and periodically depressed.

Hospital Course. The patient was first hospitalized in September, 1951, at which time he was so disturbed that he required heavy sedation and restraint. He was hallucinating and disoriented, periodically assaultive, slovenly in his personal habits, and excessively preoccupied with early childhood experiences. At times he became grandiose and euphoric.

During this hospitalization the patient received 33 electroshock treatments. He became less belligerent and neater in his personal appearance, although he remained quiet and withdrawn. Despite severe confusion and disorientation following EST, he was discharged, since he was quiet and cooperative. However, during 3 1/2 months at home the patient showed no real improvement in his behavior. Although he was less belligerent and hostile, he remained idle, seclusive, preoccupied, and hallucinating.

When the patient was rehospitalized in May, 1952, he was not assaultive or destructive, but he reported visual hallucinations, which consisted of concentric colored circles or clouds that he described as "souls." He also reported auditory hallucinations wherein male voices accused him of sexual transgressions and called him dirty names. He still seemed confused regarding temporal relationships of his previous hospitalization and treatment. Emotional responses consisted of silly, inappropriate laughter. He was apathetic, uninterested in his surroundings, and untidy and unclean in his personal habits.

Physical and Laboratory Status. Results of general physical and neurological examinations were within normal limits. Blood pressures varied from 90/74 to 140/80. Routine urine and blood findings were within normal range, as were the BUN, blood glucose, EEG, and skull and chest films.

Operation—Stimulation. June 13, 1952.

(a) Surgical techniques—Stereotaxic technique was used.

(b) Electrode placements—Six unipolar electrodes were so implanted that they could be grouped as 3 pairs. Two electrodes to make up one pair were in the caudate nucleus; two electrodes were in the rostral part of the septal region; and the other two were implanted at about the level of the anterior commissure—one in the caudal part of the septal region and the other in the rostral part of the hypothalamus.

(c) Recordings—Two EEG's made 7 and 3 days prior to operation carried the interpretation of a normal waking pattern and normal waking and sleeping patterns. On the deep recordings made prior to stimulation on the evening of operation, spikes of 100 uV. were seen in the septal leads only, intermixed with frequencies ranging from 2 to 20 seconds cycles per second. After stimulations of the septal region a delta

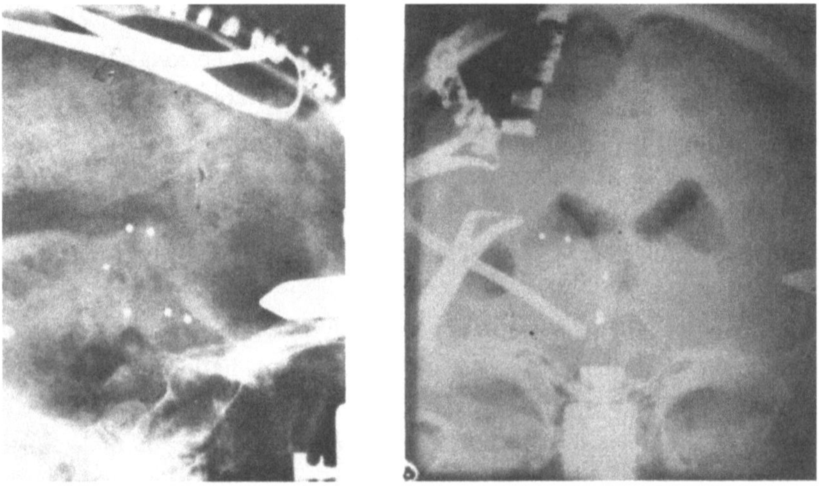

FIGURE A–1. Patient 26

wave was set up in the septal leads and remained throughout the rest of the recordings. Spiking remained in the septal leads but appeared less frequently after stimulation. Follow-up scalp recordings revealed no abnormalities.

(d) Stimulation technique—There were five stimulations to electrodes in the rostral part of the septal region (leads 13 and 14), lasting from 8 to 25 minutes at peak currents ranging from 4 to 5 ma. There was one stimulation between leads 15 and 16, one of which was in the septal region and the other in the hypothalamus. These were of 3 minutes' duration at peak currents ranging from 2 to 8 ma. The following stimulus was used: pulse repetition frequency, 100 cycles per second; pulse duration, 1 millisecond.

(e) Immediate physiological effects—Stimulation to the electrodes in the rostral part of the septal region (leads 13 and 14) had no apparent physiological effect. Septo-hypothalamic stimulation (between leads 15 and 16) produced a marked autonomic effect, with anxiety, sweating, fall in blood pressure, and shock-like appearance. Subsequent stimulations to leads 13 and 14 evoked feelings of nausea on one occasion but were consistently followed by brightening and feelings of well-being.

(f) Immediate behavioral response—During the stimulation to the rostral part of the septal region the patient perceptibly brightened, smiled, recognized a number of the doctors about him, and became more productive. When the same area was stimulated again, his voice seemed much louder as he said, "I'm starting to wake up." During the third stimulation the patient again showed progressive brightening and alertness as the current was increased. During the fourth stimulation the results were more equivocal; the patient was seemingly more productive and described a dream that indicated some of his anal preoccupation and hostility.

(g) Immediate chemical changes—Three preoperative 24-hour urine specimens were obtained on which the potassium-sodium ratio averaged 0.25 and the 17-ketosteroids 7.8 mg/24 hours. Preoperative plasma Na and K values were 137 and 4.3 meq/L., respectively. Lymphocytes were 3,046 per cu. mm., and eosinophils were 387 per cu. mm. Response to the Thorn test was a 46 per cent drop.

The first isolated stimulation of the rostral part of the septal region took place 4 days after surgery. The 17-ketosteroids rose rapidly, possibly due to the fact that the sample was obtained in the daytime (12-hour specimen). Two days later they dropped below normal values. The maximum K-Na ratio was 1.82 on the first day after stimulation. The lymphocytes rose rapidly from 1,952 to 2,366 per cu. mm., then dropped to almost prestimulation level after 19 hours. The eosinophils increased from 258 to 389 per cu. mm. at the end of 5 1/2 hours and dropped to 312 per cu. mm. after 19 hours.

The second mild stimulation to the rostral part of the septal region 10 days later showed no effect on 17-ketosteroids or plasma Na and K, but there was significant retention of K and less marked retention of Na and water. K-Na ratios were 0.54, 0.30, and 0.57.

The third stimulation was weak, with one electrode in the rostral part of the hypothalamus and one electrode in the caudal part of the septal area. On the first day following stimulation there was a high excretion of water, K, and Na. The K-Na ratio showed a marked rise on the second and third days, to 1.75 and 1.27, respectively. The eosinophils dropped from 419 (prestimulation value) to 287 per cu. mm. at the end of 3 hours. The lymphocytes dropped from 2,730 to 2,003 per cu. mm. at the end of 3 hours. The blood glucose increased from 62 to 88 mg/100 ml. in 1 hour but dropped to 70 mg/100 ml. at the end of 2 hours.

Our last stimulation (strong to the rostral part of the septal region) was followed by marked water retention. The patient was anuric for 28 hours and then excreted the most hypertonic urine we have ever analyzed (K and Na were 180 meq/L. and 131 meq/L., respectively). The K-Na ratio was 1.37. There were no changes in plasma Na and K, or 17-ketosteroids. The lymphocytes showed a slight increase, as did the eosinophils. The blood glucose increased from 52 to 72 mg/100 ml. after 2 hours.

Eight days after the last stimulation the patient was given 25 mg. of ACTH. There was no effect on plasma Na and K, but a marked increase in the K-Na ratio to 1.37 maximum occurred after 3 days. During the first 2 days after administration of ACTH the 17-ketosteroids were below normal, but on the fourth day they rose to above 12 mg/24 hours. The eosinophils dropped from 460 to 264 per cu. mm. at the end of 4 hours, a 42 per cent decrease. The lymphocytes dropped from 2,274 to 1,421 per cu. mm. after 2 hours. We have no data on the blood glucose.

(h) Complications—Twenty-one days after operation a foreign body reaction set in at the exit of the electrodes on the scalp. This cleared completely after their removal.

Follow-up Notes. On the day following the first stimulation the patient still seemed more alert and emotionally responsive. He described feeling entirely different and expressed the hope that he was going to get well. Although he still experienced hallucinations, he now expressed considerable annoyance at their presence. One week later he became quite vociferous, attempting in a rather pleading childlike way to socialize on the wards and to show the ward personnel how much he needed and liked to be helped. He expressed some despondency and discouragement over the future but would laugh appropriately when patients on the ward told jokes and, in fact, contributed two of his own. Two weeks after operation he was showing some interest in occupational therapy. He was much more friendly and cheerful. He asked for permission to go out on a pass but periodically withdrew into his room, again becoming preoccupied with his hallucinations. Three weeks after operation the patient showed more improvement, although he did express fears that he would slip back into his former illness. He still had numerous somatic complaints, but appeared to accept realistic explanations of them, recognizing that they might be due to his mental illness. One month after stimulation he left the hospital on his first overnight pass. Although he became excited at this prospect and was quite tense and anxious at home, during the following week he begged for another pass. He began expressing the idea that he would like to work. He denied daytime hallucinations, although he mentioned that he was troubled at night by frightening dreams and sometimes found it difficult to tell whether these were dreams or hallucinations. The patient was discharged from the hospital in August, 1952, to be followed in clinic.

During September and October he made a particularly good adjustment outside the hospital. He actively aided in house chores and was particularly happy when he could run errands, go to the bank, pay bills, visit relatives, drink a couple of beers in a local bar, or go to the barber shop. He was pleased with the new clothes his family provided for him and on his own initiative went to the local employment bureau, where he established contact to find a job. His main interest was to drive a truck. However, when seen in the clinic the patient seemed emotionally flat, was generally unproductive, and admitted to occasional hallucinations but refused to elaborate on them. He occasionally referred to bizarre somatic ailments. For instance, he asked the doctor if it were possible "to have snakes inside oneself." He was approached directly with this material. It was pointed out that the question probably represented some of his old "crazy" ideas returning. He seemed to accept this explanation readily but continued with numerous vague somatic complaints, particularly low back pain. Although he would read and listen to the radio, he showed little interest in world events; however, his mother reported that he had had very little interest in them for many years. Seventeen weeks after operation the patient seemed at the height of his improvement. He expressed some resentment that his mother was constantly hovering about him and was irritated because he could not get the type of job he wanted but smiled frequently and seemed to have a normal and appropriate display of emotions. He showed some initiative in periodically checking up on his applications for jobs. He objected to visiting the clinic for fear that this would interfere with his prospects of a job. When discussing his hallucinations he said, "You know, I think they are pretty weak now." No somatic delusions were present at this time. Twenty weeks after operation there seemed to be some regression. The patient would occasionally burst forth with silly, inappropriate laughter and answered "yes" when asked whether he was responding to visual hallucinations. He now had a few somatic complaints, particularly headaches. Although the visual hallucinations were present, he denied that auditory ones were. He was discouraged about this but recognized it as part of his illness, saying, "I guess it's my nerves."

In February, 1953, persecutory delusions reappeared, and the patient began looking for a gun. He was rehospitalized as an ambulatory patient and placed on sub-coma insulin therapy until May, 1953. His status on June 1, 1953, 12 months after operation, is similar to that of his previous remission. He spends weekends at home and week days in the hospital, where he receives occupational therapy.

ADDENDUM B

IMMEDIATE CHEMICAL AND BEHAVIORAL EFFECTS WITH STIMULATION OF CHRONICALLY IMPLANTED ELECTRODES IN RHESUS MONKEYS AND IN PATIENTS

ROBERT G. HEATH
BYRON E. LEACH
RUSSELL R. MONROE
WALTER A. MICKLE
FLORENCE B. STROHMEYER

The highlights of the data gathered since the original report on the immediate changes in behavior and alterations in chemistry following stimulation through chronically implanted electrodes are briefly summarized below.

ANIMAL STUDIES

CHANGES IN BEHAVIOR

Behavioral changes in a Rhesus monkey following subcortical stimulation through two hypothetical circuits, the facilitatory and the inhibitory, have been reported in Chapter 6. In the experiment described the electrodes were implanted by the open method. Since the meetings held in New Orleans in June, 1952, pairs of electrodes have been implanted by the stereotaxic method in various subcortical regions of several monkeys. The alterations in behavior observed in these animals following stimulation of the septal region and the caudate nucleus have been essentially the same as those observed in the monkey reported in Chapter 6.

Stimulation to the caudate nucleus has consistently resulted in diminution of awareness, and stimulation to the septal region has produced an alerting response. In all the animals operated upon by the stereotaxic technique, pairs of electrodes have also been implanted in the hypothalamus, hippocampus, and tegmentum of the mesencephalon and on the cortex (Figure 1).

Stimulation to each of these regions produced a different type of behavioral response. Like septal stimulation, hypothalamic stimulation produced an alerting response, but the monkeys' movements were more jittery—i.e., diffuse and meaningless. Usually dilatation of the pupils and tremor were noted. With stimulation through the more caudal region, involving the tegmentum of the mesencephalon, the monkeys often became tense; they also displayed diffuse motor behavior with even further reduction in response to outside stimuli. This jitteriness was associated with marked constriction of the pupils and occasionally some inconsistent movements of the eyes. With stimulation of the hippocampus, the monkeys displayed anxiety-like reactions, chattering and rapidly moving their heads and extremities. This was accompanied by dilatation of the pupils.

BIOCHEMICAL STUDIES WITH STIMULATION

Chemistry changes following stimulation to various regions have been quite inconsistent. Delivery of a constant stimulus to one region of the monkey brain failed to produce exactly reproducible effects from one time to the next. This was apparently related to the resting state of the total organism at the time the stimulus was administered (see page 21). Further studies are under way in an attempt to clarify this subject.

Despite these variations, however, some over-all consistencies were found. Stimulation through the midline region extending caudally from the rostral part of the septal region to the tegmentum of the mesencephalon has produced dramatic changes in those chemical constituents which are usually associated with stress. This includes marked reduction in the number of circulating eosinophils and lymphocytes, varying degrees of change in total output of urinary 17-ketosteroids, alterations in urine steroid patterns as determined by paper chromatography, alterations in serum protein and serum cholesterol. Dramatic changes of this type do not occur with stimulation of the more lateral structures—i.e., the caudate nucleus and hippocampus.

Since many of these changes are not yet clearly understood, at this time we shall not attempt to draw conclusions but instead to demonstrate some of the changes in one monkey which tend to indicate the

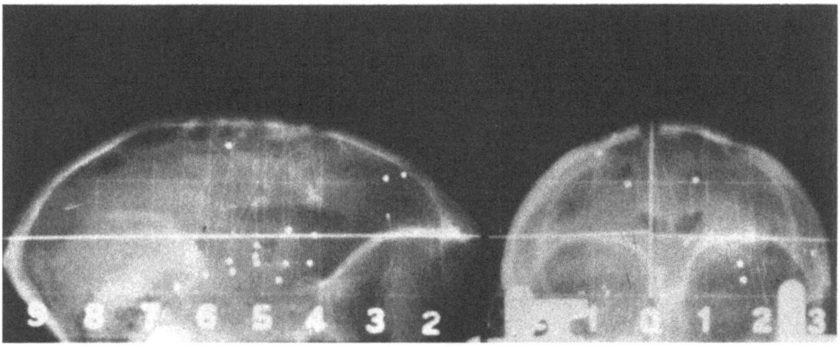

FIGURE B–1. X-ray showing sites of implantation of cortical and subcortical electrodes in the monkey brain. Some residual air remains in the ventricles

consistent differences between stimulation of the lateral structures and those obtained with stimulation of the midline structures.

In this animal we have followed blood changes and alterations in steroid excretion with stimulation of the different circuits. The data are displayed in Figure 2. Figure 3 shows the implantation of the electrodes in the different regions of the brain.

With stimulation through the septal region there was a marked increase in output of urinary 17-ketosteroids. This was accompanied by a moderate drop in circulating eosinophils and lymphocytes and a rather marked increase in the total white cell count. It is to be noted that the increased daily excretion of 17-ketosteroids continued for a rather prolonged period following this stimulation and, in fact, did not return to the prestimulation levels until after the caudate nucleus (hypothetically the inhibitory circuit) was stimulated. Immediately following this stimulation, which produced diminished awareness in the monkey (i.e., a sleeplike state), the output of 17-ketosteroids was markedly reduced. A seizure was then induced by stimulation of the cortex. The purpose of this procedure was to discover the degree to which a known type of stress would alter the blood chemistry. It is to be noted that this stimulation, in contrast to the two preceding stimulations, produced relatively little change in the output of urinary steroids. The next stimulation was applied to the hypothalamus. This produced even greater reduction in the number of circulating eosinophils and lymphocytes than septal stimulation, but a less noticeable increase in total white cells. The out-

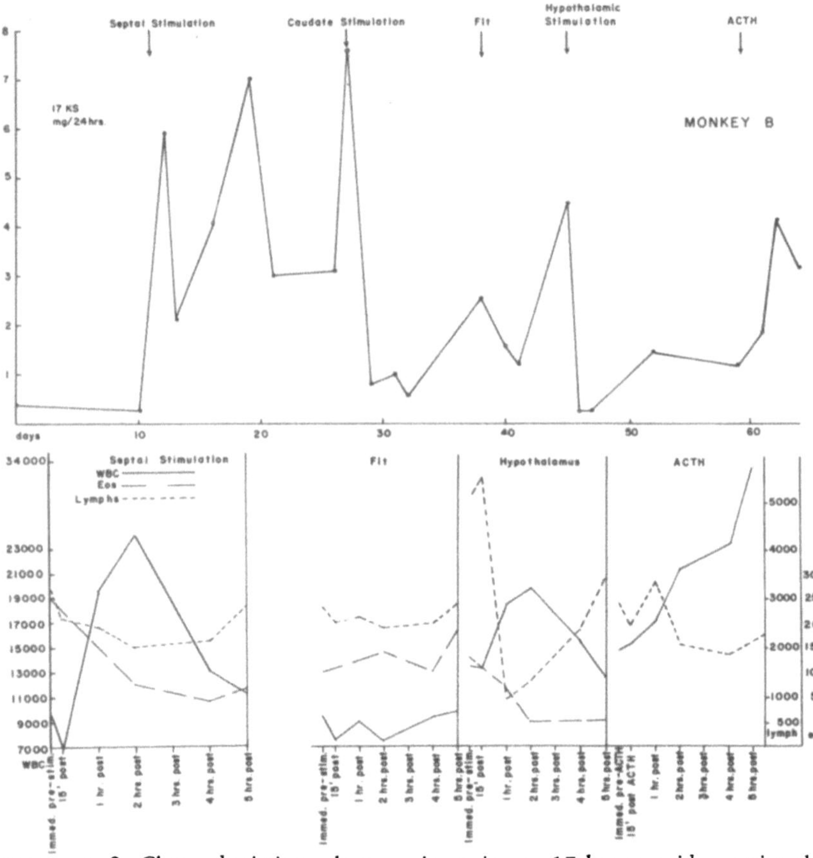

FIGURE B–2. Chart depicting changes in urinary 17-ketosteroids, eosinophil count, white cell count, and lymphocyte count with subcortical stimulation

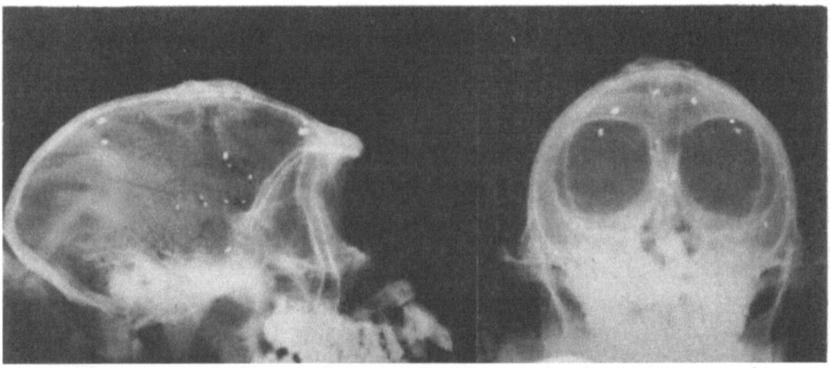

FIGURE B–3. X-rays showing position of cortical and subcortical electrodes. The faint dark lines connect the pairs of deep electrodes that were stimulated

put of urinary 17-ketosteroids was definitely reduced following this stimulation.

We were interested in comparing the changes seen following stimulation of these various regions with that which could be produced by the administration of adrenocorticotropic hormone (ACTH). A large dose of ACTH (25 mg.) was therefore administered and the same procedures followed. The monkey weighed approximately 2.8 kilograms. As indicated in Figure 2, the change in the number of circulating eosinophils and lymphocytes was quite marked, as was the increase in total white cell count. There was a significant increase in excretion of urinary 17-ketosteroids, but it was considerably less than that following a stimulation of the septal region (approximately 50 per cent) and did not persist.

SUMMARY OF CHEMICAL DATA IN MONKEY B

1. Various subcortical regions were stimulated. A seizure was induced by stimulation of the cortex, and a large dose of ACTH was administered. Metabolic changes associated with the stimuli were followed.
2. Stimulation of the septal region produced the greatest increase in excretion of urinary 17-ketosteroids. Stimulation of the caudate nucleus resulted in a marked drop in 17-ketosteroid excretion. Hypothalamic stimulation produced minimal change in excretion of urinary 17-ketosteroids. Administration of ACTH resulted in a moderate increase in 17-ketosteroid output.
3. The greatest decrease in the number of circulating eosinophils and lymphocytes appeared following hypothalamic stimulation. The greatest increase in the total white cell count followed administration of ACTH.

STUDIES WITH PATIENTS

With improved techniques of electrode implantation, which make it possible to leave electrodes in place for prolonged periods, it has been possible to separate the effects of stimulation from the effects of surgery. This has added considerably to the value of our observations on immediate behavioral changes as well as to the chemistry data. No attempt will be made to evaluate long-term therapeutic effects in the addendum series of the patient group since many are still undergoing treatment.

IMMEDIATE BEHAVIORAL RESPONSES

It has been possible to stimulate each patient several times and in several different regions. The immediate effects differ in many respects, and individual patients have differed somewhat in their responses to the same type of stimulation to the same region at different times. There were, however, some consistent findings in the sphere of affectivity.

When stimulation was applied to the more rostral midline structures (i.e., the septal region), the patients generally appeared alerted and tended to speak more rapidly. None complained of discomfort, and some have stated that they felt more comfortable. This stimulus consistently produced relief in patients suffering from intractable pain.

As the stimulus was administered more caudally, so as to involve the rostral hypothalamus, the patients tended to complain of some discomfort. The types of discomfort mentioned were those customarily associated with stimulation of the autonomics, the most frequent being abdominal discomfort, feelings of warmth, fullness in the head, pounding heart, and so forth.

Thus far only Patient A–10 has had stimulation to the tegmental region (see Addendum E, Figure 4). Intense rage developed. He became extremely restless, looked angry, and lunged out to grasp his physician, shouting, "I'll kill you." This feeling was subjectively perceived and reported as "something beyond my control." He complained of diplopia, and on examination limited conjugate eye movements, with slight internal strabismus and constricted pupils, were noted. During stimulation the patient's ability to calculate was impaired and his performance of motor tests was poor. He felt as if he were going to lose consciousness. Immediately after the stimulation was terminated the patient said that these feelings and impulses were similar to those he had felt at the time his illness began.

Stimulation to the caudate nucleus produced no complaints. Most patients exhibited a varying degree of reduction of awareness from slight drowsiness to (in one instance) a state resembling sleep.

Stimulation to the amygdaloid nucleus resulted in an intense emotional reaction. The nature of the response varied from one stimulation to the next in the same patient, although parameters of stimulation were constant. On some occasions the patient became enraged and attempted to strike out, on other occasions she became fearful and felt an impulse to run. Always the behavior was volitional and always subjectively perceived. The patient's description was, "I don't know what came over me. I felt like an animal."

One patient was stimulated in the hippocampus. He complained of marked anxiety and described a typical *déjà vu* phenomenon. During some stimulations patients have reported varying fantasies or memories, usually vivid recollections of past events in their lives. This has occurred with stimulation of the amygdaloid, the septal region, and the hippocampus. The data will be presented in detail later after more studies have been completed.

BIOCHEMICAL STUDIES WITH STIMULATION

At the time of the original presentation of biochemical data on the patient group two questions remained unanswered: (1) Whether the changes observed were definitely due to stimulation or resulted from the stress of surgery; and (2) Whether specific alterations in chemistry were elicited from stimulations of specific regions.

Improvements in operating and stimulating techniques have made it possible to clarify these points by:

1. Permitting adequate time (1 to 5 weeks) to intervene between operations and stimulations;
2. Spacing stimulations sufficiently far apart to evaluate chemical changes after each stimulation;
3. Making discrete stimulation possible through more accurate electrode placement.

Surgery has consistently been followed by the changes associated with stress. Eosinophils virtually disappear, and the lymphocyte count drops significantly with some increase in the total white cell count. The blood picture usually returns to normal by the third day.

The method of delaying stimulations beyond this period by allowing the minimum of a week between operation and stimulation and spacing the stimulations to various regions at longer intervals provided the data listed on page 562.

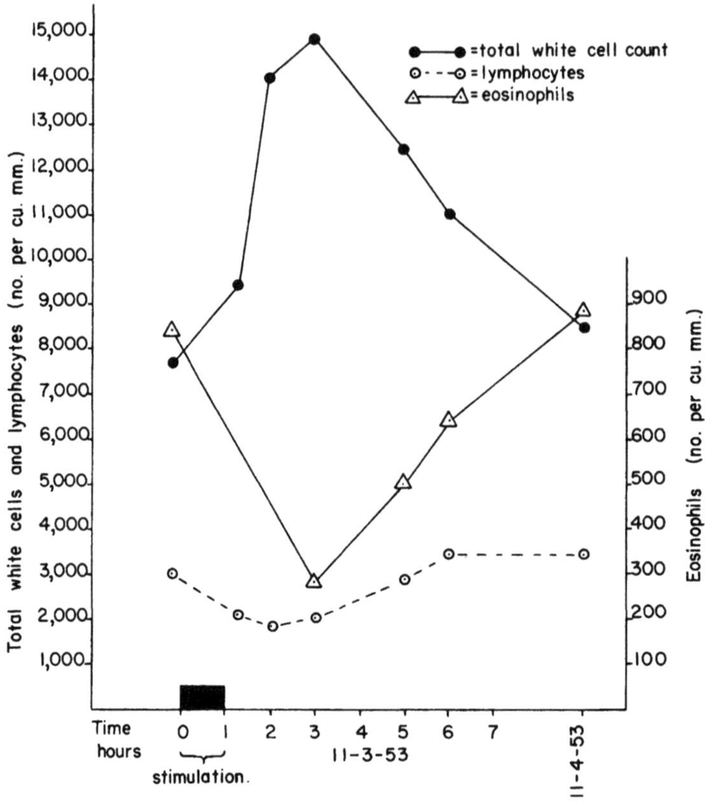

FIGURE B–4. See text

1. Stimulation through the septal region and rostral hypothalamus (facilitatory circuit) resulted in a marked drop of circulating eosinophils and lymphocytes, usually associated with a marked increase in the total white cell count and no change in the total red cell count. See the record of Patient A–10, Figure 4.
2. The same parameters of stimulation applied through the caudate region were usually associated with no eosinopenia or lymphopenia, and often a mild lymphophilia and eosinophilia resulted. A typical response is shown in the record of Patient A–4, Figure 5.
3. Changes in the number of circulating eosinophils and lymphocytes following stimulation to the more caudal midline structures (i.e., mesencephalic tegmentum) were considerably less marked than those which appeared with the septal and rostral hypothalamic stimulations. See the record of Patient A–10, Figure 6.

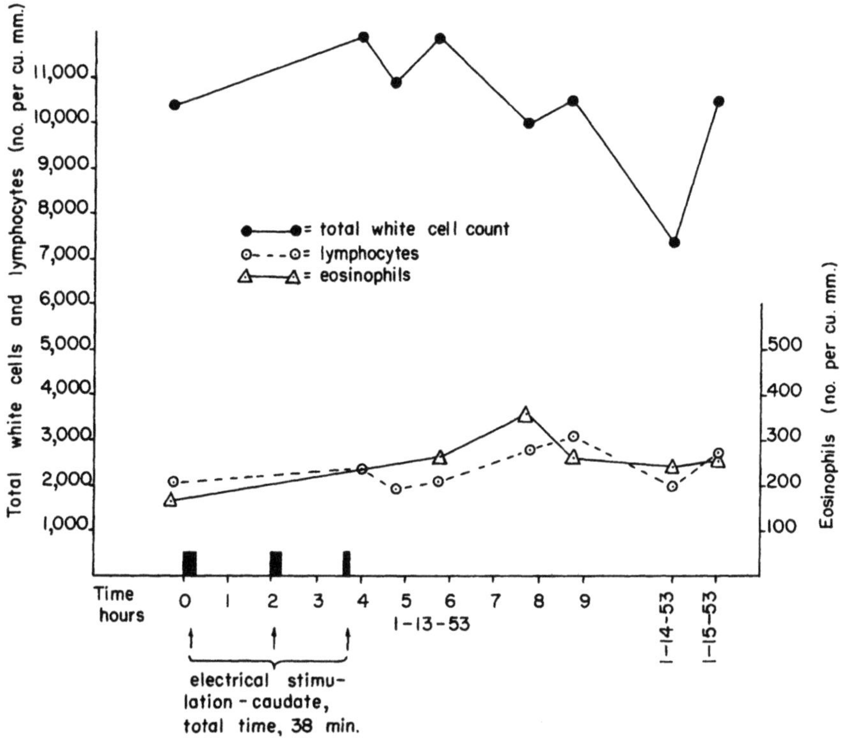

FIGURE B-5. See text

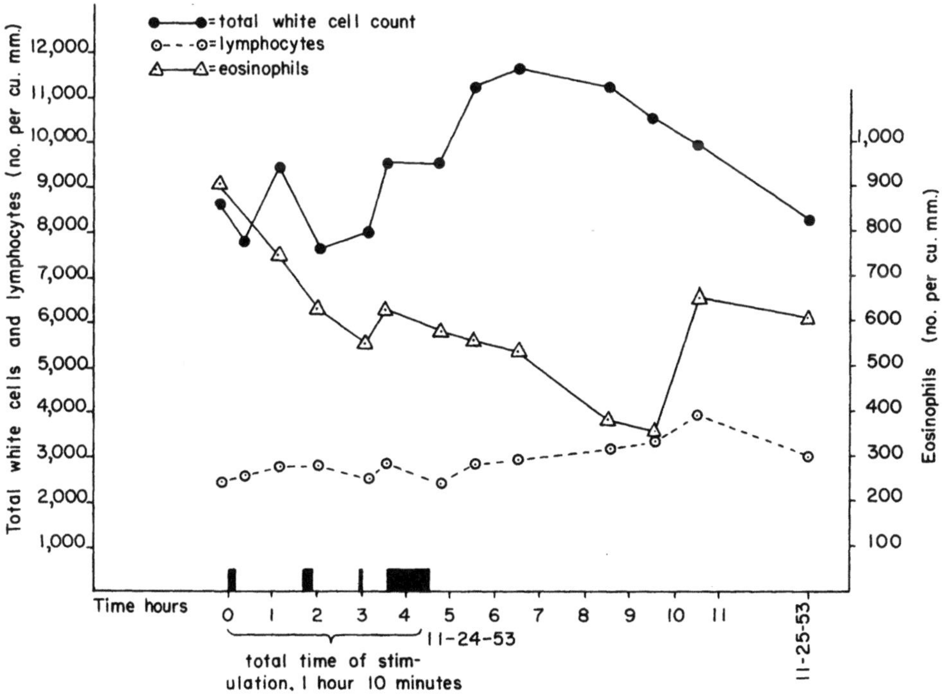

FIGURE B-6. See text

PRELIMINARY DATA OF OTHER BIOCHEMICAL STUDIES

The chemical changes found in animals following ablation and stimulation of the facilitatory region resemble those usually associated with altered function of the adrenal cortex. Likewise changes in cellular constituents of the blood like those reported above are generally interpreted as indicative of stress mediated through the adrenal cortex. For these reasons we decided to make a further investigation of the changes in steroid chemistry that accompanied stimulation in the addendum series of the patient group. With the technique of paper chromatography we have found rather striking changes in urinary steroid patterns following stimulation of the rostral midline structures (i.e., the facilitatory region). New steroids have appeared here. Caudate stimulation has consistently failed to produce alterations in the urinary steroid patterns. Although these findings are consistent, they will not be reported in detail until more data are available.

Also, in a small group of patients, consistent changes in total serum cholesterol and serum proteins have appeared following stimulation. These changes have followed stimulation through the rostral midline structures (i.e., septal region and anterior hypothalamus) and have failed to appear after stimulation of other regions. Total serum cholesterol has dropped significantly, but temporarily, in several patients after stimulation to the facilitatory regions. In Patient A–6, who received frequent stimulations over a period of several months for relief of intractable pain, a most pronounced drop in serum cholesterol occurred, the lowest reading being 29 mg. per cent. The drop began approximately 2 months after the beginning of the frequent stimulations, and the fall to this low level involved a period of 1 1/2 months.

Serum protein changes occurred after septal-hypothalamic stimulation in two patients in whom the albumin-globulin ratio was high prior to stimulation. The shift in ratio was associated with an increase in the globulin fraction to produce a normal albumin-globulin ratio.

ADDENDUM C

IMPROVEMENTS IN THE TECHNIQUE FOR IMPLANTING SUBCORTICAL ELECTRODES BY A STEREOTAXIC METHOD

HAL C. BECKER
WARREN L. FOUNDS
SAMUEL M. PEACOCK, JR.
ROBERT G. HEATH
RAEBURN C. LLEWELLYN

Although the stereotaxic method of electrode placement offers many advantages over the direct vision method, there are of course many sources of error in the use of the technique. When one is faced with the problem of placing electrodes in a given position in the human brain, it is of cardinal importance that the stereotaxic instrument be carefully aligned and continually treated with proper care, so that this initial alignment is maintained throughout each procedure and from one procedure to the next. Referring now to the specific technique reported in Chapter 10 a complete re-evaluation has been made since the June 1952 meetings in an effort to secure greater accuracy than was possible in the past. As a result, the following sources of error in placement have been found and eliminated.

One source of error was found to be the manner in which the AP and lateral cassettes containing the reference grid markings were seated in their respective cassette holders. The method of securing these cassettes has been modified, so that there is no longer any uncertainty as to how the cassettes are seated in the holders. The grids have been aligned in the vertical direction within a fraction of a millimeter and arranged so that they maintain this alignment during use. The lateral cassette holder has been fitted with a retractable index marker, so that its position on the horizontal graduated bar can be accurately determined. From this AP reference point, the AP coordinate of any target point can be calculated from the lateral x-ray.

Another, and by far the greatest, source of error in the previous placement technique was the inadequacy of the method for geometric spatial

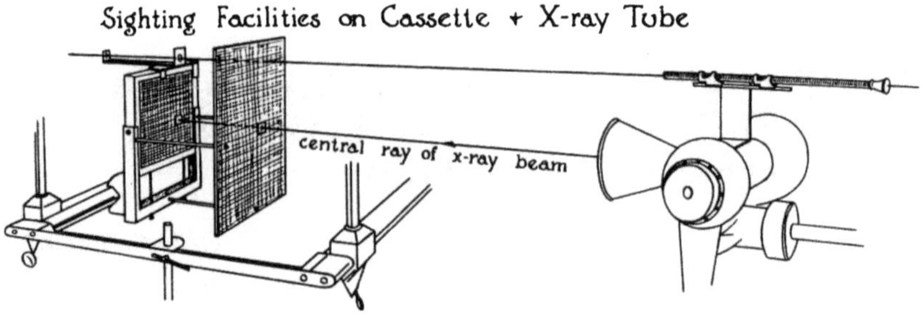

FIGURE C–1. Sighting facilities on cassettes and x-ray tube. This sketch shows ruled lucite test grid in place, with x-ray head properly sighted in to produce the test film shown in Figure 2

alignment of the central ray of the divergent x-ray beam with respect to the AP and lateral cassettes. This resulted in magnification and distortion in the mapping of anatomical structures in both the lateral and AP views, for which quantitative corrections could not be made owing to the absence of precision sighting facilities. In order to remedy this, specific sighting points at the centers of the general target areas were chosen on the lateral and AP cassettes, and a telescopic sight was mounted on the x-ray head and accurately sighted in with double sights of the peep and crosshair type (Figure 1) on both the lateral and the AP cassettes. This affords an easy and speedy method by which the central ray of the x-ray beam can be made to strike the chosen sighting point on the cassette grid at a normal angle of incidence.

The sighting problem, of course, is analogous to that of aiming a rifle so that its projectile will strike not one match at a given distance, but two matches placed a given distance apart. Thus quantitative correction factors for magnification and distortion were derived from test x-ray pictures taken with grids of ruled lucite placed 10 and 16 cm., respectively, in front of the grids held by the lateral and AP cassette holders —10 and 16 cm. being the approximate distances between the "center of gravity" of the general target areas selected and the cassettes themselves. The pictures are now taken with the x-ray head at a standard distance of 6 feet from the cassette. This distance was chosen because of spatial limitations imposed by the size of the operating room.

The x-ray map of the lines on the lucite test grid projected onto the

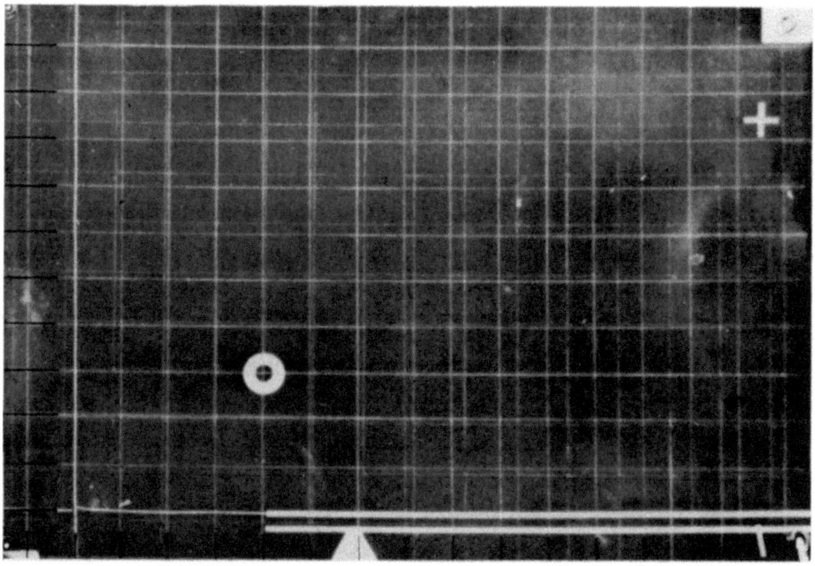

FIGURE C-2. Film showing x-ray projection of ruled lucite grid on cassette grid. See description in text. Data for this film: Distance from x-ray tube to cassette = 6 feet. The distance from the lucite test grid to the cassette face (10.8 cm.) was equal to that from the cassette to center of the patient's head

face of the grid held by the cassette is clearly shown in Figure 2. The shadow of the brass washer taped to the lucite test grid marks the approximate center of the 4 sq. cm. "area of least confusion." This is the point at which the central x-ray beam passes perpendicularly through the two parallel grids. The grid lines marked in black on the right and lower margins are shadows of the grid lines on the cassette face. The corresponding unmarked grid lines, which are superimposed on the marked ones in the "area of least confusion," are shadows of the lines on the lucite test grid. The resultant distortion and magnification (conformal mapping) of the test grid, everywhere but in the immediate vicinity of the washer, is clearly shown. Quantitative corrections for magnification and distortion in lateral and AP x-rays can be obtained from films taken in this way.

Once the x-ray pictures, both lateral and AP, have been taken with the x-ray machine carefully sighted in the manner just described, the chosen target points are then plotted from the distorted x-ray map onto linear cross-section paper, using the correction factors obtained above, to produce the new geometrically true maps. These true maps are then used in the calculations for the three coordinates necessary for accurate placement of the electrodes. This complete system will be described in detail elsewhere.

Target points chosen from air-study films are easily hit within 2 mm. by this revised method of placement. An even higher degree of accuracy can be achieved when necessary, if extreme care is taken in aligning the stereotaxic instrument, sighting in the x-ray beam, and arranging the patient so that respiratory movements, etc., influence minimally the mechanical stresses on the stereotaxic instrument.

Another ready source of error, and one which really constitutes a second phase of the electrode implantation problem, is that of maintaining the electrode in the proper target position while the guide with which it has been inserted is removed from the brain. In the past this presented a real difficulty, since there was no adequate method of keeping the electrode in place while the guide was removed except by manually holding the lead wire with forceps. Figure 3 shows the special electrode carrier which was designed to achieve this end and which is currently in use. It consists of two guide needles, one of which slides through the other as the electrode is implanted. After the electrode has been run down to the calculated depth, a clamp is attached to the carrier frame at the top of the outer guide needle in such a way that it grips the electrode lead wire firmly just above the top of this needle and presses the wire firmly against the supporting frame just behind the outer guide. When the inner guide needle is withdrawn from the brain, the column action of the captive electrode lead wire is more than sufficient to compensate for the friction of the moving guide needle on the surface of the electrode lead wire, so that the electrode remains in the calculated position while the guide needle slides over the lead wire. After the guide needle has emerged a few centimeters from the surface of the brain, the surgeon grasps the electrode lead wire very carefully at the skull level and holds it firmly while the electrode carrier is unthreaded from the lead wire and removed from the field.

A plastic skull button (Figure 4), which has previously been threaded over the guide carrier proper, is then inserted into the tapered trephine

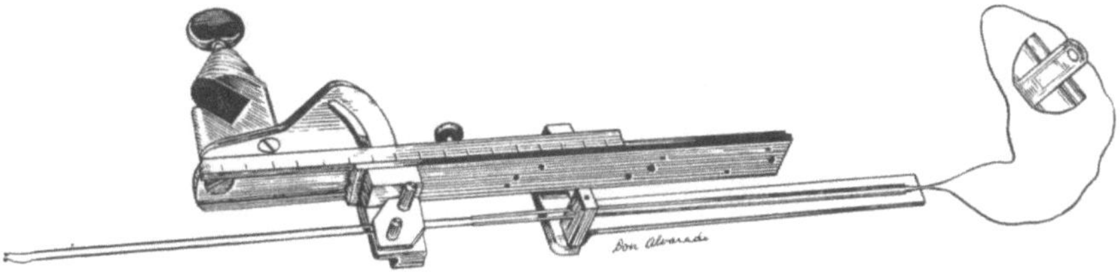

FIGURE C-3. "Trombone" electrode carrier. This sketch shows the modified electrode carrier with telescoping concentric hypodermic electrode guides as described in the text. The electrodes are shown extended about 1 cm. below the guide tubes for clarity. These silver spheres are pulled up snugly against the mouths of the guide tubes before being inserted into brain tissue

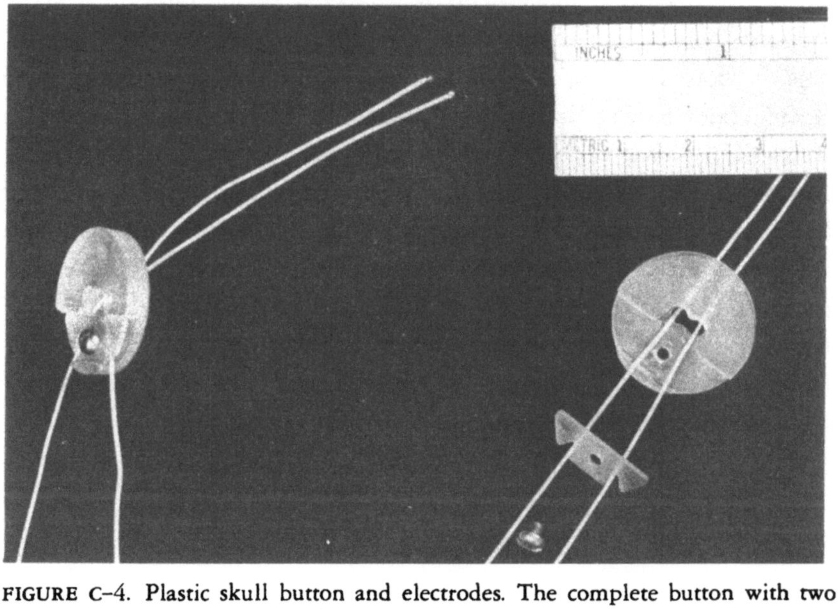

FIGURE C-4. Plastic skull button and electrodes. The complete button with two electrodes firmly held in place is shown at the left. The three parts of the button are shown in the exploded view on the right, with electrodes threaded through the button

hole and tapped solidly into place. The electrode lead wire or wires are then carefully bent at right angles at the level of the top of the skull button, and are firmly held in place by means of a thin plastic retainer plate and a stainless steel screw, as shown in Figure 4. Following the fixation of the electrode lead wires at the skull level by means of the plastic button, the electrode leads are brought out through the skin several centimeters distant from the scalp incision as described in Chapter 10. This entire technique has also been adopted for animal experimentation—the small cat-monkey stereotaxic instrument, with modifications for the addition of x-ray cassettes, now being used as an adjunct to the animal atlas.

Both the human and the animal stereotaxic instrument will shortly be modified so that the Polaroid Land one-step photographic technique can be used to produce 60-second lateral and AP x-rays.

A newer type of button has been used in animal experiments which eventually may prove more satisfactory in the human operations than the button described above. This is a tapered plastic button, of about the same outside dimensions as the one described above, with a tapered hole of about 1 cm. diameter in its center. A second plastic button with tapered sides having the proper diameter fits into this hole. Serrations are carefully made about the edge of the inner button, and these serrations are of such a size that they firmly grip the insulation of the electrode lead wires when the inner button is firmly seated in its tapered hole. The newer type of skull button has an advantage over the earlier one in that a right angle bend in the lead wires at the level of the top of the plastic button is no longer necessary, and further, that as many wires as are desired can be brought up through one burr hole without the mechanical complications found in the earlier system.

ADDENDUM D

IMPROVEMENTS IN THE TECHNIQUE OF ELECTRICAL STIMULATION

HAL C. BECKER
SAMUEL M. PEACOCK, JR.

We are currently using stimulation methods D and E. Stimulation method D has already been described in the text. Stimulation method E is identical with method A except for the addition of the stimulus monitor.

During tests using silver spherical electrodes of type 2C, with pulse repetition frequency of 100 cycles per second, pulse duration of 1 millisecond, peak currents up to 20 ma., and total durations up to 1 hour, there were no gas bubbles produced, there was no alteration in pH of physiological saline, and there was no drop in peak current as a result of polarization, when stimulation methods D and E were employed. This undoubtedly was to be explained by the vanishing of the area integral over each complete cycle of the voltage-versus-time and current-versus-time curves. By using either of these two stimulation techniques, it is therefore possible to maintain a constant amplitude current pulse throughout the train duration, and further to be reasonably assured that damage to brain tissue as a result of bubble production and alterations in pH will be minimal. Stimulation method D would also reduce to a minimum any dialysis[1] of proteins. Probably this would also apply to stimulation method E, in which depolarization takes place during the interval between pulses.

In a series of stimulations of the motor cortex in cats, no significant differences in current or Coulomb threshold between stimulation methods D and E could be found.

[1] See Chapter 12, Reference 7.

KEY TO ABBREVIATIONS IN ADDENDUM E

RC	Rostral caudate
CC	Caudal caudate
RS	Rostral septal
CS	Caudal septal
Hypo	Hypothalamic
LFC	Left frontal cortex
RFC	Right fronto-parietal cortex
S	Septal
Intraven	Intraventricular
R Hypo	Rostral hypothalamus
R Hippo	Rostral hippocampus
C Hippo	Caudal hippocampus
T	Tegmentum of mesencephalon
CA	Caudal amygdaloid
RA	Rostral amygdaloid

ADDENDUM E

ELECTROENCEPHALOGRAMS AND SUBCORTICOGRAMS RECORDED SINCE THE JUNE 1952 MEETINGS

ROBERT G. HEATH
SAMUEL M. PEACOCK, JR.
RUSSELL R. MONROE
WILLIAM H. MILLER, JR.

This is a summary of the new findings obtained on the recordings since the June 1952 meetings. Only data which help to clarify various points that were preliminary or vague at the time of the original presentation will be discussed. It was possible to gather these new data because of technical improvements in electrode implantation and stimulation described in Addenda C and D. The material will be discussed under the following headings:

- Subcortical Spikes
- Correlation of Thought Levels and Electrical Recordings
- The Slow Wave before and after Stimulation
- Correlations between Psychotic Behavior and Electrical Abnormalities
- Persisting Paroxysmal Electrical Activity in the Deep Leads after Stimulation
- The Effect on Electrical Recordings of the Administration of Drugs which Alter Levels of Awareness

Many of these new data add support to the over-all theoretical framework which postulated correlations between levels of thought and levels of physiological activity of the brain.

SUBCORTICAL SPIKES

Since the June 1952 meetings improved techniques of electrode implantation have made it possible to follow recordings for many months. We have allowed a considerably longer period between the electrode implantation and the first stimulation. Spikes have been consistently

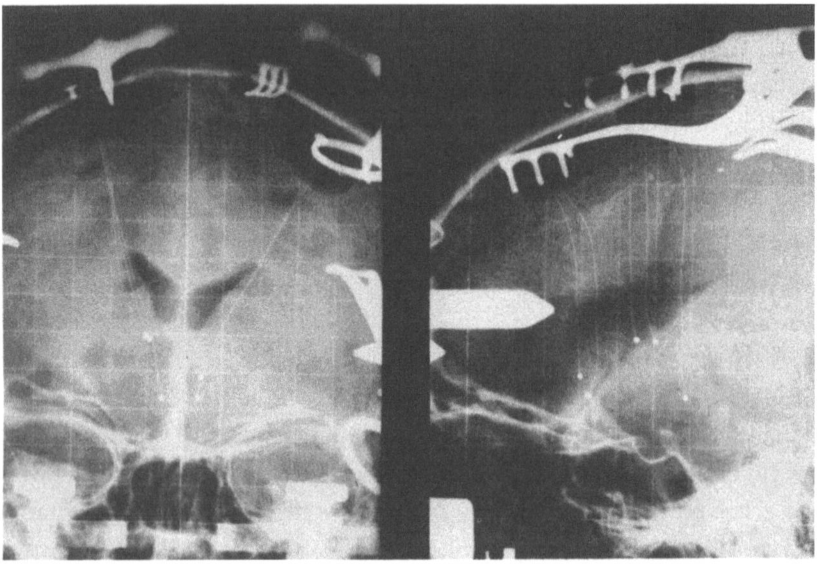

FIGURE E–1. X-rays of Patient A–4 showing electrodes in position

recorded from the septal region in the seven schizophrenic patients included in the addendum series. The spikes persist as long as the psychotic behavior is evident, thus ruling out any possibility of their being related either to anesthesia or to the temporary effect of electrode implantation. Two patients with diseases other than schizophrenia have been included in the addendum series. Neither of these patients showed spikes.

Through much greater accuracy in electrode placement we have been able to demonstrate that the spiking is recorded from a very small area within the septal region. Figure 1 is an x-ray of Patient A–4. As indicated in Figure 2, the spiking occurred predominantly from the electrode of lead 14 and to a slight extent from the electrode of lead 13, which was 3 mm. away. The electrode in the rostral part of the hypothalamus and the caudate electrodes did not show this electrical phenomenon during the 10-month period that Patient A–4 has been followed with recordings. Similar localization was present in all other patients.

At the time of the June meetings we had recorded spiking only from the septal region. Since then electrodes have been accurately implanted in many different regions of the brain in schizophrenic patients. We now have recordings from the hippocampus, hypothalamus, tegmentum of

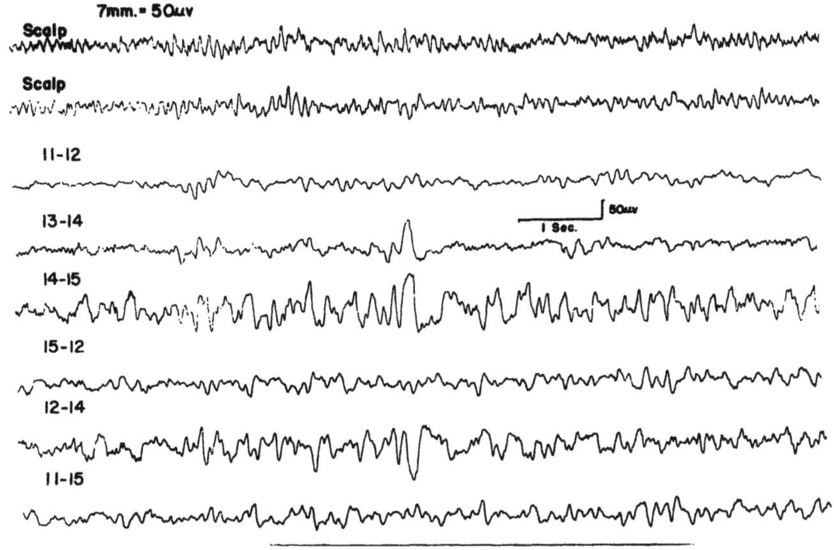

FIGURE E-2. Prestimulation record of Patient A-4. Note spiking in leads 13 and 14 (septal). Key: 11 = RC; 12 = CC; 13 = RS; 14 = CS; 15 = Hypo

the mesencephalon, caudate nucleus, thalamus, and amygdaloid nucleus, as well as from the septal region. In each case electrodes have been implanted in at least three of these sites, the septal region, caudate nucleus, and rostral hypothalamus. The only site other than the septal region from which the spiking has been obtained is the hippocampus. Hippocampal electrodes were stimulated in two patients of this series. X-rays and records will be illustrated.

When the patients were drowsy or sleepy the spiking appeared in higher amplitude and more frequently from the septal region. However, our preliminary impression is that when the patients are awake, spiking may occur more frequently from the hippocampus. Figure 3, the air study of Patient A–10, visualizes the ventricular system and demonstrates the anatomical landmarks that were used for implantation. Figure 4, an x-ray of Patient A–10, shows the electrodes in position. Figure 5, a recording from this patient, shows spikes chiefly in the septal lead but also in the hippocampal lead. It is to be noted that recordings from other regions did not show spikes. Figure 6 is a recording from various structures with the ear as an indifferent lead. The same spiking phenomenon is apparent as in Figure 5.

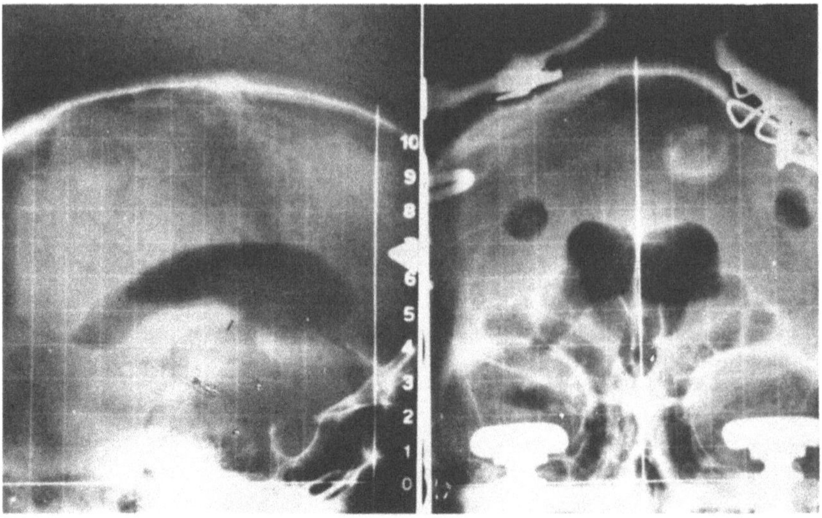

FIGURE E-3. Air study of Patient A-10 visualizing the ventricular system, including the aqueduct of the fourth ventricle. Comparison of this figure with Figure 4 demonstrates the anatomical sites in which the electrodes were implanted

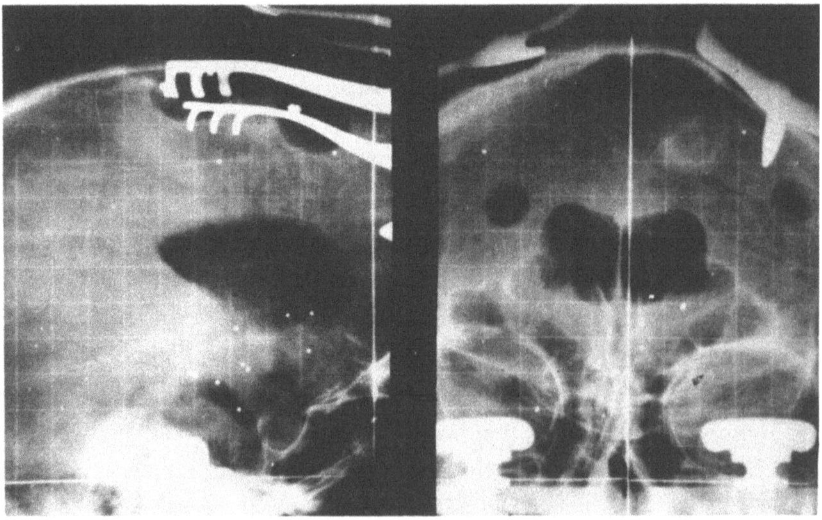

FIGURE E-4. X-rays of Patient A-10 showing electrodes in position

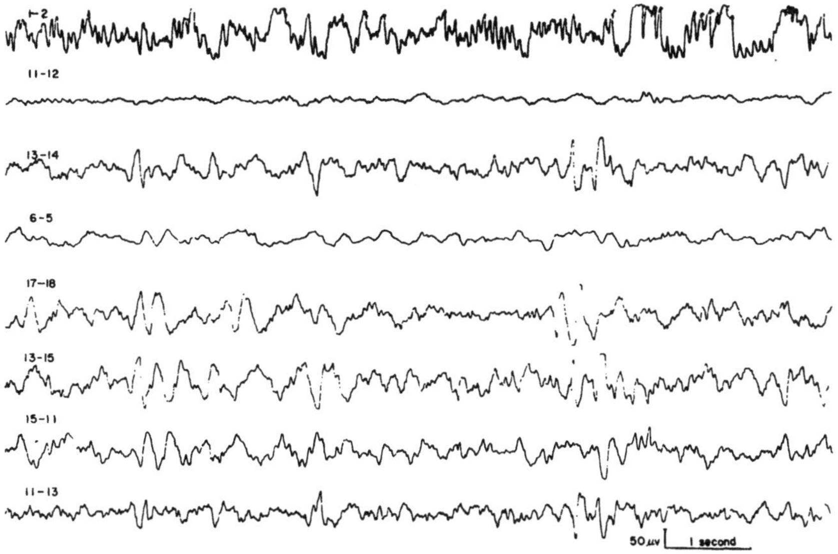

FIGURE E-5. Prestimulation recordings from Patient A-10. Note spiking in leads 13 (septal) and 17-18 (hippocampal). Key: 1 = LFC; 2 = RFC (these electrodes are placed on the arachnoid); 11 = RC; 12 = CC; 13 = S; 14 = Intraven; 5 and 6 = R Hypo (6 is the more rostral of this pair); 17 = R Hippo; 18 = C Hippo; 15 and 16 = T

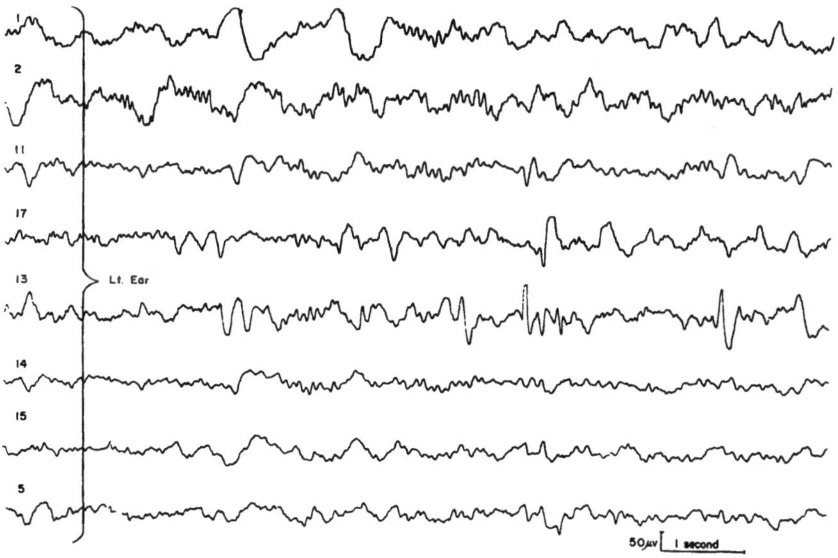

FIGURE E-6. Unipolar recordings from Patient A-10. Key: same as in Figure 5

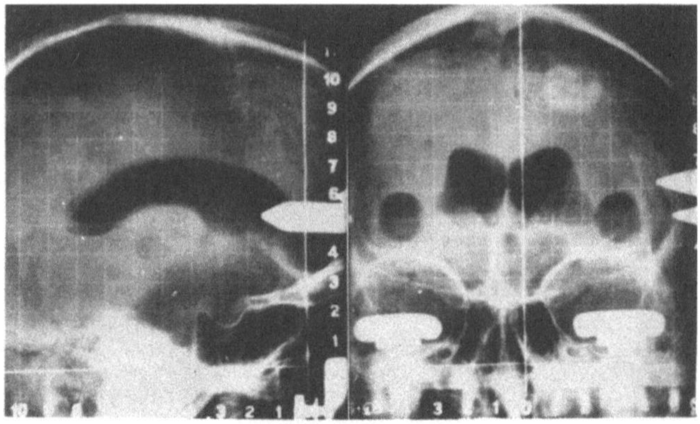

FIGURE E–7. Air studies of Patient A–11 before electrode implantation. The opaque film is an artifact from the cassette

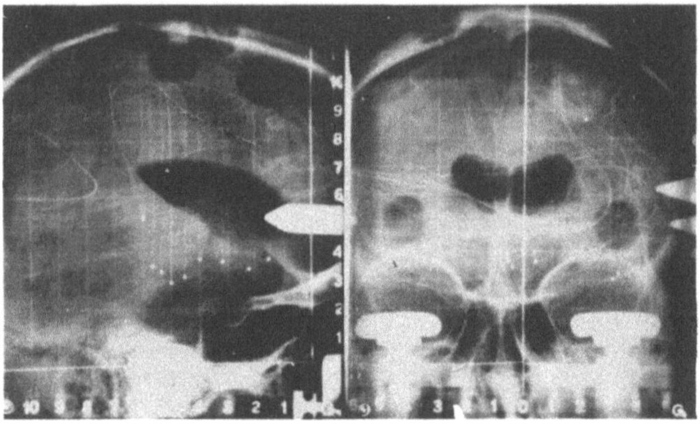

FIGURE E–8. X-rays of Patient A–11 showing electrodes in position

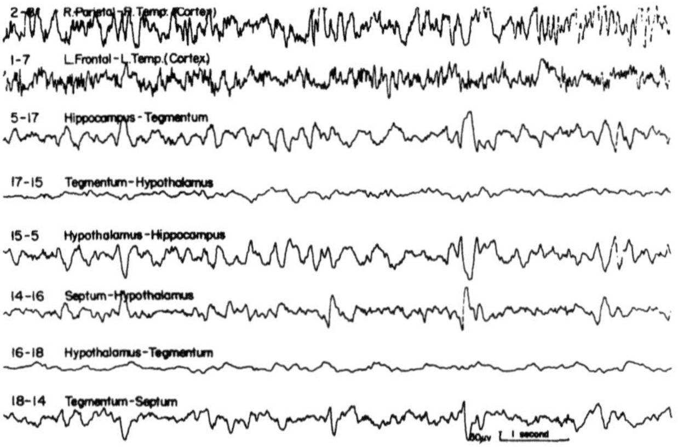

FIGURE E–9. Cortical and subcortical recordings from Patient A–11

The ventriculogram of Patient A–11 (Figure 7) shows air in the third ventricle and a slight amount in the temporal horn of the lateral ventricles. Figure 8 shows the electrodes in position. This patient had electrodes in the hippocampus and tegmentum, as well as septal region and hypothalamus. Figure 9 shows a recording from Patient A–11. Here again the spiking phenomenon is localized to the hippocampal and septal regions and is not present in leads from other structures. The spindling apparent on the cortical leads is due to barbiturates.

It seems logical that similar electrical activity should be recorded from the hippocampal and septal regions, because of the known anatomical connections. Others have reported on the similarity of electrical activity in the two structures.[1,2]

Summary. The spiking phenomenon accurately localized to the septal region is a consistent finding in the schizophrenic patients of the addendum series. In two patients spiking was also obtained from electrodes placed in the hippocampus. The spiking was not observed in the two nonpsychotic patients in this series.

CORRELATION OF THOUGHT LEVELS AND ELECTRICAL RECORDINGS

In the report made at the June 1952 meetings there was some uncertainty as to whether or not correlations could be made between the patient's thought activity and the electrical recordings. When such correlations seemed to be present, the physiological activity associated with emotionally charged thoughts appeared in the leads from the septal region.

Since making the earlier report we have continued to find many correlations between levels of thought activity and changes in electrical activity from the septal leads, but even more striking correlations have appeared in leads from the hippocampus. Sample recordings are presented to illustrate this activity (Figures 10–13).

Figure 10 shows activity recorded while the patient was more or less preoccupied with his external environment. During the time that the record in Figure 11 was taken the patient began to think spontaneously of a television program which he had seen the evening before. The theme of the show was a problem in juvenile delinquency, which initiated a

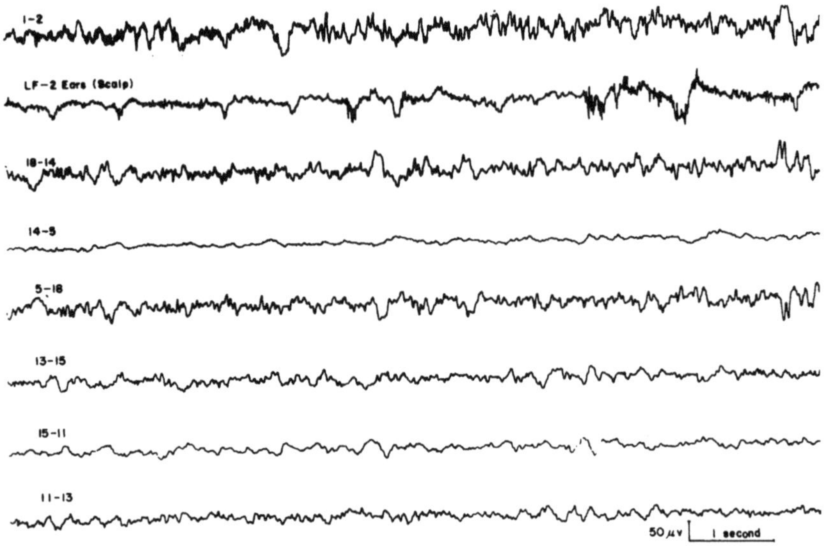

FIGURE E-10. Recordings from Patient A-10. Note that Figures 10 through 13 illustrate activity at different levels of thought (see text). Key: same as in Figure 5

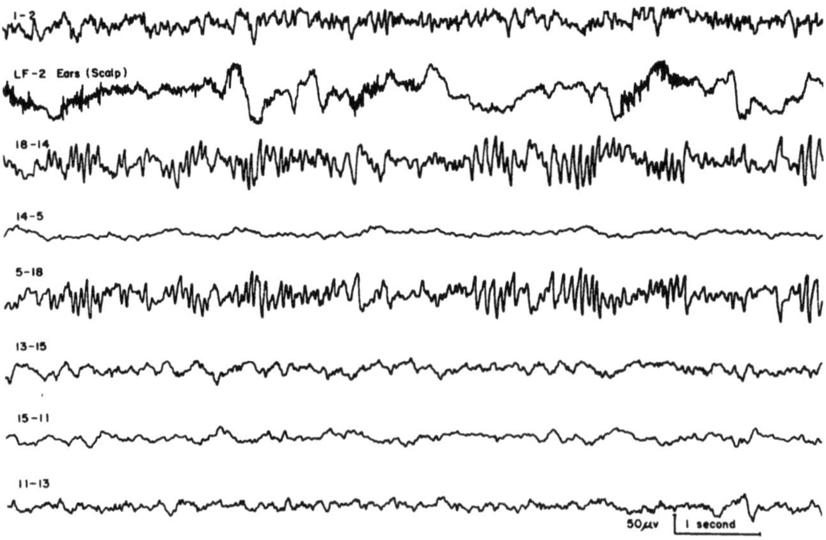

FIGURE E-11. Recordings from Patient A-10. See note above

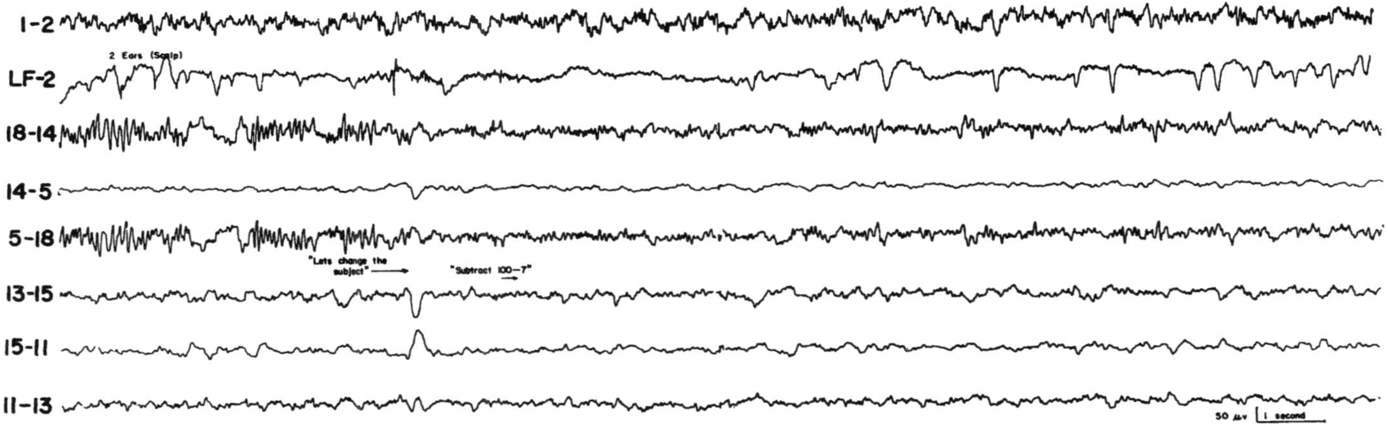

FIGURE E-12. Recordings from Patient A-10. See note under Figure E-10

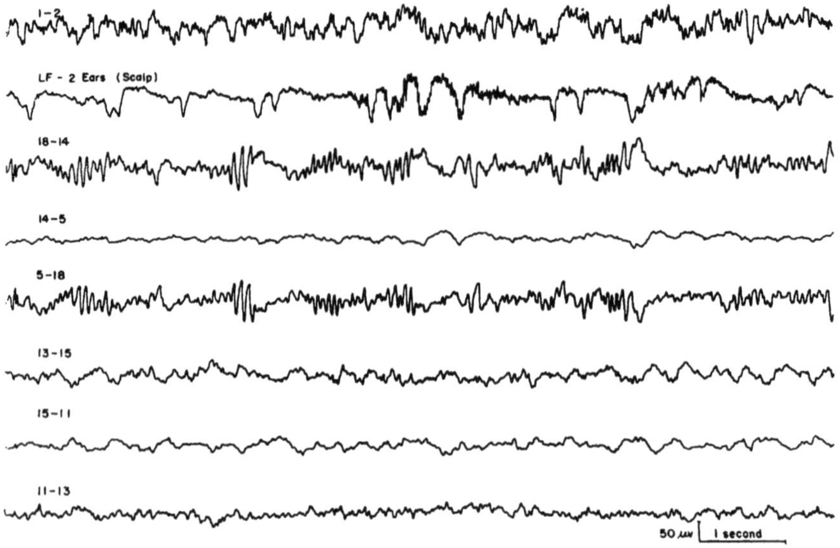

FIGURE E–13. Recordings from Patient A–10. See note under Figure 10

train of highly charged emotional associations about his own childhood. The examiner then deliberately distracted the patient by giving him a simple mathematical problem—namely, to subtract 7 from 100. The change in the recording from the hippocampal leads was immediate and dramatic (see Figure 12). Subsequently, when the emotionally charged thoughts returned, the high amplitude activity recurred in the hippocampal region (Figure 13). It was possible to change the nature of this recording repeatedly by directing the interview. The specific content has never been important in altering the electrical recordings. When changes have occurred, they have been associated with alterations in levels of thought. The high amplitude slow activity has always occurred with low level emotional thinking, whereas the faster activity of lower amplitude has been associated with higher level unemotional thinking. Recordings from leads other than the hippocampal and septal have not changed with alterations in levels of thought activity.

It is by no means implied that because of these focal findings we consider emotional phenomena to be localized to the septal region and the hippocampus. Instead we consider that this correlation of physiological activity with thought activity is a reflection of the over-all dynamic activity of the brain that can be recorded from these regions, but not from the other regions in which electrodes have been placed.

THE SLOW WAVE BEFORE AND AFTER STIMULATION

At the time of the June 1952 meetings it was noted that slow waves were usually recorded from the deep structures during the short period that intervened between operation and stimulation. It was also noted that accentuated slow wave activity consistently appeared from the poles of the electrodes that were stimulated and persisted throughout the 1 or 2 days that the electrodes remained in place after stimulation. Because the electrodes remained in place for such a short period of time it was not possible fully to evaluate the meaning of this slow wave activity. With the newer techniques of electrode implantation (see Addendum C) we have considerably lengthened the period (up to 6 weeks) between implantation and the first stimulation. The problem of the postoperative slow wave now seems to be solved.

Recordings from all patients operated upon by the newer techniques showed slow wave activity which persisted for only 1 or 2 days. We, therefore, conclude that the slow wave activity observed in the short postoperative prestimulation period in the patients of the first series was probably due to temporary edema or trauma resulting from the surgical procedure.

It was noted in the original presentation that an increase of slow wave activity appeared in recordings from electrodes stimulated after the current was applied. We could not be certain that this was caused by the stimulation until the electrodes had been left in place for longer periods after the stimulation. When this became possible, the data suggested that the persistent slow wave following stimulation may have been related to brain damage incurred as a result of the particular type of stimulation used.

The first opportunity to study these effects occurred in Patient 26, who was operated upon at the time of the meetings. Electrodes were left in place for 3 weeks following his first stimulation. Throughout this period the slow wave persisted. On the prestimulation record, the patient displayed (Figure 14) the same general findings as those seen in other schizophrenic patients. The outstanding feature was the spike confined to the septal lead. The older type of stimulus, the same as that used on Patients 3 to 25 inclusive, was administered to the septal region. Following this stimulation the record showed a high amplitude slow wave, most pronounced in the septal lead where the stimulus was administered (Figure 15). The recording made 24 hours after stimulation is shown in Figure 16. It is noted that the delta wave persisted with a maximum amount of slow activity confined to the septal leads. The spike became less frequent but persisted through the final recording, which was made 21 days after the initial stimulation and 24 hours after the last stimulation. The slow wave was present in all records, however, after the first stimulus was administered.

After obtaining this finding in Patient 26, the first patient in whom records could be followed for a long period after stimulus was administered, we assumed that damage was being done by the stimulation. Because of this the new technique of stimulation was devised (see Addendum D).

When bidirectional pulse was used instead of the old unidirectional pulse for the stimulation of subsequent patients, the persisting slow wave did not appear. The records of two patients stimulated by the new technique are presented in Figures 17–37.

The prestimulation record of Patient A–4 (Figure 17) resembled those of previous schizophrenic patients; it showed the spiking confined to the septal leads. Two weeks after operation the newer type of stimulus was administered to the caudate lead at 10 ma. for 1 hour; the record made immediately thereafter (Figure 18) did not show the slow wave.

Similarly, Patient A–8's first poststimulation record (Figure 20) shows essentially the same pattern as the prestimulation record (Figure 19); it lacks the slow wave characteristic of the poststimulation records of patients who were stimulated by the unidirectional pulse. No spikes appear in the prestimulation record chosen for illustration, since this patient demonstrated focal spiking in the septal region only when in light sleep.

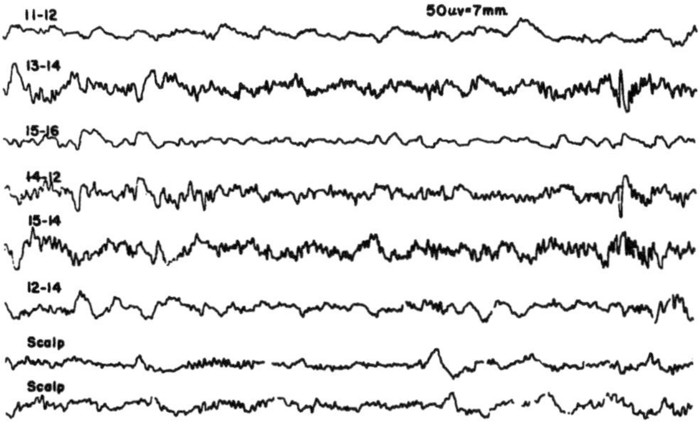

FIGURE E–14. Recordings from Patient 26 (see text). Key: 11 and 12 = RC and CC; 13 and 14 = RS and CS; 15 and 16 = R Hypo and C Hypo

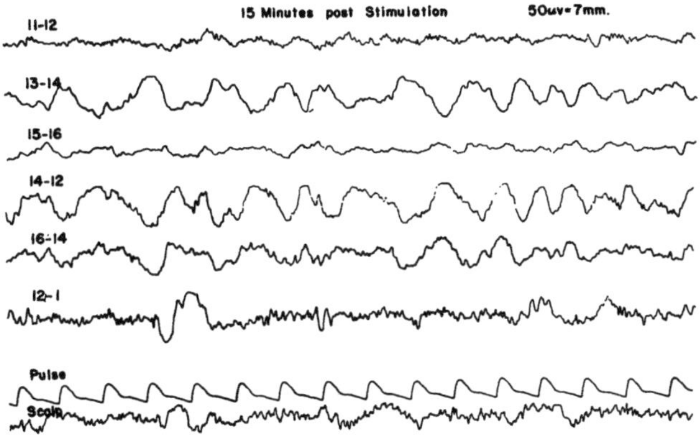

FIGURE E–15. See text. Key: same as in Figure 14 (1 = left frontal scalp)

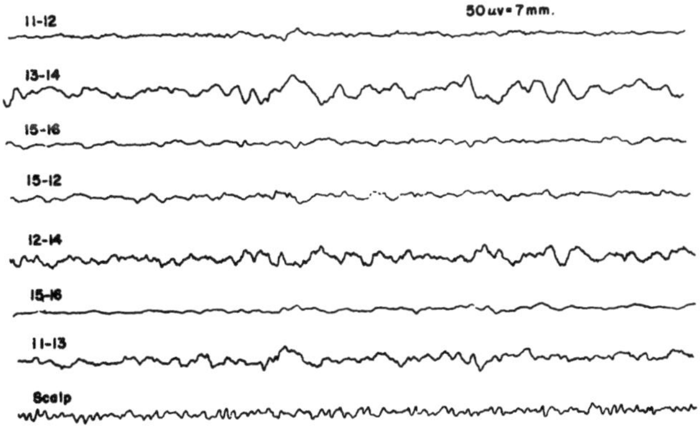

FIGURE E–16. See text. Key: same as in Figure 14

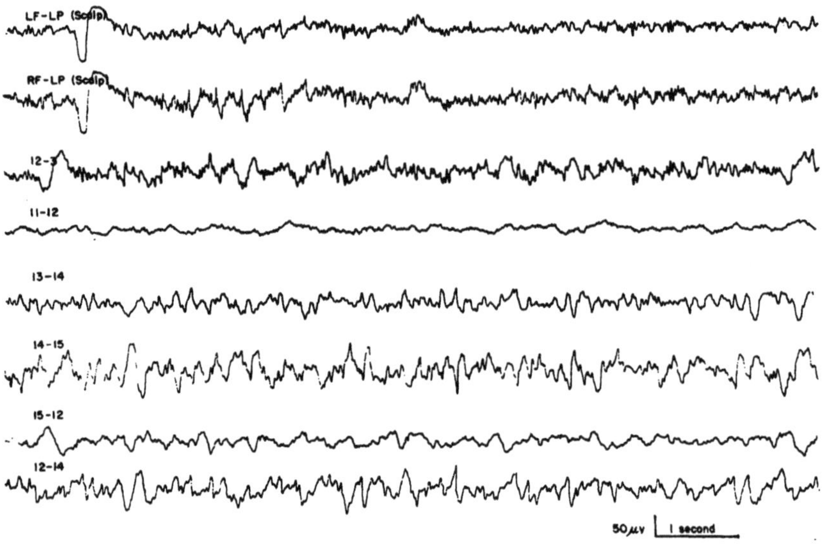

FIGURE E-17. Prestimulation record of Patient A-4. Key: 11 = RC; 12 = CC; 13 = RS; 14 = CS; 15 = Hypo

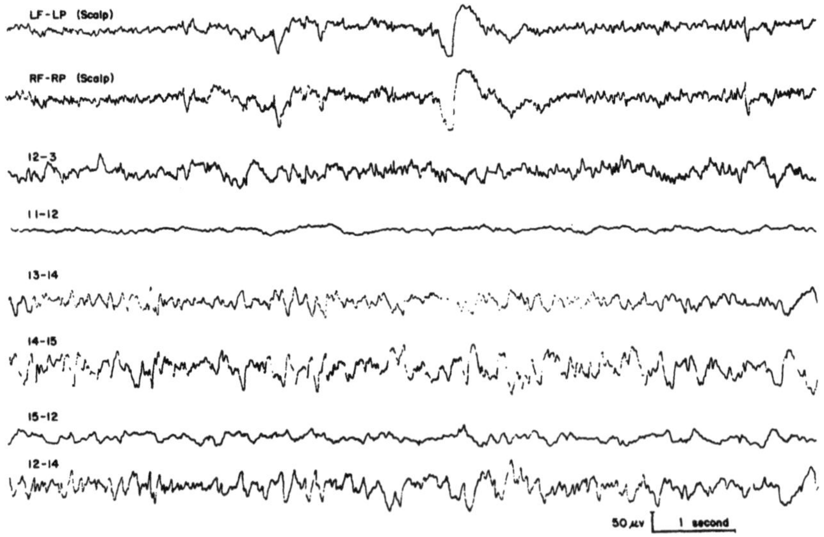

FIGURE E-18. Immediate poststimulation record of Patient A-4. Key: same as in Figure 17

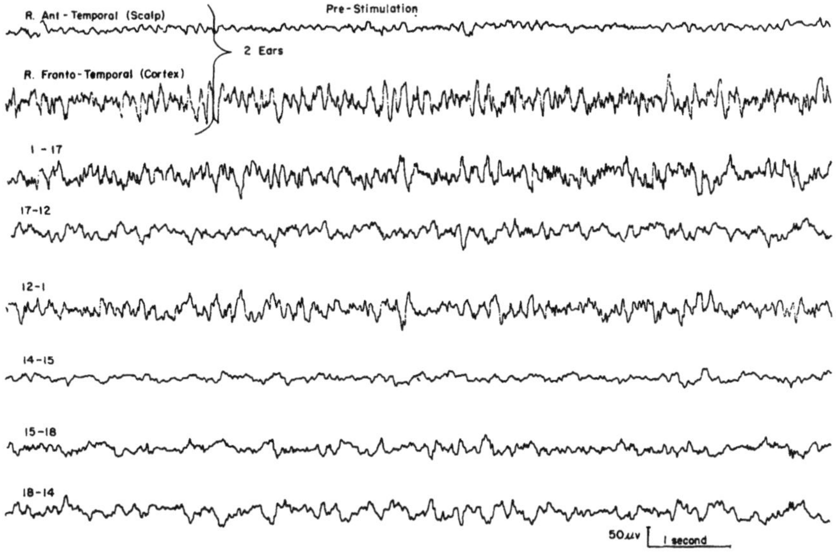

FIGURE E–19. Prestimulation record of Patient A-8. Key: 1 = LFC; 17 = CA; 12 = CC; 14 = CS; 15 = R Hypo; 18 = RA

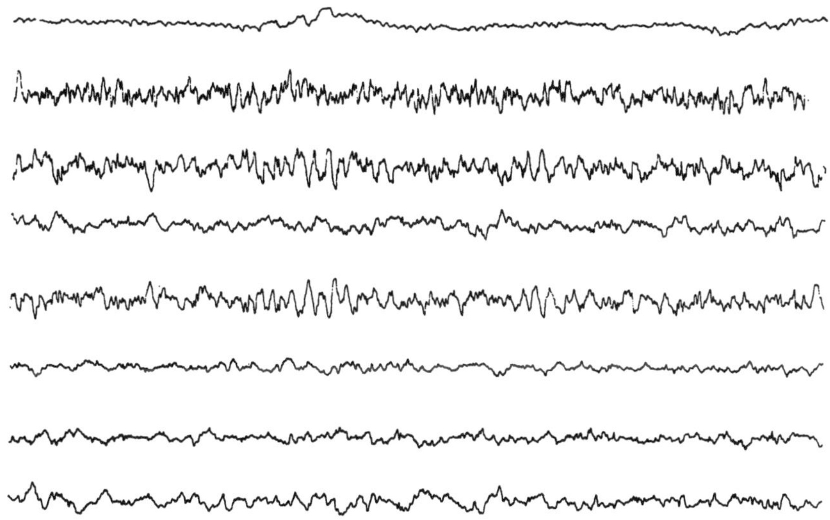

FIGURE E–20. Recordings from Patient A-8 taken immediately following stimulation to the amygdaloid nucleus over a period of 1 1/2 hours. Key: same as in Figure 19

CORRELATIONS BETWEEN PSYCHOTIC BEHAVIOR AND ELECTRICAL ABNORMALITIES

With the newer technique, in which the lead wires are soldered to a small plug that can be easily covered by conventional headdress, continuous confinement to the hospital is no longer necessary. When the patient's clinical condition permits it, he visits at home and carries on his usual social activities. This had made for more satisfactory evaluation of the patient's behavior during treatment. In several patients we have followed electrical recordings for several months, the longest period being 10 months in one patient. This patient was stimulated at various times when indicated by her behavior. Although findings on this small group of patients must be considered preliminary, there appears to be a correlation between spiking abnormalities in the septal region and overt psychotic behavior. Figure 21 is a record taken during a period of overt psychotic behavior. The record in Figure 22 was taken during a period of remission when the patient was functioning quite well at home, showing interest in her surroundings and assuming responsibility for the care of her family.

PERSISTENT PAROXYSMAL ACTIVITY IN DEEP LEADS AFTER STIMULATION

In our original report it was noted that persistent paroxysmal activity sometimes appeared in poststimulation recordings from subcortical regions. This high amplitude activity was very similar to that recorded on scalp EEG's during seizures. Sometimes it remained localized to subcortical leads and sometimes spread, after the passage of variable periods of time, to the cortex. Always, when paroxysmal activity was seen on the scalp leads, the patients developed clinical seizures. However, when paroxysmal activity was limited to the subcortical leads (always those from the septal region) there was no untoward motor response and neither clouding of consciousness nor loss of alertness occurred.

We are able now to present more data on this subject. Three of the patients of the addendum series developed persistent paroxysmal activity through the subcortical leads following prolonged stimulation. The stimulation time required to induce this activity ranged from 1 to 2 hours. Since it is impossible to record during the actual stimulation

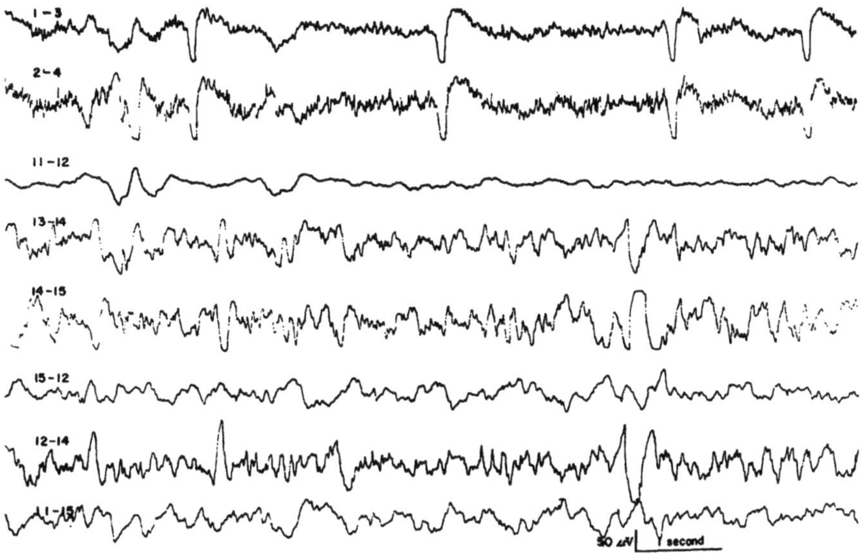

FIGURE E–21. Recordings from Patient A–4 taken during a period of overt psychotic behavior. Key: same as in Figure 17

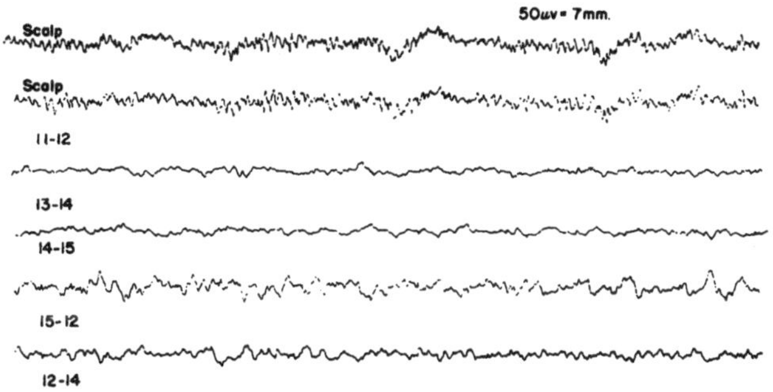

FIGURE E–22. Recordings from Patient A–4 taken during a period of remission of psychotic behavior. Key same as in Figure 17

procedure, stimulation was stopped and sample records taken at intervals of about 15 minutes. The stimulus was discontinued when the paroxysmal activity appeared. In one patient it was induced on many different occasions. This patient had terminal carcinoma of the cervix with intractable pain. Since we had noted that the pain was relieved as long

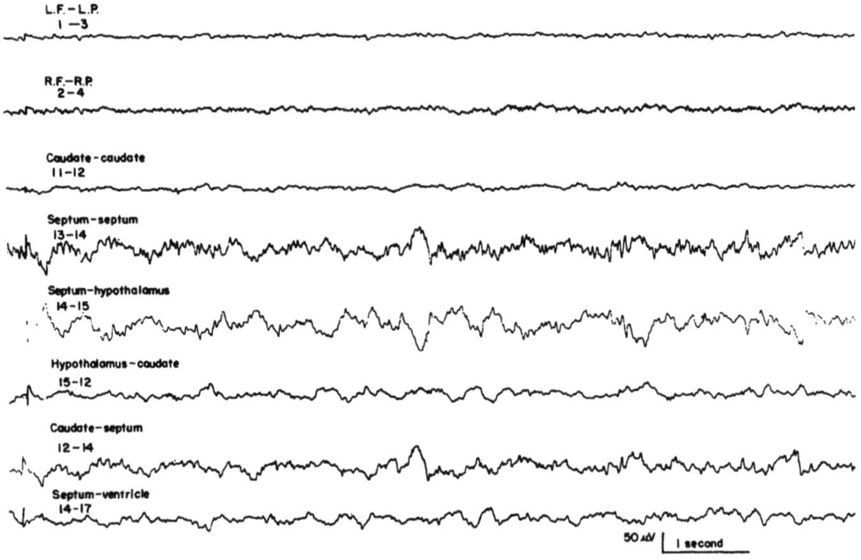

FIGURE E-23. Recordings from Patient A-6, obtained several days after multiple stimulations to the septal region. Note that Figures 24 through 30 show paroxysmal activity limited to the septal leads following stimulation to the caudal part of the septal region over a period of 2 hours. After 5 days the electrical activity returned to normal and there was a recrudescence of pain. Stimulation was at 100 c/second with a bidirectional rectangular pulse of 1 millisecond duration and a maximum current of 7 ma.

as the paroxysmal activity was present, we used its disappearance from the record as our criterion for repeating the stimulation.

The longest that this induced seizure-like type of electrical activity persisted after a single stimulation was 2 weeks. It appeared only after prolonged stimulation through the septal region, although other areas were frequently stimulated for the same periods of time. On one occasion, in the case of the patient who was repeatedly stimulated for relief of intractable pain, paroxysmal activity spread first to other deep leads and then to the cerebral cortex. When it appeared on the scalp leads, a tonic and clonic grand mal convulsion began. Figures 23–30 show induced paroxysmal activity confined to the leads stimulated (namely, those in the septal region), without involvement of other deep structures or spread to the cortex. Figures 31–37 illustrate the sequence of spread from the stimulated leads to other deep leads and then to the cortex.

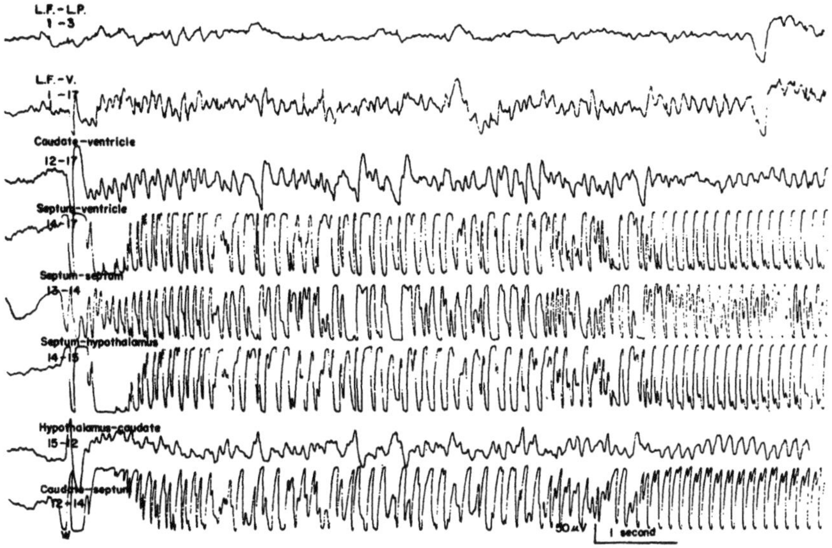

FIGURE E–24. Recordings from Patient A–6 obtained 10 seconds after prolonged septal stimulation

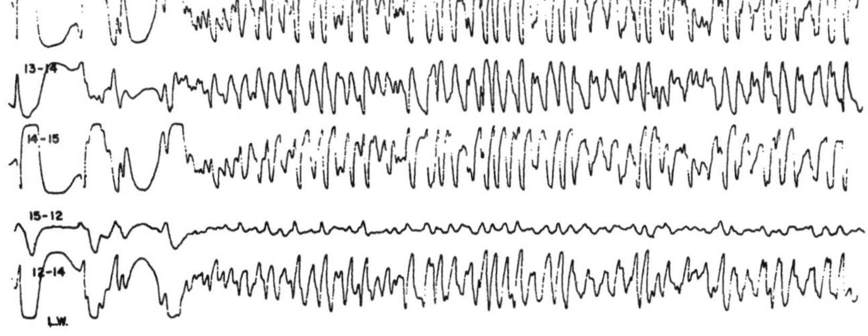

FIGURE E–25. Two minutes after septal stimulation. Note the cyclic occurrence of paroxysmal activity. The patient was well oriented and free from pain; during the time the record was made she was eating a sandwich

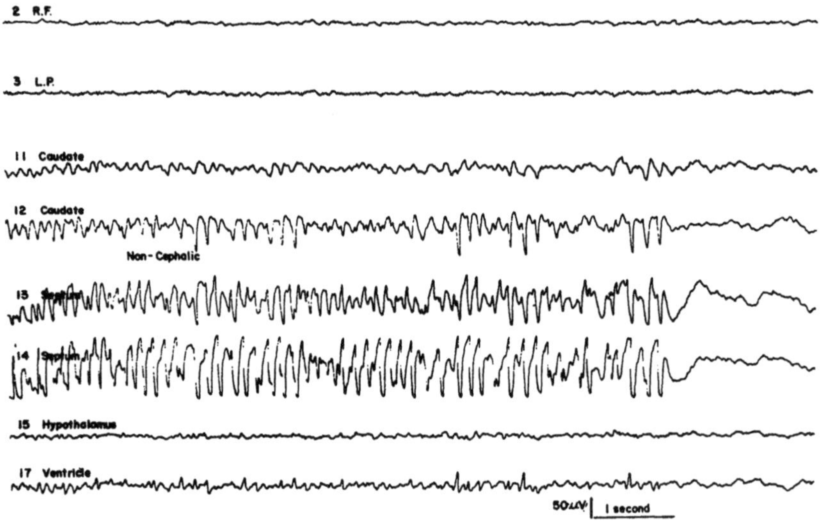

FIGURE E-26. Fifteen minutes later. Cyclic activity is still present. Unipolar recording

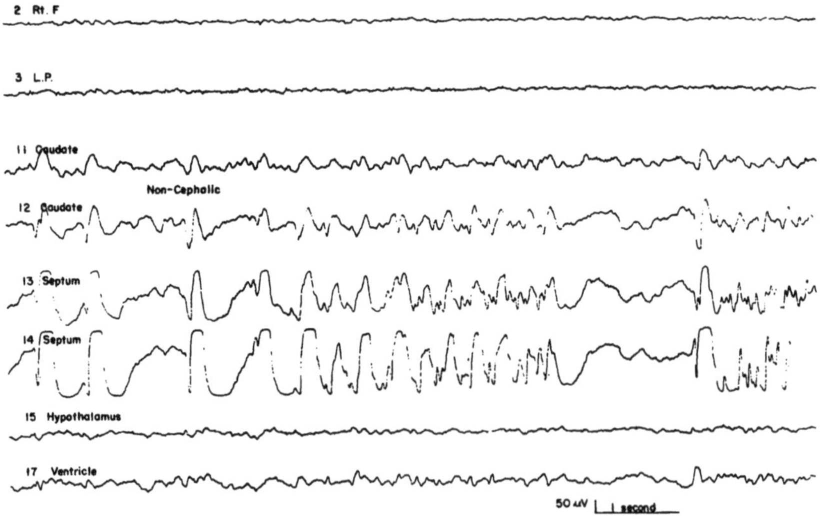

FIGURE E-27. Record obtained 15 minutes after cyclic paroxysmal activity had ceased

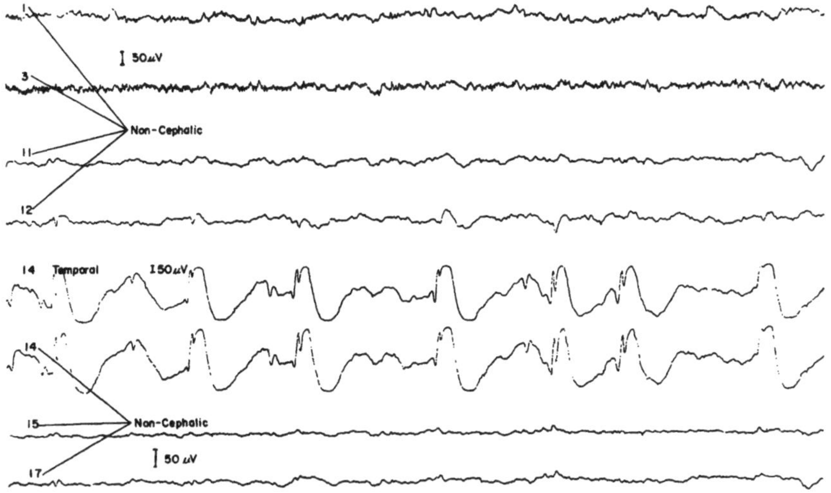

FIGURE E–28. Two hours after septal stimulation. Note abnormal activity in lead 14 (septal)

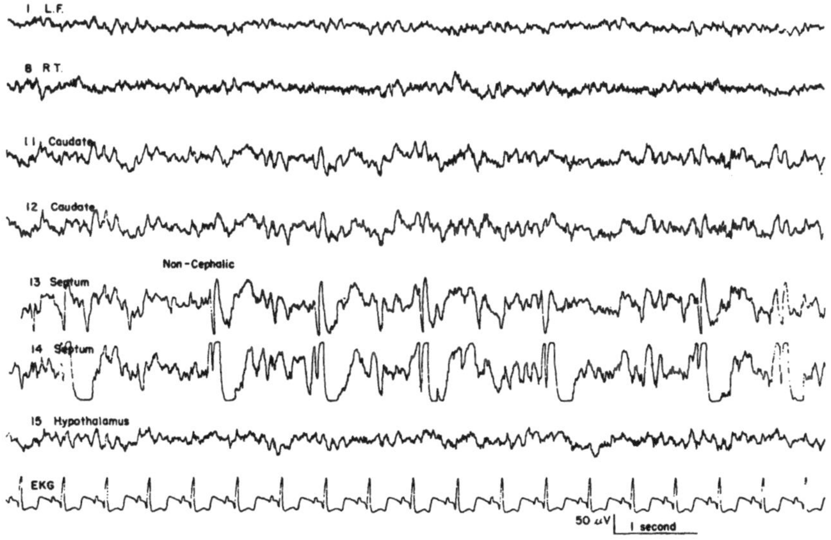

FIGURE E–29. Two days after septal stimulation. Abnormal activity is still confined to the septal leads. Unipolar recordings

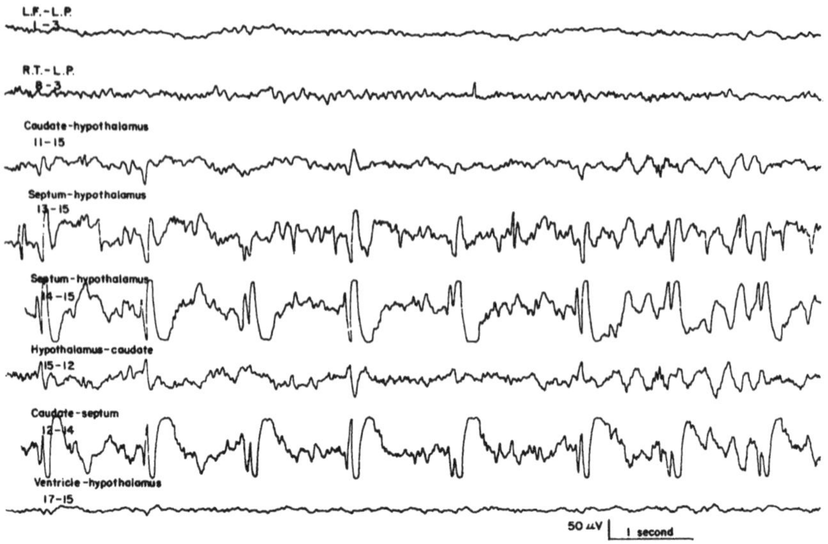

FIGURE E-30. Record obtained immediately after that shown in Figure 29. Bipolar recording

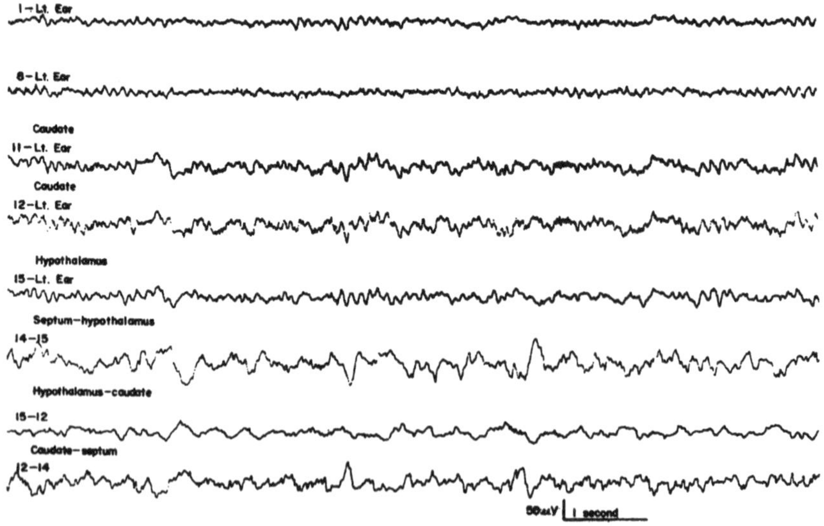

FIGURE E-31. Record obtained 8 days after that shown in Figure 23. Note that Figures 32 through 37 illustrate the spread of paroxysmal activity to the cortex after stimulation to the caudal part of the septal region. At the time that this activity began to appear in the scalp leads Patient A-6 was disoriented as to time, place, and persons and displayed bizarre movements. When the scalp leads became completely involved, she had generalized convulsions

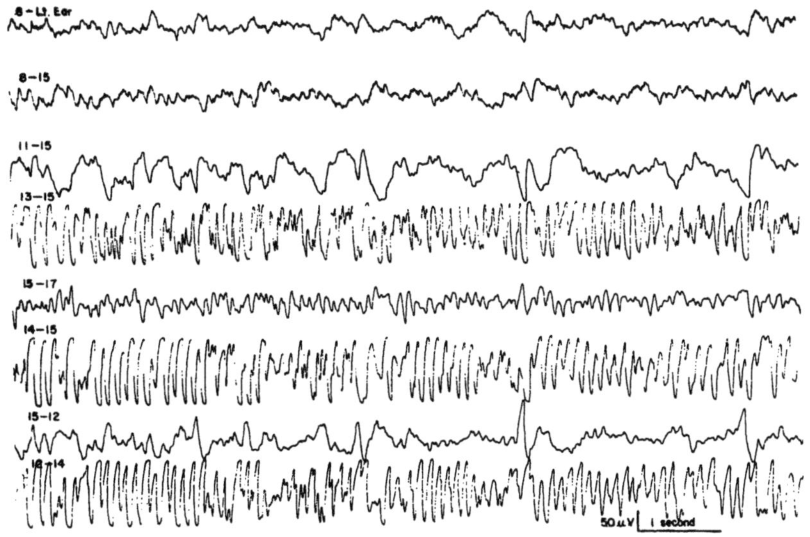

FIGURE E–32. Twenty seconds after septal stimulation over a period of 2 hours. Note the similarity of the abnormal activity in leads 13 and 14 (septal) to that in the previous records

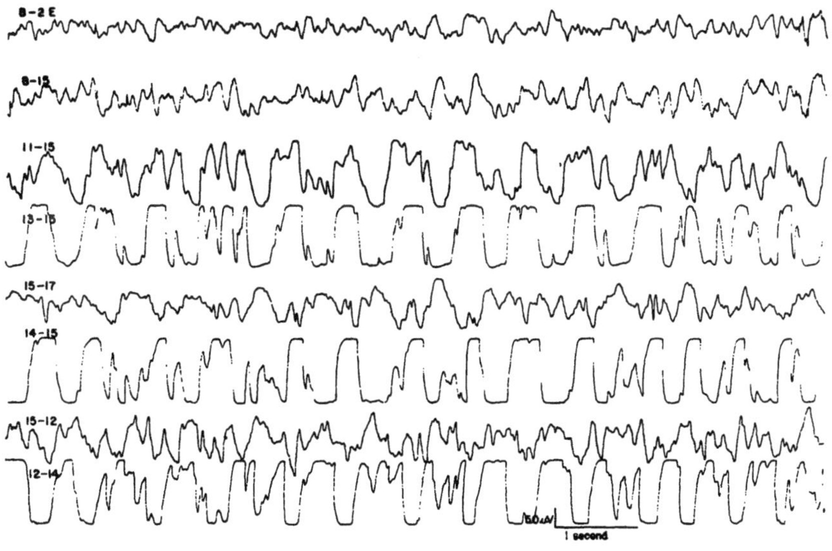

FIGURE E–33. Four minutes after septal stimulation

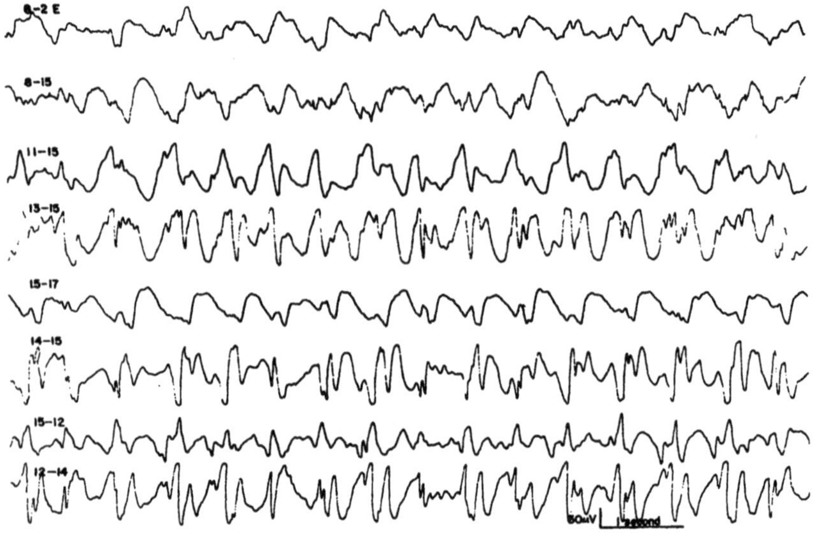

FIGURE E–34. Eleven minutes after septal stimulation. Note the spread of paroxysmal activity to the scalp leads, which coincided with the beginning of a psychomotor episode

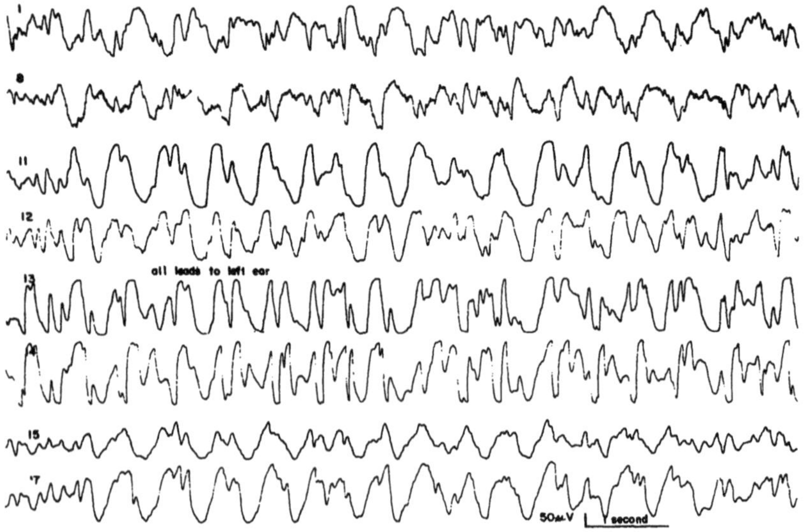

FIGURE E–35. Forty-two minutes after stimulation. Note that the paroxysmal activity in the scalp leads has increased

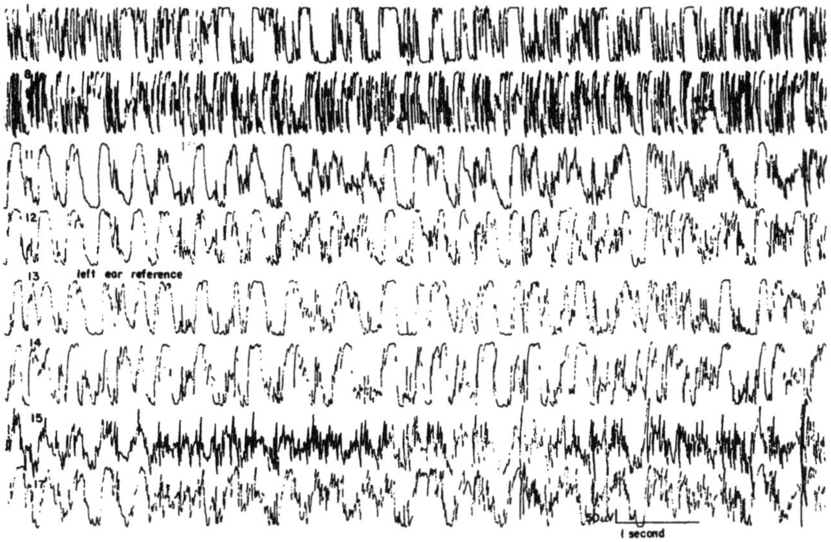

FIGURE E-36. Fifteen seconds later. The paroxysmal activity in the record was accompanied by generalized convulsions

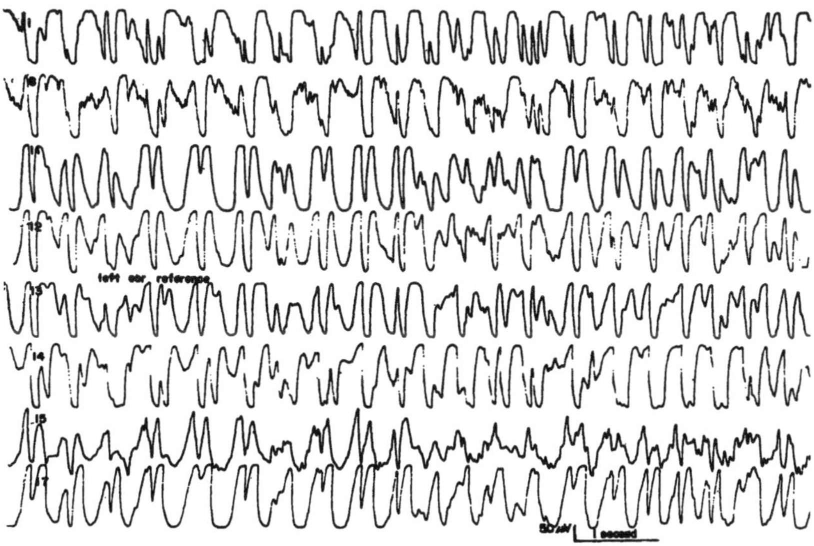

FIGURE E-37. Although abnormal activity persisted in all leads, Patient A-6 no longer displayed bizarre movements. The abnormal electrical activity ceased after intravenous administration of phenobarbital in sufficient amounts

Summary. Prolonged stimulation in the septal region has resulted in persisting paroxysmal electrical activity, usually confined to the stimulated leads. On occasion this activity has gradually spread to other deep leads and the cortex. When the cortex is implicated grand mal seizures result.*

THE EFFECT ON ELECTRICAL RECORDINGS OF DRUGS THAT ALTER LEVELS OF AWARENESS

The administration of various drugs that alter levels of awareness has been an important aspect of our studies since the introduction of our improved technique for chronic implantation of electrodes. A wide variety of such drugs has been administered to patients in the addendum series. These findings will be reported more extensively later. This is a preliminary report on some of the findings. We will consider the alterations in electrical recordings after the administration of two depressants, sodium amytal and phenobarbital, and one so-called stimulant drug, metrazol. Each patient underwent at least two tests with the same drug under similar investigative circumstances. Recordings on four patients are included in this preliminary report. All patients had electrodes implanted chronically in the septal region, caudate nucleus, and hypothalamus. One patient in addition had electrodes in the hippocampus and tegmentum of the mesencephalon. Another patient had additional electrodes in the amygdaloid nucleus. Conventional scalp recordings were taken from all patients in the group and three of the four had electrodes on the arachnoid. Both bipolar and unipolar recordings were done. Unipolar references were noncephalic and to one or both ears. Various combinations of bipolar records were obtained.

None of the patients in the group showed exactly the same findings on recordings made after administration of the drugs and the same patient showed some variations when the test was repeated. However, major consistencies were found in all patients in the group and on all tests. The procedure followed was first to administer 500 mg. of sodium amytal intravenously. After a lapse of several days from 400 to 700 mg. of sodium phenobarbital was similarly injected. The time, appearance,

*Two instances of this phenomenon were reported at the time of the June, 1952 meetings.

localization and amplitude of 20 to 25 c/second spindles were noted, as well as the patient's reaction to the injection. In all instances when the patient went into deep sleep the spindling in the records was replaced by typical sleep patterns on the EEG. Records obtained after injection of phenobarbital showed some characteristic differences from those obtained after injection of sodium amytal. These findings differed considerably from the findings obtained after the administration of metrazol.

Phenobarbital. The most consistent finding in regard to phenobarbital was its predominant effect on the cortical leads. After injection, 20 to 25 c/second spindles appeared in the cortical and scalp recordings but no striking changes appeared in the subcortical recordings. In Figures 38 and 39 the slight high amplitude of the spindles in the caudate and left parietal leads, channel 5, suggests that there may have been some spindling activity in the caudate, although there is no evidence of it in the caudate-hypothalamic lead. This is the one patient who had no cortical leads. In our experience scalp leads show only one-third the amplitude obtained from cortical leads lying directly underneath. This suggests that the high amplitude spindles would have been even more dramatic if a cortical lead had been in place. The records in Figures 40 and 41, which were obtained from Patient A–8 after administration of phenobarbital, demonstrate the high spindling in the cortical leads—predominantly those from the frontal and parietal regions. No spindles appear in the subcortical leads.

Sodium amytal. After administration of sodium amytal, spindles were clearly present in the subcortical leads, particularly those from the septal region. The amplitude in the septal spindles was at least as high as those seen on the scalp recordings (see the records of Patient A–4 in Figures 42 and 43). (One must remember, however, that the estimated amplitude from cortical leads is three times that of the amplitude demonstrated on the scalp leads.) Figures 44 and 45 demonstrate the pre- and postamytal records of Patient A–8. It is to be noted that on the preamytal record the fronto-parietal and cortical leads and to a lesser extent the frontal lead show high amplitude 6 c/second activity with superimposed 20 c/second activity. Following the administration of sodium amytal there was marked spindling in the recordings from the septal region and in those from the fronto-parietal region.

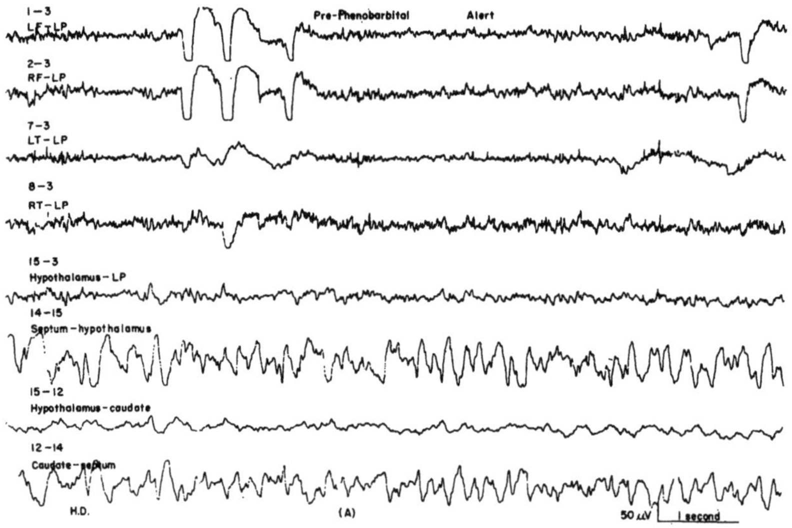

FIGURE E-38. Pre-phenobarbital record of Patient A-4

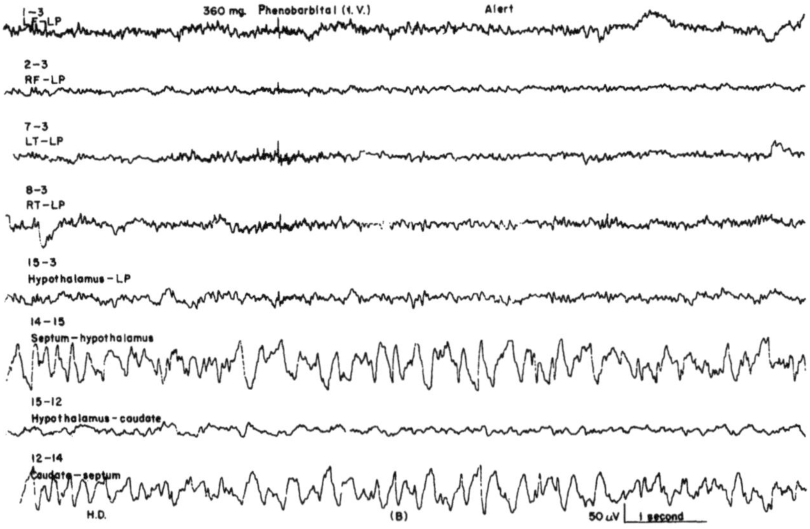

FIGURE E-39. Post-phenobarbital record of Patient A-4

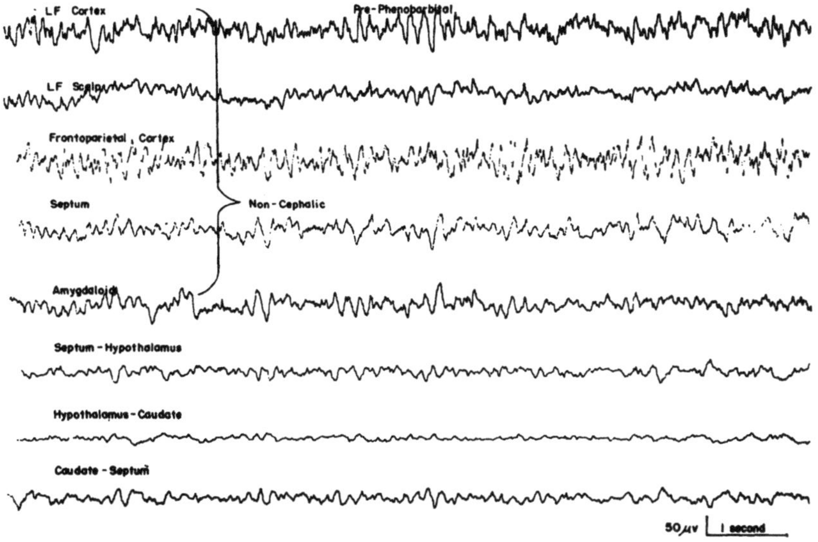

FIGURE E–40. Pre-phenobarbital record of Patient A–8. Note cortical as well as scalp recordings

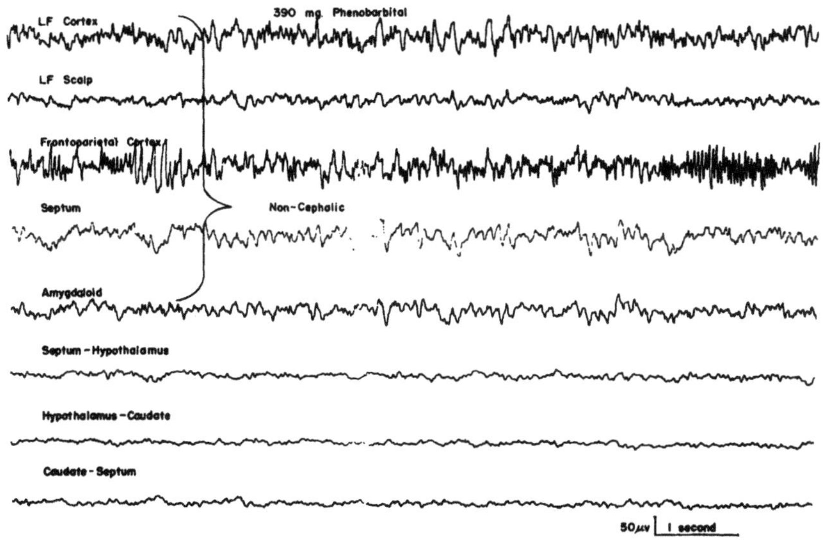

FIGURE E–41. Post-phenobarbital record of Patient A–8. Note cortical as well as scalp recordings

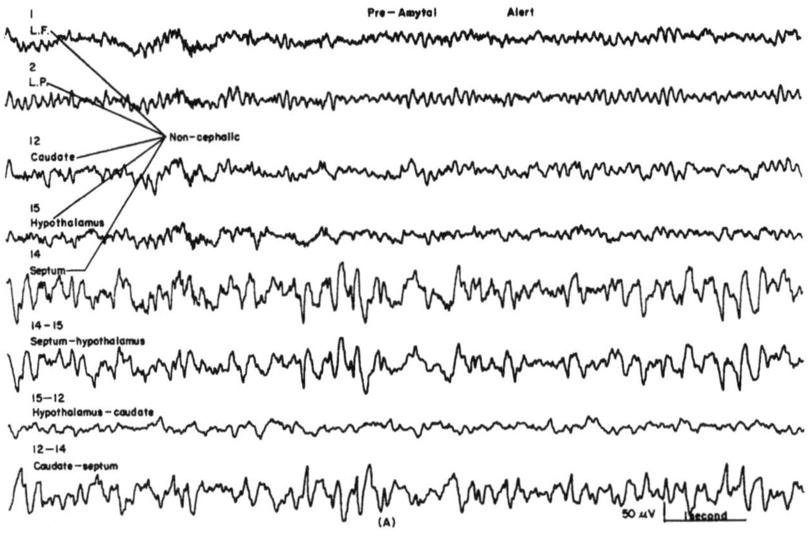

FIGURE E–42. Pre-amytal record of Patient A–4

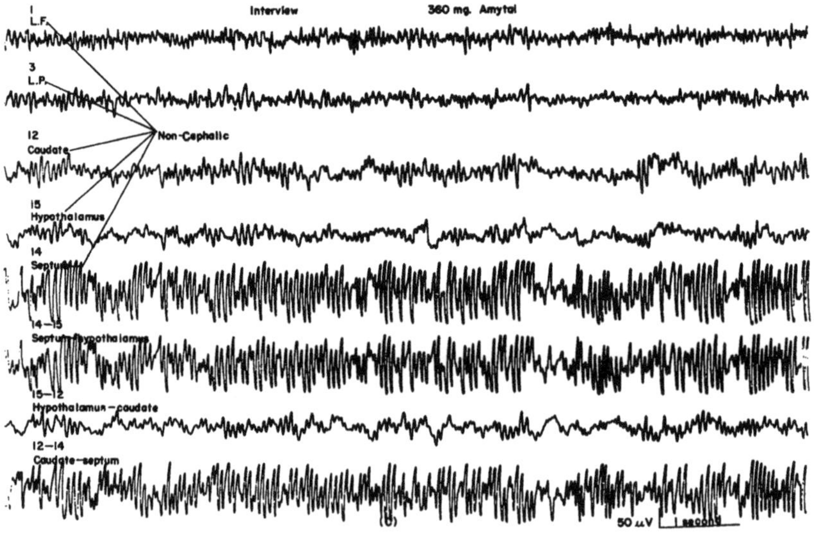

FIGURE E–43. Post-amytal record of Patient A–4

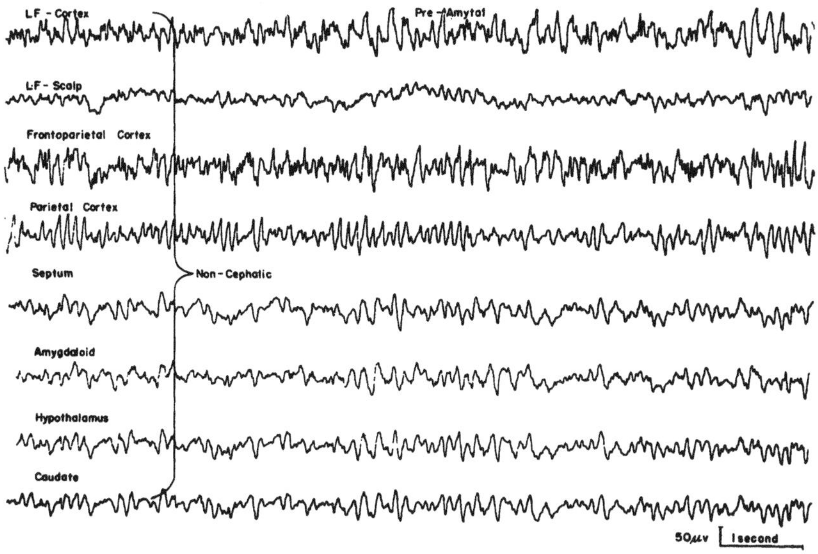

FIGURE E–44. Pre-amytal record of Patient A-8

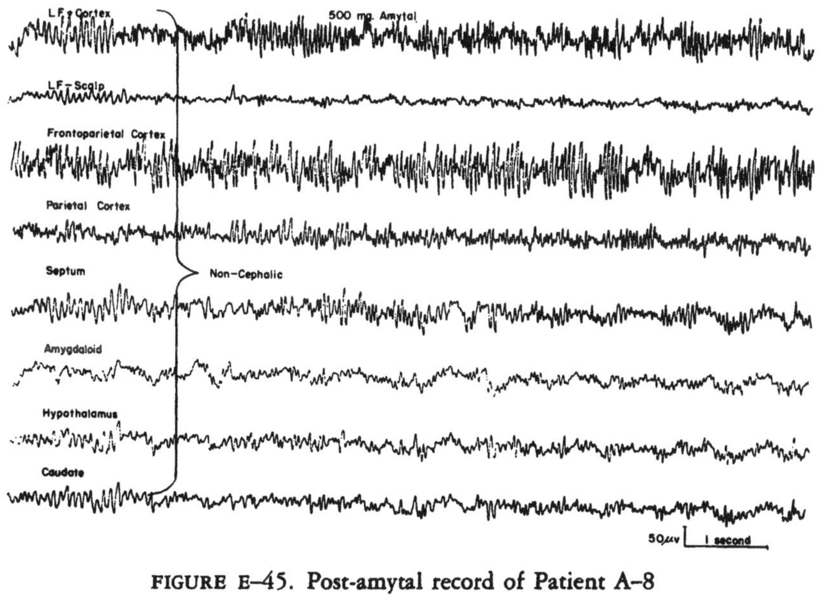

FIGURE E–45. Post-amytal record of Patient A-8

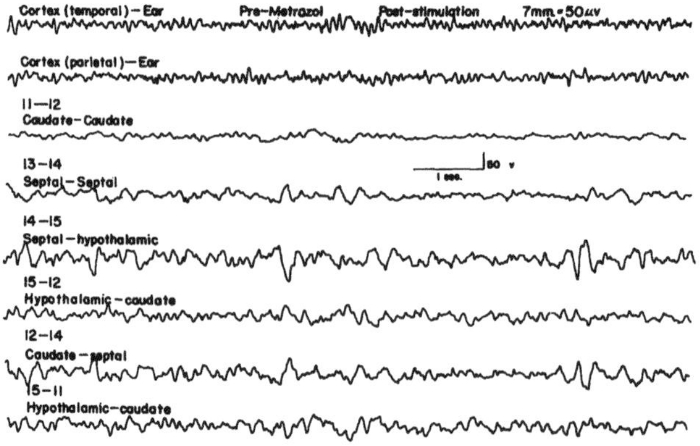

FIGURE E–46. Recordings from Patient A–4 obtained before administration of metrazol

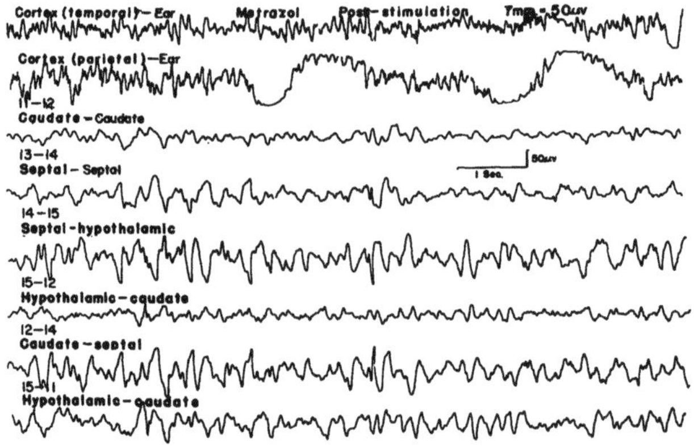

FIGURE E–47. Recording from Patient A–4 obtained after intravenous administration of subconvulsive doses of metrazol

Metrazol. Figure 46 shows a portion of a record obtained before administration of metrazol. This record illustrates the random septal spiking characteristic of schizophrenic patients. The record in Figure 47 was obtained immediately following intravenous administration of metrazol. Note the marked increase in high amplitude spiking through the septal region with occasional spread to the scalp leads. While this record was being taken the patient was very alert and fearful, and some tremor was noted in her hands. She complained that the experience was an extremely uncomfortable one.

REPEAT TESTS WITH SODIUM AMYTAL

The consistent difference between the two barbiturates was that phenobarbital had a predominant effect upon the cortical and scalp leads, whereas the sodium amytal also markedly affected the septal region and to a lesser extent other subcortical regions. There has been some variation in the findings with repetition of the tests. In a repeat test on Patient A–4 (Figure 49) 5 months following the test recorded in Figure 43, we see that, with the same technical set-up, spindling is less apparent in the septal region than it was after the first test. Cortical spindling (indicated by scalp leads) is of high amplitude, as is the spindling in the caudate and the hypothalamic leads. A repeat of the sodium amytal test on Patient A–8 (Figure 51) shows high amplitude barbiturate spindles in the lead from the frontal cortex with some difference in amplitude between these and the spindles in the fronto-parietal lead. The septal lead still shows more activity than the other subcortical leads, but the barbiturate effect is less dramatic than it was in the first test, illustrated in Figure 45.

At present we are unable to give satisfactory explanation for these variations in electrical recordings following administration of exactly the same stimulus by an identical technique. One possible explanation is that there was a difference in activity before stimulation. In comparing the preamytal records of Patient A–4, we find that the outstanding difference is the disappearance of the high amplitude slow waves in the septal lead after 5 months (see Figures 42 and 48). Comparing the preamytal records of Patient A–8, we again find a considerable difference after 2 months. Prior to the first test the fronto-parietal lead showed the predominant 6 c/second wave with superimposed 20 c/second activity (Figure 44) whereas prior to the second test the fronto-parietal lead showed a regular 10 c/second activity and irregular high voltage slow activity with superimposed fast activity in the frontal cortex (Figure 50). Possibly the site of maximal amytal activity might be influenced by the extent of the abnormal electrical activity present at the time of injection.

The principal observation—namely, that phenobarbital affects the cortex proportionately more than the deep leads, whereas sodium amytal affects subcortical leads to a greater degree—may be helpful in under-

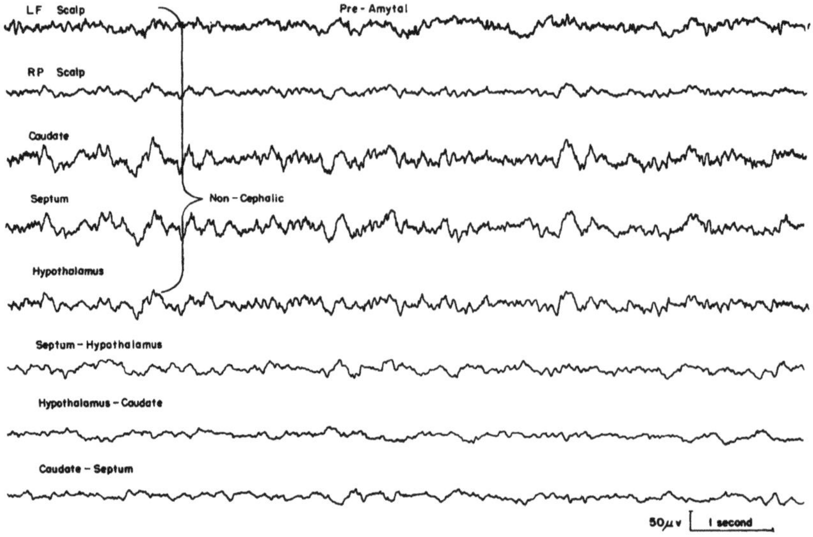

FIGURE E–48. Pre-amytal recordings from Patient A–4 obtained approximately 5 months after the recordings in Figure 42

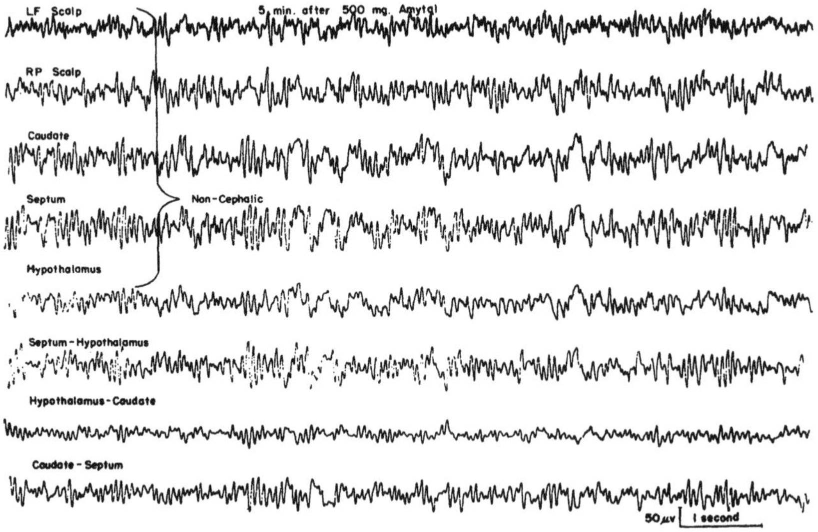

FIGURE E–49. Post-amytal recordings from Patient A–4 obtained approximately 5 months after the recordings in Figure 43

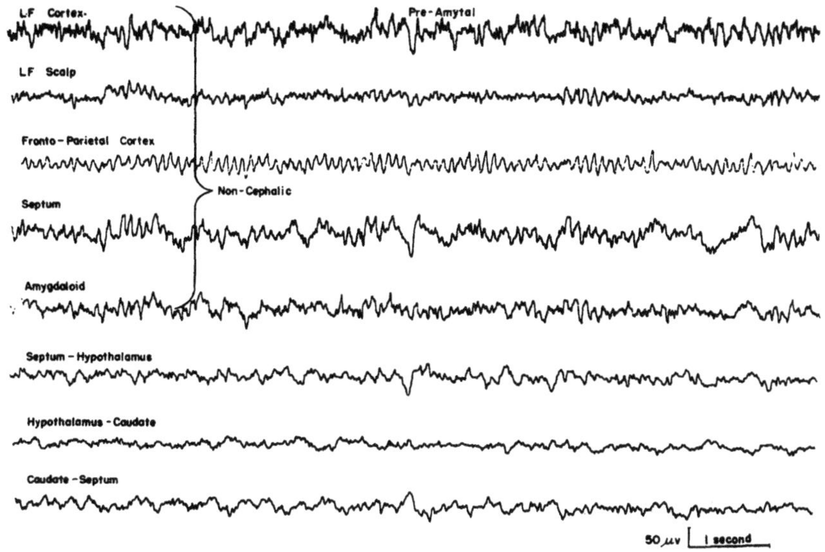

FIGURE E–50. Pre-amytal recordings from Patient A–8 obtained approximately 2 months after the recordings in Figure 44

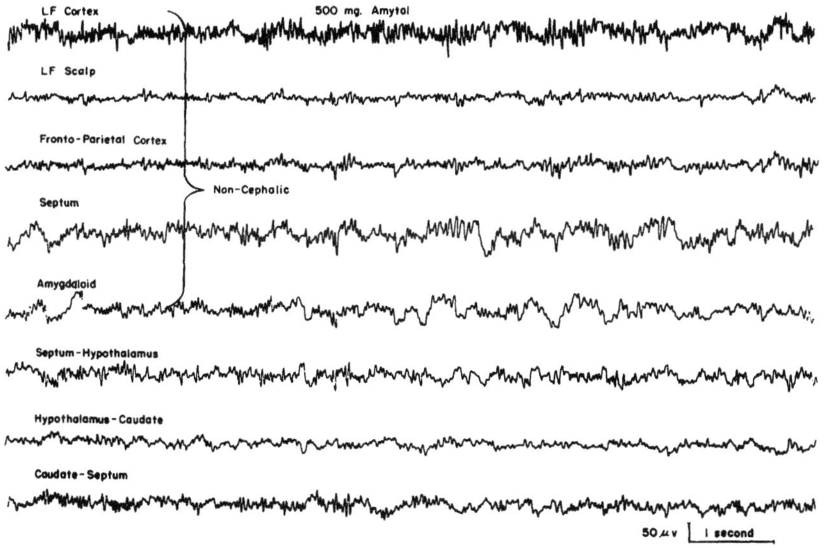

FIGURE E–51. Post-amytal recordings from Patient A–8 obtained approximately 2 months after the recordings in Figure 45

standing some long-standing clinical observations. Sodium amytal has been reported to normalize schizophrenics.[3] Phenobarbital is considerably more effective in controlling epileptic seizures. Our consistent findings in schizophrenic patients indicate an electrical abnormality throughout the subcortical region which is most profoundly affected by the administration of sodium amytal, whereas epilepsy has long been considered to be associated with a cortical dysrhythmia.

Although we have made some tentative correlations between behavior and the electrical abnormalities presented in prebarbiturate records, as well as between changes in behavior and alterations in electrical activity following administration of barbiturates, we feel that considerably more observation is necessary before these findings are finally interpreted.

REFERENCES

1. Green, J. D., and A. Arduini. Rhinencephalic responses to afferent stimulation. Abstract of a paper presented at the meetings of the International Congress of Physiology held in Montreal in 1953.
2. Creutzfeldt, O. D., and R. W. Meyer-Mickelet. Patterns of convulsive discharges of the hippocampus and their propagation. Paper presented at the meeting of the Third International Congress of Electroencephalography and Clinical Neurophysiology in 1953. *Electroencephalog. & Clin. Neurophysiol.*, Supplement 3.
3. Kalenowsky, L. B., and P. H. Hoch. *Shock Treatments and Other Somatic Procedures in Psychiatry*. Grune, New York, 1946.

ADDENDUM F

PSYCHIATRIC FOLLOW-UP

RUSSELL R. MONROE
ROBERT G. HEATH

The patients described in Sections III and IV have been followed for an additional period of 12 months. The over-all statistics are identical with those of June 1, 1952, as one patient returned to the hospital and another has been discharged. The changes that have occurred during this period are as follows:

Patient 8(15) required rehospitalization, particularly for depressive symptoms. He made an immediate response to EST and was subsequently discharged. At home the euphoria seen under EST disappeared, the patient became agitated, depressed, and paranoid. At present he remains out of the hospital on maintenance EST. Although no longer depressed, he retains numerous referential and paranoid ideas. However, he does not "act out" as he did previously.

Patient 13 continued to show improvement until November 1, 1952, when he became seclusive, manneristic, and withdrawn. He became particularly upset during the All Saints' Day religious ceremony, and 2 days later had an epileptic seizure. Since his rehospitalization he has shown vacillating but continued improvement without specific therapy. At the present time he is permitted to go home on visits and appears to be ready for discharge in the near future. Interestingly, during the recent exacerbation of his illness his EEG was normal, although previously he had shown a persistent right frontal delta (S3) focus.

Patient 16 has been going home for longer and longer visits. On the ward she is less tractable and friendly than before, showing more self-assertive behavior and frequent outbursts of rage like those shown prior to stimulation. She retains her hypochondriacal complaints and insists on remaining hospitalized, although it is felt that if she had received encouragement from the family she would have been released from the hospital by now.

Patient 18, who was in the hospital on June 1, 1952, has subsequently shown marked improvement. He was discharged October 1, 1952. Although he appears retarded and lacking in spontaneity and emotional intensity, he is making a satisfactory adjustment on the family farm. He helps with farm chores and has socialized in a limited way, going to church suppers and visiting neighbors. However, he has numerous hypochondriacal preoccupations, particularly with his bowels. He takes many cathartics and numerous antihistamines for colds and maintains himself on daily vitamins. Mild referential trends occasionally appear. Nevertheless, his family consider him markedly improved, although they recognize that he is still quite ill.

Thus, with the follow-up period now ranging from 36 to 15 months, the statistical results remain the same. Except for Patient 13, all of those who showed significant improvement are continuing to make a gradually improving social adjustment to the outside world.

INDEX

Index

Bei Fragen zur Produktsicherheit wenden Sie sich bitte an:
If you have any questions regarding product safety,
please contact:

Walter de Gruyter GmbH
Genthiner Straße 13
10785 Berlin
productsafety@degruyterbrill.com